Trends in the Biology
of Fermentations
for Fuels and Chemicals

BASIC LIFE SCIENCES

Alexander Hollaender, General Editor

Associated Universities, Inc.
Washington, D.C.

Trends in the Biology of Fermentations
for Fuels and Chemicals

Edited by

Alexander Hollaender
Associated Universities, Inc.
Washington, D.C.

and

Robert Rabson
Palmer Rogers
Anthony San Pietro
Raymond Valentine
Ralph Wolfe

PLENUM PRESS • NEW YORK AND LONDON

Library of Congress Cataloging in Publication Data

Main entry under title:

Trends in the biology of fermentations for fuels and chemicals.

(Basic life sciences; v. 18)
"Proceedings of a symposium on trends in the biology of fermentations for fuels and chemicals,
held December 7—11, 1980, at Brookhaven National Laboratory, Upton, New York"—Verso t.p.
Bibliography: p.
Includes index.
1. Fermentation—Congresses. 2. Biomass energy—Congresses. I. Hollaender, Alexander,
1898—   . II. Series.
TP156.F4T73   660.2'8449   81-5928
ISBN 0-306-40752-3   AACR2

Proceedings of a symposium on Trends in the Biology of Fermentations for Fuels and Chemicals,
held December 7-11, 1980, at Brookhaven National Laboratory, Upton, New York

© 1981 Plenum Press, New York
A Division of Plenum Publishing Corporation
233 Spring Street, New York, N.Y. 10013

Printed in the United States of America

ACKNOWLEDGEMENT

The very successful conduct of this symposium on "Trends in the Biology of Fermentations for Fuels and Chemicals" was made possible by a number of important elements. First, we are grateful for the financial support of both the Department of Energy's Division of Biological Energy Research and the National Science Foundation, and for the scientific advice and guidance of both Robert Rabson (DOE) and Oskar R. Zaborsky (NSF). We are deeply indebted to the cooperation and effort of the Biology Department (Richard B. Setlow) of the Brookhaven National Laboratory and its supporting departments, particularly for the untiring assistance of Mrs. Helen Z. Kondratuk who coordinated other staff members.

In order to publish the proceedings of a symposium within a few months of the meeting requires the cooperation of the speakers who prepared their manuscripts prior to the symposium, as well as the review and suggestions of a good editorial board. We express thanks to our editors, Ralph S. Wolfe, Palmer Rogers, Robert Rabson, Anthony San Pietro and Raymond C. Valentine, and to Willis A. Wood, who provided ad hoc comments. The major task is then to pull these papers together with transcribing, editing and production. Here, Claire M. Wilson has done a most competent job with conscientious effort and patient cooperation to guide this volume throughout its different stages. Quick publication was then made possible by the cooperation of the staff of Plenum Publishing Corporation.

Alexander Hollaender

FOREWORD

The growing concern about where energy rich chemicals for the
future will come from has stimulated a resurgence of interest in the
potentialities of microbial fermentations to assist in meeting anticipated demands for fuels and chemicals. While much attention has
been given recently to the early deployment of alcohol production
plants and similar currently available technologies, the potential
future developments have received much less attention. One of the
intentions of the present symposium was to look ahead and try to
perceive some of the prospects for future fermentation technology.
In order to accomplish this, a symposium program of sizable diversity
was developed with workers giving a representative cross section of
their particular specialty as an indicator of the status of basic
information in their area. In addition, an attempt was made to
elicit from the various participants the types of fundamental information which should be generated in the coming years to enable new
fermentation technology to proceed expeditiously. In organizing
the symposium particular effort was made to involve workers from the
academic, industrial and governmental scientific communities.

While the role of microbial conversion in the use of biomass
is considered crucial, it must never be forgotten that such conversions are a segment of an integrated system. The front end of this
system consists of the primary processes of solar conversion by
green plants to produce biomass which is the substrate for the
fermentation processes. On the other end of the system are, of
course, the engineering processes and economic factors so crucial
for the commercialization of these conversions. Neither end of the
system can be neglected; however, this symposium, in order to be
reasonable in scope in the time available, was restricted to discussions dealing only with the basic microbiological aspects of
these proposed technologies.

It is interesting to contrast this present symposium with an
an earlier one held at the Brookhaven National Laboratory in 1952
entitled "Major Metabolic Fuels". At that time the tools of radio-
isotope tracers and of enzymatic assays were just beginning to be

applied widely to chart the pathways of metabolism in microorganisms
and other biological systems. Our ideas about the general metabolic
pathways were elaborated in a relatively few years with these powerful tools. It was not long afterwards that biological research
emphases changed to studies on genetic regulation and molecular
biology. The current symposium reflects many of the spectacular
advances in our understanding of the genetics of microrganisms in
recent years and brings to bear these techniques in understanding
fermentations in much the same manner that the earlier Brookhaven
symposium highlighted isotope and enzyme methodology. What is most
significant is the opportunity now available for integrating these
approaches both for gaining a better understanding of fermentations
and for subsequently applying this knowledge.

The proceedings of the symposium contained herein attest to
the wide range of the meeting. Some of the participants commented
that one omission of the symposium was a strong effort to synthesize
the broad materials of the meeting. The recent reawakening of
interest in fermentation research should, in fact, remedy this
situation in the coming years. The reason this has not occurred
up to now is that this area has suffered neglect for a significant
period. The rapid emergence of research activity in the genetics,
biochemistry, and physiology of fermentations in the past few years
has simply not given time for synthesis and integration. The organization of this symposium is hopefully a start in this direction.

Of special note was the general tone of the symposium which
was one of optimism and enthusiasm not only about the intriguing
scientific problems themselves, but also the emerging application
of the new microbiology of producing usable energy for the future.
This in no way should be construed as indicating that the research
will be easy; rather, it will require a sizable commitment of
resources and time. As a matter of fact, the symposium pointed up
instances of virtually complete blanks in our understanding of whole
basic areas such as in methanogenesis or the genetics of anaerobic
microorganisms, attesting to the enormity of the tasks ahead. The
symposium clearly emphasized the richness of the scientific opportunities for future research contributions.

Lastly, it must be said that this symposium would not have
succeeded as it did without the efforts of a number of exceedingly
important people. These included the speakers, the chairpersons,
the panelists, the many participants, and most especially, Ms. Helen
Kondratuk of the Biology Department of Brookhaven National Laborator
and Ms. Claire Wilson of Associated Universities, Inc.   To all
these persons the organizers offer their sincere gratitude for their
undaunting and efficient efforts to make the meeting work, which
it did very well indeed.

                          The Editors

CONTENTS

POSTER ABSTRACTS

ROUNDTABLE DISCUSSION

WELCOMING REMARKS

Alexander Hollaender
Associated Universities, Inc.
Council for Research Planning
   in Biological Sciences
Washington, D. C.   20036

Welcome to the symposium to discuss the Trends in the Biology of Fermentations for Fuels and Chemicals. Fermentation by microorganisms is probably one of the oldest biological fields developed since the earliest years of civilization. It made very significant progress beginning about 140 years ago and predictable means of its application have especially advanced during the last fifty years.

The important discoveries in the genetics of microorganisms and the recent evolution of genetic engineering have compelled us to consider the present status of fermentation processes with a broad new application potential. It is hoped that the discussions following each presentation at this symposium will bring out additional scientific approaches.

Fermentation is interesting not only from a basic point of view, but its diverse and immediate application has served to bring together both academic investigators and industrial scientists. As a source of energy beginning with sunlight and the green plant, new products are created without straining our traditional energy resources.

With the cooperation of the speakers and discussants, the proceedings of this symposium will be published in early 1981, thus combining the results of our most contemporary research efforts in an important new volume.

BASIC BIOLOGY OF MICROBIAL FERMENTATION

Willis A. Wood

Department of Biochemistry
Michigan State University
East Lansing, Michigan 48824

The great majority of what we know about microbial fermentations was discovered before 1950 (See review by Wood (1)). Since then microbial and biochemical science has passed on to questions of structure and function of macromolecules, organelles and cells thought to be more intriguing or deserving of attention. Now for economic and strategic reasons, attention is once again focused on microbial fermentations for their potential to produce useful and energy-containing products from starch, waste materials or currently unusable biomass. Further, strategists in this area have a kind of tacit belief that, somewhere in the tremendous explosion of biological and chemical knowledge since 1950, there are missing pieces of information and techniques, that when capitalized upon, will propel microbial fermentations from their current state of near oblivion back to center stage, being caught up in a new wave of bioinnovation. In such a scenario the task will be to couple the new knowledge with the old science and technology of fermentation. In such a new endeavor those with the old knowledge need to know what opportunities the new knowledge makes possible, and the practitioners of new science need to know a fair amount about the old science rather than attempting to "reinvent the wheel". Lying somewhere in between is the microbial physiologist or biochemist who might be able to weave a better pattern by taking information and tricks from both the old and new.

It is clear, however, that for all the information now available, there are still large areas where specific data are needed. Most of these areas of physiological and biochemical investigation were abandoned long ago, not because they were unimportant, but rather because fashion changes, and fashion in science exists just as it does in automobiles and apparel. Thus, before any new fermentations can be developed that will constitute a significant advance

we will need to have a rather comprehensive understanding of the
various enzyme-catalyzed reactions and of the cellular environment
in which these must function. The same is also true for the transport processes that feed and relieve the enzymatic processes.

Biomass fermentation to produce liquid fuels basically amounts
to the conversion of reduced photosynthesis products to equally or
more reduced, and hence energy-containing solvents and perhaps acids
and gasses. The only reduced starting materials available to us in
significant amounts are: (a) carbohydrate homopolymers such as
starch and cellulose; (b) heteropolymers such as the hemicelluloses
(xylans and L-arabans) and lignin and; (c) the disaccharides, sucrose
and lactose. Hence certain classical and familiar fermentations of
carbohydrates offer attractive options as starting points for innova-
tions in the area of biomass fermentation.

In adapting carbohydrate fermentations to biomass utilization
major problem areas are apparent. By far the most difficult task
is the liberation of monosaccharides or disaccharides from the highly
insoluble and resistant polymers, cellulose, and hemicellulose. The
second problem area is the development of an optimal process in terms
of rate, yield and type of product(s). In seeking to solve these
problems it will be well to remember that intact cells have a different agenda than making end products on an industrial scale.
Rather their agenda is to make ATP and intermediates for cell growth
maintainance, and reproduction. Hence any manipulation of the system
for industrial purposes must successfully interface with these biological "facts of life". The fermentation products we desire are in
fact only discarded waste products from a biological viewpoint.

Fermentation Systems

The degradation of hexoses and pentoses follows three major
metabolic pathways. Figure 1 shows the well known fructose bisphosphate pathway which is the backbone system for conversion of many
monosaccharides and polyols to pyruvate. Subsequent variations in
the way pyruvate is metabolized produces several fermentation
patterns including ethanolic, lactic, solvent- and butanediol-
producing fermentations as will be described subsequently. Figure
2 outlines the hexose monophosphate pathway in three versions. In
one of these involving transaldolase and transketolase, hexonic
and ketohexonic acids and pentoses are converted to fructose-6-
phosphate and glyceraldeyhyde-3-phosphate, and these follow the
fructose bisphosphate route (Figure 1) to pyruvate. In the second
variant of this system, the heterolactic fermentation, Figures 2
and 3, xylulose-5-phosphate is cleaved by phosphoketolase to
glyceraldehyde-3-phosphate and acetyl phosphate, and these subsequently yield lactate and acetate. A third metabolic system known

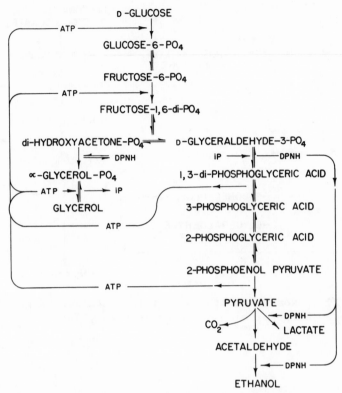

Figure 1.   Fructose bisphosphate pathway for conversion of glucose to lactate as ethanol and CO_2 (1).   Reproduced by permission of Academic Press, Inc.

as the Entner-Doudoroff pathway, Figure 4, is a hexosemonophosphate pathway variant in which 6-phosphogluconate is dehydrated to 2-keto-3-deoxy-6-phosphogluconate which is then cleaved to glyceraldehyde-3-phosphate and pyruvate.   This route is followed in the conversion of glucose to ethanol plus a small amount of lactate in *Pseudomonas lindneri* and a few other organisms.   This pathway also functions in the utilization of gluconate, 2-ketogluconate and uronic acids. From these illustrations in which the products can be the same or similar, comes the conclusion that for an unknown organism it is risky or impossible to assume that a particular pathway is responsible for the fermentation.   Further, if one keeps in mind all of these possibilities, a greater number of options become available for manipulation to achieve a desired goal.

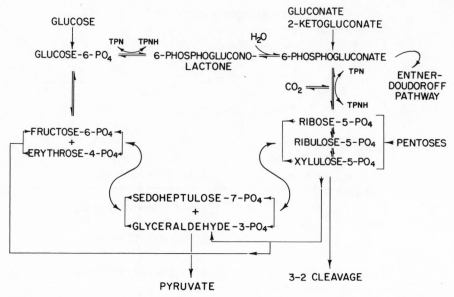

Figure 2.   Hexose monopathways for fermentation of glucose (1).
Reproduced by permission of Academic Press, Inc.

Entrance and Exit Points for Metabolic Pathways

A large number of monosaccharides and related compounds are
also utilized via the main metabolic systems. They enter the main
stream by one or a combination of: oxidation, phosphorylation,
isomerization, epimerization of a monosaccharide or related structure and phosphorolysis of glycosidic bonds. For instance, mannose
and mannitol enter the main pathway via fructose and fructose-6-
phosphate (arrow, Figure 1); the aldopentoses enter via isomerization,
phosphorylation, 3-epimerization and 4-epimerization to produce
D-xylulose-5-P (2) (Figure 5). Similarly, several of the fermentation products arise by isomerization, hydrolysis of phosphate esters
and reduction of intermediates. These include mannitol (arrow 1,
Figure 1), D-arabitol (Figure 6) and glycerol (arrow 2, Figure 1
and 6).

The main point of diversity, a virtual hub of traffic leading
to a variety of fermentation products, comes from options in pyruvate metabolism (Figure 7). These may be categorized as reductions,
carboxylations, phosphoroclastic reactions and those derived from
acetaldehyde or hydroxyethylthiamin diphosphate. The lactic,
ethanol, butanediol, acetone-butyl, acetic-butyric, propionic and
other fermentations derive from combinations of these reactions.

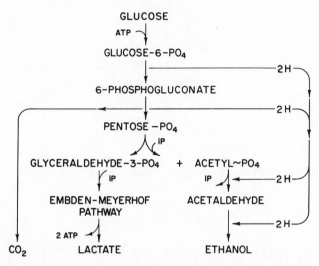

Figure 3. Heterolactic fermentation involving phosphoketolase (1).
Reproduced by permission of Academic Press, Inc.

Factors Effecting Competition at a Branch Point

The foregoing discussion indicates that a number of alternative
reactions exist for processing many of the intermediates of metabolism. It is the expression of these alternatives at branches in
the pathways that creates both diversity in fermentation products
and the opportunity for manipulation to advantage. Such branch
points in metabolism exist because more than one enzyme or enzyme
system competes for a common intermediate. A fundamental understanding of the factors involved in the competition at a branch
point has the potential for rational management of existing or
"natural" fermentations and for constructing some efficient organisms in which a favorable branch in metabolism is greatly enhanced.

One can predict many of the factors that must be considered
in determining the outcome of competition between two enzymes at
a branch point just from a general knowledge of enzyme function and
regulation. In addition there may be others that are currently
unrecognized.

In the simplest case where two enzymes compete for a metabolic
intermediate, the velocity observed in each branch is determined
by the concentration of the enzyme, its specific catalytic rate,
the K_m for the intermediate which is the substrate, and the

BACTERIAL ETHANOLIC FERMENTATION

Pseudomonas lindneri

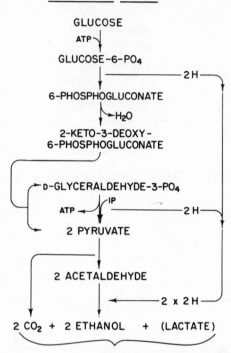

Figure 4.   Entner–Douoaroff hexose monophosphate pathway (1).
Reproduced by permission of Academic Press, Inc.

concentration of the substrate (1).   In addition, the pH of the
medium and the pH profile of the competing enzymes plays a major
role because of its effect on both the K_m values and the catalytic
mechanisms in each branch.   Further, allosteric regulation of
velocity of one or both of the competing enzymes in the simplest
case is dictated by the dissociation constant(s) for the effector,
the steady state concentration of the effector and the regulatory
constants for the enzymes involved.   These constitute an overlay
of parameters which may greatly modify the importance of primary
factors in complex ways.   Any analysis of these effects requires
considerable additional information as to the nature of the allosteric effect both qualitatively and quantitatively.   For one
kinetic analysis, see reference 3.

     Thus, competition at a branch point usually determines the
product mix.   However, in more extreme cases a new product appears,

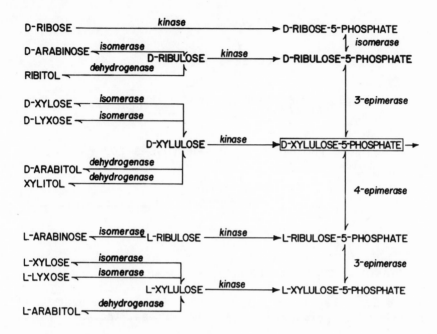

Figure 5. Aldopentose and pentitol metabolism (2). Reproduced by permission of Academic Press, Inc.

or a typical product disappears. Additionally an entirely different metabolic pathway carries out a different fermentation in each branch.

Effect of Genetic Makeup

Of course, the greatest variations in fermentation mechanism and type is conferred by the presence of structural genes coding for particular enzymes. This is exemplified by contrasting the homoethanolic fermentations by *Saccharomyces cerevisieae* and *Pseudomonas lindneri*. The yeast does not contain 6-phosphogluconate dehydrase and 2-keto-3-deoxy-6-phosphogluconate aldolase of the Entner-Doudoroff pathway (Figure 4) or lactic dehydrogenase. *P. lindneri* does not contain fructose bisphosphate aldolase, but does have the dehydrase and aldolase of the Entner-Doudoroff pathway as well as lactate dehydrogenase which gives rise to the small amount of lactate found. Similarly, *Leuconostoc mesenteroides*, which converts glucose to lactate, ethanol and CO_2 in 1:1:1 stoichiometry, does not contain fructose bisphosphate aldolase or triose phosphate isomerase and has instead a unique cleaving enzyme, phosphoketolase (Figures 2,3). Other lactics use the fructose bisphosphate route (Figure 1) to the same products in varying ratio and do not have the gene for phosphoketolase.

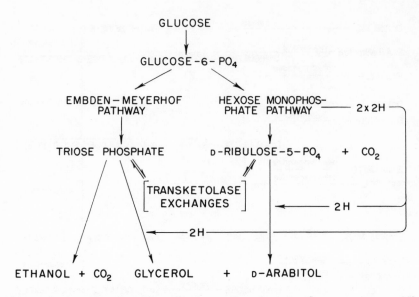

Figure 6. Ethanol and polyol production in fermentation (1).
Reproduced by permission of Academic Press, Inc.

FACTORS EFFECTING PRODUCT MIX

Carbon Chain Length

Linear C_2 to C_7 structures are fermented by a variety of organisms. This leads to entry of the substrate into various metabolic pathways at new points or to drastic alteration of the pathways and products compared to those involved with glucose fermentations. While C_6 substrates are usually converted to hexose phosphate intermediates which can enter any of the pathways, C_7, C_5, and C_4 substrates only enter the hexose monophosphate pathway (Figure 2). Thus, while glucose fermentation by some lactobacilli may yield 2 moles of lactate and by others one mole each of lactate, ethanol and CO_2, the fermentation of pentoses yields of necessity, by direct cleavage, one mole each of lactate and acetate or, via transaldolase and transketolase followed by the fructose biosphosphate pathway, 1.67 moles of lactate.

Oxidation State of the Substrate

Comparison of the fermentation of 2-ketogluconate, containing four fewer hydrogen atoms with that of glucose illustrates the role of a cosubstrate acting as a reductant in dictating the outcome of competition at a branch point. Table I shows the distribution of

TABLE I

Comparison of Products Formed by *Leuconostoc mesenteroides* from
Glucose and 2-Ketogluconate

| Product | mmoles/100 mmoles of hexose fermented | |
	glucose	2-ketogluconate
lactic acid	102	99
ethanol	112	trace
acetic acid	---	101
carbon dioxide	96	98
% carbon recovered	104	99
O/R Balance	0.86	0.98

products for glucose and 2-ketogluconate for *Leuconostoc mesente-*
roides. When glucose is utilized, NADH is generated in two steps
as is typical of the hexosemonophosphate pathway in *Leuconostoc*
(Figure 3). The available NADH reduces acetyl phosphate to ethanol.
In contrast, with 2-ketogluconate no NADH is generated because
glucose-6-phosphate is not an intermediate. The NADH required for
reduction of 2-keto-6-phosphogluconate is generated in the oxidation
of 6-phosphogluconate oxidation to ribulose-5-phosphate. Under these
conditions there is no NADH remaining for reduction of acetyl
phosphate to ethanol, hence acetate is formed by default.

In another scenario, organisms with ferredoxin and hydrogenase produce hydrogen gas during fermentation. The consequence
is that the remainder of the products are more oxidized that would
otherwise be the case. Fermentation of more oxidized substrates
diminshes hydrogen production and conditions which inhibit or repress hydrogenase result in more reduced products. In this connection, while hydrogen gas can be used as fuel, a more desirable
strategy may be either to add hydrogen gas to a fermentation to
produce more reduced products, i.e., solvents, or to coculture
organisms so that the hydrogen produced by one would be consumed
as substrate by a second organism to achieve more reduced products.

pH of Fermentation

It has long been known that altering the pH of a fermentation,

changes the distribution of products. This results from differing
pH optima of enzymes competing at a branch point. While not easily
manipulated or providing many options, pH is a factor to be remembered
in optimizing the process.

Factors Effecting Fermentation Rate

While a fermentation can be looked upon as a linear multistep
process, this is not strictly true because of the looped nature of
steps involved in ATP formation and utilization and in pyridine
nucleotide reduction and reoxidation. The oxidation-reduction steps
are self balancing in that oxidation and reduction pyridine nucleotide are linked. In contrast, more ATP is generated in all fermentation pathways than is used in forming phosphorylated intermediates.
Nevertheless, analysis of fermentation rates is facilitated by
determining the rate-limiting step or steps. Possible bottle necks
include: (a) influx of metabolites; (b) one or more enzymatic
steps in the pathway; and (c) efflux of products. Also involved are
removal of heat and products and the concentration of effectors
which alter enzyme-catalyzed reaction rates, usually at the rate
limiting steps.

While increased temperature offers promise of increasing the
rate at the rate limiting steps, elevated temperature is often used
in industrial bioprocessing for other reasons. On the other hand,
elevated temperature also increases the rates of competing side
reactions and may result in loss of membrane integrity, or decreased
half life of enzymes.

Currently, optimization of a fermentation process is approached
emperically rather than analytically. This is due to the complex
nature of the total system and the lack of specific data on each
step. With sufficient information, computer modeling of the process
should offer a rational analytical approach to optimization and
point out the rate limiting step(s). However, unknown conditions
in situ and unknown factors effecting the rate of catalysis might
well deteriorate the value of such computer-generated models. Modeling has been attempted for animal systems with limited success
primarily due to unavailability of kinetic parameters and steady
state concentrations of intermediates in the pathway. If research
could eliminate such uncertainties in modeling fermentations, genetic
manipulation could be used to increase the amount of a rate-limiting
catalyst, or substitute a catalyst with a more favorable K_m, pH
optimum, specificity, or insensitivity to a regulator. As these
rate limiters are removed, transport processes and regeneration of
ADP for use as a phosphoryl acceptor will become rate limiting. The
means to increase these rates is far from obvious and needs more
research.

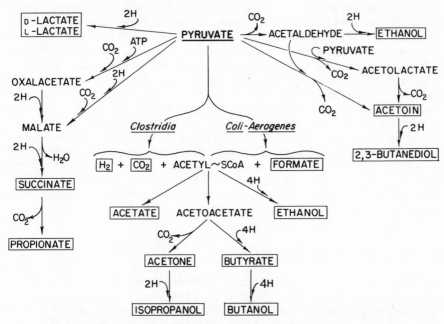

Figure 7.   Fermentation products formation from pyruvate (1).
Reproduced by permission of Academic Press, Inc.

　　　　Finally, the total fermentation process will become diffusion
limited.   It appears that most enzymes in a fermentation pathway are
present as independent, "free-swimming" molecules in the cytoplasm.
If this proves to be true, the rate of an individual first order
reaction is proportional to the concentration of enzyme and the free
concentration of the intermediate in the cytoplasm, which serves as
substrate.   However this may not be the case.   Pontremoli and
Horecker (4) showed that the overall reaction rate for transaldolase
and transketolase of liver extracts acting together to convert
fructose-6-phosphate to sedoheptulose-7-phosphate (Figure 2) was
much higher than is possible from the amount of each enzyme and the
known steady state concentrations of the substrate and intermediates.
This observation implies that a complex is formed between transaldolase and transketolase such that the intermediates produced by
transketolase and needed by transaldolase, never equilibrated with
the solvent.   Hence the local concentration of the intermediates
was higher than measured and thus the overall rate was higher. There
is evidence of this kind for sequential enzymes attached to solid
support.   Hence it appears that while diffusion-limited rates in
solution can only be improved by higher temperature and lower viscosity of the medium, entrapment or packaging of fermentation pathway
enzymes into high proximity, nonequilibrating systems may further

improve fermentation rates. This line of thinking suggests that cell-free fermentation may have some advantages worthy of further consideration. First, cell-free systems would be free of the need for entrance and exit transport systems. Second, immobilization, in addition to its usual advantages might raise the rate of the diffusion-controlled rate limiting process. The covalent attachment of sequential enzymes, the second to the first which is attached to the support and so on, can form oriented shells of pathway enzymes about the solid support. The success of this approach depends on maintaining NAD, ADP, and ATP at relatively high concentrations. Reports from the laboratory of Klaus Mossbach indicates how this might be accomplished. They have formed an active immobilized NAD-alcohol dehydrogenase compound which efficiently couples to other soluble enzymes (5,6). This approach is being studied, hence its potential has not yet been exploited.

Development of New Fermentations

The transfer of amylase into brewer's yeast is now being investigated and it is likely that an additional transfer of dextrinases will make possible the complete fermentation of starch by yeast. In practice this has the potential of dispensing with malt or malting in beer making. A similar transfer of cellulase, or hemicellulases into yeast, or bacteria, which carry out useful fermentations, would seem to offer similar advantages and enormous potential. The insoluble crystalline structure of cellulose in woody plants would still cause the availability of glucosyl units to be rate limiting for the total process as it is for all cellulytic organisms in nature. Any improvement would require a combined chemical, biochemical and microbial assault on the cellulose structure.

There is little experience to draw upon for the transfer of a structural gene into a fermenting organism of interest. However, for an exoenzyme such as cellulose, it may be predicted that its secreting mechanism, whatever it consists of, may also have to be transferred into the receptor organism.

Construction of new organisms or new fermentations will not be as simple as the transfer of the structural genes needed to create the desired catalysts. As has already been learned for the transfer of the NIF genes for nitrogen fixation, integration of new reactions into an existing metabolic pattern implies that the new genes will be sufficiently transcribed and that the transferred enzymes or systems function well in the new environment. The following questions illustrate additional concerns. Can the level of coreactants and cofactors be maintained to furnish both the new and the old reactions with active catalysts and with the needed concentrations of cosubstrates, i.e., NADH? Are the pH optima of

the new enzymes near the pH of their environment? Do the steady
state levels of intermediates interface well with the K_m values for
the new catalysts? Are the binding constants for allosteric
effectors and the steady state levels of these ligands such that the
new catalysts are active? In principle, replicon function could be
used to provide sufficient gene replication and sufficient transcription of structural genes to overcome some, perhaps considerable,
mismatch of properties. It is known, for instance, that replication of the structural gene for ribitol dehydrogenase in *Klebsiella
pneumoniae* and its transcription yields sufficient ribitol dehydrogenase, for the organism can grow on unnatural substrates such as
xylitol and L-arabitol (2,7). Ribitol dehydrogenase which provides
the first reaction, has only one thousandth the ribitol dehydrogenase
activity on L-arabitol and xylitol. However, the tolerance of
mismatch of properties, is clearly unknown territory and only time
and experimentation will tell how easy or difficult the task will be.

Desirable New Organisms

        It is entertaining to enter the fantasy world and conjure
up ideal organisms and fermentations. While in the realm of make
believe such an indulgence can yield fictional organisms which might
serve as goals for future research. My rather superficial attempt
produced the following:

Ethanol-Tolerant, Thermophilic, Cellulytic Yeast

        Clearly ethanol tolerance and thermophily are very complex
properties. Product inhibition, the effect of ethanol on pathway
enzymes and integrity of the cell membranes are possible causes.
Perhaps one could develop the desired properties in a thermophilic
yeast, by transferring in, and replicating the gene for cellulase.
One approach to ethanol sensitivity might involve ethanol removal
by continuous dialysis culture or by another continuous process
involving immobilization of the yeast and separation perhaps by
magnetic means (8).

Cellulytic, Heterotrophic, Thermophilic Methanogen

        Consolidation of the functions of a mixed culture for methane
production from carbohydrate into one organism has obvious advantages of culture stability in large scale fermentations. While not
directly of high potential for liquid fuel production, the low cost
of methane recovery, the potential for production of large amounts
from sewage and waste and its high energy content indicate that
methane should receive major attention. However desirable methane

may be, with known methanogens if one wishes to transfer in cellulytic capability, it will also be necessary to make the organism heterotrophic, that is, transfer in a portion or all of a system for conversion of glucose to any of the following: H_2, CO_2, formate, propionate, acetate, buyrate, valerate, caproate and ethanol. Alternatively, the methane generating system would have to be transferred into a cellulytic, glucose-fermenting organism. Given the poorly understood and fastidious nature of methanogens this would involve a prodigious effort at best.

Cellulytic, Thermophilic, Homobutanol Producer

Table II shows that *Clostridium butylicum* and *Clostridium acetobutylicum* ferment glucose to butyric and acetic acids, isopropanol or acetone, ethanol, butanol and large amounts of carbon dioxide and hydrogen. Figure 7 shows how these products arise. My calculations indicate that it is theoretically possible for these organisms to be homobutanol producers for the non-gaseous product.

$$C_6H_{12}O_6 \longrightarrow C_4H_{10}O + 2CO_2 + H_2O$$

glucose   butanol

In order to accomplish this, it would be necessary to eliminate the function of several enzymes to reduce the number of products. Among these are thiolase, CoA transferase, acetoacetate decarboxylase and CoA-linked aldehyde dehydrogenase. This fermentation would still not be ideal because 33% of the carbon is lost as CO_2.

TABLE II

Fermentation Balances for the Acetone-Butanol Process

Product	mmoles/100 mmoles of glucose fermented	
	Clostridium butylicum	*Clostridium acetobutylicum*
butyric acid	4.3	17.2
acetic acid	14.2	17.2
carbon dioxide	221	203.5
hydrogen	135	77.6
ethanol	7.2	---
butanol	56	58.6
acetone	22.4	---
acetoin	6.4	---
isopropanol	---	12.1
% carbon recovered	99.6	96.2
O/R Balance	1.01	1.06

While use of recombinant DNA procedures to produce new organisms seems obvious, there is every likelihood that new and very useful organisms can be found in nature, using an emperical screen approach which has been so effective in producing antibiotics and other biologicals.

If my attempt to dream up new organisms leaves you nervous or at least skeptical, then I have accomplished my purpose. Today we are nowhere near being able to accomplish any but the simplest of the above conversions. However, I am impressed by what can be done by genetic manipulation and what we can learn by investigation of relevant microbial physiology and biochemistry. The program of this meeting supports a reason for optimism. It is evident that we have the tools to begin such projects. This symposium is designed to give impetus to such an effort. And I venture to predict as experimentation proceeds with the goal of producing ultimately practical results, that many exciting new fundamental discoveries will also be made along the way.

REFERENCES

1. Wood, W.A. (1961) Fermentation of Carbohydrates and Related Compounds in Vol. II, The Bacteria. Gunsalus, I.C. and Stanier, R.Y., eds., p. 59-149, Academic Press, New York.
2. Mortlock, R.P., Fossitt, D.D. and Wood, W.A. (1965) A Basis for Utilization of Unnatural Pentoses and Pentitols by *Aerobacter aerogenes*. Proc. Nat. Acad. Sci. USA 54, 572-579.
3. Ainsworth, S. (1977) Steady State Enzyme Kinetics. p. 202-224, University Park Press, Baltimore, MD.
4. Pontremoli, S., Bonsigmore, A. Grazi, E. and Horecker, B.L. (1960) A Coupled Reaction Catalyzed by the Enzymes Transketolase and Transaldolase. J. Biol. Chem. 235, 1881-1887.
5. Mansson, M.-O., Larsson, P.-O. and Mossbach, K. (1978) Covalent Binding of an NAD Analog to Liver Alcohol Dehydrogenase Resulting in an Enzyme-Coenzyme Complex not Requiring Exogenous Coenzyme for Activity. Eur. J. Biochem. 86, 455-463.
6. Mansson, M.-O., Larsson, P.-O. and Mossbach, K. (1979) Recycling by a Second Enzyme of NAD Covalently Bound to Alcohol Dehydrogenase. FEBS Let. 98, 309-313.
7. Lerner, S.A., Wu. T.T. and Lin, E.C.C. (1964) Evolution of Catabolic Pathways in Bacteria. Science 146, 1313-1315.
8. Larsson, P.-O. and Mossbach, K. (1979) Alcohol Production by Magnetic Immobilized Yeast. Biotech. Let. 1, 501-506.

CELLULASES OF FUNGI

Karl-Erik Eriksson

Swedish Forest Products Research Laboratory
Chemistry Department
Stockholm, Sweden

One of nature's most important biological processes is the degradation of lignocellulosic materials into carbon dioxide, water and humic substances. The strong wood-degrading capability of fungi depends, in part, upon the organization of their hyphae, which gives the organisms a penetrating capacity. Different types of fungi give rise to different types of wood rot. One normally distinguishes between soft-rot, brown-rot and white-rot fungi. The blue staining fungi are also associated with wood damage. They do not, however, cause wood degradation. The morphological pattern of the attack on wood by these fungi varies. Thus, the soft-rot fungi grow in the secondary wall of the wood fiber and form cylindrical cavities with conical ends. This type of attack causes a softening of the wood surface layer which has given the name to this group of fungi.

Brown-rot and white-rot fungi normally grow in the cell lumen. Their hyphae penetrate from one cell to another through openings occurring in normal wood anatomy or by producing bore holes in the cell walls.

Not only the morphology of wood attack by the three types of rot fungi differs but also there are differences in their attack on different wood components. Thus, soft- and brown-rot fungi mainly attack the carbohydrate components, while the white-rot fungi can also degrade the lignin. In the context of biotechnical processes, a degradation of all the wood components may be of interest, thus the white-rot fungi are more suitable than other types of rot fungi.

To better understand how the wood components are degraded by
white-rot fungi on the molecular level it is important to investigate
the morphology of their attack on wood. Such studies have been
undertaken both on the micromorphological level and on the ultrastructural level using scanning electron microscopy (SEM) and transmission electron microscopy (TEM).

Before these studies were undertaken, it was important to
determine the optimal growth conditions for the fungi in wood (1).
Rypáček and Navrátilová (2) had reported earlier that the white-rot
fungus *Trametes versicolor* colonizes wood very densely. In one cubi
cm of wood up to 1300 m of fungal hyphae can be produced. This must
mean that the diffusion distances of the enzymes degrading the wood
polymers are very short. We have demonstrated that the white-rot
fungus *Sporotrichum pulverulentum* grows 1 mm per hour on a malt agar
plate surface and 0.5 mm per hour in either birch- or spruce-wood
(1). Thus, it seems likely that the rate limiting steps in fungal
degradation of wood are the enzymic reactions for degradation of the
polymeric wood components rather than the speed of growth of the
fungal hyphae. That polymer degrading enzymes diffuse from the cell
wall of white-rot fungi to attack both wood polysaccharides and the
lignin is apparent from the SEM and TEM pictures presented by
Eriksson et al. (3) and Ruel et al.(4). It can be seen in Figure 1
that the thin surface layer, most likely of hemicellulosic nature,
has been eroded at a distance of 3-4 μm from the fungal wall. This
shows that enzymes attacking wood components diffuse from the fungal
cell wall out into the surrounding medium.

It is apparent from the TEM studies by Ruel et al. (4) that
lignin also can be morphologically changed at a distance from the
fungal cell wall (Figure 2). The fungus is the white-rot fungus
S. pulverulentum. The enzymes attack the lignin causing a change
in pattern from a layering in the wood to aggregates in the form
of granula. As far as is known this is the first case where lignin
modifying enzymes have been visibly shown to diffuse from fungal
cell walls. That the lignin barriers in the wood fiber wall are
destroyed is important, since this allows the polysaccharide degrading enzymes such as cellulases and hemicellulases to diffuse
more freely in the wood.

Mutants of microorganisms have been widely used for metabolic
studies. However, to my knowledge fungal mutants have never been
utilized in morphological studies of wood degradation. We therefore
undertook a study with both SEM- and TEM-techniques to determine the
difference in the attack on wood by the wild-type and a cellulase-
less mutant, Cel 44, of the white-rot fungus *S. pulverulentum* (3,4).
The most striking differences obtained were the following: while the
wild-type can grow through the fiber cell walls, mainly the S_2-
layer, the mutant cannot. The capacity of the wild-type fungus to

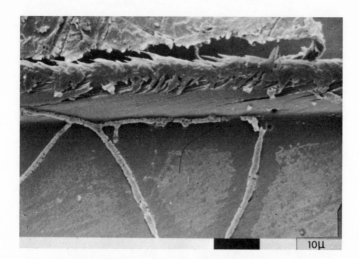

Figure 1.   A substance, most likely of hemicellulosic nature, has disappeared up to a distance of 3 to 4 μm from the cell wall of the white-rot fungus *Phlebia radiata* due to the action of diffusing, extracellular enzymes.   From Eriksson et al.(3).

bore holes in the fiber cell walls must be related to the ability of the wild-type fungus to attack cellulose.   It is clear from (4) that the mutant has mainly attacked the boundary layer between S_1 and S_2. In the transition layers the cellulose microfibrills change direction.   This seems to make these boundary layers more susceptible to attack by the mutant.   However, the transition layers are easier to degrade for both wild-type and cellulase-less mutant.   The transition layer between S_2 and S_3 is also easily degraded while the S_3- layer itself is surprisingly resistant to attack by *S. pulverulentum*. Our studies (4) have clearly demonstrated that the most resistant parts to microbial attack are the S_3-layer and the middle lamella.

ENZYME MECHANISMS INVOLVED IN FUNGAL CELLULOSE DEGRADATION. *S. PULVERULENTUM* AND *T. REESEI*

The enzyme mechanisms involved in cellulose degradation have been particularly well studied in two fungi, namely the white-rot fungus *S. pulverulentum* (5) and the mould *Trichoderma reesei* (6) (the fungus *T. viride* QM 6a and strains derived from it are now referred to as *T. reesei*).

At the end of the sixties and the beginning of the seventies it was generally accepted that the hydrolytic attack on cellulose was carried out by three different types of enzymes, namely endo- and

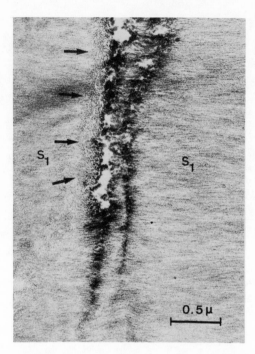

Figure 2. Lignin lamellae are changed in pattern from a layering
in the wood to aggregates in the form of granula. The changes are
seen to take place at a distance from the cell wall of the white-
rot fungus *Sporotrichum pulverulentum*.   From Ruel et al.(4).

exo-1,4-β-glucanases and by 1,4-β-glucosidases. Since then no
really striking changes in our conception of enzymic cellulose
hydrolysis has taken place. For the fungi *S. pulverulentum* and
T. reesei the pattern of attack on cellulose may be summarized as
follows: The fungus *S. pulverulentum* in hydrolyzing cellulose
produces: a) five different endo-1,4-β-glucanases which attack at
random the 1,4-β-linkages along the cellulose chain; b) one exo-1,
4-β-glucanase which splits off cellobiose or glucose units from the
non-reducing end of the cellulose; c) two 1,4-β-glucosidases which
hydrolyse cellobiose and water-soluble cellodextrins to glucose
and cellobionic acid to glucose and gluconolactone (5)

     It has been generally accepted that essentially the same
picture is also true for cellulose hydrolysis by *T. reesei* (7).
However, a few differences have been recognized including the numbe
of the various hydrolytic enzymes and the degree to which the β-
glucosidase activity is bound to the fungal cell wall. The action
of the exo-glucanase in *S. pulverulentum* differs from the action of

the corresponding enzymes in *T. reesei* in that the exo-glucanase
from *S. pulverulentum* splits off both glucose and cellobiose, while
the exo-glucanases from *T. reesei* only split off cellobiose (5,6).

Amorphous cellulose is degraded by both endo- and exoglucanases
separately (5,6). To degrade crystalline cellulose, however, a co-
operative action between these two types of enzymes seems necessary,
since crystalline cellulose is not attacked by either of these
enzymes alone. It is of particular interest in this context that
the exo-1,4-β-glucanase produced by one fungus can act synergistically with the endo-1,4-β-glucanase synthezised by another in
degrading highly crystalline cellulose. However, it has recently
been shown by Wood (8) that the extent of co-operative action shown
by mixtures of these enzymes can vary considerably. Thus, the endo-
and exo-glucanases from the fungi *Trichoderma koningi, Fusarium
solani* and *Penicillium funiculosum* can be interchanged and give rise
to an extensive solubilization of highly ordered cellulose. In
contrast, when the exoglucanases of these fungi are mixed with endo-
glucanases of the fungi *Myrothecium verrucaria, Stachybotrys atra,
Memmoniell echimata* or *Gliocladium roseum* only a small potentiation
in activity is obtained. There is a striking difference in the
cellulase systems of these two groups of fungi, in that exo-1,4-β-
glucanases have not been isolated from cultures of the last four,
while such enzymes have been isolated from the first group of fungi.
Where the exoglucanase has been isolated a synergistic action
between mixtures of endo- and exo-glucanases was observable.

The conclusion drawn by Wood (8) is that "cross-synergism" is
best between endo- and exo-glucanase components of fungi that freely
release exoglucanases into the culture medium. The question of
why all endoglucanases are not completely compatible in their activity is also discussed by Wood (8). He discusses several possibilities but suggests that the problem of an exoglucanase attack
can be a stereochemical one. Wood suggests that the configuration
of the non-reducing end of the chain may not fit with the enzyme
since the reducing end can have two different configurations,
Figure 3. If the endoglucanase cleaves the cellulose chain in one
way, it may be that the resulting configuration of the non-reducing
end does not fit the active site of an exoglucanase from another
fungal origin.

In a recent paper by Gritzali and Brown (9) a much simpler
enzymic pattern, particularly of the number of endo-glucanases
obtained from the fungus *T. reesei* QM9414, has been suggested,
compared with that previously found (7). Using a different cultivation technique, only one endoglucanase and two exoglucanases were
obtained (9). Instead of cellulose, glucose was used as carbon
source for the fungus. After washing, the glucose grown cells were
transferred to a buffer where the hydrolytic cellulose degrading

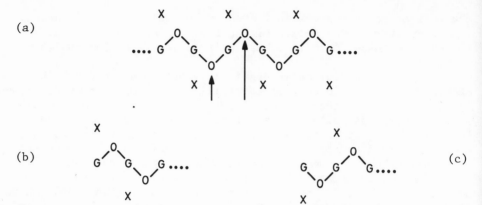

Figure 3. (a) Cleavage of a cellulose chain by endo-1,4-β-glucanase
can give rise to two sterically different end groups. (b) Non-reducing end group type I.   (c) Non-reducing end group type II.   It is
suggested by Wood (8) that if end group type I is attacked by an
exo-1,4-β-glucanase, end group type II may not be

enzymes were induced by the addition of sophorose. Polyacrylamide
gel electrophoresis of the concentrated culture solution revealed
a fewer number of cellulases in the sophorose induced cultures than
in cultures grown on cellulose. One possible reason for the apparent
multiplicity of cellulases in the cellulose culture can be protein
modification by proteases. Indeed, Nakayama et al. (10) reported
that partial proteolysis of an endo-glucanase from *T. viride* yielded
enzymes with changed substrate specificity and protein structure.
In *S. pulverulentum* the five endo-glucanases are very similar in
molecular weight, amino acid composition, etc. However, they differ
somewhat in function (11).

     Recent investigations of culture solutions after growth of
S. pulverulentum on cellulose have demonstrated the existence of
two different proteases, one of carboxy-peptidase and the other of
chymotrypsin type. These enzymes seem to influence the release
of endo 1,4-β-glucanases from the fungal cell wall and also appear
to modify the fungal cell wall (12). Whether or not these enzymes
are responsible for the multiplicity of endo-glucanases in *S.
pulverulentum* is not known. However, the recent findings of
Gritzali and Brown (9) concerning the very simple enzyme picture
in *T. reesei* QM9414 when the cellulases are induced by sophorose
in a short term culture point to this possibility. An investigation
of the effect of similar cultivation conditions on the endo-glucanase pattern in *S. pulverulentum* will be undertaken.

     In *S. pulverulentum* an oxidative enzyme of importance for
cellulose degradation has been discovered in addition to the hydrolytic enzymes described above (13). The enzyme has been purified

and characterized and found to be a cellobiose oxidase, which oxidizes cellobiose and higher cellodextrins to their corresponding onic acids using molecular oxygen. The enzyme is a hemoprotein and also contains a FAD group. It is not yet known whether this enzyme also oxidizes the reducing end group formed in cellulose, when 1,4-β-glucosidic bonds are split through the action of endo-glucanases. It was recently reported by Vaheri (14) that cultures of *T. reesei* grown on cellulose also contained gluconolactone, cellobionolactone and cellobionic acid. These findings indicate that *T. reesei* also produces an oxidative enzyme involved in cellulose degradation. However, further confirmation of these observations is necessary.

Cellobiose is one of the principal products of the combined action of endo- and exo-glucanases and as this product accumulates, the enzyme action is inhibited. It was reported by Wood and McCrae (15) that cellobiose at a concentration of only 0.01% is enough to cause 79% inhibition of the co-operative attack on cotton cellulose by the endo- and exo-glucanases from *T. koningi*. Glucose is also a potent inhibitor of these enzymes but the inhibition caused by glucose at the same concentration is only 45% (15). Thus, the rate of hydrolysis of cellulose is carefully regulated by the products of the reaction.

By the production of the enzyme cellobiose oxidase *S. pulverulentum* seems to have an important mechanism to prevent enzyme inhibition by cellobiose. The importance of cellobiose oxidase in *S. pulverulentum* is reflected by a considerable increase in the solubilization of cotton fiber under aerobic conditions, under which this enzyme is active, compared to the situation under a nitrogen atmosphere, where cellobiose oxidase is inactive. The same conditions applied to *T. koningi* shows only a slightly enhanced degradative action in an oxygen atmosphere compared to a nitrogen atmosphere (15).

The importance of cellobiose as an inhibitor of cellulose degradation is probably demonstrated by the fact that the fungus *S. pulverulentum* has several different pathways to metabolize cellobiose. The most important degradation is through the two β-glucosidases (16) but in addition breakdown occurs through the action of the most abundant of the endo-1,4-β-glucanases produced by *S. pulverulentum* (11). Three of the five endo-glucanases in *S. pulverulentum* also have a synthetic activity and produce cellotriose with cellobiose as substrate (11). Another pathway for cellobiose conversion is through the already described enzyme cellobiose oxidase and still another is through the enzyme cellobiose:quinone oxidoreductase (17-19). This enzyme is of importance for the degradation of both cellulose and lignin. Although the enzyme seems to be involved in both lignin and cellulose degradation, the highest enzyme production was reached when cellulose powder was used as a carbon source. In *S. pulverulentum* development

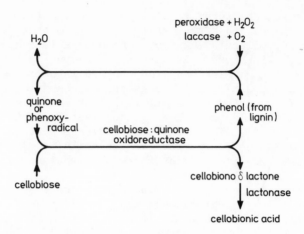

Figure 4. Reaction mechanism of the enzyme cellobiose:quinone oxidoreductase of importance for the degradation of both cellulose and lignin. From Westermark and Eriksson (18).

of cellobiose:quinone oxidoreductase activity and cellulolytic activity occur simultaneously. The oxidoreductase is relatively specific for its disaccharide substrate, while the specificity for its quinone substrates is much less. The enzyme is able to reduce both ortho- and para-quinones. A reaction scheme for the enzyme is presented in Figure 4 and a total reaction scheme for cellulase degradation in *S. pulverulentum* is given in Figure 5. However, the cellobionic acid formed by *S. pulverulentum* through the enzymes cellobiose oxidase and cellobiose:quinone oxidoreductase is subsequently cleaved by the 1,4-β-glucosidase enzymes into glucose and gluconolactone (5). Gluconolactone is a very powerful inhibitor of the β-glucosidases as evidenced by recent studies in our laboratory (16). The extracellular 1,4-β-glucosidase activity in *S. pulverulentum* can be split into two main peaks. The K_i-values for gluconolactone inhibition of the two β-glucosidases are 3.5×10^{-7} and 15×10^{-7}M, respectively. The corresponding K_i-value for the *T. reesei* QM9414 1,4-β-glucosidase was found to be 3.2×10^{-5}M. The K_i-value for inhibition of the same enzyme with glucose is 1×10^{-3} M (9).

Regulation of endo-1,4-β-glucanase production in the white-rot fungus *S. pulverulentum* has recently been investigated using a newly developed sensitive method (20). The method is based upon the viscosity lowering effect of endo-1,4-β-glucanases in solutions of carboxymethyl cellulose (CMC). The effect of inducers and repressors can be determined with the method as well as whether the enzyme are localized on cell wall surfaces or actively released into the surrounding medium. The results show that cellobiose causes induction of endo-1,4-β-glucanases at concentrations as low as 1 mg/l.

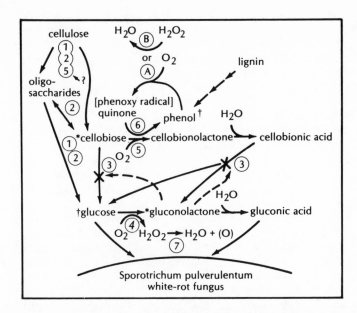

Figure 5. Enzyme mechanisms for cellulose degradation and their extra-cellular regulation in *Sporotrichum pulverulentum*. From Eriksson (5). The following enzymes are involved in the reactions: 1. endo-1,4-β-glucanases; 2. exo-1,4-β-glucanase; 3. β-glucosidases; 4. glucose oxidase; 5. cellobiose oxidase; 6. cellobiose-quinone: oxidoreductase; 7. catalase. Enzymes involved in lignin degradation A. laccase; B. peroxidase. *Products regulating enzyme activity, gluconolactone inhibits (3) cellobiose increases transglycosylations. †Products regulating enzyme synthesis glucose, gluconic acid → catabolite repression; phenols → repression of glucanases.

It was also shown that glucose causes catabolite repression of enzyme formation at concentrations as low as 50 mg/l. Mixtures of inducer and repressor give rise to a delayed enzyme production compared with solutions of inducer only.

Studies of the mould *T. reesei* QM6a using the same technique show that cellobiose under our conditions was not an inducer of endo-1,4-β-glucanases. However, sophorose causes induction of endo-1,4-β-glucanases at a concentration of 1 mg/l. This has recently been confirmed in studies by Sternberg and Mandels (21).

The comparison between the regulation of endo-1,4-β-glucanase production in the two fungi also demonstrates several other impor-tant differences. For example, a solution of CMC alone induces enzyme formation in *S. pulverulentum* but not in the *T. reesei* strain. Under our experimental conditions no endo-1,4-β-glucanases were actively excreted into the solution by *T. reesei*. This had

previously been reported also by Berg and Pettersson (22), although
they used cellulose as a carbon source. The enzymes were bound to
the cell wall. However, *S. pulverulentum* released the enzymes into
the medium although they first appeared bound to the cell wall.
However, it was recently shown (9,21) that sophorose gives rise to
active excretion of endo-1,4-β-glucanases into the culture solution
of *T. reesei* QM9414. The differences in the results of these studie
must be due either to the differences in the fungal strains or in
cultivation conditions [the same strain was used in the studies
reported in (20) and in (22)].

    The production of cellulases in fungi can also be hampered by
factors other than catabolite repression. Thus, it was demonstrated
by Váradi (23) that a wide variety of phenols repress the production
of both cellulases and xylanases in the fungi *Schizophyllum commune*
and *Chaetomium globosum*. At concentrations of less than 1 mM,
vanillic acid, vanillyl alcohol and vanillin considerably repressed
the production of these enzymes. Studies in our laboratory (24)
have furthermore demonstrated that in a phenol oxidase-less mutant
(Phe 3) of *S. pulverulentum* the production of endo-1,4-β-glucanases
was drastically repressed in the presence of kraft lignin and
phenol at a concentration of 10^{-3} M. However, both the wild-type
(WT) and a phenol oxidase-positive revertant (Rev 9) of the same
fungus produced the endo-glucanases without significant repression
by phenols. Furthermore, if a highly purified laccase preparation
was added to the growth medium of Phe 3 in the presence of phenols,
the endo-1,4-β-glucanase production reached normal levels. These
results indicate that kraft lignin and phenols decrease endo-1,4-
β-glucanase synthesis in Phe 3 due to the absence of phenol-oxidizing enzymes. Phenol oxidases may thus function in regulating the
production of cellulases by oxidizing lignin-related phenols which
act as repressors of enzyme production when *S. pulverulentum* is
growing on wood.

CELLULOSE DEGRADATION BY BROWN-ROT FUNGI

    Brown-rot fungi, which extensively degrade cellulose, seem
to utilize entirely different mechanisms than those described
above for the white-rot fungus *S. pulverulentum* and the mould *T.
reesei*. Brown-rot fungi produce endo-1,4-β-glucanase activity
but lack the exo-1,4-β-glucanase activity (25). Crystalline
cellulose is thus not degraded by a synergistic action between
endo- and exo-glucanases. Still, brown-rot fungi depolymerize
cellulose rapidly during early stages of wood decay contrary to
white-rot fungi which depolymerize cellulose in wood more slowly.

    Koenigs (26) offers the explanation that the initial attack
on crystalline cellulose by brown-rot fungi is via an H_2O_2/Fe^{++}
system. He founds that brown-rot fungi are strong producers of

H_2O_2- much more so than white-rot fungi (27). Koenigs also found (26) that the effect of H_2O_2/Fe^{++} on cellulose is similar to that caused by brown-rot fungi. This kind of mechanism would be oxidative. It has been reported by several authors that brown-rot fungi do oxidize cellulose (26). It is an attractive hypothesis that the initial attack on the cellulose takes place via a chemical agent of low-molecular weight origin that can easily diffuse through the wood fiber walls rather than an enzyme with limited diffusibility. In the case of white-rot fungi it seems to be necessary at least to morphologically modify the lignin barriers in wood to allow diffusion of enzymes attacking the polysaccharides (4). A brown-rot attack on wood is characterized by a gradual thinning of the fiber cell walls as the polysaccharides are digested leaving a framework of lignified tissue (28). It was demonstrated in a scanning electron microscope study by Blanchette et al. (29) that typical brown-rot decay of wood was evident in tracheids occupied by hyphae as well as in tracheids distal to the fungus. Decay caused by white-rot fungi characteristically takes the form of erosion troughs closely associated with the hyphae (3,29).

It was found by Highley (30) that the brown-rot fungus *Poria placenta* was unable to utilize cellulose unless placed in contact with wood. Nilsson (31) found no morphological change on cotton fibers placed between brown-rot inoculated wood pieces but reported that after this exposure no tensile strength was left in the cotton fibers, indicating attack by the brown-rot fungus. These studies suggest that when cultured on wood, fungi produce a factor able to diffuse into the pure cellulose and depolymerize it. In a more recent study, Highley (32) found that when other carbohydrate supplements such as cellobiose, glucose and mannan are added to cellulose this results in the depolymerization of cellulose by *P. placenta*. However, although xylan in wood is utilized by this fungus (33) and although xylanases are produced in cultures (34), cellulose was not utilized by *P. placenta* in the presence of xylan (32). Taking all this information into account it seems possible that a hexose such as glucose or mannose must be present to induce glucose oxidase. When a hexose is oxidized by this enzyme, H_2O_2 is formed as a byproduct. This H_2O_2 in combination with Fe^{++} may well start the initial attack on crystalline cellulose, which can then be degraded to glucose and water-soluble cellodextrins by endo-1,4-β-glucanases – the only type of cellulases produced by brown-rot fungi. If this hypothesis holds true, the reason why the brown-rot fungus can start its attack on crystalline cellulose with not only glucose as "starter" but also with cellobiose and mannan must be that β-glucosidase- and endo-1,4-β-mannanase enzymes respectively convert these compounds into their hexose monomers which function as substrates for H_2O_2 producing oxidases.

HOW IS CELLULOSE BEST SACCHARIFIED TO GLUCOSE BY ENZYMES?

For enzymic saccharification of cellulose to glucose mainly the *T. reesei* endo- and exo-glucanase enzyme system has hitherto been considered. The reason for this is that the enzyme mechanisms of cellulose saccharification utilized by this fungus are fairly well known but also that *T. reesei* produces the enzymes in higher amounts than other, so far studied, organisms. The enzyme producti can also be increased by mutations in accordance with well known an tried techniques (35). In spite of this we know that the costs for the enzymic hydrolysis of cellulose to glucose are high, actually s high that it can be questioned if, or at least when, it will be economically feasible. It seems, at this point, necessary to con- sider if there are other possibilities for enzyme production and enzymic saccharification than through the *T. reesei* enzyme symstem. I would therefore suggest that the brown-rot fashion of decreasing cellulose crystallinity and DP is investigated in more detail to allow an evaluation if the system employed by these organisms can be technically and economically feasible. There are, of course, other, mechanical and chemical, means to destroy crystallinity. The final saccharification of the amorphous cellulose can then be carried out by only an endo-glucanase in combination with a heat- stable, matrix-bound β-glucosidase to convert water-soluble cello- dextrins to glucose. If *in vitro* saccharification of cellulose with fungal cellulases in the long run can compete with the similtaneous saccharification and ethanol production obtained when utilizing anaerobic bacteria is, of course, an entirely different story.

REFERENCES

1.   Eriksson, K. -E., Grünewald, A. and Vallander, L. (1980),
      Biotechnol. Bioeng. 22, 363.
2.   Rypáček, V. and Navrátilová, Z. (1971), Drev. Výskum 16, 115.
3.   Eriksson, K.-E., Grunewald, A., Nilsson, T. and Vallander, L.
      Holzforschung. In press.
4.   Ruel, K., Barnoud, F. and Eriksson, K.-E. Holzforschung.
      In press.
5.   Eriksson, K.-E. (1978), Biotechnol. Bioeng. 70, 317.
6.   Ryu, D.D.Y. and Mandels, M. (1980), Enzyme Microb. Technol.
      2, 91.
7.   Emert, G.H., Gum, Jr., E.K., Lang, J.A., Lin. T.H. and Brown,
      Jr., R.D. (1974), Adv. Chem. Ser. 136, 76.
8.   Wood, T.M. (1980) in Collogue Celluloyse Microbienne, CNRS,
      Marseille, p. 167.
9.   Gritzali, M. and Brown, Jr., R.D. (1979), Adv. Chem. Ser. 181
      237.
10.   Nakayama, M., Tomita, Y., Suzuki, H. and Nisizawa, K. (1976),
      J. Biochem. 79, 955.

11.   Streamer, M., Eriksson, K.-E. and Pettersson. B. (1975),
       Eur. J. Biochem. 59, 607.
12.   Eriksson, K.-E., von Hofsten, A. and Pettersson, B.   To be
       published.
13.   Ayers, A.R., Ayers, S.B. and Eriksson, K.-E. (1978), Eur. J.
       Biochem. 90, 171.
14.   Vaheri, M. (1980), Report at Nordforsk's Workshop. May, 6-7,
       VTT Biotechnical Laboratory, Helsinki, Finland.
15.   Wood, T.M. and McCrae, S.I. (1977), Ed. T.K. Ghose, Proc.
       Bioconversion Symp. IIT, Delhi, p. 111.
16.   Deshpande, V., Eriksson, K.-E. and Pettersson, B. (1978),
       Eur. J. Biochem. 90, 191.
17.   Westermark, U. and Eriksson, K.-E. (1974), Acta Chem. Scand.
       B 28, 204.
18.   Westermark, U. and Eriksson, K.-E. (1974), Acta Chem. Scand.
       B 29, 419.
19.   Westermark, U. and Eriksson, K.-E. (1975), Acta Chem. Scand.
       B 29, 419.
20.   Eriksson, K.-E. and Hamp, S.G. (1978), Eur. J. Biochem. 90,
       183.
21.   Sternberg, E. and Mandels, M. (1979), J. Bacteriol. 139, 761.
22.   Berg, B. and Pettersson, G. (1977), J. Appl. Bacteriol. 42, 65.
23.   Váradi, J. (1972), in "Biodeterioration of Materials" 2, 129.
       Eds. A.H. Walters and E.H. Hueck-van der Plas, London: Appl.
       Science Publishers.
24.   Ander, P. and Eriksson, K.-E. (1976), Arch.Microbiol. 109, 1.
25.   Highley, T.L. (1975), Wood and Fiber 6, 275.
26.   Koenigs, J.W. (1974), Wood and Fiber 6, 66.
27.   Koenigs, J.W. (1972), Phytopathology 62, 100.
28.   Jutte, S.M. and Sachs, 1.B. (1976), IIT Research Institute/
       SEM, Chicago, 111., Vol. 11, 535.
29.   Blanchette, R.A., Shaw, C.G. and Cohen, A.L. (1978), SEM
       Vol. 11, 61.
30.   Highley, T.L. (1975), For. Prod. J. 25, 38.
31.   Nilsson, T. (1974), Material u. Organismen 9, 173.
32.   Highley, T.L. (1977), Material u. Organismen 12, 25.
33.   Cowling, E.B. (1961) U.S. Dep. Agric., For. Serv. Techn.
       Bull. 1258, 79 p.
34.   Highley, T.L. (1976), Material u. Organismen 11, 33.
35.   Monenecourt, B.S. and Eveleigh, D. E. (1977), Appl. Environ.
       Microbiol. 34, 777.

DISCUSSION

Q.   LADISCH: In electron micrographs of the wall were dark lines
      which were microfibrils, these in turn were surrounded by
      lignin and hemicellulose especially in certain types of wood.
      Do your microorganisms attack this particular lignin as well?

A.   ERIKSSON: Yes, they do and thereby cause a swelling of the
      secondary wall. However, the cellulaseless mutants cannot
      degrade wood in a direction across the cellulose microfibrils.

Q.   BANDURSKI: When the strain of fungus which lacks the cellulas
      alters the physical state of lignin, does it incorporate eithe
      deuterium or oxygen from heavy water? I'm curious whether the
      phyenyl propanoid matrix is somehow altered.

A.   ERIKSSON: We have not investigated that. What we see is
      probably a change in the morphology caused by depolymerization
      or polymerization caused by phenol oxidase. I dare not say
      that what we have encountered by this granular formation is
      actually lignin degradation. It may well be that lignin de-
      gradation cannot take place other than in a direct physical
      contact between the lignin and the fungal cell wall, whereas
      obviously changes in the morphology of the lignin can take
      place at a distance from the fungal wall.

Q.   BROWN: Cellobiose is an inducer with a *Sporotrichum pulveru-
      lentum* and sophorose is not an inducer, is that correct?

A.   ERIKSSON: Sophorose is an inducer also in *S. pulverulentum*.
      However, the induction time is longer for sophorose than for
      cellobiose.

Q.   BROWN: Do you recall whether or not the endoglucanase cleaves
      sophorose since it apparently does cleave cellobiose which is
      a bit unusual?

A.   ERIKSSON: We have not studied that.

Q.   REILLY: I was very interested by your statement that the
      lignolytic enzyme system may be diffusing like the other
      enzyme system. Is that correct? You said that this was the
      first time that it has been shown that the lignin digesting
      enzyme should be diffusing?

A.   ERIKSSON: I did not say lignin digesting enzyme. I said
      that enzymes that change the lignin morphology in wood seem
      to diffuse and that I interpreted these enzymes to be phenol
      oxidases.

Q.   REILLY: OK, but you are not talking about depolymerization
      of lignin then?

A.   ERIKSSON: What changes the morphology of the lignin in wood
      may be depolymerization but it may also be polymerization.

REGULATORY CONTROLS IN RELATION TO OVER-PRODUCTION OF FUNGAL CELLULASES**

B.S. Montenecourt, S.D. Nhlapo, H. Trimiño-Vazquez,
S. Cuskey, D.H.J. Schamhart,* and D.E. Eveleigh

Department of Biochemistry and Microbiology, Cook College
Rutgers - The State University of New Jersey
New Brunswick, New Jersey 08903

INTRODUCTION

A growing trend in the development of viable processes for the conversion of renewable cellulosic biomass to glucose is the use of microbial cellulases as biological catalysts. Unfortunately, the cost of the cellulase enzymes has been prohibitive for large scale industrial application in saccharification of cellulose. The high cost of cellulase is due largely to the low yield and to the low specific activity of enzymes from the available microbial strains. Improvement of the cellulolytic microbial strains can be considerably enhanced through selective screening programs. However, the rationale for selection and the chance of isolation of more useful strains are hampered by our lack of understanding of mechanisms controlling the synthesis and secretion of cellulase. Successful genetic cloning and expression of the cellulase genes from *Trichoderma* or any other cellulolytic microorganism is similarly dependent upon a sound basic knowledge of the control mechanisms. *Trichoderma* genetics is an unexplored abyss. Although *Trichoderma* is reported to have a sexual stage, in the *Hypocrea* (1,2) mating types are generally unavailable. Thus, traditional methods of delineating genetic linkages are elusive. We have therefore initiated studies to unravel the complexities of synthesis and secretion of cellulase by the cellulolytic fungus *Trichoderma reesei* through comparison of the wildtype strain QM6a with several high yielding mutant strains. Elucidation of

---

* Present address: Department of Molecular Cell Biology, State University of Utrecht, The Netherlands.

** A journal paper of the New Jersey Agricultural Experiment Station.

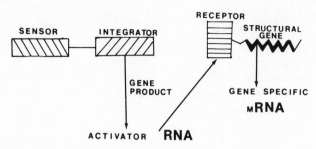

Figure 1. Model of control protein synthesis in eukaryotic cells
proposed by Davidson and Britten (5).

physiologic differences between the strains may shed light on the
regulatory controls governing cellulase biosynthesis. The data will
be interpreted in the light of current theories regarding the
mechanisms controlling the synthesis and secretion of proteins in
eukaryotic and prokaryotic organisms.

MODELS FOR CONTROL OF EUKARYOTIC AND PROKARYOTIC PROTEIN SYNTHESIS

A brief review of current genetic models controlling eukaryotic and prokaryotic protein synthesis is given below. It is
intended to familiarize the reader with concepts of control mechanisms and provide a basis for interpretation of observations on the
synthesis of fungal cellulases. Reviews of current concepts in
gene expression have been compiled by Lewis (3) and (4).

Generalized Model for Control of Eukaryotic Protein Synthesis

A current model advanced by Davidson and Britten (5) for the
control of synthesis of proteins in eukaryotic organisms is outlined in Figure 1. A structural gene, analogous to that in the
bacterial system, codes for the functional protein. The control
function resides in a series of sites each comprised of a sensor
and an integrator sub-site. Inducers or other regulatory molecules
interact with the sensor site to cause stimulation of the integrator
gene which presumably translates an activator RNA. This activator
RNA finds its corresponding receptor site(s) which is located
adjacent to the structural gene(s) and thus initiates messenger RNA
synthesis. Many aspects of this model are analogous to the proposed
mechanism of negative control in prokaryotes. A major distinction
is the role of an RNA molecule as the activator rather than a protein. As the genetic functions of eukaryotes are clearly organized
in a discrete nuclear region, while the majority of protein synthesis occurs on the endoplasmic reticulum, it is difficult to envision
a telegraphic protein synthesized in the cytoplasm traveling freely
between the nucleus and the cytoplasm to perform a regulatory

function. However, nuclear proteins could function in this capacity.
To account for the co-ordinate control of the number of unrelated
genes by a single environmental stimulus, Britten and Davidson proposed that integrator and receptor sites are redundant and multiple
copies of any one integrator or receptor sequence may be found in
a genome and can be simultaneously activated. Thus the structural
genes for a group of enzymes such as comprise fungal cellulase,
which are required to interact synergistically, may be located in
widely separated sites on the genome but could be coordinately
controlled if each possessed a copy of the same receptor sequence.

Control of Catabolite Repressible Enzymes in Prokaryotes

Since fungi represent a separate kingdom of relatively un-
differentiated eukaryotic cells (6), the machinery for control of
protein synthesis may not be as highly evolved as that proposed for
differentiating animal cells (Davidson-Britten model). However, a
clear distinction is the presence of the nuclear membrane, present
in fungi and absent in bacteria; and this barrier must be penetrated
to effect expression of a given gene. Bacteria exhibit both positive
and negative control of protein synthesis. In general, genes which
are closely related in a metabolic pathway are located adjacent to
each other and are under a common regulatory gene. An example of
negative control in prokaryotes is the lactose operon in *E. coli*,
and of positive control, the arabinose operon. Since the cellulase
genes of cellulolytic fungi have not been mapped, it is not known
if they are located in adjacent genes or even if they are on the
same chromosome.

Regulation of catabolite repressible enzymes in bacteria is
through an additional control involving the levels of cyclic adenine
monophosphate (cAMP) in the cell. The cAMP binds with a CAP protein
(cyclic AMP binding protein or catabolite-gene activator protein).
In the absence of cAMP the CAP protein is inactive. In the presence
of cAMP, a CAP·cAMP complex is formed which interacts with the
catabolite sensitive operon and RNA polymerase to initiate transcription. The levels of cAMP in the cell are mediated by adenyl-
cyclase and phosphodiesterase. When the metabolic activity of the
cell is high, as would be the case during growth on readily metabolizable substrates, levels of cAMP are low, and synthesis of catabolite repressible enzymes is halted. However, when the available
energy in the cell is depleted, cAMP levels become elevated in the
cell. Expression of catabolite repressible enzymes in bacteria is
a consequence of both the metabolic activity of the cell as well
as the genetic regulatory mechanisms.

Secretion of Extracellular Proteins

Control of cellulase production in fungi goes beyond transcription and translation of the structural genes. The vast majority

of fungal cellulases (endoglucanases and exoglucanases) are reported
to be extracellular proteins. Thus overproduction of cellulases wil
be a result of both hypersynthetic capacity as well as a superior
ability to transport the proteins to the external environment.

    Little is known about the mechanism of secretion of proteins
in filamentous fungi. Our basic knowledge has been derived from
studies with bacteria and specialized animal cells. Exportable
proteins are synthesized on membrane bound ribosomes in the rough
endoplasmic reticulum. They are recognized as exportable by a
specific sequence (signal sequence) present in the mRNA. A series
of elaborate processing steps have been proposed as the secretory
pathway of proteins in specialized animal cells (for detailed review
see references 7,8 and in bacteria (9). These steps include glycosylation, packaging into secretory vesicles, movement to the site
of exportation and discharge to the environment. Since fungi are
eukaryotic cells, the tendency has been to suggest that their
secretory mechanisms are comparable to mammalian cells. However,
it should be noted that the basic subcellular structures required
for processing extracellular mammalian proteins (e.g. Golgi apparatus) are frequently absent in fungi (10,11). Since extracellular
enzymes and metabolites produced by fungi are of great industrial
interest, there is a basic need to identify the subcellular structures and the sequence of processing events involved in their
synthesis and transportation to the external environment.

Current Knowledge of the Control of Cellulase Synthesis in Fungi

    Cellulase synthesis in _Trichoderma_ is inducible and can be
effected by cellulose, lactose, cellobiose and sophorose (12-14).
Presumably, the natural inducer of cellulase is cellulose. However,
it is not known how an insoluble macromolecule unable to obtain
entry into the cell can effect regulation of gene expression. It
has been proposed that physical contract between the cell and the
insoluble inducer (cellulose) must occur for induction to take
place (15,16). This suggests that there may be some recognition
site on the cell surface which triggers activation of the cellulase
synthetic machinery. An alternative suggestion alluded to by many
workers in the field but unsubstantiated by experimentation, is
that _Trichoderma_ synthesizes basal levels of cellulase constitutively. It is the activity of this enzyme on the cellulose which
produces the true inducer of cellulase in _Trichoderma_. Sophorose,
(glycosyl β-(1→2)-glucose) is by far the most potent soluble induce
of cellulase in _Trichoderma_ (12,17,18). Sophorose as well as other
disaccharides of glucose can be formed from cellobiose by transglycosylation reactions (13,14,19,20). _Trichoderma_ has been shown
to have low levels of constitutive β-glucosidases which are bound
to the cell even during growth on non-inducing substrates glycerol
(21) and glucose (see below). These constitutive β-glucosidases

could be the key enzymes in the formation of the natural inducer
from the environment or a yet unidentified enzyme could be involved.
It should be noted that although sophorose is an excellent cellulase
inducer in *Trichoderma* (12,17,18,22,23) and in bacteria (24,25) other
cellulolytic fungi such as *Phanerochaete* do not respond to sophorose
(26). In addition, other glucosyl disaccharides are not efficient
inducers (17).

The cellulases of *Trichoderma* have long been known to be
subject to repression by glucose or other readily metabolizable
substrates (17,27,29). Growth of *Trichoderma* QM9414, a mutant
derived from *Trichoderma* QM6a (30), in the presence of 5% glycerol
(repressor) and 1% cellulose (inducer) yielded no measurable extracellular cellulase activity (31). A similar effect of catabolite
repression has been shown with other cellulolytic fungi (26) and
with bacteria (25). The precise mechanism of catabolite repression
in fungi is not known. Nisizawa (29) has suggested that catabolite
repression in *Trichoderma* occurs at the translational level rather
than the transcriptional level based on studies employing actino-
mycin D and puromycin. However, the precise molecular biology of
catabolite repression in fungi is not known.

Comparative physiological studies of highly cellulolytic
mutant strains of *T. reesei* and the wild type QM6a were performed
in order to give greater insight into mechanisms controlling induction, synthesis and secretion of cellulase. These studies include
the role of cAMP, the location of the enzyme in relation to the
inducing substrate, the effect of catabolite repressors on extracellular enzyme production and ultrastructural observations.

RESULTS

Effect of Sophorose on Induction of Cellulase and Intracellular
Cyclic AMP Levels in *Trichoderma*

In an effort to elucidate the mechansism of catabolite repression of cellulases in *Trichoderma*, intracellular cAMP levels
were determined during growth of *T. reesei* QM6a on cellobiose (1%)
(Figure 2). Relatively high levels of intracellular cAMP were
present in the germinating spores and these levels decreased during
the rapid phase of growth. There was no apparent correlation
evident between the cAMP level of the mycelium and the specific
activity of the cellobiase (intracellular plus mycelial bound
activity).

Since sophorose is reported to be the most potent soluble
inducer of cellulase (endoglucanases and cellobiohydrolase) the
effect of sophorose on intracellular cAMP levels was examined

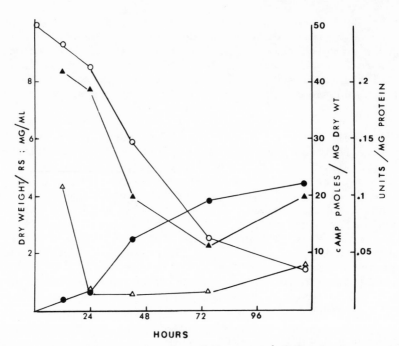

Figure 2. Mycelial cAMP levels of *T. reesei* QM6a during growth
on cellobiose (1%) and Vogels medium (31). Symbols: (o————o),
reducing sugar in extracellular culture fluid; (●————●), dry
weight; (△————△), mycelial β-glucosidase/mg protein; (▲————▲),
mycelial cAMP.

(Figure 3). Young mycelia grown on glucose were washed, resuspended
in the induction medium (22) containing sophorose and the synthesis
of endoglucanase in relation to intracellular cAMP levels was
observed. During the period of endoglucanase induction following
exposure to sophorose, no dramatic differences in intracellular
cAMP levels of the induced and control cultures were observed. Thus,
in *Trichoderma*, the synthesis of one catabolite repressible enzyme,
endoglucanase, appears to be unrelated to intracellular cAMP levels.
The results are consistent with the observations of Nisizawa and
co-workers (29) that catabolite repression of inductive cellulase
formation in *Trichoderma* occurs primarily at the translation level.
This data does not, however, rule out the possibility that another,
as yet unidentified compound, may interact with the sensor gene
and thus establish control at the transcriptional level.

Cellulase Biosynthesis in the Wild Type Strain *T. reesei* QM6a

        Detailed studies on cellulase biosynthesis (location and yield)

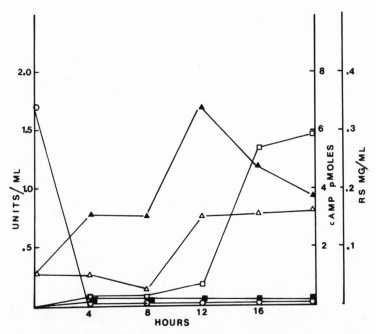

Figure 3.   Mycelial cAMP levels of *T. reesei* QM6a in relation to
extracellular endoglucanase production.   Spores were germinated on
the medium of Borgia and Sypherd (32) containing glucose (0.3%.
Mycelial mats were washed and resuspended in the above medium
containing sophorose (1 mM).   Symbols: (o———o), sophorose in the
medium; (▲———▲), cAMP control (-sophorose); (△———△), cAMP induced
(+ sophorose); (□———□), endoglucanase induced; (■———■),
endoglucanase control.

have focussed on comparison of the wild *T. reesei* strain QM6a with
hypercellulolytic mutant strains QM9123 and QM9414 (21,33). We have
selected additional high yielding strains, RUT-NG14 and RUT-C30, each
exhibiting an identifying characteristic with respect to the pattern
of cellulase synthesis (Figure 4).   Their biosynthesis of cellulase
is now compared to the wild type strain QM6a.   The location and
distribution of the endoglucanase, cellobiase, filter paper degrading activity and aryl-β-glucosidase activity of the wild type QM6a
during growth on cellulose (Figure 5) indicate that the endoglucanase
and FPase are principally extracellular throughout the fermentation
while the cellobiase and aryl-β-glucosidase appear to be equally
distributed between particle-bound enzyme and free extracellular
enzyme.   There are small but detectable levels of "intracellular"
endoglucanase and cellobiase activity.   Whether these are true
intracellular or nascent enzymes, or periplasmically located forms
which have been solubilized during breakage of the mycelium is not
known.   The location and yield of endoglucanase and cellobiase
during growth on glucose, a soluble "noninducing" substrate, yields

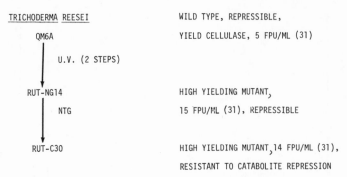

Figure 4. Genealogy of *T. reesei* mutants. Symbols: (U.V.), ultraviolet light; (NTG), nitrosoguanidine; and (FPU/ML), filter paper
units per ml. assayed according to ref. 31.

a strikingly different pattern. Barely detectable levels of endoglucanase activity are evident extracellularly, intracellularly or
cell bound during growth on glucose (less than 0.02 units). (Data
not shown). However, substantial amounts of cellobiase activity
are found in the particulate fraction during growth on glucose
(Figure 6A) which is equivalent to the amount of bound activity
of the cellulose grown culture (Figure 5B). Little if any cellobiase activity is found in the supernatant broth under these
conditions.

      During growth on cellobiose (1%), a soluble but weak cellulase
inducer (Figure 6B), a pattern similar to the glucose grown cultures
is apparent. Cellobiase activity remains bound to the particulate
fraction with extremely low levels of activity found in the extracellular fluid. Barely detectable levels of endoglucanase activity
are found in any location. It is clear (Figures 5 and 6) that the
basal level of cellobiase activity which is bound to the mycelium
remains relatively constant and independent of the growth substrate.
Whether this bound cellobiase activity is identical to or biochemically distinct from the activity induced and secreted extracellularly during growth on cellulose is currently under investigation in our laboratory.

Yield and Location of Cellulase Activity in Mutant Strains of *T.*
reesei

      RUT-NG14 is a high cellulase yielding mutant derived in two
steps from QM6a (Figure 4). The total yield and the distribution
of various cellulolytic activities are shown in comparison to the
wildtype when grown on cellulose (Table I). RUT-NG14 secretes
substantially higher amounts of extracellular protein (0.843 mg/ml
as compared to 0.548 mg/ml). All of the activities associated with

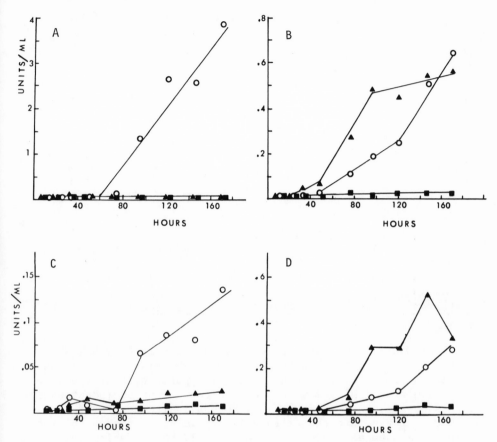

Figure 5. Location of the cellulase enzymes of *T. reesei* strain QM6a during growth on 1% Avicel PH 101. A. Endoglucanase. B. Cellobiase. C. Disc activity (34). D. Aryl β-glucosidase. Symbols: (o———o), extracellular enzyme; (▲———▲), mycelial bound enzyme; (■———■), intracellular enzyme.

saccharification of cellulose are elevated 3-5 fold in this mutant. In addition to cellulolytic activities, acid phosphatase, trehalase and laminarinase levels are also increased in this mutant. A second striking difference is the distribution of the activities among the subcellular fractions. As much as 80% of the cellobiase activity is extracellular in RUT-NG14 in comparison to a 50-50 distribution in the wild type. The percentage extracellular disc activity is also increased from 80% to 95%. Since there is no apparent shift in the location of endoglucanase activity, the increase is presumably due to release of cellobiohydrolase. In comparison trehalase, a physiologically intracellular/bound enzyme, though increased in yield, shows no change in the proportion of intra and extracellular components.

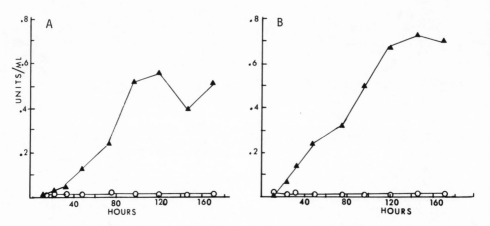

Figure 6. Location of cellobiase activity of *T. reesei* strain QM6a
(A) Glucose (1%) grown; (B) cellobiose (1%) grown; symbols as in
Figure 5.

Synthesis of the Cellulase Enzymes by RUT-C30 Under Induced and Repressed Conditions

RUT-C30 is a mutant strain derived directly from RUT-NG14
(Figure 4) and selected on the basis of its resistance to catabolite
repression of the cellulase enzymes. The pattern of synthesis of
extracellular cellulases under various conditions of induction and
repression are shown (Figure 7-9). Overall, it is evident that
RUT-C30 secretes into the extracellular fluid, components of the
cellulase system regardless of the solubility of the inducer
(cellulose, lactose, cellobiose 7A, 8A, 9A) and in the presence
of high levels of a catabolite repressor (5% glycerol) (Figures
7B, 8B, 9B). In addition, measurable amounts of endoglucanase
(1 U/ml) are secreted by RUT-C30 during growth on cellobiose (Figure
9). In comparison, QM6a produces an extracellular complex only
when grown on an insoluble inducer cellulose (Figures 5 and 6 and
see above). A further distinction is that cellulases are formed
extracellularly by RUT-C30 following growth on glycerol as the
sole carbon source (Figure 9C). In this instance, although the
absolute levels of the enzymes are reduced in comparison to cellulose or lactose grown cultures, they are clearly present in the
extracellular fluid (Figure 9C). Thus RUT-C30 appears capable of
constitutive cellulase synthesis during growth on glycerol. The
extracellular location of these RUT-C30 enzymes contrasts with the
recent report of Vaheri and co-workers (21) studying *T. reesei*
strain QM9414. They found low levels of filter paper (FP) hydrolyzing activity but no endoglucanase activity in this strain during
growth on glycerol but the FP activity was solely located in the

TABLE I

Yield And Distribution Of Enzymes In
T. Reesei Strains QM6A and RUT-NG14[a].

	STRAIN QM6A				STRAIN NG-14			
	TOTAL U/ML	% E	% I	% MB	TOTAL U/ML	% E	% I	% MB
ARYL-β-GLUCOSIDASE[b]	0.643	65.3	3.9	30.8	1.952	84.0	3.8	12.2
CELLOBIASE	0.707	57.4	4.5	38.1	2.080	80.1	4.0	15.9
ENDO-β-GLUCANASE[c]	4.200	96.2	2.0	1.8	22.947	99.3	0.7	0
DISC ACTIVITY[d]	0.110	80.9	00	19.1	0.588	94.7	1.0	4.3
XYLANASE	8.749	95.4	4.0	0.5	19.402	97.0	2.5	0.5
TREHALASE	0.199	19.6	7.0	73.4	0.467	19.9	7.5	72.6
ACID PHOSPHATASE	0.176	69.3	16.5	14.2	0.415	75.7	17.8	6.5
LAMINARINASE	0.965	75.0	5.0	20.0	1.79	80	5.0	15.0
α-MANNANASE	0.019	0	15.8	84.2	0.016	0	12.5	87.5
	MG/ML				MG/ML			
PROTEIN	0.548	36.5	3.3	60.2	0.843	66.8	2.3	30.8

[a]AFTER SEVEN DAYS OF GROWTH WITH 1% CC41 (WHATMAN MICROSCRYSTALLINE CELLULOSE)
E (EXTRACELLULAR); I (INTRACELLULAR); MB (MYCELIAL BOUND) ENZYME ACTIVITIES WERE
DETERMINED.

[b]ENZYME ACTIVITY MEASURED WITH pNITRO PHENYL-β-GLUCOSIDE AS SUBSTRATE

[c]ENZYME ACTIVITY MEASURED WITH CARBOXYMETHYL CELLULOSE (7L) AS SUBSTRATE

[d]MEASURED ACCORDING TO METHOD DESCRIBED IN REFERENCE 34.

particle bound fraction of the cell. No detectable levels of either endoglucanase or exoglucanase activity were found free in the medium.

A further illustration of the tendency to resistance to catabolite repression by RUT-C30 but with respect to glucose is shown in Table II. When QM6a and RUT-C30 are grown on low levels of lactose (0.4%) and lactose (0.4%) plus glucose (5%) and the levels of a variety of catabolite repressible enzymes measured, clear distinctions can be made between RUT-C30 and QM6a. When QM6a is

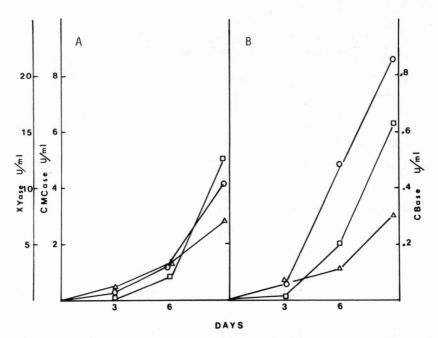

Figure 7. Extracellular cellulase production by strain RUT-C30. Panel A: Growth on Avicel PH 105 (1%). Panel B: Growth on Avicel PH 105(1%) plus glycerol (5%). Symbols: (o———o), CMCase, endoglucanase; (□———□), XYase, xylanase; (△———△), CBase, cellobiase.

grown in the presence of glucose, the levels of all enzymes studied are repressed except amylase, acid protease and proteolytic activity. More striking, is the repression of extracellular protein synthesis in general (0.37 mg/ml versus 0.04 mg/ml). In contrast, RUT-C30 shows equivalent or enhanced levels of all of the enzymes and substantially increased levels of extracellular protein (0.71 mg/ml versus 1.08 mg/ml). Thus a mutation in a generalized regulatory function of either protein synthesis or secretion may be present in RUT-C30, in addition to changes in catabolite repression.

Ultrastructural Observations of QM6a and RUT-C30

Preliminary electron micrographs of QM6a and RUT-C30 during growth on cellulose (Figure 10) point out dramatic morphological differences between the strains. A distinct rough endoplasmic reticulum is present in both organisms; smooth endoplasmic reticulum appears lacking. However, the amount of rough endoplasmic reticulum found in RUT-C30 is markedly increased in comparison to QM6a. Small

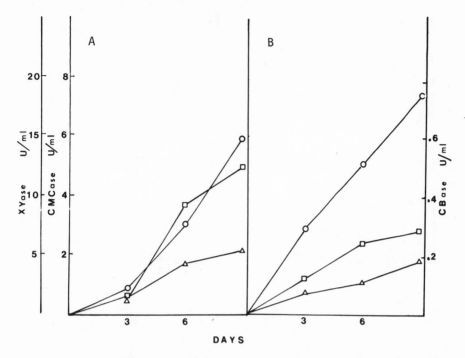

Figure 8.   Extracellular cellulase production by strain RUT-C30,
Panel A: Growth on lactose (1%).   Panel B: Growth on lactose (1%)
plus glycerol (5%).   Symbols as in Figure 7.

vacuoles, perhaps lomasome-like structures, are seen budding from
the rough endoplasmic reticulum and in close association with the
plasma membrane.   It would appear that in RUT-C30 the machinery
for general synthesis and secretion of extracellular proteins has
been enhanced. Neither strain appears to have a recognizable
Golgi apparatus.

Discussion

     We are still far from obtaining even a rudimentary under-
standing of the molecular events controlling the expression and
secretion of the cellulase enzymes in *Trichoderma*. We have presented here only a few isolated pieces in the complex puzzle.
Cellulases, although catabolite repressible enzymes, do not appear
to be under the same type of cAMP control demonstrated in bacteria.
However, these results are initial and should not be taken as
conclusive.   Control may be mediated through subtle changes in
cAMP levels which are undetected due to the cAMP assay method.
Additionally, within the scope of the Britten-Davidson model, the

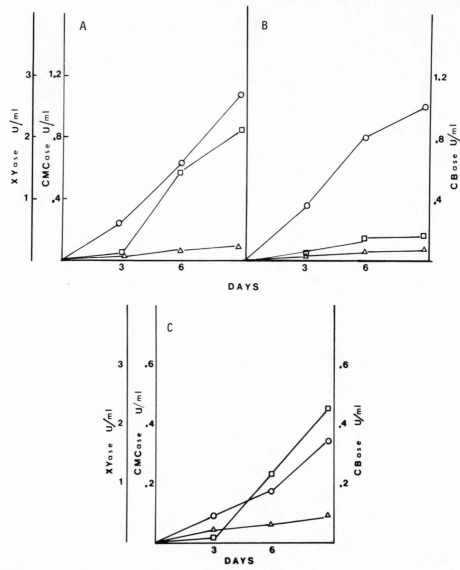

Figure 9. Extracellular cellulase production by strain RUT-C30.
Panel A: Growth on cellobiose (1%). Panel B: Growth on cellobiose
(1%) plus glycerol (5%). Panel C: Growth on glycerol (1%).
Symbols as in Figure 7.

location of the sensor site is within nucleus. Dramatic changes
in cAMP levels may be occuring within the nucleus and would not
be reflected in total cell cAMP. Definitive proof of the role of
cAMP must await demonstration of its envolement in *in vitro*
experiments.

TABLE II

Activities of a Number of Enzymes of *T. reesei* strain, (QM6A) and a Catabolite Repression Resistant, Hypercellulolytic Strain (RUT-C30).

| | ENZYME ACTIVITY IN CULTURE FILTRATE (UNITS/ML) | | | |
| | STRAIN QM6A | | STRAIN RUT-C30 | |
ACTIVITY TESTED	CONTROL[a]	5% GLUCOSE[a]	CONTROL[a]	5% GLUCOSE[a]
DISC ACTIVITY	0.11	ND[b]	0.18	0.17
ENDO-β-GLUCANASE	3.89	0.10	12.07	10.36
CELLOBIASE	0.06	ND	0.27	0.19
ARYL β-GLUCOSIDASE	0.28	ND	0.50	0.76
XYLANASE	1.11	0.08	1.65	1.10
LAMINARINASE	0.50	0.06	0.37	3.76
AMYLASE	0.26	1.56	0.44	2.99
ACID PHOSPHATASE	0.40	0.41	0.32	0.44
PROTEOLYTIC ACTIVITY	0.16	0.08	0.04	0.50
EXTRACELLULAR PROTEIN (MG/ML)	0.37	0.04	0.71	1.08

[a]AFTER GROWTH WITH 0.4% LACTOSE (CONTROL) OR WITH 0.4% LACTOSE PLUS 5% GLUCOSE, THE CULTURE FILTRATES WERE TESTED FOR THE ENZYME ACTIVITIES SHOWN.

[b]ND: NONE DETECTABLE

Major physiological differences between the wild type *T. reesei* QM6a and the hypercellulolytic mutants RUT-C30 and RUT-NG14 have been demonstrated. The mutant strains (RUT-C30 and RUT-NG14) show a greater yield as well as enhanced release of extracellular proteins in general, including enzymes of the cellulase complex as well as unrelated enzymes (amylase and acid phosphatase). In addition, RUT-C30 shows dramatic ultrastructural changes which suggest that the machinery for protein synthesis and/or secretion have also been enhanced in this mutant. Within the context of the Davidson-Britten model for control of eukaryotic protein synthesis, the data suggest that perhaps all extracellular proteins share a common regulatory mechanism such as redundant receptor sites. Whatever stimulates transcription appears to be present in elevated concentrations and effecting a wide range of structural

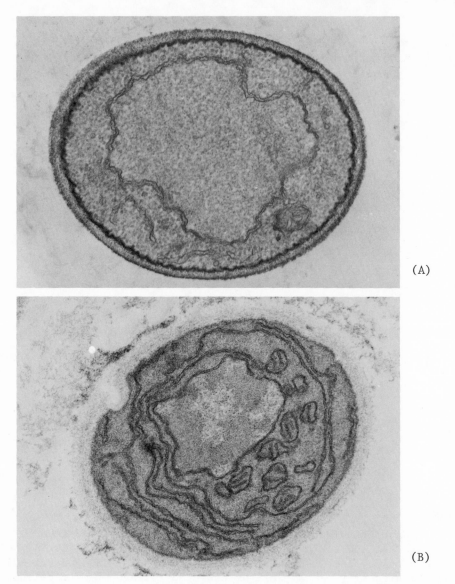

Figure 10. Ultrastructure of *T. reesei* QM6a (A) and RUT-C30 (B).
A. QM6a: Cross section of 4 day old mycelium after growth on 1%
Avicel PH 105, double aldehyde fixation; 47,500X. B. RUT-C30: Cross
section of 4 day old mycelium after growth on 1% Avicel PH 105,
permanganate fixation; 26,000X.

genes. Resistance to catabolite repression, here measured by the
ability of the mutant strains RUT-C30 to synthesize cellulases
during growth on an inducing substrate (cellulose or lactose) in

the presence of repressor (glucose or glycerol), appears to be independent from the control of general protein synthesis. The intermediate mutant RUT-NG14 shows greater yield and release of extracellular proteins but is still suceptible to repression by glucose or glycerol. This would suggest that, as in bacteria, additional controls function to regulate the synthesis of catabolite repressible proteins.

ACKNOWLEDGEMENTS

The authors wish to thank Drs. B. K. Ghosh and A. Ghosh, Dept. of Physiology and Biophysics, Rutgers Medical School for the electron microcopsy, T. Garrett, T. Spohn and H. Peled for their technical assistance and T. Chase, Jr. for his helpful criticism of the manuscript. This work was supported by the U.S. Department of Energy contract No. ET-78-S-02-4591-A000 and the New Jersey Agricultural Experiment Station. D.H.J.S. was supported by a NATO Post doctoral fellowship sponsored by Z.B.O., the Hague, the Netherlands. S.D.N. was supported by a Fulbright-Hays Scholarship. H.T.-V. was supported by LASPAU and the Universidad Nacional (Costa Rica).

REFERENCES

1.   Webster, J. 1964. Trans. British. Mycol. Soc. 47:75.
2.   Doi, Y. 1968. Bulletin National Science Museum, Tokyo. 11:185.
3.   Lewin, B. 1980. Gene Expression Vol. 2. John Wiley and Sons, London, England.
4.   Watson, J.D. 1976. Molecular Biology of the Gene. W.A. Benjamin, Inc., Menlo Park, CA.
5.   Davidson, E.H. and R.J. Britten. 1979. Science. 204:1052.
6.   Whittaker, R.H. 1969. Science 163:150.
7.   Palade, G.E. 1975. Science, 189:347.
8.   Hopkins, C.R. 1979. XXXIII Symposium of the Society for Experimental Biology, Secretory Mechanisms, Cambridge University Press, Cambridge, England.
9.   Davis, B.D., and P.-C. Tai. 1980. Nature 283:433.
10.   Berg, B. and A. Hofsten. 1976. J. Appl. Bacteriol. 41:395.
11.   Handley, D.A. and B.K. Ghose. 1980. J. Bacteriol. 141:521.
12.   Mandels, M., F.W. Parrish and E.T. Reese. 1962. J. Bacteriol.
13.   Reese, E.T. and A. Maguire. 1971. Dev. Indust. Microbiol. 12:212.
14.   Reese, E.T. and M. Mandels. 1970. J. Bacteriol. 79:816.
15.   Berg, B. and G. Pettersson. 1977. J. Appl. Bacteriol. 42:65.
16.   Binder, A. and T.K. Ghose. 1978. Biotechnol. Bioeng. 20:1187.
17.   Nisizawa, T., H. Suzuki, M. Nakayama and K. Nisizawa. 1971. J. Biochem. 70:375.
18.   Nisizawa, T., H. Suzuki, and K. Nisizawa. 1971. J. Biochem. 70:387.

19. Gritzali, M. and R.D. Brown. 1979. Adv. Chem. Ser. 181:237.
20. Okada, G. and K. Nisizawa. 1975. J. Biochem. 78:297.
21. Vaheri, M.P., M.E.O. Vaheri and V.S. Kauppinen. 1979. Eur.J.
     Appl. Microbiol. Biotechnol. 8:73.
22. Steinberg, D. and G. Mandels. 1979. J. Bacteriol. 139:761.
23. Loewenberg, J.R. and C.M. Chapman. 1977. Arch. Microbiol.
     113:61.
24. Yamane, K., H. Suzuki, M. Hirotani, H. Ozawa and K. Nisizawa.
     1970. J. Biochem. 67:9.
25. Stewart, B.J. and J.M. Leatherwood. 1976. J. Bacteriol. 128:
     609.
26. Eriksson, K.-E. and S.G. Hamp. 1978. Eur. J. Biochem. 90:183.
27. Mandels, M., 1975. Biotechnol. Bioeng. Symp. 5:81.
28. Peitersen, N. 1978. Bioconversion of Cellulosic Substances
     into Energy, Chemicals and Microbial Proteins (Ghose, T.K.,
     ed.) Indiana Institute of Technology, Delhi, India.
29. Nisizawa, T., H. Suzuki and K. Nisizawa. 1972. J. Biochem.
     71:999.
30. Mandels, M., J. Weber and R. Parizek. 1971. Appl. Microbiol.
     21:152.
31. Montenecourt, B.S. and D.E. Eveleight. 1977. Appl. Environ.
     Microbiol. 34:777.
32. Borgia, P. and P.S. Sypherd. 1977. J. Bacteriol. 130:812.
33. Ryu, D. and M. Mandels. 1980. Enzyme Microb. Technol. 2:91.
34. Montenecourt, B.S., D.E. Eveleight, G.K. Elmund and J.
     Parcells. 1978. Biotechnol. Bioeng. 20:297.

DISCUSSION

Q.   MANDELS: First of all we agree enthusiastically that your
     NG-14 and C-30 mutants are excellent, useful, and greatly
     improved over the wild strain. However, I really can't agree
     with you that they are derepressed. The data that you showed
     on enzyme production on sugars or on glycerol is really only
     1% of what you would get on cellulase. There is perhaps a
     constitutive level there; but I would hardly say they were
     derepressed. In our hands, we never see any enzyme until
     glucose (which we usually add as a repressor) is consumed;
     and, if we add glucose to a culture growing on cellulose, that
     is producing cellulase, we see an immediate cessation of
     cellulase production until the glucose is consumed.

A.   MONTENECOURT: I agree. I think we have to qualify things
     when we say repression. We observe a slight repression which
     can be relieved by adjusting C/N ratios. But what we were
     trying to demonstrate today is, that, if you grow the wild-
     type strain and the mutant strain with an inducing substrate
     (cellulose or lactose) in the presence of a repressor (glucose

or glycerol), the response of the two organisms is completely different. We have been discussing control mechanisms today and not industrial productivity, although the two have to go hand in hand. We can increase our industrial productivity, if we learn more about what is controlling the synthesis and secretion of these enzymes. What I wanted to demonstrate is that there appear to be differences in the two strains. Why there are differences is unclear since the molecular biology of control of cellulases is unknown.

Q.　MANDELS : Secondly, I would like to comment on the difference involving all of the mutants we've seen at Natick. We feel that probably the cellulase genes themselves are not effected at all. There seem to be entirely quantitative differences; you get more enzyme, maybe more readily released, but the actual properties and ratios of the components of the enzymes are not significantly changed in the various mutants compared to the wild strain.

A.　MONTENECOURT: I agree with you 100%. I think anybody involved in strain development should seriously look into the specific activity of the enzymes. The specific activity of all the mutants are identical-about 1 unit/milligram protein. Amylases, on the other hand, have a specific activity of about 80 u/mg - a 100 fold difference. If we could find out why we need so much protein in this system to do so little work, this would go a long way toward improving the industrial application of cellulases.

Q.　SHOEMAKER: Have you shown that RUT C-30 produces cellulase on glucose alone, and, if so, what amount of enzyme activity do you obtain?

A.　MONTENECOURT: We are currently determining the response of RUT C-30 on glucose.

Q.　LEDBETTER: How do the growth rate and the cell yield of the mutant compare to the wild type?

A.　MONTENECOURT: The cell yield within a given substrate is approximately the same. Also the intracellular protein levels and dry weights are about the same so the amount of extracellular protein being synthesized cannot be ascribed simply to an increase in growth rate. We do find major differences and, I think these have been confirmed at Natick, in the cell yield at the end of the fermentation. QM6$\hat{\text{a}}$ and QM9414 are completely autolized and the mycelium have all lysed at the end of the fermentation. In our hands, we do have viable RUT C-30 cells at the end of a fermentation.

They can be subcultured and appear to be a lot healthier than the other mutants or the wild-type strain .

Q.   WOODWARD: Although the RUT C-30 organism is not repressed by glucose, do you agree that the enzyme itself can still be inhibited by glucose?

A.   MONTENECOURT: I can only speculate. We have not looked at end product inhibition of the beta-glucosidase from RUT C-30 using glucose as an inhibitor, primarily because it is very difficult in the absence of the proper equipment to do such product inhibition studies using cellobiose as a substrate. Certainly, when we use high levels of glucose as an end-product inhibitor and the product is also glucose, we have to be able to demonstrate high enough activity above the initial inhibitor glucose concentration to be able to do kinetic analysis. We have done some preliminary experiments using p-nitrophenyl-glucoside (PNPG) as a substrate and we all know that results are not comparable. We cannot use PNPG or any aryl-substrate and predict that our results will be the same as if we use the natural substrate cellubiose. If we take the RUT C-30 enzyme and carry out kinetic studies using glucose as an end product inhibitor and p-nitrophenyl-glucoside as substrate, we find that this enzyme is more resistant to glucose end-product inhibition than is RUT NG-14 or QM9414. We have not done the experiments with the wild-type organism. You, I understand, find similar results. But we have not done the absolute kinetics using cellobiose as substrate because of the difficulty of doing the kinetics with high concentrations of glucose. We hope to be able to do this. We now have an HPLC system set up which will allow us to look at cellobiose degradation and increases in glucose level. The system is very sensitive and we should be able to quantitate the kinetics in this fashion. We also have an active program to isolate mutants of *Trichoderma* whose beta-glucanases are specifically resistant to end-product inhibition by glucose and we have been quite successful. We've been able to change the Ki for glucose to values about 4 or 5 times greater in these mutants. So, I think there's really hope in overcoming this problem.

Q.   TSUCHIYA: I'm interested in your work and I have some questions. The first concerns your mutant which shows some resistance to repression by glucose and glycerol. At what concentration do they act as repressors?

A.   MONTENECOURT: In the last slide which showed the effects of glucose and lactose, we were using a soluble inducer. In that case, the medium contained 5% glucose which was still detectable at the end of the fermentation. In the case of glycerol we were using 5% glycerol plus 1% soluble inducer.

Q.   TSUCHIYA: Was washed mycelia used to study the effect of the
      repressors on the production of cellulase?

A.   MONTENECOURT: We have not done those experiments. We have
      simply grown the organisms in the presence of both a repressor
      and an inducer and looked at the synthesis and release of the
      enzymes. Experiments showing the effect of exogenous re-
      pressor on actively synthesizing cells will be useful.

Q.   TSUCHIYA: I think if you use the washed mycelia to study the
      effect of repressors, it is more reliable. We compared the
      mutants and the wild strain and we used washed mycelia to
      study this effect. We incubated the mycelia with sophorose
      for about three hours during which time cellulase is produced.
      We then washed the mycelia and resuspended it in fresh medium.
      About 38 minutes after we added a repressor, the synthesis of
      cellulase was inhbited. After a longer time, the glucose or
      glycerol actually stimulated cellulase production.

A.   MONTENECOURT: In our sophorose experiments, the mycelia were
      washed. In the catabolite repression experiments, the mycelia
      were actually grown with repressors. As I mentioned earlier,
      we have been trying to understand the controls. Our approach
      now is to compare mutants with wild type. It certainly will
      be interesting to look at some of these mutants under your
      experimental conditions. I do agree.

Q.   BROWN: In line with the last question, I'd like to make a
      comment. There seems to be a lot of uncertainty as to the
      physiological state of cellulase-producing cells - that is,
      whether they're growing or resting cells. It's our experience
      that if we do the necessary experiment of growing *T. Reesei*
      QM9414 on sophorose as sole carbon source, they produce
      essentially no cellulase. One would expect then, that with
      an adequate source of a metabolizable carbohydrate, repression
      would dominate.

CELLULASE KINETICS

Michael R. Ladisch[1,2,3], Juan Hong[1], Marcio Voloch[1,3], and George T. Tsao[3]

Laboratory of Renewable Resources Engineering[1]
Department of Agricultural Engineering[2], and
School of Chemical Engineering[3]
Purdue University, West Lafayette, Indiana 47907

INTRODUCTION

The production of fermentable sugar from biomass is the first step in obtaining liquid fuels and chemicals from renewable resources by fermentation processes. Biomass materials include corn residue, small grain residues (straws), sugarcane bagasse, forages and forestry residues. It is estimated that these sources alone could yield up to 40 billion gallons of ethanol/year (1,2).

The primary constituents of biomass are hemicellulose, cellulose, and lignin in a ratio of ca 3:4:3 (3). While the hemicellulose is readily hydrolyzed to pentoses by weak acid hydrolysis (4,5), the cellulose is protected by its crystalline structure and lignin seal (3). These factors impede hydrolysis of cellulose both by acid (4) and enzyme (6).

The major product from hemicellulose hydrolysis is xylose. Until recently, this sugar was not easily fermented to ethanol and hence, was of limited value. However, Gong et al. (7) reported that glucose (xylose) isomerase could be combined with ordinary brewer's yeast to ferment xylose to ethanol in high yield.

The major product from cellulose hydrolysis is glucose. A variety of pretreatments have been proposed to make cellulose more susceptible to either acid or enzyme hydrolysis. These pretreatments include mechanical techniques (8,9,19), chemical methods (10-14), or a combination of the two (15,16). The pretreatment of cellulose improves the rate and extent of hydrolysis by cellulase enzymes (10,13,16). However, the activities of commercially available cellulase enzymes are still several orders of magnitude less than

commercially available amylases (17) which are widely used to sac-
charify starch. Thus, significant improvements in cellulase activity
are needed. It is in this context that the study of cellulase
kinetics is important.

BACKGROUND

The *Trichoderma sp.* cellulolytic micro-organisms appear to
produce three primary cellulase components: 1,4-β-D-glucan glucanohydrolase (EC 3.2.1.4), 1,4-β-D-glucan cellobiohydrolase (EC 3.2.1.
91) and β-glucosidase (EC 3.2.1.21) (19-23). These components are
sometimes referred to as endoglucanase (C_x), exoglucanase (C_1) and
cellobiase, respectively. While there is agreement that a multiplicity of each of these primary components exists (19,24-26), the
source of this multiplicity is a subject of discussion. There is
some evidence that multiplicity may be due to post translational
modification (19,45).

The primary functions of the three enzymes are described as
(24,27,30,32-37):

1) endoglucanase (C_x)-random scission of cellulose chains
   yielding glucose, cellobiose, and cellotriose;

2) exoglucanase (C_1)-end-wise attack on the non-reducing end
   of cellulose with cellobiose as the primary product; and

3) β-glucosidiase (cellobiase)-hydrolysis of cellobiose to
   glucose with high activity.

Figure 1 gives a schematic diagram of these actions. Reese
proposed in 1952 that C_1 causes a disruption in cellulose hydrogen
bonding and that C_x then hydrolyzes this accessible cellulose (31).
He later modified this scheme to give C_1 both disruptive and hydrolytic activity (22). While the exact mechanism is still being
discussed, there seems to be agreement that the C_1 and C_x components
exhibit synergism (19,22,26,31,36).

All three components hydrolyze soluble cellodextrins as well
as cellulose. Both endoglucanase and cellobiase hydrolyze cellobiose
to glucose (24,28-30,38,39). However, cellobiase has a much higher
activity with respect to cellobiose than does endoglucanase (39).
Cellobiohydrolase also hydrolyzes soluble cellotriose and cellotetraose to give cellobiose and glucose, or cellobiose, respectively,
as products (24,40). The soluble products, cellobiose and glucose,
have been reported to be inhibitors of the cellulase complex (41-44)
and of the individual enzyme components endoglucanase (35,39),
cellobiohydrolase (40), and β-glucosidase (26,28-30). Furthermore,

β-glucosidase is also inhibited by its substrate, cellobiose (28,36, 38). Thus, the kinetics of cellulase enzymes can be complex since both inhibition and activity with respect to multiple substrates must be considered.

METHODS

There are several ways in which cellulase kinetics can be studied. A cell-free cellulase enzyme preparation can be combined with cellulose and the disappearance of substrate and/or appearance of sugars can be measured. Alternatively, the endoglucanase, exo-glucanase and β-glucosidase components of the cellulase system can be separated and purified and their individual activities quantitated with respect to defined substrates. This approach is perhaps more definitive in obtaining an idea of the mode of action and mechanisms of cellulase enzymes.

Experimental

The separation of cellulase enzymes into pure components is the subject of much literature (for example, references 19,20,21,24,30, 32-35,37-40). Characterization of the kinetics of these enzymes components requires: 1) cellulose of a known degree of polymeriza-tion having a well defined crystalline or amorphous character; and/or 2) pure component cellodextrins (water soluble oligomers of cellulose, cellohexaose through cellobiose). While cellobiose is commercially available, the other cellodextrins are not, and hence, must be made and separated on a preparative scale in the laboratory (40,46,47).

The hydrolysis of celluloses and cellodextrins by pure component cellulases may yield a multiplicity of products (19,24). In this case, it is desirable to be able to separate and quantitate these products. Rapid liquid chromatography (LC) instruments, which have become available to many laboratories within the last seven years, are able to separate soluble sugars without prior derivatization. Two LC techniques have been used in studying hydrolysis catalyzed by cellulases: reverse phase chromatography (RPC) with acetonitrile: water as eluent (24,48,49) and chromatography over ion exchange resin using water as the eluent (50,51,52). The latter method stemmed from earlier work with aqueous LC (53,54,55) and is the method of choice in our laboratory for reasons discussed elsewhere (39,52). When glucose is the only product (such as in cellobiose hydrolysis) or when a hydrolysis reaction gives a predictable ratio of glucose to higher molecular weight product, the use of an automated glucose analyzer is convenient (28). In certain instances, only the total sugars formed need be determined. Colorometric assays such as the Nelson-Somogyi method (56-59), the phenol sulfuric assay (60), and the anthrone method (61,62) are then applicable.

TABLE I

Summary of Optimum Conditions

COMPONENT	pH	TEMPERATURE °C	REFERENCE
Glucan-glucanohydrolose	4.8	40	39
Cellobiohydrolase	4.8	50	40
β-Glucosidase	4.75	50	28,29

The kinetics of an enzyme are usually measured at optimum pH and temperature. These are summarized in Table I for cellulase components from *Trichoderma*. These values, determined in our labora tory, are in general agreement with conditions reported by other researchers (25,30,32,35,38,63).

Kinetic Studies on Soluble Substrates

Studies on the hydrolysis of soluble substrates have been carried out with derivatized celluloses such as carboxy-methyl-cellulose (CMC) and water-soluble cellulose acetate (WSCA)(64); p-nitrophenyl glucosides (30,36); and oligosaccharides of cellulose (cellodextrins) having a DP of 6 or less (47). The results from studies with cellodextrins are perhaps the most interesting since cellodextrins represent potential intermediate products, and there-fore, substrates,for the cellulase enzymes. Studies with soluble cellodextrins are limited to a DP $\leq$ 6, since at DP $\geq$ 7, the cello-dextrins become sparingly soluble in water (see Table II).

Studies with purified cellulase components from *Trichoderma viride* carried out with cellodextrins are summarized in Table III. In all cases the classical Michaelis-Menten type kinetics were used to model the kinetics. In this type of approach, the kinetics for the cellodextrins shown followed combinations of the reaction equations given below:

$$S + E \underset{k_{-1}}{\overset{k_1}{\rightleftharpoons}} SE \overset{k_2}{\longrightarrow} P + E \tag{1}$$

$$SE + P \underset{k_{-3}}{\overset{k_3}{\rightleftharpoons}} SEP \tag{2}$$

TABLE II

Solubility of Cellodextrins *

COMPOUND	MOLECULAR WEIGHT	WATER SOLUBILITY** mg/ml	mM
Cellobiose	342.3	125 to 147	360 to 429
Cellotriose	504.45	"very soluble"	---
Cellotetraose	666.59	78	117
Cellopentaose	828.73	<40	<48
Cellohexaose	990.86	<10	<10.1
Celloheptaose	1152.90	1	0.87

* A detailed listing of other properties is given in Ref. 47

** at 25°C

$$E + P \xrightleftharpoons[k_{-4}]{k_4} EP \tag{3}$$

$$SE + S \xrightleftharpoons[k_{-5}]{k_5} SES \longrightarrow SE + P \tag{4}$$

where S represents substrate, E represents enzyme, and P represents product. General forms of initial rate expression and integrated rate equations for competitive inhibition (corresponding to reaction Eqs. (1) and (3), non-competitive inhibition (Eqs. (1) to (3)), non-competitive with substrate inhibition (Eqs. (1) to (4)), and no inhibition (Eq. (1)) are summarized in Table IV (Eqs. A.1-A.3, B.1-B.3, C.1-C.3, and D.1-D.3).

The general technique used for β-glucosidase and glucanohydro-lase (28,29,39,65) was to obtain initial rate date, to plot it on a Lineweaver-Burke plot, and to postulate a model based on the observed initial rate inhibition patterns. A model consistent with the initial rate patterns was then developed and kinetic constants were determined from the initial rate data using these equations. The constants obtained include: the Michaelis constant, K_m ($=(k_{-1} + k_2)/k_1$), which is the concentration of substrate giving half maximal velocity; and dissociation constants, $K_{i,1}$ ($= k_{-3}/k_3$), $K_{i,2}$ ($= k_{-4}/k_4$), and K_s ($= k_{-5}/k_5$) which give a measure of affinity of inhibitors (product or substrate) for the enzyme. Complete details on this type of kinetics are given in the textbooks (67,68).

While correlation of initial rate patterns with initial rate equations is often used as the criteria for determining a model for

TABLE III

Summary of Kinetic Studies with Cellodextrins
For Cellulase Components from *Trichoderma viride*

COMPONENT	SUBSTRATE(S) STUDIED	REFERENCE
β-glucosidase	cellobiose	28,29,30,65
(cellobiase)	cellotriose	
Glucan glucanohydrolase	cellobiose	39
(endoglucanse,	cellotriose	} 66
or C_x)	cellotetraose	
Cellobiohydrolase	cellobiose	
(exoglucanase,	cellotriose	} 40
or C_1	cellotetraose	

enzyme action, a further check on consistency can be provided by
integrating the initial rate expression and comparing the fit to
timecourse data.   Thus, the model and the constants determined at
low conversion (ca. 2% to 10%) are extrapolated to higher conversions (up to 90%).   If the postulated model accurately reflects
the mode of enzyme action, the integrated rate expression should
follow the trend of timecourse data to high conversions.   The
integrated rate expressions can not, however, be used at complete
conversion since the pseudo-steady-state assumption used in
deriving the equations does not hold at complete conversion for
irreversible hydrolysis.

Initial rate kinetics have a disadvantage in that many replicate data points are required and relatively small changes in
substrate or product levels must be measured. While improved
methods of determining initial rates have been proposed (69-71),
accuracy still requires many data points. In some cases an alternate approach using an integrated rate equation may be used.

Foster and Nieman developed a graphical method for determining
kinetic constants based on an integrated rate equation for competitive inhibition (72). This method assumes knowledge of the mechanis
and is based upon Michaelis-Menten kinetics. Hsu, et al. (40),
used this type of approach for hydrolysis of cellotriose and cellote
traose by cellobiohydrolase, and which is competitively product
inhibited by both glucose and cellobiose.

Kinetic Studies on Insoluble Substrates

The hydrolysis of cellulose by cellulase is of obvious significance. The measurement of the kinetics of cellulose hydrolysis
is complicated by the factor that the reaction is heterogeneous
since a solid substrate is involved. An early attempt to model
cellulose hydrolysis resulted in the "Shutz Law" (73):

$$P = kt^{1/2} \tag{5}$$

and modification

$$P = kt^{n} \tag{6}$$

where P is the fraction of substrate hydrolyzed, t is reaction time,
k is the hydrolysis rate constant, and n an exponent which is
function of the nature of the cellulose and cellulase. These expressions are not adequate for extended reaction times so other
suggestions have been made.

King proposed (74):

$$\frac{dA}{dt} = k' (S_o)^2 \tag{7}$$

where A is substrate surface destroyed, S_o is substrate surface
available, and k' is the rate constant. Equation (7) reflects
King's observation that the rate of the crystalline substrate surface destroyed is a linear function of the surface area available.

The factor of surface area in cellulose hydrolysis was further
developed by Maguire (75), Whitaker (76), Huang (82) and Humphrey
(77). In these cases an adsorption isotherm was combined with a
rate equation to model the system. Maguire (75), using an expression derived by McLaren and Packer (78) for the action of soluble
enzymes on insoluble substrates, analyzed the kinetics of C_1 action
on cellulose. The equation used was:

$$v = k' \left(\frac{a}{A_E}\right) \tag{8}$$

where v is the rate of hydrolysis, a is the surface area occupied
by enzyme, and A_E is the area occupied by a mole of adsorbed enzyme.
Assuming a mono-layer of enzyme is absorbed at equilibrium, the
Langmuir adsorption isotherm:

$$\frac{a}{A} = \frac{K_L E}{1 + K_L E} \tag{9}$$

TABLE IV

Summary of Kinetic Equations For Soluble Cellodextrins

TYPE OF INHIBITION	REACTION EQUATIONS	INITIAL RATE PATTERNS	INITIAL RATE EXPRESSION	
None	[1]	$\frac{1}{v}$ vs $1/s$	$v = \frac{dP}{dt} = \frac{VS}{K_m + S}$	(A.1)
Competitive	[1],[3]	$\frac{1}{v}$ vs $1/s$, increasing P	$v = \frac{VS}{K_m(1 + \frac{P}{K_{i,2}}) + S}$	(B.1)
Non-Competitive	[1],[2] [3]	$\frac{1}{v}$ vs $1/s$, increasing P	$v = \frac{VS}{K_m(1 + \frac{P}{K_{i,2}}) + (1 + \frac{P}{K_{i,1}})(S)}$	(C.1)
Non-Competitive with Substrate Inhibition	[1],[2] [3],[4]	$\frac{1}{v}$ vs $1/s$, increasing P	$v = \frac{VS + v'S^2/K_s}{K_m(1 + \frac{P}{K_{i,2}}) + (1 + \frac{P}{K_{i,1}})S + \frac{S^2}{K_s}}$	(D.1)

[†] For cellobiose hydrolysis. S_o = cellobiose; P = glucose; $S = S_o - P/2$
  Substrate and product equations are in molar concentrations.

(+) Expression which gives indicated initial rate pattern.

can be combined with Eq. (4) to give:

$$v = \frac{k'Ak_L E}{A_E(1 + K_L E)} = \frac{k'E_o A}{A_E E_o + (A_E/k_L) + (A - a)} \qquad (10)$$

where E is the concentration of enzyme in solution, K_L is the equilibrium constant, A is total surface area, E_o is total enzyme concentration, E_a is adsorbed enzyme, and $E_o = E + E_a$. Using this approach with purified enzyme, Maquire (75) showed that when the C_1 enzyme concentration is large, the initial rate is proportional to surface area. At large E_o, Eq. (10) reduces to:

$$v = k'(A) \qquad (11)$$

and hence, predicts this behavior.

Whitaker (76) in a similar approach, used the Freundlich isotherm:

$$\frac{a}{A} = kE^n \qquad (12)$$

$$\frac{1}{v} = \frac{K_m}{V} \cdot \frac{1}{S} + \frac{1}{V} \qquad (A.2)$$

$$Vt = P - 2K_m \ln(1 - \frac{P}{2S_0}) \qquad (A.3)$$

$$\frac{1}{v} = \frac{K_m(1 + \frac{P}{K_{i,2}})}{V} \cdot \frac{1}{S} + \frac{1}{V} \qquad (B.2)$$

$$Vt = (1 - \frac{2K_m}{K_{i,2}})P + 2K_m(1 + \frac{2S_0}{K_{i,2}})\ln(\frac{S_0}{S_0 - P/2}) \qquad (B.3)$$

$$\frac{1}{v} = \frac{K_m(1 + \frac{P}{K_{i,2}})}{V} \cdot \frac{1}{S} + \frac{(1 + P/K_{i,1})}{V} \qquad (C.2)$$

$$Vt = \frac{P^2}{2K_{i,1}} + (1 - \frac{2K_m}{K_{i,2}})P - 2K_m(1 + \frac{2S_0}{K_{i,2}})\ln(1 - \frac{P}{2S_0}) \qquad (C.3)$$

$$\frac{1}{v} = \frac{K_m(1 + \frac{P}{K_{i,2}})}{V + V'S/K_s} \cdot \frac{1}{S} + \frac{(1 + P/K_{i,1})}{V + V'S/K_s}$$
$$+ \frac{1}{V + V'S/K_s} \cdot \frac{S}{K_s} \qquad (D.2)$$

$$0.5t = \frac{K_s}{V'}\left[1 + \frac{V_{max}}{V'}(\frac{K_s}{0.5\,K_{i,1}} - 1) - \frac{K_m}{0.5K_{i,2}} \cdot S_0(\frac{1}{0.5K_{i,1}}\right.$$
$$\left. - \frac{K_m V}{0.5K_{i,2}K_s V_{max}}) - \frac{K_m V'}{K_s V_{max}}\right] \times \ln\left[\frac{V_{max} + \frac{V'}{K_s}S_0}{V_{max} + \frac{V'}{K_s}(S_0 - 0.5\,P)}\right]$$
$$+ \frac{0.5P}{V'}(1 - \frac{K_s}{0.5K_{i,1}}) + \frac{K_m}{V_{max}}(1 + \frac{S_0}{0.5K_{i,2}})\ln(\frac{S_0}{S_0 - P/2}) \qquad (D.3)$$

He then obtained the equation:

$$v = k'AKE^n \qquad (13)$$

where $n = 0.66$ for cellulose and $n = 0.77$ for swollen linters.

Huang (82) derived an equation comparable to equation (10) which included competitive product inhibition. In this case, cellulase enzyme having high levels of C_1 and C_x and a low level of β-glucosidase was postulated to follow the reaction scheme:

$$E + S \underset{k_{-1}}{\overset{k_1}{\rightleftarrows}} X_1 \qquad (14)$$

$$X_1 \overset{k_2}{\longrightarrow} E + P \qquad (15)$$

$$E + P \underset{k_{-3}}{\overset{k_3}{\rightleftarrows}} X_2 \qquad (16)$$

The enzyme was assumed to be rapidly adsorbed on cellulose (S) to form a complex (X_1) which yields products (P) in an irreversible manner. The products, cellobiose and glucose, then reversibly combine with enzyme to give complex X_2. Huang combined the Langmuir isotherm:

$$\frac{X_1}{X_{1_M}} = \frac{k_L E}{1 + k_L E} \tag{17}$$

with the pseudo-steady state assumption and a conservation of enzyme equation:

$$(E)_o = (E) + (X_1) + (X_2) \tag{18}$$

to obtain the rate equation:

$$v = \frac{dP}{dT} = k_2 X_1 = \frac{k_2 X_{1_M} K_L (E)(S)}{1 + K_L(E)} = \frac{k_2 X_{1_M} K_L (E)_o (S)}{1 + K_3(P) + K_L (E)_o + K_L (S)[X_{1_M} - X_1]} \tag{19}$$

where K_3 is the dissociation constant, k_3/k_{-3}.

Actually, the number of sites available to enzyme changes as hydrolysis proceeds. This is reflected by the "shrinking site model" recently suggested by several investigators (79-81) and described by Humphrey (77). In this approach, the disappearance of cellulose is assumed to follow the steps:

$$S \xrightarrow[\quad(C_1, C_X)\quad]{E} S_2 \xrightarrow[\quad(\beta\text{-Glucosidase})\quad]{E_2} S_1 \tag{20}$$

where S, S_2, and S_1 represent cellulose, cellobiose, and glucose, respectively. The enzymes E and E_2 were assumed to be subject to simple, non-competitive inhibition. Hence, the disappearance of cellulose was written as:

$$\frac{dS}{dt} = KE_{ads} S \frac{K_{i,2}}{K_{i,2} + S_2} \tag{21}$$

where K is the reaction rate constant, E_{ads} is grams enzyme adsorbed/gram of cellulose, and $K_{i,2}$ is a cellobiose inhibition constant. The enzyme adsorbed, assuming a Langmuir isotherm, is

$$E_{ads} = E_M \left[\frac{K_L E}{1 + K_L E} \right] \tag{22}$$

by equation (9). E_M represents the maximum amount of enzyme which can be adsorbed on the cellulose surface and is proportional to the surface area susceptible to hydrolysis:

$$E_M = kS^{2/3} \tag{23}$$

where k is a proportionality constant. Combination of equations (21), (22), and (23) gives an expression for the disappearance of cellulose as:

$$\frac{dS}{dt} = -kKS^{5/3} \left[\frac{K_L E}{1 + K_L E} \right] \times \left[\frac{K_{i,2}}{K_{i,2} + S_2} \right] \tag{24}$$

This model was extended to the microbial hydrolysis of cellulose by accounting for the generation of the enzymes as the organism grows and the repression of enzyme production to glucose.

Another type of model has been reported by Okazaki and Moo-Young (83). This generalized mechanistic model included the action of three enzyme components, defined to have the activities:

1) E_1 - forms an enzyme-substrate complex with cellulose (S_i) having DP $\geq$ 3, and then hydrolyzes it randomly to cellobiose and glucose;

2) E_2 - forms a complex with the non-reducing end of the cellulose molecule, and then hydrolyzes it endwise to produce cellobiose;

and

3) β-glucosidase - hydrolyzes cellobiose to glucose.

These enzymes were assumed to be inhibited by glucose (E_1, E_2, and β-glucosidase), cellobiose (E_1 and E_2), and products from random cleavage (E_1). Simple non-competitive (i.e., inhibition constants have the same value) and competitive inhibition mechanisms were considered. The equations obtained (see ref. 83) were solved by computer with the assumptions that the Michaelis inhibition, and maximum velocity constants are independent of cellulose chain length. Calculations with this model showed that apparent synergism between E_1 (endoglucanase) and E_2 (exoglucanase) is affected by product inhibition, the DP and type of cellulose, the enzyme concentration at a constant E_1/E_2 ratio, and also by the ratio of E_1/E_2.

In some earlier work, Howell and Stuck (41) examined cellulose hydrolysis with a less complex model which included non-competitive product inhibition and ignored the possibility of multiple substrates. Both competitive and non-competitive inhibition were examined. The non-competitive model gave the best fit to the data (obtained with unpurified enzyme) with the equation:

$$Vt = K_S \left(1 + \frac{S_o}{K_i}\right) n \; \frac{S_o}{S - P} + \left(1 - \frac{K_s}{K_i}\right) P + \frac{P^2}{2K_i} \tag{25}$$

where V is the maximum reaction velocity, S_o is the initial cellulose substrate expressed as mol of polyanhydrocellobiose, P is product expressed as cellobiose, K_S and K_i are dissociation constants for enzyme-substrate and enzyme-product complexes, and t is time. This model gave a good fit of the data up to 65% conversion and predicted the trend in the timecourse hydrolysis data. An interesting conclusion made from this study is that excess substrate (cellulose) causes inhibition of the enzyme. The authors reported this finding to be consistent with work done earlier by Van Dyke (81).

RESULTS AND DISCUSSION

Kinetic constants for glucanohydrolase, cellobiohydrolase, and β-glucosidase determined by Michaelis-Menton kinetics are summarized in Tables V, VI, and VII respectively. Trends in these constants are helpful in describing the hydrolytic behavior of these cellulsase components which were purified at least to the point of being free of competing activities. The reader is referred to the references cited for details.

The data for glucanohydrolase (Table V) shows that this component hydrolyzes cellobiose (G_2), cellotriose (G_3), and cellotetraose (G_4) with a generally increasing maximum velocity. The K_m's for this enzyme are on the magnitude of order of 1. The hydrolysis of cellobiose is competitively product inhibited by glucose. The enzyme is also apparently subject to substrate inhibition at 10 x K_m according to Shoemaker and Brown (24).

The hydrolysis of cellulose by glucanohydrolase has also been studied. The limited hydrolysis of phosphoric acid swollen cellulose at pH 4.5 and 40°C with endoglucanose gives G_1, G_2, and G_3 as products (24). Cellodextrin production was also observed in our laboratory for Avicel[R] (micro-crystalline cellulose) for glucanohydrobose at pH 4.8 and 40°C was shown in Figure 2. The hydrolysis of cellobiose (39), cellotriose (24,66), cellotetraose (24,66), and cellopentaose (24) has been reported to result in small quantities of higher oligosaccharides. This indicates that hydrolysis of soluble cellodextrins is reversible to a small extent.

TABLE V

Kinetic Constants For Glucanohydrolase
(Endoglucanase) From *Trichoderma*

SUBSTRATE	ASSAY CONDITIONS		V/E_{tot} $\frac{\mu moles}{min \cdot mg\ protein}$	K_m mM	$K_{i,2}$[**] mM
	Temp °C	pH			
Cellobiose	40	4.8	0.58[*]	1.6	0.98
	40	4.5	0.498[≠,a]	1.03	----
			3.65[≠,b]	(162.)[+]	----
			0.301[≠,c]	1.26	----
Cellotriose[≠]	40	4.5	1.22[a]	0.339	----
			24.4[b]	2.65	----
			0.957[c]	0.279	----
Cellotetraose[≠]	40	4.5	66.7[b]	1.33	----
			14.1[c]	2.13	----

[**] Competitive Inhibition constant for product inhibition by glucose

[*] Data from Ladisch, Gong, and Tsao (39)

[≠] Data from Shoemaker and Brown (24), with values for T. underline viride
        [a] "Endoglucanase II"
        [b] "Endoglucanase III"
        [c] "Endoglucanase IV"

+ Estimate

In comparison, cellobiohydrolase catalyzed hydrolysis of G_2 G_3, and G_4 is not reversible (40). As shown in Table VI, cellobio-hydrolase has no activity with respect to cellobiose. The activity with respect to G_3 and G_4 is competitively product inhibited by cellobiose and glucose (40). The inhibition by cellobiose is much stronger (K_2 = 0.2 mM) than for glucose (K_1 = 2.1 mM). The inhibition by glucose of both cellobiohydrolase and glucanohydrolase is of the same magnitude of order (compare Table V and VI). In comparison cellobiose inhibition is significantly stronger than glucose inhibition of gluconohydrolase. The activity of cellobio-hydrolase seems to be somewhat lower with respect to G_3 and G_4 compared to glucanohydrolase. The K_m's of cellobiohydrolase appear to significantly decrease with increasing molecular weight of the

TABLE VI

Kinetic Constants For Cellobiohydrolase
(Exoglucanase) From *Trichoderma*

SUBSTRATE	ASSAY CONDITIONS		V/E_{tot} μmoles min·mg protein	K_m mM	K_{G1}[**] mM	K_{G2}[***] mM
	Temp °C	pH				
Cellobiose[≠]	50	4.8	No Activity	--	--	--
Cellotriose[≠]	50	4.8	0.1	0.2	2.1	0.2
Cellotetraose[≠]	50	4.8	2.7	0.08	--	0.4
Fibrous α-cellulose[*]	25	5.2	0.0071[++]	--	--	1.13
Bacterial cellulose[+]	37	4.8	---	<0.01[+++]	--	0.06

[≠] Data from Hsu, Gong, and Tsao (40), T. reesei.

[*] Data from Maguire (75), T. viride.

[+] Data from Halliwell and Griffin (35), T. koningi; significant inhibition also also caused by carboxy-methyl cellulose.

[++] $V = 0.118 \frac{\mu mole}{\ell \; sec} \cdot \frac{60 \; sec}{min} \cdot \frac{1 \; \ell}{1000 \; ml} \cdot \frac{10 \; ml}{10 \; mg \; protein}$

[+++] Calculated from data of Halliwell and Griffin assuming cellulose DP > 30 (MW > 4860).

[**] Competitive inhibition constant for glucose.

[***] Competitive inhibition constant for cellobiose.

substrate. Cellobiohydrolase hydrolyzes micro-crystalline celluose giving cellobiose and glucose as the sole products (see Figure 2).

The hydrolysis of both α-cellulose and bacterial cellulose is strongly inhibited by the product cellobiose. Thus when cellobiose is combined with cellobiohydrolase an apparent improvement in activity is observed (19,85). This synergistic effect can be explained by the partial relief of cellobiose product inhibition when cellobiose is hydrolyzed to glucose. While glucose also inhibits cellobiohydralase, its dissociation constant is 10 times larger than that for cellobiose (40). Hence, the inhibition effect of glucose is lower than cellobiose and the net effect is relief of inhibition.

Another interesting finding reported for cellobiohydrolase is that it is also strongly inhibited by carboxy-methyl cellulose (35).

TABLE VII

Kinetic Constants for β-Glucosidase
(Cellobiase) From *Trichoderma*

SUBSTRATE	ASSAY CONDITIONS		V/E_{tot} μmoles min·mg protein	K_m mM	$K_{i,1}$[*] mM	$K_{i,2}$[**] mM	K_s[***] mM
	Temp °C	pH					
Cellobiose [‡]	50	4.8	116	2.5	16.4	1.22	inh. noted[‡]
Cellobiose [+]	25	4.94	---	2.68	---	inh. noted	---
Cellobiose [++]	50	5.0	---	1.5	---	---	inh. noted
Cellobiose [x]	40	5.0	33	1.5	---	---	inh. noted
Cellobiose [xx]	Not given. Probably similar to conditions above.		97	1.8	---	---	31.5
Cellotriose [xx]			185	0.22	---	---	26.6
Cellotetraose [x]	40	5.0	(19)	(0.35)	Cellotetraose causes strong inhibition		

[‡] Data from refs. 28, 29; *T. viride*.

[+] Data from Maguire (30); *T. viride*.

[++] Data from Sternberg (84); *T. viride*.

[x] Data from Berghen and Pettersson (38); *T. viride*.

[xx] Data from Brown (36).

[*] Noncompetitive glucose inhibition constant.

[**] Competitive glucose inhibition constant.

[***] Substrate inhibition constant.

This seems to be consistent with the observation of Howell and Stuck (41) who reported substrate inhibition by cellulose for a crude cellulase preparation from *T. viride*. In the context of inhibition by insoluble substrates, it is interesting to speculate that part of the C_1-C_x synergism may reflect the relief of C_1 inhibition by the action of C_x. This would be analogous to the stimulating effect observed when β-glucosidase is added to a cellulase preparation (85) to enhance the hydrolysis of cellobiose which inhibits cellobiohydrolase.

The properties of β-glucosidase are summarized in Table VII. This enzyme has a much higher apparent maximum velocity towards cellobiose than do the other cellulase components with repect to their substrates. β-Glucosidase is subject to non-competitive product inhibition (28,29,65) and substrate inhibition (36,65). The

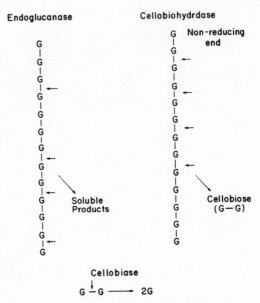

Figure 1.   Schematic representation of action of cellulase components.

competitive part of glucose inhibition (represented by $Ki_{,2}$) is the
most pronounced inhibition, with uncompetitive product inhibition
($K_{i,1}$) being less and substrate inhibition (K_s) being the least.
While β-glucosidase has very high activity with respect to cellobiose (hence, the term "cellobiase"), some β-glucosidases have also
been found to exhibit significant activity with respect to cello-
troise (36) and cellotetraose (38).   Berghem and Petterson also
reported that cellotetraose strongly inhibits β-glucosidase.

For cellobiase enzymes exhibiting non-competitive product
inhibition, it is relevant to note an interesting artifact reported
by Segal for non-competitive type inhibition (ref. 68, pg. 149).
The undetected contamination of substrate by small amounts of
product can give a Lineweaver-Burke plot which indicates substrate
inhibition.   This arises from the mathematical form of the kinetic
equation for non-competitive inhibition.   Hence, when measuring
the kinetics of β-glucosidase using purchased cellobiose, it is
probably prudent to check for glucose contamination before doing
initial rate assays.

Using that data in Table V to VII, some kinetic characteristic
of the three components can be described.

(1) The apparent maximum velocities for individual cello-
    biose hydrolase and glucanohydrolase components are
    low while the velocity for β-glucosidase is high.

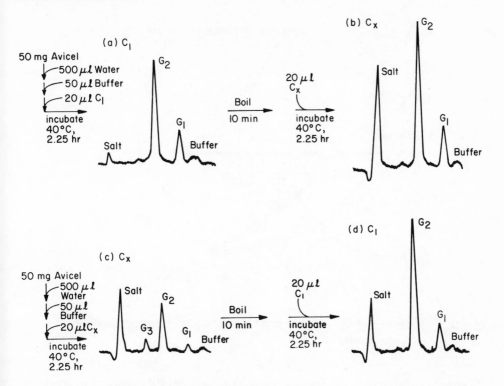

Figure 2. Chromatograms showing action of C_1 and C_X components from
T. reesei. C_1= 10 mg protein/ml. C_X = 1.75 mg protein/ml. C_1,C_X
purified as indicated in ref. 19.

(2) All three components are product inhibited. The
    magnitude of glucose inhibition for all three
    components is similar. The cellobiose product
    inhibition of cellobiohydrolase is about 5 times
    stronger than the glucose product inhibition of
    cellobiase. This may explain why cellobiose
    product inhibition in culture filtrates seems more
    prominent than glucose inhibition.

(3) All three enzyme components show substrate inhibi-
    tion. Substrate inhibition with respect to soluble
    cellodextrins is weak and occurs at relatively high
    substrate concentrations.

(4) Cellobiohydrolase and β–glucosidase do not appear
    to catalyze a reversible reaction. Glucanohydro-
    lase shows a small extent of reversible hydrolysis.

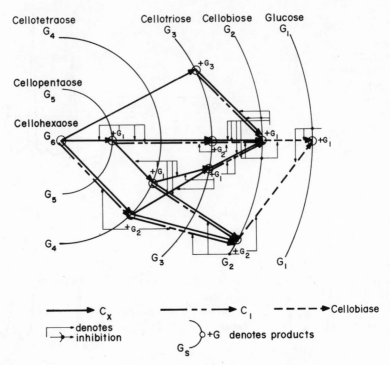

Figure 3. Schematic diagram summarizing possible reaction pathway for cellulase components acting on soluble substrates. Detailed explanation of figure is given in text.

Additional studies on hydrolysis of cellodextrins by pure component endo- and exo-glucanases from *T. viride* and other sources have also been reported. The trends observed and kinetics constants obtained are similar to those in Table V to VII. These results, which include the work of Whitaker, Nisizawa and collegues, Li, Flora, King, and others, are given in a comprehensive review by Nisizawa (44) on the mode of action of cellulases and hence are not discussed here.

The diagram in Figure 3 attempts to summarize the possible hydrolysis pathways leading to complete conversion that a molecule of G_6 could follow according to the discussion and data presented thus far. This scheme includes consideration of glucanohydrolase (C_x) and cellobiohydrolase (C_1) having activity with respect to the same substrate, product inhibition by glucose, substrate and product inhibition by cellobiose, and the multiplicity of products possible. Reversible reactions are assumed to be small, and hence, are not included here although they could affect apparent rates of hydrolysis at intermediate conversions. Substrate inhibition by G_3 through G_6 is not included since these components are not

TABLE VIII

Pathways Represented in Figure 3[#]

$\underline{G_6}$ 6 → 5 → 4 → 3 → 2 → 1

6 → 5 ————→ 3 → 2 → 1

6 → 5 → 4 ————→ 2 → 1

6 ————→ 4 → 3 → 2 → 1

6 ————→ 4 ————→ 2 → 1

6 ————————→ 3 → 2 → 1

$\underline{G_5}$ 5 → 4 → 3 → 2 → 1

5 ————→ 3 → 2 → 1

5 → 4 ————→ 2 → 1

$\underline{G_4}$ 4 → 3 → 2 → 1

4 ————→ 2 → 1

$\underline{G_3}$ 3 → 2 → 1

$\underline{G_2}$ 2 → 1

[#]Numbers indicate DP of product or substrate.

readily soluble (47) to the extent necessary for strong substrate inhibition.

This diagram is helpful in discussing the qualitative aspects of soluble cellodextrin hydrolysis. The curves in the figure represent potential products (or substrates), as indicated by G_n (n = 1 to 6). The circled (ϕ) intersections represent product arising from a particular path. The information of two different products is inicated by a circle (ϕ) for the one product and a (+G_2) for cellobiose or (+G_1) for glucose, which are the other possible products. The possible pathways represented if Figure 3 are summarized in Table VIII. Some of these pathways are duplicated in Figure 3 for the purposes of clarity. Two further examples comparing this scheme to literature results are given below.

The action of endoglucanases from *T. viride* (86) shows $G_2:G_1$ product ratios (86) of about 1:1 for G_3 hydrolysis 2:1 for G_4, 1.5:1

(with some G_3 product) for G_5 hydrolysis, and 1.8:1 (with some G_3 and G_4 product) for G_6 hydrolysis. Based on careful biochemical studies, the authors concluded that their enzyme was not acting randomly. Figure 3 indicates that if the endoglucanase (C_x) were strictly random, mole product ratios of about 1:1 for G_6, G_5, and G_3 and 1.5:1 for G_4 should be observed. These are not observed, and hence, the prediction from Figure 3 is consistent with the data. It should be noted that other researchers have also reported less than random action for endoglucanase from *T. viride* (24) and *Cellivibrio gilvus* (87).

The activity of cellobiohydrolase (C_1) is defined to be sequential with hydrolysis is progressing from the non-reducing end of cellulose or cellodextrin. Consequently, there is only one pathway by which each particular substrate reacts. Substrate G_n will give $(n - 1)/2$ moles G_2 to each mole of G_1 if n is odd, and $n/2$ moles G_2 (with no G) if n is even. The product distribution is again consistent with experimental data (40).

The results from kinetic studies using solid substrate are helpful in explaining some of the observed synergistic effects reported for cellulases. In this context the work of Moo-Young (83) is interesting. Their mechanistic model describes synergism as enzyme E_1 (endoglucanase) randomly attacking cellulose and "opening up" non-reducing ends in the cellulose structure which can be attacked by E_2 (exoglucanase). Their model predicts that an E_1/E_2 ratio of between 0.01 and 0.1 gives the optimum degree of synergism depending on the molecular weight of the cellulose substrate. In a careful study of relative quantities of protein in *T. reesei*, Gong et. al. (19) found the endo: exo (i.e., E_1/E_2) ration to be 0.12. This is within the range predicted. Thus, according to Okazaki and Moo-Young's model further improvement should be observed if the amount of E_2 (cellobiohydrolase) is increased. The effect should be especially pronounced if higher DP cellulose is being hydrolyzed.

The interpretation of synergism observed experimentally is made more difficult by the strong product inhibition of exoglucanase (C_1) by cellobiose. Thus, while synergistic effects may increase with C_1 concentration, the greater production of cellobiose will also increase the inhibitory effect on C_1.

Figure 2 shows results from an experiment in which C_1 and C_x were added sequentially with the enzyme being inactivated inbetween steps without removing the product. When C_1 was added first the products were G_2 and G_1. When C_x was added first the products were G_3, G_2, and G_1 which indicated random action. However, in both cases the final products are G_2 and G_1. In the case of C_1 action this is expected. However, in the case of C_x (Figure 2(b)) a product distribution which includes significant G_3 would be expected just as was observed in Figure 2(c). Considering that less than 10% of the substrate was hydrolyzed, this result is somewhat surprising and difficult to explain.

An important aspect of cellulose hydrolysis is the measurement of what changes occur to the cellulose itself upon enzymatic attack. Gel permeation chromatography of native cotton, swollen cotton, and rayon after incubation with an unspecified fungal cellulase showed an 18% drop in the number average molecular weight (M_n) for native cotton, a 14 fold drop in M_n for swollen cotton and little change in rayon (88). In all cases "significant" solubilization was obtained. These data indicate that the cellulose surface area is an important parameter to enhancing the action of cellulases. Further results on morphological changes of cellulose have been reported by Tsao and Chang (89). They reported that phosphoric acid treated cotton linter having an initial DP of 2000 attained a DP of 40 as hydrolysis with *T. viride* cellulase proceeded. Untreated linters incubated with the same enzymes changed from 2000 DP to 150 DP.

Both these results indicate that accessibility of substrate affects efficiency of enzyme hydrolysis. With this in mind, Zabriskie et al. (64) tested the hydrolysis of water soluble cellulose acetate (WSCA) with *T. reesei* cellulase. The activity observed for WSCA was almost 20 times higher than that observed with Solka Floc at the same incubation conditions. This experiment gives an indication of the maximum rate which could be expected if impediments to hydrolysis due to cellulose crystalline structure are removed. Hence, there seems to be an incentive for quantitatively examining the question of accessibility along with that of synergism.

CONCLUSIONS

The study of cellulase kinetics is helpful together with other data in developing a better understanding of cellulase action. The kinetics reported thus far appear to fall into the categories of Michaelis Menten (MM) type kinetics, non MM kinetics, and a combination of the two. The analytical solution of rate equations and the determination of rate constants is complex even when single substrates are considered because of the product and substrate inhibition characteristics of cellulase enzymes. Despite this, Michaelis constants have been reported for the cellodextrins for all three cellulase components. Other kinetic (inhibition) constants are also slowly being reported in the literature.

The modeling of enzyme hydrolysis of solid substrates is also being examined. The heterogeneous nature of the reaction system requires consideration of enzyme adsorption, surface area, and diffusion phenomena. Much work still remains to be done in this area.

Future research on cellulase kinetics will have to deal with the combination of cellulase action on both cellulose and soluble cellodextrins. Thus GPC will probably become a useful tool in studying the changes of the solid cellulose substrate upon C_1 and C_x action. One of the challenges in this research will be in obtaining the definitive experimental data which will be needed (1) to develop models of cellulose hydrolysis, and (2) to determine the kinetic constants. One of the objectives of this work should be to develop sufficient understanding of the system to identify the rate limiting steps. Then simplifying assumptions could be made to reduce the complexity of the mathematical form of the kinetics. The objective should then be to obtain equations which are sufficiently sophisticated to accurately extrapolate trends in cellulose hydrolysis from a minimum of data, yet simple enough to be useful.

ACKNOWLEDGEMENT

The efforts of Dr. C. S. Gong in purifying the cellulase components and the many helpful suggestions he had during the preparation of this manuscript are gratefully acknowledged. The authors are also grateful to the Department of Energy, Basic Sciences Division, for their support of this research through grants DE-AC02-78CS40071 and DE-AS02-76ER02755.

REFERENCES

1. Tyner, W.E., Biotechnol. Bioeng. Symp. No. 10, C.D. Scott, ed., 81 (1980).
2. Bellamy, W.D., Biotechnol. Bioeng., XVI, 869 (1974).
3. Tsao, G.T., Process Biochemistry, 13 (10), 12 (1978).
4. Ladisch, M.R., Process Biochemistry, 14(1), 21 (1979).
5. Wenzel, H.F., The Chemical Technology of Wood, Academic Press, N.Y., 157 (1970).
6. Cowling, E.B. and W. Brown, Adv. Chem. Series No. 95, Am. Chem. Soc., Washington, DC, 152 (1969).
7. Gong, C.S., C.S. Chen, L.G. Chiang, M.C. Flickinger, and G.T. Tsao, "Production of ethanol from D-xylose using D-xylose isomerase and yeast," Appl. Environ. Microbiol., in press (1981).
8. Nystrom, J., Biotechnol. Bioeng. Symp. No. 5, 221 (1975).
9. Han, Y.W., W.P. Chen, and T.R. Miles, Biotechnol. Bioeng, XX, 567 (1978).
10. Sasaki, T., T. Tanaka, N. Nanbu, Y. Sato, and K. Kainuma, Biotechnol. Bioeng., XXI, 1031 (1979).
11. Dunning, J.W. and E.C. Lathrop, Ind. Eng. Chem., 37, 24 (1945).
12. Millett, M.A., A.J. Baker, and L. T. Saffer, Biotechnol. Bioeng. Symp. No. 5, 193 (1975).

13. Ladisch, M.R., C.M. Ladisch, and G.T. Tsao, _Science_, 201, 743 (1978).

14. Sakai, Y., _Bull. Chem. Sco._ (Japan), 38(6), 863 (1965).

15. Uskov, Yu. N., and N.V. Chalov, _Gidr. i. Lesokhimi. Promylshl._ (USSR), 8 1 (1979).

16. Detroy, R.W., L.A. Lindenfelser, G. St. Julian, Jr., and W.L. Orton, _Biotechnol. Bioeng. Symp. No. 10_, 135 (1980).

17. Chang, M. Laboratory of Renewable Resources Engineering, Personal Communication (1980).

18. Millett, M.A., M.J. Effland, and D.F. Caulfied, _Adv. Chem. Ser. No. 181_, Am. Chem. Soc., Washington, D.C. 71 (1979).

19. Gong, C.S., M.R. Ladisch, and G.T. Tsao, op. cit., p. 261.

20. Gritzali, M. and R.D. Brown, _Adv. Chem. Ser. No. 181_, Am. Chem. Washington, D.C., 237 (1979).

21. Montenecourt, B.S., and D.E. Eveleigh, _Adv. Chem. Ser. No. 181_, Am. Chem. Soc., Washington, D.C., 181 (1979).

22. Wood, T.M., and S.I. McCrae, _Adv. Chem. Ser. No. 181_, Am. Chem. Soc., Washington, D.C., 181 (1979).

23. Mandels, M., R. Andreotti, and C. Roche, _Biotechnol. Bioeng. Symp. No. 6_, 21 (1976).

24. Shoemaker, S.P., and R.D. Brown, Jr., _Biochimica et Biophysica Acta._, 523, 133 (1978).

25. ibid., p. 147.

26. Wood, T.M. and S. I. McCrae, _Symposium on Enzymatic Hydrolysis of Cellulose_, M. Bailey, T.M. Enari, and T.M. Linko, eds., Helsinki, Finland, 231 (1975).

27. Berghem, L.E.R., and L.G. Pettersson, _Eur. J. Biochem._, 37, 27 (1973).

28. Ladisch, M.R., C.S. Gong, and G.T. Tsao, _Dev. Ind. Microbiol._, 18, 157 (1977).

29. Gong, C.S., M.R. Ladisch, and G.T. Tsao, _Biotechnol. Bioeng._ 19, 959 (1977).

30. Maguire, R., _Can. J. Biochem._, 55, 19 (1977).

31. Reese, E.T., R.G.H. Siu, and H.S. Levin, _J. Bacteriol._, 59 485 (1950).

32. Selby, K. and C.C. Maitland, _Biochem. J._, 104, 716 (1967).

33. Erickson, K.E., and B. Petterson, _Eur. J. Biochem._ 51, 193 (1975).

34. ibid., p. 213.

35. Halliwell, G. and M. Griffin, _Biochem. J._, 135, 587 (1973).

36. Emert, G.H., E.K. Gum, Jr., J.A. Lang, T.H. Lin, and R.D. Brown, Jr., _Adv. Chem. Ser. No. 136_, Am Chem. Soc., Washington, D.C., 79 (1974).

37. Wood, T.M. and S.I. McCrae, _Biochem. J._, 128, 1183 (1972).

38. Berghem, L.E.R., and L.G. Pettersson, _Eur. J. Biochem._, 46, 295-305 (1974).

39. Ladisch, M.R., C.S. Gong, and G.T., Tsao, _Biotechnol. Bioeng._ XXII, 1107 (1980).

40. Hsu, T.A., C.S. Gong, and G.T. Tsao, _Biotechnol. Bioeng._, XXII, 2305 (1980).

41. Howell, J.A., and J.D. Stuck, Biotechnol. Bioeng. XVII, 873 (1975).

42. Katz, M. and E.T. Reese, Appl. Microbiol., 16 (2), 419 (1968).

43. Ghose, T.K., Adv. In Biochem. Eng., 6, T.K. Ghose, A. Fiechter, N. Blakebough, eds., Springer-Verlag, Berlin, 39 (1977).

44. Nisizawa, K., J. Ferment. Technol., 51 (4), 267 (1973).

45. Nakayama, M., Y. Tomita, H. Suzuki, and K. Nisizawa, J. Biochem., 79, 955 (1976).

46. Miller, G.L., J. Dean, and R. Blum, Arch. Biochem. Biophys., 91, 21 (1960).

47. Huebner, A., M.R. Ladisch, and G.T. Tsao, Biotechnol. Bioeng. XX, (10), 1669 (1978).

48. Gum, E.K., Jr., and R.D. Brown, Jr., Anal. Biochem., 82 372 (1977).

49. Palmer, J.K., Appl. Polym. Symp. No. 28, 237 (1975).

50. Ladisch, M.R., A.L. Huebner, and G. T. Tsao, J. Chromatog., 147, 185 (1978).

51. Ladisch, M.R., and G.T. Tsao, J. Chromatog. 166, 85 (1978).

52. Ladisch, M.R., A.W. Anderson, and G. T. Tsao, J. Liq. Chromatog., 2 (5), 745 (1979).

53. Brobst, K.M., H.D. Scobell, and E. M. Steeler, Proc. Am. Soc. Beer Brewing Chemists, 43 (1973).

54. Jandera P., and J. Churacek, J. Chromatog., 98, 55 (1974).

55. Saunders, R.M., Carbohydr. Res. 7, 76 (1968).

56. Shaffer, P.A. and A.F. Hartman, J. Biol. Chem., 45, 349 (1921).

57. Shaffer, P.A. and M. Somogyi, J. Biol. Chem., 100, 695 (1933).

58. Somogyi, M., J. Biol. Chem., 70, 599 (1926); 117, 771 (1937); 160, 61, 69 (1945); 195, 19 (1952).

59. Nelson, N., J. Biol. Chem., 153, 375 (1944).

60. Dubois, M., K.A. Gilles, J.K. Hamilton, P.A. Rebers, and F. Smith, Anal. Chem., 28, 350 (1956).

61. Viles, F.J., Jr., and L. Silverman, Ind. Eng. Chem., Anal. Ed., 21, 950 (1949).

62. Dreywood, R., Ind. Eng. Chem., Anal. Ed., 18, 499 (1946).

63. Mandels, M., R. Andreotti, and C. Roche, Biotechnol. Bioeng. Symp. No. 6, 21 (1976).

64. Zabriskie, D.W., Syed A.S.M. Qutubuddin, and K.M. Downing, Biotechnol. Bioeng. Symp. No. 10, 149 (1980).

65. Hong, J., M.R. Ladisch, C.S. Gong, P.C. Wankat, and G.T. Tsao, Biotechnol. Bioeng. submitted.

66. Ladisch, M.R., PhD Thesis, Purdue University, 1977.

67. Plowman, K.M., Enzyme Kinetics, McGraw-Hill, NY (1972).

68. Segal, I.H., Enzyme Kinetics, Wiley-Interscience, NY (1975).

69. Cornish-Bowden, A., Biochem. J., 149, 305 (1975).

70. Eisenthal, R. and A. Cornish-Bowden, Biochem. J., 139, 715 715 (1974).

71. de Miguel, M., Biochem. J., 143, 93 (1974).

72.   Foster, R.J. and C. Nieman, Proc. Nat. Acad. Sci., 39, 999
      (1953).
73.   Dixon, M. and E. C. Webb, in The Enzymes, Academic Press, NY,
      69 (1958).
74.   King, K.W., Biochem. Biophys. Res. Com., 24 (3), 395 (1966).
75.   Maguire, R.J., Can. J. Biochem., 55, 644 (1977).
76.   Whitaker, D.R., in Biological Degradation of Cellulose, J.A.
      Gascoigue, and M.M. Gascoigue, ed., Butterworths, London, 161
      (1960).
77.   Humphrey, A.E., in Adv. Chem. Ser. 181, Am. Chem. Soc.,
      Washington, D.C., 25 (1979).
78.   McLaren, A.D. and L. Packer, Adv. Enzymol. Related Subj.
      Biochem., 33, 245 (1970)
79.   Humphrey, A.E., E.R. Moreira, W.B. Arminger, and D. Zabriskie,
      Biotechnol. Bioeng. Symp. No. 7, 45 (1977).
80.   Lee, S.E., PhD Thesis, University of Pennsylvania (1977).
81.   Van Dyke, B.H., Jr., PhD Thesis, Massachusetts Institute of
      Technology (1972).
82.   Huang, A.A., Biotechnol. Bioeng., XVII, 1421 (1975).
83.   Okazaki, M. and M. Moo-Young, Biotechnol. Bioeng. XX, 637
      (1978).
84.   Sternberg, D., Appl. Environ. Microbiol., 31 (5) 648 (1976).
85.   Bissett, F. and D. Sternberg, Appl. Environ. Microbiol., 35
      (4) 750 (1978).
86.   Okada, G. and K. Misizawa, J. Biochem., 78, 297 (1975).
87.   Cole, F.E. and K.W. King, Biochimica et Biophysica Acta, 81,
      122 (1964).
88.   Rinardo, M., F. Barnard, and J.P. Merle, J. Polym. Sci.,
      Part C, No. 28, 197 (1969).
89.   Tsao, G.T. and M.M. Chang, Colloque Celluloyse Microbienne,
      Centre National de la Recherche Scientifique, (Marseille), 93
      (1980).

DISCUSSION

Q.   DETROY: Mike, I wanted to ask if you have done any work with
      xylan for a possible binding affinity against your three
      enzymes?

A.   LADISCH: No, I haven't done any work with xylan.

Q.   MANDELS This is more in the nature of a question going on
      from where you stopped. It seems to me that in cellulase
      kinetics, you're faced with a tremendous dilemma. You have
      a laboratory world in which you look at initial rates and
      collect kinetic constants and inhibition constants and so
      forth but this leaves you to deal with the purest possible
      enzyme and the simplest possible substrate - ultimately with
      soluble cellodextrins and purified components. Yet, what

we're headed for is a real world in which we hope to get 50% or more conversion of a very concentrated cellulose slurry. It seems to me the kind of kinetics you're talking about downplays a factor in which you are obviously tremendously interested because Purdue is doing so much work on pre-treatment. Obviously the crystallinity of the substrate is an extremely important factor in your cellulase kinetics and related to that is this whole nature of synergism and this dilemma: As a biochemist you want to work with a purified component and yet if you use β-glucosidase alone, endo-B-glucanase alone, or exo-B-glucanase alone, with cellulose you get essentially no activity and the purer the component the less the activity. So obviously the synergism is, like crystallinity, a very overriding factor. Now, I don't know how we go about looking at this in a biochemical way but certainly in the real world way, we have to look at these under real use conditions. Is it possible, if in fact Tom Wood is right, that we have to have the two components there together, that you get a kind of activation when the two components are individually adsorbed and should we be looking in this direction too?

A.   LADISCH: Well, I'll answer your second question first. If I remember your first question, I'll try to answer that too. Anyhow, yes, adsorption might be the key factor in synergism, but what we're saying is that when an enzyme adsorbs to some component in your system and does not produce product, by a kineticist's definition this is inhibition, and so I guess again I think the essentially same thing is being said. I think its a very important factor to consider that you do need the enzyme components together to have very high activity. Now I think that ties in very strongly with the cellulase work. Several years ago we did and we're still doing very strong work in our lab on the effect of pre-treatment on cellulose hydrolysis and with culture filtrates from QM-9414 we found that by pre-treating cellulose with a solvent known as cadoxen we could get, for instance with Avicel, which is a microcrystalline cellulose having an average DP of about 200, close to full solubilization in a matter of three hours. Except for the little bit of inhibition of the cellobiase by the glucose formed, we could get up to 90% conversion within 10 hours to glucose. This same Avicel incubated under the same conditions with no pre-treatment gave, I think, 15% conversion after 24 hours, so indeed by dissolving the cellulose and reprecipitating it we greatly increase the amorphous character of the cellulose. At that time I think Dr. Tsao and Dr. Chang felt it had something to do with the cellulose structure, with which I agree.

If you look at the material which is pre-treated you will find that you can take an amount of Avicel which you can place on

the tip of your fingernail, and put it in a test tube
containing two milliliters of liquid. Finally you end up
with a test tube containing two milliliters of water, in
which this cellulose, upon pretreatment, will form a very
flocculant material which will fill the entire 2 milliliters.
In looking at that I think also what has been done is that
we greatly increase the surface area and that ties in with
synergism because Dane Zabrisky, when he was at Buffalo, (he's
now with Biochem technology), did a very interesting study
with water-soluble cellulose acetate. In this case he prepared a cellulose acetate which was verified to have high
activity with respect to hydrolysis by $T.$ $reesei$ again. He
prepared it in such a way that it dissolved in water. When
he did this and incubated it with the enzyme, he found the
solubilizing activity and reducing sugar activity increased
by a factor of 20. When he did the same thing with solka
floc and used the $T.$ $reesei$ cellulase he found that on a
relative basis his activity was one. I think that sort of
experiment is very interesting to an engineer anyhow because
it indicates the maximum improvement in activity one could
possibly expect if the enzyme, which is a fairly large molecule, had complete access to the cellulose.

This brings to mind Moo Young's work. I think this was the
most advanced model that we found in the literature including
this article and Nisizawa's article which thoroughly reviews
cellulase kinetics prior to 1973. The former model, with a
minimum of data, predicted that the optimum ratio of C_x to C_1
should be between 0.1 to 0.01. It turns out that some people
(Dr. Brown, our group, and others) now have done some very
careful work to provide a mass balance for the cellulase
protein. We find that the ratio of these two enzymes is
between 1:10 and 1:30. Thus, this particular model indicates
that synergism is very important. The synergistic effects
were described mathmatically by assuming there is a changing
surface area and that some of the products which are formed
and which are not soluble are indeed very strong inhibitors
of the complex. So tying these things together I think shows
that synergism exists and perhaps we're all describing the
same thing. Like the analogy of the elephant and a lot of
people who can't see. You know you feel the tusk and you say,
"Well, it's smooth," and you feel its leg and it's kind of
wrinkled, someone else feels the body and says "Well, it's
really solid." What I think exists in the literature if you
look really close is a lot of things now coming together into
a unified theory. I think this theory is necessary if we are
going to be able to intelligently improve the activities of
cellulases through genetic engineering or other means.

Q.   WOODWARD: Mike, I was wondering if you could comment on
      McGuire's data, I think it came out in 1977. He showed activa
      tion of β-gucosidase by glucose. That's rather intriguing, I
      was wondering if you could say a few words about that?

A.   LADISCH: He found that at very low glucose concentrations –
      I think it was less than 0.1 milligram – you do indeed have
      activation of the enzyme. We are aware of this data but we
      did not address this because, as engineers, what we are
      interested in doing is getting the glucose concentrations as
      high as possible in the final liquid solution. That's why we
      concentrate on the glucose inhibition itself.

      In the paper that goes with this talk you'll find an equation
      which I think is about 6 lines long and the only thing that
      it describes is inhibition by product and substrate. If we
      are to add the activation effect I think the equation would
      become too long to be useful and this is the reason we ignored
      it. The other point to bring out in the kinetics is that,
      due to the fact that you have non-competitive inhibition, if
      you ignore these particular activation affects, you can get a
      Lineweaver-Burk plot that resembles substrate inhibition. If
      there's a small amount of glucose contaminating your substrate
      (and indeed we found certain commercial preps did contain
      glucose) one does get something that resembles substrate inhi-
      bition far below the substrate level that was predicted by our
      data and Dr. Brown's data. This particular effect has been
      described by Segal in his textbook. So there are several fine
      points here that we didn't cover. What I tried to do was sort
      out the two fine points from what I thought were the more
      important things in our work.

Q.   BROWN: The methodology that you and we employ when we look at
      these oligosaccharides usually is HPLC and that, alone, often
      forces us to use substrate concentration ranges that we might
      not wish otherwise to have to use. I wonder if you believe
      that it's possible that by using some of these higher concen-
      trations we may be forcing the appearance of competitive or
      noncompetitive inhibition?

A.   LADISCH: I think that's true and I think, historically, if
      you look at it the first thing that was noticed was cellubiose
      inhibition. The reason for this is the K_S is about 30 to 40
      as opposed to glucose where the K_i is about 1. It's only
      since we've had the sensitive techniques which include an
      analytical glucose analyzer made by Beckman and HPLC that
      we've been able to get into the lower ranges and it's only
      recently that we have been able to detect sugars down in the
      hundred ppm level. It's this level that you need to accurately

model inhibition (if it exists) of higher cellooligosaccharides in the same quantitative manner that you do for cellobise. So I think it's a very important consideration.

Q.   BROWN: Of course, nature solves these problems by getting rid of the "end product" because that's the real beginning for metabolism. In cases where one ferments these products, for example to ethanol, some of our work has shown that you are not out of the woods yet because the ethanol at appreciable concentrations will serve as an acceptor for transglycosylation both by the endoglucanase and by the β-glucosidase.

A.   LADISCH: Another problem I think we will run into later is the same problem one has with starches. You get non-specific reversion products which, from our point of view, aren't good for fermentation. They're not suitable substrates and they don't yield alcohol. Consequently that may be the problem we'll talk about two years from now.

MICROBIAL ENZYMES ATTACKING PLANT POLYMERIC MATERIALS

Mary Mandels

U. S. Army Natick R&D Laboratories

Natick, Massachusetts

This symposium is good evidence of the current interest in utilization of renewable resources via fermentation. For substrates, various forms of plant biomass are available in large quantities or may be produced on energy farms. Solar energy is fixed by photosynthesis of green plants initially as small molecules, but these are rarely available in high concentrations or large quantities. Most of the excess over immediate metabolic requirements are rapidly converted into more complex molecules which are utilized by the plants as reserve foods or as structural materials. Most of these are polymers that are awkward to use for chemical or biological processes because they are chemically and physically complex and are attacked only by limited groups of specialized organisms that do not normally produce high levels of fermentations products of commercial interst. Therefore, we would like to convert these polymers back to the more usable monomers. An exception to the above is sucrose, a non-polymeric plant reserve food which is a simple soluble molecule, readily separated from plant juices in a high degree of purity. Not surprisingly, sucrose molasses is the basis for many industrial fermentations, notably the production of ethanol by yeasts. Since there is not enough sucrose available to support our expanded ambitions, we must resort to the more difficult polymers and learn to depolymerize them by physical, chemical, or biological (enzymatic) processes.

The topic for this session is enzymes and it is probable that in the long run, at least for the carbohydrates, these will be the catalysts for the most successful processes, although initially acid processes may be easier. Limitations of the acid process increase as the substrates become more insoluble, crystalline, and resistant, and include degradation of the products, interactions of acid with impurities in the substrate, and corrosion of equipment, resulting in low yields, impurities in the syrups, and high capital costs. The hemicelluloses are fairly easily hydrolyzed by dilute acids and this may remain the method of choice, even used as a pretreatment before enzymatic hydrolysis of cellulose (1). The starch hydrolysis process has already moved from the acid to the enzymatic phase. For cellulose, the problems for either acid (2) or enzymatic processes are much more difficult. Advantages for the enzymatic processes include their greater specificity and moderate reaction conditions, resulting in cleaner syrups and much higher yields. The chief disadvantages of enzymes are higher costs for the catalysts and the necessity for more precise process controls. Lignins are not susceptible to acid hydrolysis.

The apparent chemical simplicity of the polymers we will discuss today is deceptive because we are not dealing with soluble defined compounds, where the chemical reactions are known, and where biochemists understand most of the rules of enzyme action. These polymeric compounds have indefinite molecular structure and size, are often branched or substituted in an irregular manner, and the physical interactions between chains dominate the properties of the substrate, and greatly affect enzyme:substrate interactions (3). Because of this, the polymers are attacked by enzyme complexes which are a series of enzymes containing at least endo-enzymes which attack the polymer chains in a random fashion, exo-enzymes which remove monomers or dimers successively from the non-reducing chain ends, and glycosidases which hydrolyze oligosaccharides to monomers. These enzymes interact with each other, synergistically as is the case for the endo- and exo-glucanases of the cellulase complex, or sequentially as when one enzyme produces the substrate for a second enzyme. The action of one enzyme may favor the action of a second enzyme, either by removal of inhibitory products as is the case for β-glucosidases in the cellulase system (4), or by removing substances that hinder access of a second enzyme to its substrate as is the case for the hemicellulases (5) or lignolytic enzymes in the cellulase system. On the other hand, the action of one enzyme may be unfavorable when it produces products inhibitory to a second enzyme or even acts directly on a second enzyme as may occur with proteolytic enzymes. The kinetics of such systems are difficult to study; complex, yet fascinating. How are Michaelis Menten kinetics to be applied when the substrate is insoluble so that available surface becomes a much more meaningful term than substrate concentration? The usual approach is to study the hydrolysis of soluble oligosaccharides, but it is a giant step to apply the result to a real life substrate and to an understanding of synergism.

This morning we heard three papers on cellulases and this afternoon we will have a fourth. This is a reflection of the present very active state of cellulase research due to the abundance of cellulose, and the lure of cheap glucose to be used as food for man and animals and as the basis for useful fermentations. The synergistic action of the enzymes of the cellulase complex has been recognized since the classic paper of Reese, Siu, and Levinson in 1950 (6) and has been frequently affirmed and clarified by a number of researchers. Nevertheless our understanding is still incomplete. Unravelling of this enigma is a fascinating challenge that provides much of the fun of cellulase research.

The second paper in this session will be on xylanases. These enzymes are important because of the abundance of xylan in natural cellulosics, the need to find uses for the large quantities of xylose that will be present in saccharification syrups, and the realization that removal of hemicellulose may increase availability of the glucans to cellulase. There are interesting questions of cross specificities or the absence thereof between cellulases and xylanases (7) and the roles of the various xylanases and xylosidases in xylan breakdown.

The third paper will be on lignin, which is second only to cellulose in abundance, and is by far the most difficult problem for a conversion process. Even the microbes cannot attack lignin anaerobically, which is fortunate for us, since our civilization depends on fossil fuels derived from the lignins of yesteryears. Can we define and trap a useful intermediate from lignin degradation and so obtain a useful product from all those phenolic rings? We are at least beginning to understand some of the steps by which lignin is degraded and depolymerized.

The last paper this afternoon is on amylases. The starch conversion process is the model the rest of us are attempting to imitate. Here we have a successful enzymatic conversion of biomass to produce food grade glucose, and more recently liquid fuel from domestic crops even though at least two or three enzymes from two or three different microorganisms are required (8). One of the big advantages of the amylase system is the relatively high specific activity of the glucoamylase, at least 100 times the specific activity of presently available cellulase, resulting in moderate enzyme costs for the starch process. Starch, a reserve food, is a less recalcitrant more digestible substrate than the more insoluble, more recalcitrant cellulose which plays a structural role in the plant.

REFERENCES

1. Knappert, D., H. Grethlein, and A. Converse. 1980. Partial Acid Hydrolysis of Cellulosic Materials as a Pretreatment for Enzymatic Hydrolysis. Biotechnol. Bioeng. 22: 1449-1463.
2. Saeman, J. F. 1945. Kinetics of Wood Saccharification. Hydrolysis of Cellulose and Decomposition of Sugars in Dilute Acid at High Temperature. Ind. and Eng. Chem. 37: 43-52.

3.   Reese, E. T.   1977.   Degradation of Polymeric Carbohydrates
     by Microbial Enzymes.   Recent Advances in Phytochemistry 11:
     311-367.
4.   Sternberg, D., P. Vijayakumar, and E. T. Reese.   1977.   β -
     Glucosidase: Microbial Production and Effect on Enzymatic
     Hydrolysis of Cellulose.   Can. J. Microbiol.   23: 139-147.
5.   Ghose, T. K. and V. S. Bisaria.   1979.   Studies on the Mech-
     anism of Enzymatic Hydrolysis of Cellulosic Substances.
     Biotechnol. Bioeng.   21: 131-146.
6.   Reese, E. T., R. G. H. Siu, and H. S. Levinson.   1950.   The
     Biological Degradation of Soluble Cellulose Derivatives and
     its Relationship to the Mechanism of Cellulose Hydrolysis.
     J. Bact.   59: 485-497.
7.   Toda, S., H. Suzuki, and K. Nisizawa.   1971.   Some Enzymatic
     Properties and the Substrate Specificities of *Trichoderma*
     Cellulases with Special Reference to their Activity toward
     Xylan.   J. Fermentation Technology (Japan)   49: 499-521.
8.   Underkofler, L. A.   1969.   Development of a Commercial Enzyme
     Process: Glucoamylase.   Adv. Chem. Series   95: 343-358.

CELLULASES: DIVERSITY AMONGST IMPROVED *TRICHODERMA* STRAINS

S.P. Shoemaker, J.C. Raymond and R. Bruner

Cetus Corporation

Berkeley, CA 94710

BACKGROUND

In natural, mixed-culture fermentations of cellulose as well as in multistep conversion of cellulose to glucose, the depolymerization step seems rate limiting. Improvements in rate and yield of glucose from cellulose could greatly affect process economics (1-2). Indeed significant improvements have been achieved through pretreatment (2-5), better strains (6-10), and process integration (11-12). As part of the Biomass Program at Cetus, we have attempted to increase the rate at which cellulose is utilized in fermentation processes by isolating organisms deregulated in the production of cellulase. For this work we have selected one of the most thoroughly studied of the cellulolytic organisms, *Trichoderma reesei*. This paper will focus on a few of our strains in order to illustrate their diversity both in the control of cellulase production and in the types and levels of the individual enzyme components. The data should give further support for the existence of multiple levels of control in *Trichoderma*. Finally, as a separate topic, cellulase productivity data will be presented for one of our best strains.

The cellulase system of *T. reesei* comprises three classes of enzymes: endoglucanases, exo-cellobiohydrolases and β-glucosidases (13). The endoglucanases attack internal cellulosic linkages; the exo-cellobiohydrolases cleave cellobiosyl units from the non-reducing end of cellulose polymer chains; and the β-glucosidases specifically cleave glucosyl units from the non-reducing end of cellooligosaccharides. It is generally accepted that the endoglucanases and the exo-cellobiohydrolases act cooperatively and synergistically in depolymerizing cellulose to glucose and oligosaccharides, which then are converted by β-glucosidase to glucose. (see Eriksson, this vol.)

Cellulase synthesis in *Trichoderma* is under multiple regulatory control of induction and repression (6,14-15). From the work at the Natick Laboratory (16) and Rutgers Laboratory (14) and our own, it is highly probable that β-glucosidase is controlled separately from endoglucanases and exo-cellobiohydrolases. The latter enzymes may be coordinately controlled. In addition, it has been well established by the work of Sternberg (15) that β-glucosidase is limiting in standard *Trichoderma* cultures. Addition of exogenous β-glucosidase to these cultures greatly improves the rate at which cellulose is converted to glucose. In this paper, the term cellulase will refer to endoglucanases and exo-cellobiohydrolases; β-glucosidase will be referred to separately.

MUTANT SELECTION

A geneology chart summarizing the results of a series of our mutation and selection steps is shown in Figure 1. For mutagenesis, spores were treated with 8-methoxypsoralen, then illuminated with near UV light to give 90-99% kill (17). The first selections were based on high β-glucosidase production in a glucose-containing medium. This selection gave strain 144, which appeared to be constitutive for β-glucosidase. Strain 144 did not require addition of any known cellulase (or β-glucosidase) inducers, such as cellobiose or lactose, for production of β-glucosidase. It did not concomitantly produce endo- or exo-glucanases when grown on glucose. Thus, the next generations were selected for high cellulase production on glucose and on cellulose. The most interesting strains from this selection were L21, L25, L27, and L65. All strains isolated after 144 contained levels of β-glucosidase elevated over QM9414, even with cellulose as carbon source. A final generation of mutants, including L77, were selected from L27 as constitutive cellulase strains on plates. This paper will focus on the characterstics of strains 144, L25, L27, L65 and L77.

CELLULASE PRODUCTION BY MUTANT STRAINS GROWN ON SOLUBLE CARBOHYDRATES

The diversity among these strains for cellulase production is illustrated in Table I. These results are based on kinetic studies in shake flasks using the indicated carbon sources. No attempt is made here to quantify volumetric activities and there is a wide range in activities. This table clearly points out differences among these strains. QM9414 gave the expected result in producing significant amounts of cellulase only when grown on cellulose. Strain 144 behaved like QM9414 except that, as discussed before, it produced β-glucosidase alone when grown on glucose. Members of the next generation of strains, L25, L27 and L65, were quite different. L27 produced cellulase well when grown on glucose, less well on galactose

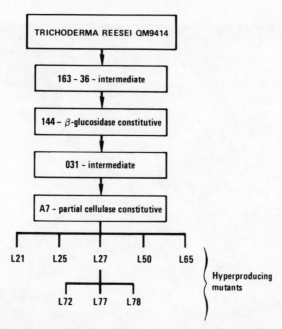

Figure 1. Genealogy of Cetus mutants. All mutagenesis was performed with NUV-MOPS, as described in the text.

and xylose (and only in presence of an inducer), and did not produce on glycerol. L25 produced cellulase on glycerol. L65 is a strain interesting because of its poor production of cellulase on cellulose and its high cellulase production on other carbon sources. L77 produces very high levels of cellulase on glucose and cellulose and detectable levels on most of the other carbon sources tested. Strains L25, L27 and L77 all produced at least 2 $g \cdot l^{-1}$ of extracellular protein in 2-3 days when grown in a medium containing 2% glucose. L25 produced 2-4 $g \cdot l^{-1}$ of protein in 2-3 days when grown on 4% glucose. L27 and L77 gave the highest volumetric activities on cellulose.

Strains L27 and L25, which were obtained from the same generation, illustrate well the differences in cellulase production on plates. (Figure 2a and 2b). The strains were grown at 30° on Nuclepore filters overlayed on growth media containing the indicated carbon sources. After 5 days, the filters were lifted and transferred to cellulose-agar plates, then incubated for one day at 40°C. Cellulase activity was evaluated by the clearing. In order to view the clearing more easily, part of the filter on the right half of the plates has been cut away; thus colonies can be viewed on the left half of each plate and clearing on the right half. Plate tests are much more sensitive than corresponding flask tests and results sometimes differed between plates and flasks. In this test, L27

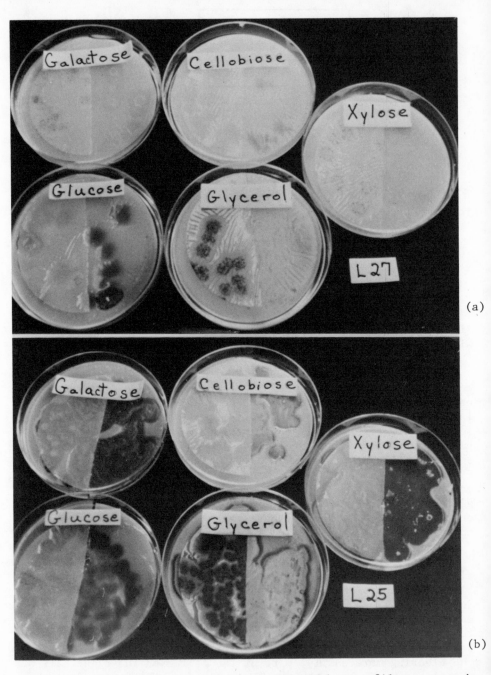

Figure 2. (a) PSC plates overlayed with Nuclepore filters containing colonies of strain L27 grown on indicated carbon sources. The
right half of each filter has been cut away. (b) Plates of strain
L25, prepared as described for Figure 2(a).

TABLE I

Cellulase Production on Selected Carbon Sources

Strain	Cellulose	Lactose	Glucose	Galactose	Xylose	Glycerol
QM9414	+	±	−	−	−	−
144	+	±	−	−	nd	−
A7	+	+	+	I_D	I_L	−
L25	+	+	+	±, I_D	±, I_D	±, I_D
L27	+	±	+	I_D	±, I_D	−
L65	±	nd	−	+	nd	+
L77	+	nd	+	±	nd	±

Symbols: +, Production of cellulase; ±, Low or late production of cellulase; −, No production of cellulase; I_D, Production only in presence of inducer; I_L, Low or late production in presence of inducer; and nd, Not determined.

cleared well on glucose and cellobiose, less well on galactose and xylose, and failed to clear on glycerol. In flasks, production was low or required inducer on galactose or xylose. L25, in comparison to L27, gave much larger clearing zones on all substrates. L25 consistently performed better on plates than any of our other strains. In flasks, other strains have produced higher levels of protein and cellulase unless the conditions were optimized for production by L25.

Strains L27 and L25 were also different in their response to increasing concentrations of glucose (Figure 3). Glucose showed some repressive effects on L27 at concentrations greater than 2%. Glucose, however, did not show any repressive effects on L25 at concentrations less than or equal to 4%. At 6 and 8% glucose, high cellulase titers were still reached after some of the glucose was utilized.

ENZYME COMPOSITION OF MUTANTS GROWN ON GLUCOSE OR CELLULOSE

The strains also differed in the ratios of individual cellulase components which they produced. We have characterized the proteins by isoelectric focusing (IEF), high performance liquid chromatography (HPLC), and activity on various carbon sources. For these studies, strains were grown in an optimized medium containing either cellulose (Avicel) or glucose. Cellulose-containing cultures also contained corn steep liquor instead of the peptone normally used in glucose-containing media. At early times in the fermentation less total extracellular protein was found, but the

TABLE II

Major Cellulase Components of Cetus Strains

	pI	Enzymic Activity (U mg^{-1})		
		PSC	CMC	PNPG
1. Exo-cellobiohydrolases				
— CBH I	4.0	0.2	0.03	0.00
— CBH II	5.9	3.5	0.95	0.00
2. Endoglucanases				
— EG I	4.4	26.0	27.00	0.02
— EG II	5.2	4.1	30.00	0.00
— EG III	7.4	2.5	8.60	0.10
3. Beta-glucosidase				
— BG I	> 8.2	2.0	0.33	14.40

Values were obtained using purified enzyme fractions. Abbreviations are described in the text.

types and ratios of individual proteins were similar to those found at later times. In addition, no extracellular protease activity was observed. Therefore, we took samples near the peak of production. At 3 days the glucose-grown and at 8 days the cellulose-grown cultures were harvested and the extracellular broth concentrated and dialyzed against 40mM sodium acetate buffer (pH 4.8).

Purification of the major components from these crude enzyme preparations allowed a good comparison of strains. Individual cellulases were characterized by their isoelectric points and specific activities on phosphoric acid swollen cellulose (PSC), carboxymethylcellulose (CMC) and p-nitrophenyl-β-D-glucoside (PNPG) (Table II). Activity on CMC was measured as a decrease in viscosity using a rotating viscometer. CBH I and II appear similar to the exo-cellobiohydrolases described by Gritzali and Brown (13). Note the significantly higher activity on PSC by CBH II. The endoglucanases also appear to have different modes of action. Our EG I has many of the characteristics of the EG III purified from a commercial cellulase preparation (18-19). Our EG III may be similar to a low MW endoglucanase reported by Hakansson et. al. (20). We have isolated one aryl-glucosidase from *T. reesei*. It has pI greater than 8.2 and has been hard to keep in aqueous solution.

IEF has given the best resolution of the individual enzyme components. Figures 4 and 5 illustrate the separation of components on wide (pH 3.5 - 9.5) and narrow (pH 4.5 - 6.5) range gels, respectively. Glucose- and cellulose-grown cultures differed in

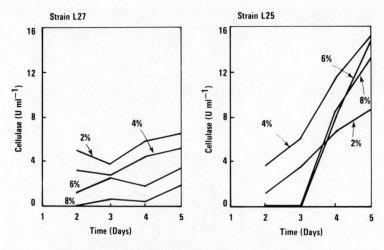

Figure 3. Kinetics of cellulase production by strains L27 and L25 in cultures with 2,4,6 or 8% glucose. Activity with PSC.

the following:

1. The β-glucosidase was found in higher proportion in glucose-grown cultures.

2. EG III and CBH II were more abundant in cellulose-grown cultures.

3. A new and distinct band was found primarily in glucose-grown cultures.

Some strains also differed in the relative amounts of individual enzymes they produced. Strains 144, L77 and L27 contained more CBH II and higher proportions of EG II. Strain L27 grown on cellulose contained a higher proportion of EG I, the most active cellulase. Strain 144, when grown on glucose, gave two major bands which are still being characterized. In most strains, the bands which are slightly more acidic than CBH I are likely to be exo-cellobiohydrolases.

An HPLC technique was used to quantify amounts of individual components identified by IEF. Activity of individual peaks also could be checked after collection of eluted peak fractions. We compared various anion exchange columns and found that the column manufactured by Synchrom has the highest column capacity. Although the selectivity was slightly different with this column compared to glycophase columns, the same general elution pattern was observed. Elution of protein was achieved by a convex gradient of 0 to 0.25M NaCl in 40 minutes. Under these conditions β-glucosidase was found to be associated with the first peak and CBH I was found to be

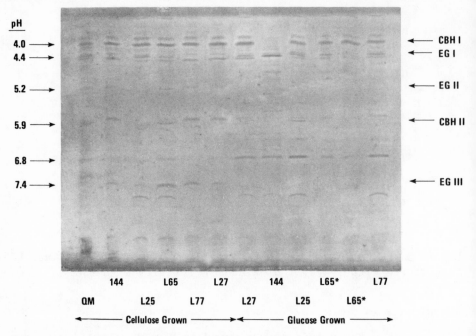

Figure 4. Analytical isoelectric focusing of extracellular proteins
in a ready-made polyacrylamide gel slab. Carrier ampholytes in the
range pH 3.5 - 9.5 were used together with an LKB Multiphor electrophoresis apparatus. Samples of approximately 45 µg each were applied
directly on the gel surface and run for 1.5 hour at 10ºC. The final
voltage was 1200V. Gels were stained for protein with Coomassie
brilliant blue. The lanes are identified in the bottom margin; QM
represents QM9414. The identity and corresponding pH values are
given on the side margins; these were determined separately, using
purified components.

associated with the final peak. Sometimes the exo-cellobiohydrolase
peak split into two peaks but separate analysis of these peaks by
polyacrylamide gel electrophoresis or cellulase activity gave similar
components and activities. Endoglucanases were found to elute before
the CBH I. EG II eluted with the first peak, EG I eluted at about
33 minutes (Figure 6).

A comparison of chromatograms of equal amounts of total protein from 4 strains grown on cellulose illustrates some differences
in the enzyme preparations. The peaks in the middle region of the
QM9414 (Fig. 6) chromatogram appear not to be cellulases based on
activity studies. The HPLC profiles for L27 and L77 look very similar. Differences in enzyme levels on L27 grown on cellulose and
on glucose are seen in Figure 7. The peak at 23 minutes, usually
seen only in cultures grown on glucose, corresponds to a single

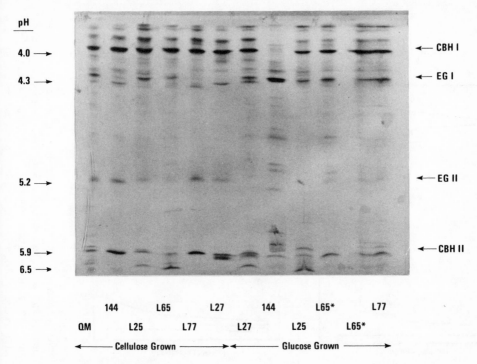

Figure 5.   Analytical isoelectric focusing in a ready-made polyacrylamide gel slab.   Carrier ampholytes in the range pH 4.5 - 6.5
were used.   Samples were run for 2.5 hour at 10°C.   The final
voltage was 1200V.   Description of samples and staining were as
described for Figure 4.

protein with a pI of about 4.3.   Unlike L27, strain L25 produced
this protein on both glucose and cellulose (Figure 8).   Some
cellulase activity was associated with this protein and we are
still examining its significance.

        From the IEF gels it appears that strain L27 has a higher
ratio of EG I to CBH I than the other strains.   An attempt to
determine the ratio of endoglucanase to exo-cellobiohydrolase from
HPLC data is shown in Table III.   This data should be viewed with
caution since endoglucanase peak areas were very small.   Still,
the higher ratio of EG I to CBH I protein in the case of L27 is
probably significant.

        A comparison of specific activities (at 40°) supports the
gel and HPLC data (Table IV).   The substrates and assays are the
same as described earlier.   In part, the higher specific activities
on PSC of culture broths from mutant strains compared to QM9414
reflect elevated levels of β-glucosidase.   CMC activity specifically

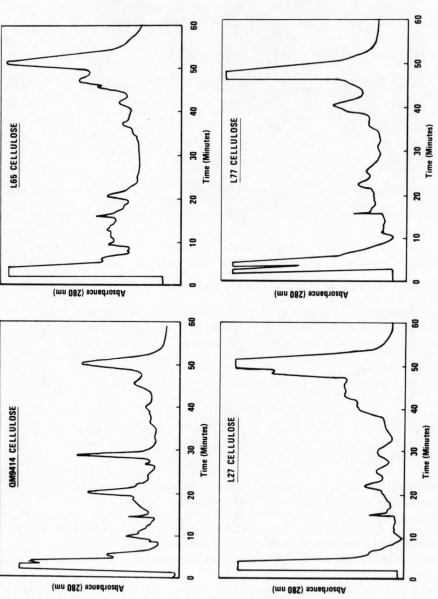

Figure 6. High performance liquid chromatographic separations of extracellular proteins from indicated strains using a Synchropak anion exchange column (250 x 4.1mm I.D.). Samples from cellulose grown cultures containing 1mg protein each were eluted by a 40 minute convex gradient (Waters 660 solvent programmer, curve 5) running from 0 to 0.25M sodium chloride in a 20mM potassium phosphate

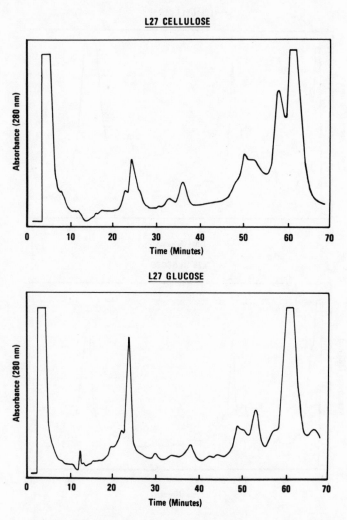

Figure 7. High performance liquid chromatographic separations of extracellular proteins from strain L27 grown on cellulose or glucose. Chromatographic conditions were the same as detailed for Figure 6.

reflects endoglucanase activity and PNPG activity specifically reflects aryl-glucosidase activity. Note that, when grown on cellulose, the improved strains produced higher specific activities of aryl-glucosidase and cellulase than QM9414. QM9414, of course, did not produce aryl-glucosidase or cellulase activity when grown on glucose.

The differences in protein composition observed among these strains are reflected in their enzyme activities.

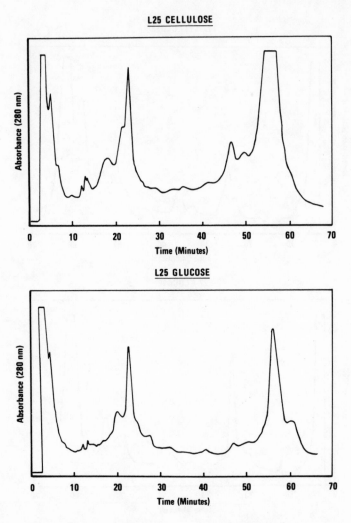

Figure 8. High performance liquid chromatographic separations of extracellular proteins from strain L25 grown on cellulose or glucose. Chromatographic conditions were the same as detailed for Figure 6.

1. Strain 144 grown on glucose produced only β-glucosidase; the culture broths were not active toward CMC or PSC.
2. Strain L25 had a relatively high activity on PNPG reflecting its higher level of β-glucosidase. Its relatively low activity on CMC and PSC reflects a lower level of endoglucanase.
3. Strain L27 had one of the highest activities on CMC, reflecting its higher level of endoglucanse (especially EG 1);

TABLE III

Ratio of Endoglucanase I to Exo-cellobiohydrolase I
in Improved Strains.

Strain	Growth substrate for cellulase production	Ratio of EG I to CBH I
QM9414	Cellulose	0.020
144	Cellulose	0.020
L25	Cellulose	< 0.005
	Glucose	0.040
L27	Cellulose	0.080
	Glucose	0.090
L77	Cellulose	< 0.005
	Glucose	0.020

Values were derived from HPLC peak areas corresponding to endoglucanase I and exo-cellobiohydrolase I as determined using purified
enzymes as standards.

    4.   L65 produced a high level of β-glucosidase; and
    5.   Strain L77 was similar to L27.

The correlation between the high activities on PSC for strains 144,
L27 and L77 grown on cellulose and the higher levels of CBH II
found in these strains may be important. Specific activities (on
PSC) for these strains were all about twice that of QM9414. Thus,
although cellulases tended to be produced together, different
strains appeared to control the ratios produced differently. In
addition, different ratios were produced on different substrates.

    Culture broths of these strains were further compared for
their abilities to produce soluble reducing sugar from PSC and
cotton linters at 50°C (Figure 9). On the basis of known protein
components and specific activity data, we might have predicted
strains 144 (grown on cellulose), L77 and L27 to be the most active
on PSC. The data given in Figure 9 support this prediction. In
order to get a more complete picture of the products formed, we
measured production both of glucose and reducing sugar. The amount
of reducing sugar (calculated as glucose) for the 24 hr time point
illustrates differences among strains in amount of β-glucosidase
(Figure 10). Consistent with previous findings, practically all
of the reducing sugar from strain L65 was glucose. In addition,
a higher proportion of glucose was seen with strain L25, which tends
to produce a higher ratio of β-glucosidase to cellulase

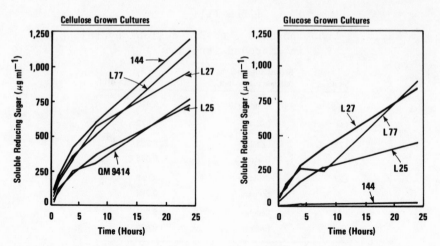

Figure 9. Comparison of kinetics of hydrolysis of 1% PSC by extracellular preparations derived from cellulose- and glucose-grown
cultures of various strains. Protein concentration (2.44 μg · ml^{-1})
was the same for each strain.

Figure 11 shows the identical experiment with cotton linters as substrate. In these experiments we added 100 μg enzyme per reaction
tube. Again strains 144, L77 and L27 gave the highest activities.
Note the enhanced levels of reducing sugar produced by strain L77

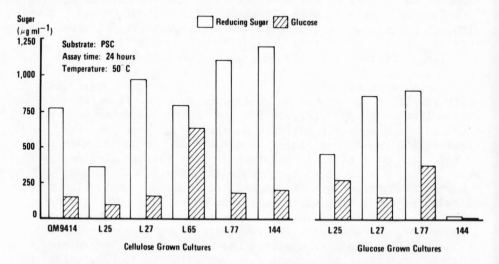

Figure 10. Production of soluble reducing sugar and glucose from
1% PSC by selected cellulase preparations derived from cellulose- and
glucose-grown cultures. Conditions are as described for Figure 9.

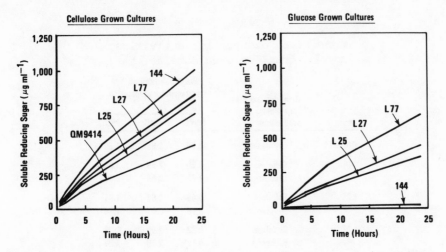

Figure 11. Comparison of kinetics of hydrolysis of 1% cotton linters by extracellular preparations derived from cellulose- and glucose-grown cultures. Protein concentration $(24.4 \mu g \cdot ml^{-1})$ was the same for each strain.

on glucose compared to the other two strains. In this case, as expected, we see a much higher proportion of glucose due to the higher β-glucosidase produced by this strain (Figure 12). For strains L25 and L65 grown on cellulose, and strains L25 and L77 grown on glucose,

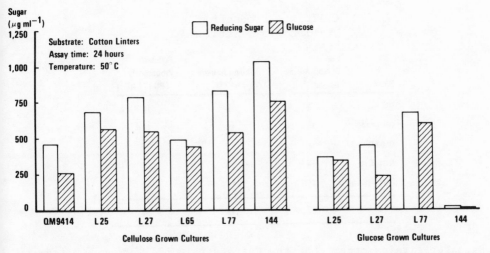

Figure 12. Production of soluble reducing sugar and glucose from 1% cotton linters by selected cellulase preparations derived from cellulose- and glucose-grown cultures. Conditions are as described for Figure 11.

TABLE IV

Comparison of Specific Activities
from Improved Strains.

Strain	Growth substrate for cellulase production	Specific activity of extracellular preparation (U mg^{-1})		
		PNPG	CMC	PSC
QM 9414	Cellulose	0.08	1.90	1.80
144	Cellulose	0.26	2.69	3.65
	Glucose	1.73	0.05	0.07
L 25	Cellulose	0.46	0.97	1.81
	Glucose	0.76	0.67	1.44
L 27	Cellulose	0.32	3.59	2.99
	Glucose	0.17	2.76	3.09
L 65	Cellulose	0.99	1.65	2.32
	Glycerol	0.65	1.28	2.09
	Galactose	0.50	1.45	2.07
L 77	Cellulose	0.30	3.57	3.41
	Glucose	0.26	1.76	2.40

The substrates and assays are described in the text.

TABLE V

Cellulase Production by
Trichoderma Strains.

Strain	Soluble Protein (mg ml^{-1})	Cellulase Activity (FPU ml^{-1})	Cellulase Productivity (FPU l^{-1} h^{-1})
QM 6a	7	5	15
QM 9414	14	10	30
QM-MCG-77	16	11	33
RUT-C30	19	14	42
RUT-NG14	21	15	45
L 27	22	18	94

Data for strains other than the Cetus strain L27 were taken from a
recent article by Ryu and Mandels (6).

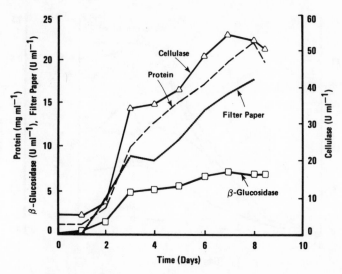

Figure 13. Fermentation kinetics for strain L27 grown on 8% Avicel. Protein was measured by the method of Peterson (21). Cellulase was measured in terms of soluble reducing sugar from PSC (22-23). Filter paper activity was measured according to the standard assay developed at Natick (24). β-glucosidase was measured as p-nitrophenol release from PNPG (25).

almost all of the reducing sugar was glucose. Here all mutants performed better than QM9414, both in specific activity and glucose produced over time.

Thus, using a variety of techniques, we have partially characterized several of our mutant strains. Correlations between proteins produced by these strains and enzyme activities have been made and are consistent. In our strategy, β-glucosidase was decontrolled first (Strain 144) and separately from that of the exo- and endo-glucanases. In the work of Natick labs, β-glucosidase was decontrolled after the exo- and endo-glucanases (16). Our results, thus, support and add further evidence for independent control of β-glucosidase. Exo- and endo-glucanases may be coordinately controlled. However, we also have shown proof for the operation of a finer level of control among strains, reflected in the different levels of some of the proteins. The varieties of control of enzyme production found among these mutants is as great as might be found among a number of independent isolates from nature.

PRODUCTION OF CELLULASE BY L27 IN A FERMENTOR WITH MEDIA CONTAINING GLUCOSE OR CELLULOSE.

For a practical estimate of improvement we obtained cellulase

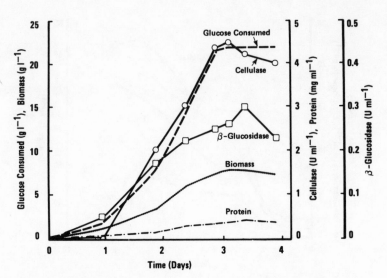

Figure 14.   Fermentation kinetics for strain L27 grown on 2% glucose.
Biomass was measured as dry cell weight.   Residual glucose was
measured using YSI glucose analyzer.   Protein, cellulase and β-
glucosidase were measured as described for Figure 13.

productivity information on one of our best strains, which at that
time had shown the highest levels of protein and volumetric activity
in shake flasks.   In the first experiment, we followed cellulase
production of strain L27 on 8% Avicel under controlled fermentor
conditions (Figure 13).   At 8 days, the extracellular protein concentration was 22 $g \cdot 1^{-1}$ and filter paper (FP) activity was 18
$FPU \cdot ml^{-1}$.   Cellulase productivity after 8 days was 94 FPU 1^{-1}.

For comparison, results for strain L27 grown on 2% glucose
are shown in Figure 14.   Here the fermentation time was 4 days and,
as expected, lower levels of protein and activity were found. Still,
this is the first demonstration we know of for *Trichoderma* cellulase
production on glucose alone.   Cellulase productivity, measured at
4 days, was found to be 32 $FPU \cdot 1^{-1} \cdot h^{-1}$.   This is slightly better
than the value given for QM9414 grown on cellulose, due mostly to
the shorter fermentation time (6).   As strain L27 produces more
activity than QM9414 when it is grown on cellulose, presumably the
productivity of strain L27 on glucose can be improved by the same
proportion.   A comparison between L27 and other improved *Trichoderma*
strains (6) is given in Table V.   The comparison is not under
identical conditions: values for strains other than L27 were based
on 14-day fermentation using 2-roll milled cellulose.   According
to Dr. Mandels, 2 roll-milled cellulose gives higher activities with
these strains than does solka floc or Avicel.   Thus, strain L27

appears as good or perhaps better than other strains in terms of extracellular protein production and cellulase activity. Productivity appears dramatically in favor of strain L27, because of the shorter fermentation time. However, higher productivity values for Rut-C30, of about 75 $FPU \cdot 1^{-1} \cdot h^{-1}$, using other conditions, have been quoted. Regardless, strains L27 and Rut-C30 are different. At this time, we are continuing process development work on several of our improved strains, such as L25, which have not as yet been tested in a fermentor.

ACKNOWLEDGEMENTS

The authors would like to acknowledge the excellent technical assistance of D.L. Bugawan, L.S. Chang, R.V. Cox, F.J. Fago, M.S. Pemberton, B.A. Shepanek, L.S. Strehl, and G.R. Takeoda.

REFERENCES

1. Mandels, M. and Andreotti, R.E. (1978). Problems and Challenges in Cellulose to Cellulase Fermentation. Process Biochem. May, 7-13.
2. Ladisch, M.R. (1979). Fermentable Sugars from Cellulosic Residues. Process Biochem. January, 21-25.
3. Tassinari, T., Macy, C. and Spano, L. (1980). Energy Requirements and Process Design Considerations in Compression-Milling Pretreatment of Cellulosic Wastes for Enzymatic Hydrolysis. Biotech. Bioeng. XXII, 1689-1705.
4. Marchessault, R.H., Coulombe, S., Hanai, T. and Morikawa, H. (1979). Monomers and Oligomers from Wood. In Proceedings Canadian Wood Chemistry Symposium, pp. 103-107, Harrison Hot-Springs, British Columbia.
5. Knappert, D., Grethlein, H. and Converse, A. (1980). Partial Acid Hydrolysis of Cellulosic Materials as a Pretreatment for Enzymatic Hydrolysis. Biotech. Bioeng. XXII, 1499-1463.
6. Ryu, D.D.Y. and Mandels, M. (1980). Cellulases: Biosynthesis and Applications. Enzyme Microb. Technol. 2, 91-102.
7. Andreotti, R.E., Mediros, J.E., Roche, C., Mandels, M. (1980). Effects of Strain and Substrate on Production of Cellulases by *Trichoderma reesei* Mutants. Second International Conference on Cellulose Bioconversion, New Delhi, India.
8. Montenecourt, B.S. and Eveleigh, D.E. (1978). Hypercellulolytic Mutants and Their Role in Saccharification. In Second Annual Fuels from Biomass Symposium, pp. 613-625. Edited by W. Schuster. Troy, NY: U.S. Department of Energy.
9. Garcia-Martinez, D.V., Shinmyo, A., Madia, A. and Demain, A.L. (1980). Studies on Cellulase Production by *Clostridium thermocellum*. Eur. J. Appl. Microbiol. Biotechnol. 9, 189-197.

10. Gray, P.P., Choudhury, N., Haggett, K.D. and Dunn, N.W. (1980).
     Saccharification Using Mutants of a *Cellulomonas* species.
     Presented at Second International Conference on Cellulose Bio-
     conversion, New Delhi, India.

11. Takagi, M., Abe, S., Suzuki, S., Emert, G.H. and Yata, N.
     (1977). A Method for Production of Alcohol Directly From
     Cellulose Using Cellulase and Yeast. Proc. Bioconv. Symp.,
     IIT Delhi, 551-571.

12. Wang, D.I.C., Biocic. I., Fang, H.Y. and Wang, S.D. (1979).
     Direct Microbiological Conversion of Cellulosic Biomass to
     Ethanol. In Third Annual Biomass Energy Systems Conference
     Proceedings, SERI: U.S. Department of Energy.

13. Gritzali, M. and Brown, R.D., Jr. (1979). The Cellulase System
     of *Trichoderma*. In Hydrolysis of Cellulose: Mechanisms of
     Enzymatic and Acid Catalysis. Edited by Brown, R.D., Jr. and
     Jurasek, L. Adv. Chem. Series, Vol. 181, pp. 237-260, ACS,
     Washington, D.C.

14. Montenecourt, B.S., Schamhart, D.H.J., and Eveleight, D.E.
     (1979). Mechanism Controlling the Synthesis of the *Tricho-
     derma reesei* Cellulase System. In Microbial Polysaccharides
     and Polysaccharases. Edited by Berkeley, R.C.W., Gooday,
     G.W. and Ellwood, D.C., pp. 327-337. Academic Press, NY.

15. Sternberg, D. and Mandels, G.R. (1980). Regulation of the
     Cellulolytic System in *Trichoderma reesei* by Sophorose:
     Induction of Cellulase and Repression of β-glucosidase. J.
     Bacteriol. 144, 1197-1199.

16. Mandels, M., Weber, J. and Parizek, R. (1971). Enhanced
     Cellulase Production by a Mutant of *Trichoderma viride*. Appl.
     Microbiol. 21, 152-154.

17. Scott, B.R. and Alderson, T. (1971). The Random (Non-Specific)
     Forward Mutational Response of Gene Loci in *Aspergillus*
     Conidia After Photosensitisation to Near Ultraviolet Light
     (365 nm) by 8-Methoxypsoralen. Mutation Res. 12, 29-34.

18. Shoemaker, S.P. and Brown, R.D., Jr. (1978). Enzymic Activities
     of Endo-1, 4-β-D-Glucanases Purified From *Trichoderma viride*.
     Biochim. Biophys. Acta 523, 133-146.

19. Shoemaker, S.P. and Brown, R.D., Jr. (1978). Characterization
     of Endo-1, 4-β-D-Glucanases Purified from *Trichoderma viride*.
     Biochim. Biophys. Acta 523, 147-161.

20. Hakansson, U., Fagerstam, L., Pettersson, G. and Andersson,
     L. (1978). Purification and Characterization of a Low Mole-
     cular Weight 1, 4-β-Glucan Glucanohydrolase From the Cellulo-
     lytic Fungus *Trichoderma viride* QM9414. Biochim. Biophys.
     Acta 524, 385-392.

21. Peterson, G.L. (1977). A Simplification of the Protein Assay
     Method of Lowry et al. Which is More Generally Applicable.
     Anal. Biochem. 83, 346-356.

22. Nelson, N.J. (1944). A Photometric Adaptation of the Somogyi
     Method for Determination of Glucose. J. Biol. Chem. 153, 375-
     380.

23.   Somogyi, M.J. (1952). Notes on Sugar Determination. <u>J</u>. <u>Biol</u>.
      <u>Chem</u>. 195, 19–23.
24.   Mandels, M. and Sternberg, D. (1976). Recent Advances in
      Cellulase Technology. <u>J</u>. <u>Ferment</u>. <u>Technol</u>. 54, 267–286.
25.   Emert, G.H. (1973). Purification and Characterization of
      Cellobiase from *Trichoderma viride*. Ph.D. Dissertation, VPI
      & SU, Blacksburg, Virginia.

DISCUSSION

Q.   LADISCH: I'd just like to ask you one question. Do you have
      any idea what the comparison is for soluble carbohydrate pro-
      duction either as glucose, cellobiose or higher oligosaccha-
      rides? That is, you showed filter paper units and this
      measurement includes the reducing ends in cellulose which are
      not appearing as soluble sugars.

A.   SHOEMAKER: In the slides illustrating fermentation kinetics
      I also showed cellulase activity in terms of soluble reducing
      sugar from PSC for strain L27.

Q.   LADISCH: Also, in the terms of your last figure, how does
      that value compare between QM 9414, Rut C-30, C-30 and L27?

A.   SHOEMAKER: We have not tested QM 9414 or Rut C-30 under the
      same controlled fermentor conditions. We do not have Rut C-30
      in our laboratory. However, under comparable conditions, L27
      shows 2 to 3 times the amount of soluble reducing sugar from
      PSC as QM 9414.

XYLANASES: STRUCTURE AND FUNCTION

Peter J. Reilly

Department of Chemical Engineering
Iowa State University
Ames, Iowa 50011

INTRODUCTION

A number of papers in this seminar are devoted to the production and characterization of cellulases. This is proper, since the
use of cellulases is perhaps the most feasible method of converting
cellulose to products that may be used for fuels and chemicals.
However, all celluloses from hardwoods and grasses are associated
with significant amounts of xylan, a hemicellulose possessing a
β-1,4-linked xylose backbone, with branches containing xylose and
other pentoses, hexoses, and uronic acids (Figure 1).

Xylan hydrolysis has been studied less than cellulose hydrolysis. This is largely because the products of xylan breakdown are
less valuable than the glucose that is produced from the breakdown
of cellulose. In addition, because xylan is chemically heterogeneous,
no yield of any single substance can be obtained. Nevertheless, in
a process where cellulose is converted to products, xylan must be
converted also. Otherwise, the cost of the raw material becomes so
high, because of the large amount of unused xylan, that the products
of cellulose breakdown are not competitive with the same products
from other sources.

As with cellulose, there are two ways to hydrolyze xylan: by
acid and by use of enzymes. Again, as with cellulose, acidic hydrolysis was the first to be used on an industrial scale. This method
is quick and easy, and if conditions are sufficiently mild, xylan
may be hydrolyzed in the presence of cellulose without significant
attack on the latter. However, acidic hydrolysis is not specific;
therefore many products, difficult to separate, issue from the acidic

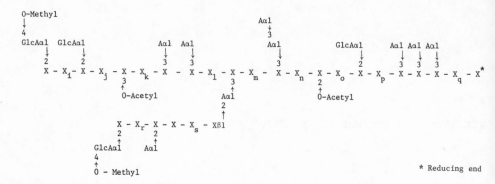

Figure 1.   Hypothetical structure of xylan, showing bonds found in
major quantities in different types of plants.   Adapted from Northcote (1).   Symbols: A , L-arabinofuranosyl residue; GlcA , Glucur-
nic acid residue; X_j , D-xylopyranosyl residue; Subscripts: i, j,
k,... number of D-xylopyranosyl residues linked to each other by
β-1,4 bonds.

hydrolysis of xylan.   In addition, breakdown is rarely complete and
the conditions necessary for significant hydrolysis in a reasonable
time are sufficiently rigorous that byproducts occur.

Enzymic hydrolysis is not used industrially at present, because
research on the enzymes necessary for the process is still at a
rudimentary stage.   Without further research, enzyme cost would be
high, yield would be low, and products would be mixed.   These are
the same drawbacks encountered with acidic hydrolysis, except the
cost would be higher.   However, because enzymic hydrolysis is by
nature a more specific process, it holds out the hope that xylose
could be obtained free of other monosaccharides.   Use of properly
chosen xylanase mixtures could lead to the production of xylose
mixed with large residual fragments, from which xylose could be
easily separated.   Also, because conditions under which enzymic
hydrolysis occurs are milder than those of acidic hydrolysis, byproduct formation would be decreased.

Despite the advantages of the enzymic hydrolysis of xylan, it
is not at all clear that it will eventually be the preferred process.
After all, xylan can be hydrolyzed more easily by acid than can
cellulose, while there is no assurance yet that enzymic hydrolysis
of xylan will be easier than that of cellulose.   Without further
research to discover and characterize all the enzymes that take part
in xylan hydrolysis, we really will not know if hydrolysis with
xylanases will be feasible in the future.   To determine future
research directions, it is instructive to consider the process that
has already been made in the study of the xylanase family of enzymes.

OVERVIEW OF THE XYLANASE FAMILY

Before discussing the xylanases, several points need to be made. First, with the exception of β-xylosidase, only research dealing with homogeneous enzymes will be discussed. Work with xylanase mixtures is too open to misinterpretation to be useful.

Second, as previously mentioned, there are many different types of xylanases. They are produced by many different fungal species and by some animal, plant and bacterial species. Very few species are likely to produce all the different types of xylanases.

Third, many xylanases are isozymes of each other. They have similar specificities but differ in amino acid or carbohydrate content. This leads to differences in isoelectric point, relative stability and in the optimum pH for activity and stability for the different isoenzymes. What portion of these differences in composition is caused by differences in genetic coding and what portion by attack of other enzymes during production or purification is not yet known.

Fourth, the xylanase family may be compared to two other major hydrolase families that are being discussed in this seminar: the cellulases and the amylases. While there are many similarities, there are also some differences between the xylanases and the other two families. The differences are caused by the greater structural and chemical heterogeneity of xylan compared to cellulose and starch. While starch is branched and cellulose is partially crystalline, they are at least composed completely of glucose. Xylan, on the other hand, is branched and is composed of several monomers. As most hydrolases are very specific as to the bonds they attack, it might be expected that there would be more xylanases than amylases or cellulases. In fact, to this point xylanases of at least six types have been described by us and others:

1.) β-Xylosidases, which break down short xylooligo-saccharides to xylose, and have substantial transferase activity;

2.) Exo-xylanases, producing xylose at high rates from xylan, but only at low rates from short oligosac-charides. These enzymes invert product configuration unlike β-xylosidase, and have little or no transferase activity. As yet there is no conclusive evidence of an exo-xylanase that produces mainly xylobiose;

3.) Endo-xylanases of four types:
   a.) Those that cannot cleave L-arabinosyl initiated

branch points, and produce mainly xylobiose and
xylose as final products. They are generally
active on xylooligosaccharides as short as xylotriose, but at much lower rates than on larger
substrates.

b.)   Those that cannot cleave branch points and
produce mainly oligosaccharide fragments larger
than xylobiose. They are generally inactive on
xylotetraose and smaller substrates.

c.)   Those that can cleave branch points and produce
mainly xylobiose and xylose.

d.)   Those that can cleave branch points and produce
mainly xylooligosaccharides of intermediate size.

These different xylanases will be discussed in turn in the
sections that follow. Results will be both from the published
literature and from our own as yet unpublished work. There will
be many gaps, because even after roughly thirty years of research,
much remains to be done.

β-XYLOSIDASES

Many different enzymes labelled as β-xylosidase have been
described. However, some appear to be xylose-producing exo-
xylanases, and they will be covered in the following section. In
addition, though extensive research has been conducted on animal
and plant β-xylosidases, it is unlikely that they will be of
industrial importance. Therefore, they will not be dealt with here.

There is no complete survey of the incidence of β-xylosidase
throughout the microbial kingdom, but Reese et al. (2) found a
large number of producers in five genera of fungi: *Aspergillus,
Botryodiploidia, Penicillium, Pestalotia* and *Trichoderma*. β-xylosidase has also been found in various species of *Absidia, Mucor,
Rhizopus, Thermoascus* and *Thermomyces* (3), in the yeast genus
Cryptococcus (4), in various strains of *Bacillus* (5), and in
some plant pathogenic members of the bacterial genera *Agrobacterium,
Corynebacterium, Erwinia, Flavobacterium, Pseudomonas* and *Xantho-
monas* (6).

β-Xylosidase from rumen bacteria (7,8), *Aspergillus niger* (9-15),
Coniophora cerebella (16), *Chaetomium trilaterale* (17), and *Penicillium wortmanni* (18) have been purified to a sufficient degree
that enzyme properties could be determined. The enzyme is active
on small xylooligosaccharides (7,12), aryl-β-D-xylopyranosides (7,
10,11,17-19), alkyl-β-D-xylopyranosides (2,11,13,18,20), aryl-α-L-
arabinopyranosides (11,18), aryl-β-D-glucopyranosides (11),

aryl-β-D-quinovopyranisides (11), xylobiitol (13), xylotriitol (2, 13), and L-serine xylopyranoside (2). With increasing xylooligo-saccharide chain length, β-xylosidase activity decreases (7,13). Xylose is an inhibitor with a K_i between 2.5 mM (19) and 5.0 mM (15). Xylonolactone (2,19), γ- and δ-gluconolactone (19), alkyl-1-thio-β-D-xylopyranosides (18-20), and TRIS (8) are also inhibitors.

β-Xylosidase attacks from the nonreducing end of the chain (13, 18) with the products retaining configuration (18,21). The reaction appears to proceed by a concerted attack of an electrophile in the active center on the anomeric oxygen atom and of a nucleophile, also in the active center, on the nonreducing C-1 atom, with heterolysis of the glycosyl-oxygen bond. This is followed by nucleophilic attack of an acceptor molecule like water on the C-1 atom (22). Transfer reactions occur to give substantial yield losses with acceptors other than water, such as the substrate itself (12,13,18,20) and aliphatic and polyhydric alcohols (11,12, 15,18,20). Both β-1,3 and β-1,4 bonds are formed (11,21).

Only the *P. wortmanni* β-xylosidase has been purified to homogeneity (18). It has a molecular weight of 102,000, a pI of 5.0, 23% carbohydrate, and an amino acid profile high in aspartic acid, glutamic acid, alanine, serine, and glycine and low in cysteine, tryptophan, methionine and histidine (18). There are no metals, sulfhydryl groups or histidine in the active center (18).

The β-xylosidase from *A. niger* has a pI of 4.3 - 4.6 and a molecular weight greater than 200,000 (11). The large difference in molecular weight between the *P. wortmanni* and *A. niger* enzymes may be caused by subunit deaggregation, which occurs at high ionic strengths (14).

Activity of *A. niger*, *P. wortmanni* and *Botryodiploida* β-xylosidases on aryl- and alkyl-β-D-xylopyranosides is highest around pH 3 (2, 11,13-15) while the *C. trilaterale* enzyme had an optimum pH for activity of 4.5 (17). Optimum pH for stability is between 4 and 5 for the *A. niger* and *Botryodiploidia* enzymes (2,13,15) and somewhat higher for the *C. trilaterale* (17) and *P. wortmanni* (18) β-xylosidases. *A. niger* β-xylosidase is very stable, optimum termperatures in a 15- or 20-minute assay being near 70°C (12,13, 15). It has a half-life at 65°C and pH 4.2 buffer of about 75 h (15). The *C. trilaterale* enzyme appears to be only slightly less stable (17). Activation energy on aryl-β-D-xylopyranosides is near 13 kcal/mol (15,22).

β-Xylosidase has evidently been immobilized twice. Puls et al. (23) attached it to alkylamine porous glass or silica with glutaraldehyde, a carbodiimide, or $TiCl_4$, while Oguntimein and Reilly (14) tested Enzorb-A (a phenoxyacetyl cellulose), four Enzacryls, Sepharose CL 4B-200 with CNBr, alkylamine Bio-Gel P-2

and porous silica with glutaraldehyde, and stainless steel and
alumina with $TiCl_4$. The former authors achieved highest immobilized
activities with a carbodiimide link to porous glass and silica gel,
lower activities with glutaraldehyde, and lowest with $TiCl_4$ (23).
The latter, on the other hand, did best with $TiCl_4$ and alumina (14).
In neither case was immobilized activity high enough to be industrially feasible, however.

β-Xylosidase when immobilized had roughly the same properties
as when in free form. There is some disagreement over the pH
optima for activity and stability of the immobilized enzyme and
whether immobilization causes an increase or decrease in stability
(15,23), but in any case the pH optima remain very acid.

It appears that β-xylosidase is not a good candidate for the
industrial production of xylose. The greatest problem is the high
level of transferase activity; and in order to avoid this, very
low substrate concentration would be required. In addition, the
rather low K_i of xylose necessitates its removal as soon as it is
formed. Furthermore, β-xylosidase is not formed by microorganisms
in very high activities. Immobilization often counters this
problem by allowing an enzyme to be used over long periods. However
in the case of β-xylosidase, immobilization does not give high
activities and may, in fact, cause a decrease in stability.

XYLOSE-PRODUCING EXO-XYLANASES

Several enzymes, commonly called β-xylosidases but having
significanly different properties, have been purified and studied
since 1969. The most thorough work has been conducted on two
enzyme preparations, one from *Bacillus pumilus* and the other from
Malbranchea pulchella. In addition, a less studied enzyme from
A. niger appears to have similar properties and will be discussed
here also.

The *B. pumilus* enzyme is active only on β-1,4-xylooligo-
saccharides and aryl-β-D-xylopyranosides (24,25). Unlike β-xylosidase, it has no transferase activity (24,25) and anomeric configuration of the products is inverted (25,26). Xylose is a
competitive inhibitor but with a much higher K_i (26.2 mM) than
is measured with β-xylosidase (24). Many other sugars, synthetic
substrates and divalent cations also inhibit this enzyme (24).
Cysteine is a component of the active center (24,27,28) along with
perhaps histidine (28), but no metals appear to take part in the
catalytic reaction (24). The main binding is between the enzyme
and the glycon while aglycon binding is weak and nonspecific (29).
The enzyme is found in dimeric and tetrameric forms (30-32), the
latter being formed at higher protein concentrations and ionic
strengths (33). Monomeric molecular weight is 60,000. The enzyme

is high in glutamic acid, aspartic acid and leucine; it is low in methionine, cysteine and tryptophan; and it has less than 0.5% carbohydrate (32). The pI is 4.4 (24). This exo-xylanase appears to be rather unstable, especially in dilute solutions (29). It is stabilized by ethylene glycol and sucrose, but not by cysteine or EDTA (29). Optimum pH for activity is 7.3 - 7.4, while that for stability is higher (29).

The enzyme from *M. pulchella* is almost equally active on xylobiose through xylopentaose, giving only xylose and the next shortest oligosaccharide. It is active on xylan and aryl-β-D-xylopyranosides. There is no activity on β-1,2 or β-1,3 linkages. No transfer products are formed from 2% xylobiose (34). The *M. pulchella* exo-xylanase is inhibited by many divalent cations. A sulfhydryl group appears to be part of the active center (34). The molecular weight is 26,000. pH optima for activity and stability are near 6.5. In a short assay, the optimum temperature is 50°C (35).

The third apparent exo-xylanase from, *A. niger*, hydrolyzes arabinoglucuronoxylan and methyl-β-D-xylopyranoside to yield xylose. It gives xylose, xylobiose, xylotriose and a higher oligosaccharide from xylotriose and xylose, xylobiose, and a higher oligosaccharide from xylobiose. The pI is 4.6 and the molecular weight is 30,000. The optimum pH on methyl-β-D-xylopyranoside is 3.0 (36).

The exo-xylanases from *B. pumilus* and *M. pulchella* enzymes differ from the β-xylosidases described in the previous section in their ability to attack xylan and long xylooligosaccharides, their lack of transferase activity, their more limited substrate specificity, and the sulfhydryl group in the active center. The *A. niger* enzyme can attack xylan, but differs from the others in that it apparently has transferase activity and can cleave alkyl-β-D-xylopyranosides. It, however, has a molecular weight far below that of the regular β-xylosidase from *A. niger*. It appears, at least until further information is available, to occupy an intermediate postion between β-xylosidases and xylose-producing exo-xylanases.

If an exo-xylanase that produced xylose could be found with stability greater than that exhibited by the *B. pumilus* and *M. pulchella* enzymes, it would be a prime candidate for industrial use. The absence of transferase activity and the low inhibition by the product, xylose, would lead to higher yields and, at equal activities, to lower required reactor volumes for equivalent conversions. The ability of these enzymes to attack larger xylooligosaccharides than can the β-xylosidases is also an advantage. This enzyme class deserves more emphasis than it has so far received.

ENDO-XYLANASES

Endo-hydrolases as a class do not engage in endwise attack on
polymers, but instead cleave bonds throughout the molecule. Attack
is not random, as often stated. On the contrary, the bonds most
likely to be broken are determined by the length of the substrate,
its degree of branching, the presence of substituents, and the subsite pattern of the hydrolases. Obviously, many enzymes with different specificities must take part in the breakdown of a substrate
as chemically and structurally heterogeneous as xylan. Insufficient
research has been conducted for us to be able to identify all of
the different endo-xylanases that do exist. Undoubtedly, many
xylanases have not yet been discovered, and of those that have been
studied, often a complete picture of their specificities has not
emerged.

It is convenient to divide the endo-xylanases by the products
they form. Two ways of dividing the enzymes are obvious. First,
a division may be made between those xylanases that produce xylose
and xylobiose and those that produce longer oligosaccharides, and
secondly, between those xylanases that cleave at an L-arabinosyl-
initiated branch point, producing L-arabinose by itself and in
longer chains, and those that do not. Further research may well
indicate that the first division is not absolute, in that there may
well be endo-xylanases that produce mainly xylobiose and xylotriose,
and therefore debranch chains of more than one unit length only,
without ever producing L-arabinose itself. However, at present our
knowledge is not sufficiently broad to make these distinctions; so
I will press on with the four categories just identified.

Non-Debranching Xylobiose and Xylose Producers

Endo-xylanases that do not produce L-arabinose but give mainly
xylobiose and xylose from xylan are excreted by *Aspergillus* (10,
36-46), *Schizophyllum* (47,48), *Sterium* (49), *Trametes* (50-52), and
Streptomyces (53-55).

The *A. niger* enzyme has a pI of 6.7 (42,46), a molecular weight
of 22,000 (42,46), an optimum temperature in a short assay of about
55°C (42,46), and a pH optimum for activity near 5 (37,42,46). The
optimum pH for stability is also near 5 (46). The enzyme is high in
glycine, glutamic acid and aspartic acid and low in methionine,
cysteine and phenylalanine, and has a carbohydrate content of 34%
(46).
Activity on xylan and large oligosaccharides is high, decreasing
as the chain length decreases below 6. Xylotetraose is hydrolyzed
mainly to xylobiose, with some xylose and xylotriose, and the product
have inverted configuration (46). Activity on xylotriose is very low
and the enzyme is inactive on xylobiose (46). It has high affinity

for linkages near an L-arabinosyl branch, leaving X_2A and X_3A (38) (see Figure 1). With glucuronoxylans the main products are xylobiose, xylose and 4-0-methylglucuronoxylotriose (43).

Another *A. niger* endo-xylanase that produces xylobiose and xylose appears somewhat different than that just described. It has a molecular weight of 24,000-33,000, 20% carbohydrate and an amino acid profile high in glycine, threonine, aspartic acid and serine, and low in cysteine, valine, histidine and methionine (44). The pI is 4.2 and the optimum temperature in a short assay is $50^{\circ}C$ (44). There appears to be some transferase activity and a slight tendency to liberate L-arabinose from arabinoglucuronoxylan (45).

Turning to other species, the *Schizophyllum* xylanase has a pH optimum for activity of 5 and for stability of 6-8, and an optimum temperature of $50-55^{\circ}C$ (47,48). Its molecular weight is 31,000-33,000 (48), and it is not a glycoprotein (47,48). It is high in glycine, serine and aspartic acid and low in methionine, histidine and cysteine.

The enzyme from *Trametes* is most active at pH 5-5.5 and is most stable in a pH range centered on 6 (51). Its molecular weight is 22,000-24,000 (50). Michaelis constants decrease and maximum rates increase with chain length for the xylanase from *Trametes*, with activity on X_3 being very low and that on X_2 nonexistent (52). The preferred cleavage point on reduced xylooligosaccharides is the bond β to the former reducing end, except for X_3 where it is α (52).

The *Stereum* enzyme has a molecular weight of 22,000-24,000 and is high in serine, threonine and glycine and low in arginine, methionine, histidine and cysteine (49).

The only xylanase of this type from a nonfungal source, that from *Streptomyces*, has a temperature optimum of $60^{\circ}C$ and an optimum pH for activity and stability of 6 (53,54). Its pI is 7.3 and its molecular weight is 40,000 (54). K_m's vary erratically, but V_m's increase with increasing chain length (54). Surprisingly, the amino acid profile is closer to that of the first *A. niger* endo-xylanase than any of those determined from xylanases of fungal origin (54). Attack on xylan initially yields X_3 and X_4 in largest amounts, followed by production of xylose and X_2. Larger xylooligosaccharides are preferentially hydrolyzed to X_3,and X_2 is very slowly broken down to xylose (55).

These endo-xylanases are all relatively small and appear to be most stable at a pH equal to or above that optimal for activity. Though the information is scattered, the first *Aspergillus* enzyme appears similar to those from *Stereum* and *Trametes*, while the other *Aspergillus* enzyme differs in amino acid profile, transferase activity and pI. The *Schizophyllum* xylanase is not a glycoprotein but nevertheless has a higher molecular weight, while the *Streptomyces* xylanase has a higher pI and molecular weight. Whether further differences will appear awaits further research into this potentially very valuable enzyme group.

Non-Debranching Xylooligosaccharide Producers

A number of enzymes that do not produce L-arabinose from xylan but do produce mainly xylooligosaccharides have been described. Four of these are xylanases from *A. niger* studied in our laboratory (56-58); others are from *Cephalosporium* (59,60) and *Trichoderma* (61.

One *A. niger* xylanase has an isoelectric point of 3.75 and a molecular weight of 26,5000 to 28,000. It is active on soluble xylan but on insoluble xylan only if arabinosyl-initiated branches are first cleaved by gentle acid hydrolysis. Soluble and debranched insoluble xylan yield large oligosaccharide fragments and tri-, penta-, hexa-, tetra-, and disaccharide in descending amounts. This xylanase is also active on an X_5-X_9 mixture, but not on X_2, X_3, or X_4. In a 20 min assay, maximum activity occurs at 42°C. The optimum pH for activity and stability is near 5.0. Carbohydrate content is 22% and the enzyme is high in serine, glycine and glutamic acid and low in cysteine, arginine and methionine (56).

A second *A. niger* xylanase has an isoelectric point of 4.5 and a molecular weight of 12,000. Like the enzyme just described, this one is active on an X_5-X_9 mixture, but not on X_2, X_3, or X_4. It breaks down soluble xylan but not insoluble xylan even when debranched. Products in descending order are large fragments or unreacted xylan and penta-, tri-, di-, hexa-, and tetrasaccharides but not xylose. The amino acid profile is similar, though not identical, to the previous xylanase, and the carbohydrate content is 10.9%. Maximum activity in a 25 min assay occurs at 45°C. The optimum pH for activity is 4.8, while that for stability is approximately 5.6 (57).

The third and fourth *A. niger* xylanases have isoelectric points of 8.5 and 9.0 and molecular weights of 12,500. Both attack insoluble xylan much more completely than soluble xylan, giving unreacted xylan and xylooligosaccharides, but no xylose. Only substrates larg than X_4 are attacked. The optimum pH for activity is between 5 and 6, while both xylanases have maximum activities in a 20 min assay near 50°C. The two enzymes have amino acid profiles somewhat simila to each other but different from the other three xylanases described being high in glycine, glutamic acid, serine and alanine, and low in cysteine, methionine, histidine and tyrosine. They each have carbohydrate contents of 5% or less (58).

It appears that the first two *A. niger* xylanases are isozymes of each other, being significantly different only in pI, molecular weight and carbohydrate content. The third and fourth are even more similar to each other, differing only in pI. The first two are different from the second two in their pIs and in their specificities, the first two being active chiefly on soluble rather than insoluble xylan and having low pIs.

Among xylanases from species other than *A. niger*, the *Cephalosporium* xylanase has a pI of 6.0, an optimum pH for activity of 6.5, an optimum temperature of 37°C, and a molecular weight of 9,500. It produced, in descending order, X_2, X_3, X_4, AX_3, AX_4, and xylose (59,60). The *Trichoderma* xylanase produced an X_2-X_5 mixture but no xylose and had a pI of 9.6 and a molecular weight of 15,000 by SDS-gel electrophoresis and 20,000-22,000 by sucrose density gradient ultracentrifugation (61). This group of enzymes, which produce xylooligosaccharides but not xylose or arabinose from xylan, would be very useful industrially if forms that were sufficiently stable could be found. To this point, however, none seems to be.

Debranching Endo-Xylanases

Much less is known about xylanases that can release L-arabinose from xylan than those that cannot. Enzymes of this type have been purified from cultures of *Aspergillus* (10,36-39,62), *Ceratocystis* (59,63), *Cephalosporium* (59,60), *Trichoderma* (41-43), and *Oxiporus* (41-43).

The six xylanases from *A. niger* purified by John et al. (62) have molecular weights from 30,000 to 50,000 and pH optima for activity that range from 4 to 6.5. Major products vary from enzyme to enzyme; some of the enzymes are active on microcrystalline cellulose (62). Other debranching *A. niger* xylanases can attack arabinoxylan less completely than can a xylanase from the same culture that does not release L-arabinose (37,39). One enzyme can hydrolyze X_2A to L-arabinose and xylobiose, and X_3A to L-arabinose, X_2, X_3, and xylose. This enzyme exhibits a higher affinity for xylosidic linkages near the α-1,3 L-arabinose to xylose bond than it shows for these linkages when the L-arabinose is not present (38). The pH optima for activity and stability are in the acid range (10).

Two enzymes from *Ceratocystis paradoxa* and *Cephalosporium sacchari* similar to those just described also are most active at an acidic pH (59,60,63). They have very high pIs, 9.17 and 9.4 respectively, and neither is very stable. The former enzyme attacks X_4 and longer products, and it gives L-arabinose, X_2, and xylooligosaccharides from AX_2, AX_3, and longer substrates (59,63). The *C. sacchari* enzyme, which has a molecular weight of 10,000, gives primarily X_2 and AX_3, but also X_3, AX_4, xylose, and L-arabinose from xylan (59,60).

Finally, the *Trichoderma* and *Oxiporus* homogeneous enzymes, each purified from many other xylanases (41), have molecular weights of 18,000 and 37,000 and pIs of 9.2 and 6.2 respectively (42). They each give X_2, xylose and 4-O-methylglucuronoxylotriose from hardwood xylan and release L-arabinose from softwood xylan (43).

MISCELLANEOUS ENZYMES

Three enzymes not previously discussed are worthy of brief mention here. A supposed *A. niger* β-xylosidase purified by John et al, (62) is more active on X_3 than X_2 and appears to have a sulf-hydryl group in the active center, both typical traits of the xylose-producing exo-xylanases discussed earlier. Its molecular weight and stability are both lower than that of the standard *A. niger* β-xylosidase (10,14), and more in line with what has been determined for the exo-xylanase. Further information will allow its proper identification.

A *Bacillus* xylanase has alkaline pH optima for activity and stability and gives large amounts of xylobiose but no xylose from xylan (64). It may be the xylobiose-producing exo-xylanase that is expected by analogy with the cellulases and amylases, but not yet found. However, no further work has been conducted to prove this.

The third enzyme was not discussed before this point because it is slightly contaminated with an invertase, and therefore did not meet the requirement for homogeneity imposed on the xylanases presented previously. It is an endo-xylanase from *C. paradoxa* that preferentially hydrolyzes xylosyl bonds near L-arabinose and uronic acid residues (65). It produces X_2, X_3, AX_2, and AX_3 from AX_3 and longer chains, but unlike the products from a similar enzyme from *A. niger* (38), the arabinose in the produce is linked α-1,3 to the nonreducing end of the xylosyl chain (66). It is a very stable enzyme with an optimum temperature of 80°C in a short assay at pH 5.5 (65), which is extremely high for a xylanase. Xylose is an inhibitor of this enzyme.

CONCLUSION

All reviews of this type end with a statement that more research needs to be conducted, and this review ends in the same fashion. While β-xylosidase has been characterized extensively, its properties are such that it may not be acceptable for industrial use. A more attractive enzyme for this purpose is what appears to be a xylose-producing exo-xylanase produced by *Bacillus pumilus* and *Malbranchea pulchella* and perhaps by *Aspergillus niger*. It has less tendency to form transfer products and therefore decrease the yield of xylose; it is also less inhibited by xylose and can attack longer substrates than can β-xylosidase. However, all forms so far tested are insufficiently stable for industrial use, and it is imperative that enzymes of this type with greater stability be found.

Data on the endo-xylanases are copious but widely scattered. In this review these enzymes have been divided into four classes, based on their ability to cleave L-arabinose from xylan and their propensity to produce xylose and xylobiose or, on the other hand, larger oligosaccharides. Within these divisions there are undoubtedly subdivisions, but as yet, given the widely varying studies that have been conducted, these are not apparent. Missing is work on the subsite structure of different endo- and exo-xylanases, so that they can be differentiated more surely from each other. There has been only one reported study of this sort (52). Also lacking are studies where all the xylanases produced by one strain are purified and characterized. As with the exo-xylanases, evidence is missing for highly stable enzymes suitable for use outside the laboratory.

Hydrolysis of xylan by a method that is reasonably inexpensive and gives high yield is essential to the success of industrial processes that utilize cellulosic residues. Whether the method of choice will be enzymic or acidic hydrolysis is not yet clear. The further research suggested here should clarify that decision.

REFERENCES

1. Northcote, D.H., 1972, Chemistry of the plant cell wall, An. Rev. Plant Physiol., 23: 113.
2. Reese, E.T., Maguire, A., and Parrish, F.W., 1973, Production of β-D-xylopyranosidases by fungi, Can. J. Microbiol., 19:1065.
3. Flannigan, B. and Sellars, P.N., 1977, Amylase, β-glucosidase and β-xylosidase activity of thermotolerant and thermophilic fungi isolated from barley, Trans. Brit. Mycol. Soc., 69, Pt. 2:316.
4. Notario, V., Villa, T.G., and Villanueva, J. R., 1976, β-Xylosidase in the yeast *Cryptococcus albidus* var. *aerius*, Can. J. Microbiol., 22:312.
5. Lajudie, J. and de Barjac, H., 1976, Search of some glycosidases in 22 species of *Bacillus*, An. Microbiol. (Paris), 127A: 317.
6. Hayward, A.C., 1977, Occurrence of glycoside hydrolases in plant pathogenic and related bacteria, J. Appl. Bacteriol., 43:407.
7. Howard, B.H., Jones, G., and Purdom, M. R., 1960, The pentosanases of some rumen bacteria, Biochem. J., 74:173.
8. Walker, D.J., 1967, Some properties of xylanase and xylobiase from mixed rumen organisms, Austral. J. Biol. Sci., 20:799.
9. Loontiens, F.G. and De Bruyne, C.K., 1963, Separation of β-D-xylosidase and β-D-glucosidase present in commerical

hemicellulase by column electrophoresis on Sephadex G25, Naturwiss., 19:614.

10. Fukuomoto, J., Tsujisaka, Y., and Takenishi, S., 1970, Studies on the hemicellulases. Part I. Purification and some properties of hemicellulases from *Aspergillus niger* van Tieghem sp., Nippon Nogeikagaku Kaishi, 44:447.

11. Claeyssens, M., Loontiens, F.G., Kersters-Hilderson, H., and De Bruyne, C.K., 1971, Partial purification and properties of an *Aspergillus niger* β-D-xylosidase, Enzymologia, 40:177.

12. Sasaki, T., 1971, Xylanases produced by *Aspergillus niger*, with emphasis on β-xylosidase, Mem. Coll. Agric. Ehime Univ., 15:71.

13. Takenishi, S., Tsujisaka, Y., and Fukumoto, J., 1973, Studies on hemicellulases.IV. Purification and properties of the β-xylosidase produced by *Aspergillus niger* van Tieghem, J. Biochem., 73:335.

14. Oguntimein, G.B. and Reilly, P.J., 1980, Purification and immobilization of *Aspergillus niger* β-xylosidase, Biotechnol. Bioeng., 22:1127.

15. Oguntimein, G.B. and Reilly, P.J., 1980, Properties of soluble and immobilized *Aspergillus niger* β-xylosidase, Biotechnol. Bioeng., 22:1143.

16. King, N.J. and Fuller, D.B., 1968, The xylanase system of *Coniophora cerebella*, Biochem. J., 108:571.

17. Kawaminami, T. and Iizuka, H., 1970, Studies on xylanase from microorganisms. V. Purification and some properties of β-xylosidase from *Chaetomium trilaterale* strain no. 2264. J. Ferment. Technol., 48:169.

18. Deleyn, F., Claeyssens, M., Van Beeumen, J., and De Bruyne, C.K. 1978, Purification and properties of β-xylosidase from *Penicillium wortmanni*, Can. J. Biochem., 56:43.

19. Claeyssens, M. and De Bruyne, C.K., 1965, D-Xylose-derivatives with sulfur or nitrogen in the ring: Powerful inhibitors of glycosidase-activities, Naturwiss., 52:515.

20. Kersters-Hilderson, H., Claeyssens, M., Loontiens, F.G., Krýnski A., and De Bruyne, C.K., 1970, Chain length effects of n-alkyl 1-oxygen- and n-alkyl 1-thio-β-D-xylopyranosides on β-D-xylosidases, Eur. J. Biochem., 12:403.

21. Claeyssens, M., Van Leemputten, E., Loontiens, F. G., and De Bruyne, C. K., 1966, Transfer reactions catalysed by a fungal β-D-xylosidase: Enzymatic synthesis of phenyl β-D-xylobioside, Carbohydr. Res., 3:32.

22. Van Wijnendaele, F. and De Bruyne, C.K., 1970, The enzymic hydrolysis of substituted phenyl β-D-xylopyranosides, Carbohydr. Res., 14:189.

23. Puls, J., Sinner, M. and Dietrichs, H.H., 1977, Hydrolysis of hemicelluloses by immobilized enzymes, Trans. Tech. Sect. Can. Pulp Paper Assoc., 3:TR64.

24. Kersters-Hilderson, H., Loontiens, F.G., Claeyssens, M., and De Bruyne,C.K., 1969, Partial purification and properties of

an induced β-xylosidase of *Bacillus pumilus* 12, Eur. J. Biochem. 7:434.

25. Van Doorslaer, E., Kersters-Hilderson, H., and De Bruyne, C.K., 1976, Mechanism of action of β-xylosidase from *Bacillus pumilus*, Arch. Internat. Physiol. Biochim., 84:198.

26. Kersters-Hilderson, H., Claeyssens, M., Van Doorslaer, E., and De Bruyne, C.K., 1976, Determination of the anomeric configuration of D-xylose with D-xylose isomerases, Carbohydr. Res. 47: 269.

27. Samen,E., Claeyssens, M., and De Bruyne, C.K., 1975, *Bacillus pumilus* β-D-xylosidase: Study of the thiol groups, Biochem. Soc. Trans., 3:998.

28. Samen, E., Claeyssens, M., and De Bruyne, C.K., 1978, Study of the sulfhydryl groups of β-D-xylosidase from *Bacillus pumilus*, Eur. J. Biochem., 85:301.

29. Kersters-Hilderson, H., Van Doorslaer, E., and De Bruyne, C.K., 1978, β-D-xylosidase from *Bacillus pumilus* PRL B12: Hydrolysis of aryl β-D-xylopyranosides, Carbohydr. Res., 65:219.

30. Claeyssens, M., Kersters-Hilderson, H., Van Wauwe, J.-P., and De Bruyne, C.K., 1970, Purification of *Bacillus pumilus* β-D-xylosidase by affinity chromatography, FEBS Lett., 11:336.

31. Claeyssens, M., Samen, E., and DeBruyne, C.K., 1975, *Bacillus pumilus* β-D-xylosidase: Dimeric-tetrameric structure elucidated by cross-linking studies, Biochem. Soc. Trans., 3:999.

32. Claeyssens, M., Samen, E., Kersters-Hilderson, H., and De Bruyne, C.K., 1975, β-D-xylosidase from *Bacillus pumilus*. Molecular properties and oligomeric structure, Biochim. Biophys. Acta, 405:475.

33. Claeyssens, M. and De Bruyne, C.K., 1978, Binding of 4-methylumbelliferyl β-D-ribopyranoside to β-xylosidase from *Bacillus pumilus*, Biochim. Biophys. Acta, 533:98.

34. Matsuo, M., Yasui, T., and Kobayashi, T., 1977, Studies on xylanase system of thermophilic fungi. Part III. Enzymatic properties of β-xylosidase from *Malbranchea pulchella* var. *sulfurea* No. 48, Agr. Biol. Chem., 41:1601.

35. Matsuo, M., Yasui, T., and Kobayashi, T., 1977. Studies on xylanase system of thermophilic fungi. Part II. Purification and some properties of β-xylosidase from *Malbranchea pulchella* var. *sulfurea* No. 48, Agr. Biol. Chem., 41:1593.

36. Rodionova, N.A., Gorbacheva, I.V., and Buivid, V.A., 1977, Fractionation and purification of endo-1,4-β-xylosidases of *Aspergillus niger*, Biokhimiya, 42:659 (Biochemistry (USSR), 42:505).

37. Tsujisaka, Y., Takenishi, S., and Fukumoto, J., 1971. Studies on the hemicellulases. II. The mode of action of three hemicellulases produced from *A. niger* van Tieghem sp., Nippon Nogeikagaku Kaishi, 45:253.

38. Takenishi, S. and Tsujisaka, Y., 1973, Studies on hemicellulases. V. Structures of the oligosaccharides from the enzymic hydrolyzate of rice-straw arabinoxylan by a xylanase of *A. niger*,

Agr. Biol. Chem., 39:2315.

40. Sinner, M., and Dietrichs, H.H., 1975, Enzymatische Hydrolyse
von Laubholz-Xylanen. I. Untersuchung von Pilzenzym-Handelspräparaten auf Xylanen und andere polysaccharid-spaltende
Enzymen, Holzforschung, 29:123.

41. Sinner, M., and Dietrichs, H.H., 1975, Enzymatische Hydrolyse
von Laubholz-Xylanen. II. Isolierung von fünf β-1→4-Xylanasen
aus drei Pilzenzym-Handelspräparaten, Holzforschung, 29:169.

42. Sinner, M., and Dietrichs, H.H., 1975, Enzymatische Hydrolyse
von Laubholz-Xylanen. III. Kennzeichnung von fünf isolierten
β-1→4-Xylanasen, Holzforschung, 29:207.

43. Sinner, M., and Dietrichs, H.H., 1976, Enzymatische Hydrolyse
von Laubholz-Xylanen. IV. Abbau von isolierten Xylanen, Holzforschung, 30:50.

44. Gorbacheva, I.V., and Rodionova, N.A., 1977, Studies on xylan-
degrading enzymes. I. Purification and characterization of
endo-1,4-β-xylanase from *Aspergillus niger* str. 14., Biochim.
Biophys. Acta, 484:79.

45. Gorbacheva, I.V. and Rodionova, N.A., 1977, Studies on xylan-
degrading enzymes. II. Action pattern on endo-1,4-β-xylanase
from *Aspergillus niger* str. 14 on xylan and xylooligosaccharides,
Biochim. Biophys. Acta, 484:94.

46. Frederick, M.M., Frederick, J.R., Fratzke, A.R., and Reilly,
P.J., Purification and characterization of a xylobiose- and
xylose-producing endo-xylanase from *Aspergillus niger*, submitted for publication.

47. Váradi, J., Nečesaný, V., and Kovács, P., 1971, Cellulase and
xylanase of fungus *Schizophillum commune*. III. Purification
and properties of xylanase, Drevársky Výskum, 3:147.

48. Paice, M.G., Jurasek, L., Carpenter, M.R., and Smillie, L.B.,
1978. Production, characterization and partial amino acid
sequence of xylanase A from *Schizophyllum commune*, Appl. Env.
Microbiol., 36:802.

49. Eriksson, K.-E., and Pettersson, B., 1971, Purification and
characterization of xylanase from the rot fungus *Stereum san-
guinolentum*, Internat. Biodeterior. Bull., 7:115.

50. Kubačková, M., Karácsonyi, Š., and Toman, R., 1976, Purification of xylanase from the wood-rotting fungus *Trametes hirsuta*,
Folia Microbiol., 21:28.

51. Kubačková, M., Karácsonyi, Š., Bilisics, L., and Toman, R.,
1978, Some properties of an endo-1,4-β-xylanase from the
ligniperdous fungus *Trametes hirsuta*, Folia Microbiol., 23:202.

52. Kubačková, M., Karácsonyi, Š., Bilisics, L., and Toman, R.,
1979, On the specificity and mode of action of a xylanase from
Trametes hirsuta (Wulf) Pilát, Carbohydr. Res., 76:177.

53. Iizuka, H., and Kawaminami, T., 1965, Studies on the xylanase
from *Streptomyces*. I. Purification and some properties of
xylanase from *Streptomyces xylophagus* nov. sp., Agr. Biol.
Chem., 29:520.

54. Kusakabe, I., Kawaguchi, M., Yasui, T., and Kobayashi, T.,

1977, Studies on xylanase system of *Streptomyces*. VII. Purification and some properties of extracellular xylanase from *Streptomyces* sp. E-86, Nippon Nogeikagaku Kaishi, 51:429.

55. Kusakabe, I., Yasui, T., and Kobayashi, T., 1977, Studies on xylanase system of *Streptomyces*. VIII. The action of *Streptomyces* xylanases on various xylans and xylooligosaccharides, Nippon Nogeikagaku Kaishi, 51:439.

56. Fournier, A.R., Frederick, M.M., Frederick, J.R. and Reilly, P.J., unpublished research.

57. Shei, J.C., Fratzke, A.R., Frederick, M.M., Frederick, J.R., and Reilly, P.J., unpublished research.

58. Frederick, M.M., Kiang, C.-H., Frederick, J.R., and Reilly, P.J., unpublished research.

59. Dekker, R.F.H., Richards, G.N., and Shambe, T., Comparative properties and action patterns of the hemicellulases from the phytophathogens *Ceratocystis paradoxa* and *Cephalosporium sacchari*, Biochem. Soc. Trans., 3:1081.

60. Richards, G.N., and Shambe, T., 1976, Studies on hemicellulases, V. Production and purification of two hemicellulases from *Cephalosporium sacchari*, Carbohydr. Res. 49:371.

61. Baker, C.J., Whelan, C.H. and Bateman, D.F., 1977, Xylanase from *Trichoderma pseudokoningii*: Purification, characterization, and effects on isolated plant cell walls. Phytopath., 67:1250.

62. John, M., Schmidt, B., and Schmidt, J., 1979, Purification and some properties of five endo-1,4-β-D-xylanases and a β-D-xylosidase produced by a strain of *Aspergillus niger*, Can. J. Biochem., 57:125.

63. Dekker, R.F.H., and Richards, G.N., 1975, Studies on hemicellulases. II. Purification, properties,and mode of action of hemicellulase I produced by *Ceratocystis paradoxa*, Carbohydr. Res. 39:97.

64. Horikoshi, K., and Atsukawa, Y., 1973, Production of enzymes by alkalophilic microorganisms. VII. Xylanase produced by alkalophilic *Bacillus* no. C-59-2, Agr. Biol. Chem., 37:2097.

65. Dekker, R.F.H., and Richards, G.N. 1975, Studies on hemicellulases. III. Purification, properties, and mode of action of hemicellulase II produced by *Ceratocystis paradoxa*, Carbohydr. Res., 42:107.

66. Dekker, R.F.H., and Richards, G.N., 1975, Studies on hemicellulases. IV. Structures of the oligosaccharides from the enzymic hydrolysis of hemicellulose by a hemicellulase of *Ceratocystis paradoxa*, Carbohydr. Res., 43:335.

DISCUSSION

Q.   WOODWARD: Is β-xylosidase a glycoprotein?

A.   REILLY: Yes.   The *Penicillum wortmanni* β-xylosidose is a glycoprotein and very recent work from Bratislava suggests the *Cryptococcus albidus* β-xylosidase is also.

Q. WOODWARD: I was interested in the fact that when you immobilize that enzyme it becomes less stable. Do you know whether the sugar moiety is essential for stability?

A. REILLY: With most glycoproteins, it is; I'm not sure about this one.

Q. WOODWARD: I'd like to suggest that perhaps it could be immobilized using the sugar moiety. Since a protein is stabilized by its amino acid interactions, this may prevent loss of stability.

A. REILLY: I think that's possible. Certainly some of the methods we used would have formed bonds between the carbohydrate and the carrier. I'd like to add a point to that. I think when people first started to immobilize enzymes there was the general belief that immobilization stabilized enzymes. I think that most people have gotten away from that belief now and understand that immobilization results are random. Some are stabilized and some are destabilized and, in addition, some are immobilized easily and some are not immobilized easily. We seem to have the worst of both worlds here, in that β-xylosidase is not immobilized easily, at least not by the methods we in the United States and Puls, Sinner and Dietrichs in Germany have used. It also doesn't seem to be quite as stable when immobilized, although in that regard we and they disagree.

Q. ERIKSSON: Do you think that the reason why an exo-xylanase that releases xylose is not as sensitive to inhibition by this xylose as a β-xylosidase would be is that the exo-enzymes cause an inversion of configuration of the related products? As you know, exo-glucanases release glucose or cellobiose with reversion of configuration. Might this reversion of configuration be involved as a regulatory phenomenon?

A. REILLY: I suppose it might be. It certainly is a good observation.

Q. ERIKSSON: I wasn't aware, as a matter of fact, that there was such a thing as exo-xylanase, since to degrade xylan it would not to be necessary to have both an endo- and an exo-system for xylan degradation, as xylan is not crystalline in nature, different from cellulose.

A. REILLY: Of course, there are both exo- and endo-amylases. In fact, there are two exo-amylases.

Q.   ERIKSSON: I certainly think it is a possibility that exo-
glucanases and now also this exo-xylanase release their products
with reversion of configuration might be involved in regulation.

A.   REILLY: And we have to extend that to suggest that this is
true of the amylases also, as both glucoamylase and β-amylase
invert configuration. Of course, product configuration is
not always constant for a single enzyme. A recent paper from
Japan reported that product configuration for an amylase
changed with reaction conditions and reactant substituents.

ERIKSSON: That would be consistent with my idea.

Q.   TSUCHIYA: I have a very simple question: What is the source
of the xylanase you spoke about, *Aspergillus* and *B. pumilus*
and so forth?

A.   REILLY: Our xylanase is from a commercial preparation from
Rohm and Haas called "Rhozyme HP-150 Concentrate", which is
a very crude *Aspergillus niger* mixture that contains many
different xylanases.

Q.   TSUCHIYA: A crude mixture of what?

A.   REILLY: Of everything. There is not a single hydrolase that
we ever assayed for that has not been present. It's very
crude.

TOWARD ELUCIDATING THE MECHANISM OF ACTION

OF THE LIGNINOLYTIC SYSTEMS IN BASIDIOMYCETES

T. Kent Kirk

Forest Products Laboratory, Forest Service
U. S. Department of Agriculture
Madison, Wisconsin 53705

The fact that this lecture is scheduled between lectures on xylanases and amylases perhaps illustrates the common misconception that the ligninolytic system bears a close biochemical similarity to other common biopolymer-degrading microbial systems. It does not. It is a most unusual system which has not yet been defined biochemically. However, recent studies, which I shall review here, have resulted in progress toward this end.

In terms of global importance to the carbon cycle, lignin bio-degradation is of significance not only because lignin is second only to cellulose in abundance among renewable organic materials, but also for two often less appreciated reasons: (1) Lignin physically pro-tects most of the world's cellulose and hemicelluloses from enzyma-tic attack, and the lignin barrier must be disrupted before the polysaccharides can be biologically processed or digested; and (2) lignin's carbon content is 50% higher than that of the polysac-charides, making lignin relatively more abundant as a carbon/energy repository than its weight would indicate.

The relationship of lignin to the subject of this conference is in its potential as a source of chemicals and fuels, in the necessity to remove or modify it prior to enzymatic processing of most available biomass and in the fact that it will be a high volume byproduct of most currently envisioned biomass-processing schemes. Evolution has, of course, resulted in the development of micro-organisms that efficiently biodegrade lignin. It is hoped that we can learn from what evolution has provided and use this knowledge to increase the number of options available for the processing of biomass.

Lignin is a variable polymer of p-hydroxyphenylpropane units which are connected by C–C and C–O–C linkages. The immediate biosynthetic precursors of the polymer are p-coumaryl-, coniferyl-, and sinapyl alcohols (4-hydroxy-,4-hydroxy-3-methoxy-, and 4-hydroxy-3, 5-dimethoxy-cinnamyl alcohols, respectively). Peroxidase-catalyzed single-electron oxidation at the phenolic hydroxyl groups in these compounds produces free radical species which exist in mesomeric forms and which couple with each other non-enzymatically. Phenolic groups in the oligomeric products are also oxidized, and polymerization involves primarily the coupling of single units to the growing polymer. A variety of inter-phenylpropane linkages results, and a polydisperse, 3-dimensional plastic is formed. This mode of polymerization means that lignin is optically inactive and that all asymmetric carbons (C_α- and C_β [carbon designations: Table I, structure A]) are mixed R and S forms. The major interunit linkages and their frequencies in representative gymnosperm (spruce) and angiosperm (birch) woods are illustrated in Table I; several other quantitatively less important linkages also occur. The relative proportion of the three cinnamyl alcohol precursors incorporated into lignin varies with the plant species, tissues and even location in cell walls. In general, gymnosperm lignin is made from coniferyl alcohol and angiosperm lignin from mixtures of coniferyl and sinapyl alcohols. Most lignins contain only a small proportion of p-coumaryl alcohol, so that the methoxyl content of lignins is usually 14 to 22% of the weight.

Lignin exists in lignocellulosics primarily as an interpenetrating matrix with hemicelluloses, to which covalent linkages, of as yet imprecisely understood chemistry, exist. The lignin-hemicellulose matrix surrounds the cellulose fibrils. Lignin is found in high concentration between contiguous cells. The reader is referred to Adler (1), Freudenberg (2) and Sarkanen and Ludwig (3), for further details about lignin structure.

The microbiology of lignin biodegradation has been substantially clarified in recent years. The complex polymer is completely metabolized by pure cultures of various higher fungi, primarily basidiomycetes, and is substantially degraded by some ascomycetes and imperfect fungi (4). It is partially degraded by axenic cultures of certain actinomycetes (5). Undoubtedly, it is degraded—albeit slowly—by the mixed microbial populations of many soils (6-9). It is probably not degraded to volatile products in anaerobic environments (10), but whether it is structurally modified in the absence of O_2 is not yet known—nor in fact has this been investigated. Zeikus (11) has recently summarized the microbial ecology of lignin biodegradation.

Little is known about the chemistry and biochemistry of lignin metabolism by microbes other than white-rot wood-decay fungi, which are primarily basidiomycetes, although actinomycetes *(Streptomycetes,*

TABLE I

Frequencies of Major Interunit Linkages in Lignin
(adapted from ref. 1).

Substructure type	Proportions (% of total C_9-units)	
	Spruce	Birch
A	48	60
B	9-12	6
C	9.5-11	4.5
D	6-8	6-8
E	7	8
F	3.5-4	6.5

nocardias) and imperfect fungi (*fusaria*) are being studied currently in several laboratories. This lecture is limited to the white-rot fungi, and will briefly summarize the current understanding of the physiology and chemistry of their action. In keeping with the assigned subject, I shall speculate about the indicated biochemistry of lignin polymer degradation. Recent reviews can be consulted for detailed coverage of particular points (4,5,11,12).

PHYSIOLOGICAL FEATURES

     During the past 5 years we have optimized the nutritional and
environmental culture parameters for lignin degradation for a selec
white-rot fungus (13). These investigations were conducted with
Phanerochaete chrysosporium Burds., chosen for its rapid growth and
rapid degradation of lignin, its prolific conidiation, its unusuall
high temperature optimum of 40°C and its low phenol-oxidizing enzym
activity. Finding all these traits in a single species is unusual,
and makes *Phanerochaete chrysosporium* [=Sporotrichum pulverulentum
Nov. (14)] attractive for study. As an assay for biodegradation we
used conversion of synthetic ^{14}C-lignins (labeled in the prophyl si
chains, in the methoxyl groups or in the aromatic nuclei) to CO_2.
These were prepared *in vitro* by the peroxidase-catalyzed oxidation
of labeled coniferyl alcohols (15). Empirical studies with *P.
chrysosporium* and the radiochemical assay have now permitted the
description and optimization of the culture parameters influencing
the rate of lignin degradation; some parameters that are optimal
for lignin degradation are not optimal for growth (Table II). Certa
of the factors critical for the oxidation of lignin to CO_2 by *P.
chrysosporium* are unusual, and as a result their discovery was un-
anticipated. They clearly establish the uniqueness of lignin metab
olism among biopolymer degradations. Here I want to draw particula
attention to the lack of inducibility of the ligninolytic system by
lignin, the requirement for lignin degradation of a growth substrat
other than lignin, and the strong influence of nutrient nitrogen on
lignin degradation rates.

     These three unusual features are closely interrelated and hav
been rationalized in the conclusion that lignin degradation is a
secondary metabolic ["idiophasic" (25)] event (13). That lignin de
gradation is a secondary metabolic is supported by the observations
that: (a) Its appearance in cultures is triggered by nitrogen-,
sulfur- or carbohydrate starvation (20); (b) it is temporally separated from primary growth (17,20,21); and (c) it occurs in N-limite
cultures, together with the biosynthesis of a typical secondary
metabolite, 3,4-dimethoxybenzyl alcohol [from glucose via phenylalanine (26,27)]. The separation of lignin degradation from primary
growth and the lack of inducibility of the ligninolytic system show
that the energy stored in lignin is not of much importance to the
organism. We have suggested that lignin is at best only a marginal
energy/carbon source for maintenance metabolism (20). Indirect
evidence indicates that lignin carbon does enter central metabolic
pathways (13,26), although attempts to demonstrate lignin-derived
carbon in TCA cycle intermediates were not successful (Kirk and
Zeikus, unpub.).

     Further studies of the physiology of lignin metabolism (lig-
non→CO_2) have examined ligninolytic cultures limited for nitrogen

TABLE II

Culture Parameters Important for Growth and Lignin Degradation by *Phanerochaete chrysosporium*

Parameter	Influence	References
Nutritional		
Lignin	Does not influence appearance or titer of ligninolytic system: does not serve as growth substrate.	16,17
Carbon source (growth substrate)	Required for growth; not clear if lignin can support its own degradation; cellulose, glucose, xylose, glycerol, succinate, etc., are suitable carbon sources; carbon limitation can trigger ligninolytic activity.	16,18-20
Nutrient nitrogen	Cultures must be nitrogen-starved for sustained degradation of lignin; amino nitrogen, NH_4^+ are best sources for growth, although NO_3^- will serve.	17,21-23
Other nutrients	Thiamine required for growth; balance of trace metals is important for lignin degradation; sulfur but not phosphorus limitation can trigger ligninolytic activity.	20-22
Oxygen	High concentration in culture fluid stimulatory to both development and activity of ligninolytic system.	21-23, S. S. Bar-Lev and T. K. Kirk, unpublished.
Environmental		
pH	pH control important; optimum pH 4-4.5 for lignin degradation, probably broader for growth; certain buffers inhibit ligninolytic activity.	21,24
Temperature	Optimum for growth near 40°C; influence on ligninolytic activity not studied.	14
Agitation	Growth is good in agitated or stationary cultures; agitation resulting in pellet formation strongly suppresses lignin degradation; agitation of pre-grown mats does not affect lignin degradation.	21,23

or carbohydrate (20,26,28). The oxidation of lignin to CO_2 in nitrogen-limited cultures is sharply suppressed by addition of certain nitrogenous compounds. Of various compounds tested, glutamic acid was the most suppressive. Investigations indicated that nitrogen addition stops the regenerative synthesis of some component(s) of the ligninolytic system--i.e. that the effect is biochemical repression. Recent results show that lignin degradation can be made to occur with renewal of primary growth by addition of non-repressive amounts of NH_4^+, which causes only a fraction of the suppression exhibited by glutamate. In carbohydrate-starved, nitrogen-rich cultures, lignin metabolism begins after carbohydrate depletion and is accompanied by autolysis. Autolysis apparently provides carbon and energy for cell maintenance and lignin degradation ceases when autolysis does. Addition of extra carbohydrate stops (temporarily) lignin degradation. Interestingly, glutamate at concentrations supplying negligible carbon strongly suppresses lignin metabolism in carbohydrate-limited cultures, as it does in nitrogen-limited cultures; NH_4^+ is without effect under the former conditions. This and other observations have led us to speculate that glutamate metabolism might play a role in the regulation of lignin degradation as a part of secondary metabolism in P. chrysosporium.

In any case, these unusual physiological features indicate that lignin is degraded almost passively, or incidentally, which leads to interesting questions and speculation about the evolution of the ligninolytic system (4,11,13).

A drawback to the physiological studies is the assay, lignin→ CO_2, which is too crude for definitive studies. Research on the chemistry of lignin metabolism, however, is beginning to point to specific reactions, which will make it possible eventually to pinpoint the basis for the physiological features. The chemical studies are indicating a low degree of specificity of the ligninolytic system which is in accord with its "passive" physiological nature. Having specific assays will allow answering the old question of whether lignin-degrading catalysts diffuse away from the hyphae, as microscopic studies of wood decay indicate (29), or whether they are closely associated with the hyphae, as chemical studies indicate (30).

CHEMISTRY OF LIGNIN BIODEGRADATION

Model compound studies. Because lignin is a heterogeneous polymer with chemically resistant and varied interunit linkages, its chemical characterization has been exceptionally challenging -- from the pioneering work of Freudenberg (2) and Adler (1) on its structure, to current attempts to describe its biodegradation, the nature of the lignin-hemicellulose linkages, and other features. Progress in all areas of lignin chemistry has relied heavily on the use of low molecular weight substructure model compounds-usually "dimers" containing important interunit linkages.

Early studies of the metabolism of such model compounds by various white-rot fungi defined a number of reactions and degradative pathways. However, these studies were frustrated by the observations that some reasonable model compounds were not degraded, and that some of the observed reactions were of questionable relevance to lignin metabolism (4). It is now clear that most of those early studies--including our own--employed culture conditions good for growth but not for lignin degradation. Recent studies have taken advantage of the findings discussed above (Table II) and have been conducted with ligninolytic nitrogen-starved cultures. Enoki et al. (31) and we (unpub.) have shown that several relevant model compounds are metabolized by *P. chrysosporium* only during secondary metabolism. Enoki et al. (31) have shown that one compound is degraded differently in the primary and secondary metabolic phases (Figure 1). Thus whether any of the early work with model compounds is significant to lignin degradation is not clear at this time.

Recent work with model compounds has defined several reactions in ligninolytic cultures of *P. chrysosporium*, and a number of additional reactions have been established, but not yet published, by us and by several other groups (K.-E. Eriksson et al.; M. Gold et al.; and T. Higuchi et al., pers. comm.). Figures 1 and 2 show the fate of two lignin substructure model compounds established quite recently (31,32). Studies like these are rapidly defining specific reactions. Demonstration that the identified specific degradative reactions are catalyzed only during secondary metabolism will help establish their relevance to ligninolytic activity; determination that the catalyst(s) is (are) extracellular will indicate the possible activity against the polymer.

Lignin Polymer Studies. A more direct approach to defining the chemistry of lignin biodegradation is the characterization of the partially degraded polymer isolated and purified from white-rotted wood (see 4, for review). Various chemical and spectroscopic techniques have been used to compare degraded and sound lignins, and the following conclusions can be reached concerning the degradative reactions in the polymer: (a) They are primarily oxidative; (b) demethylation (or demethoxylation) occurs; (c) side chains are oxidized at C_α; (d) side chains are cleaved between C_α and C_β; and (e) aromatic nuclei are oxidatively cleaved. Recent comparisons of sound and white-rotted (polymeric) lignins with ^{13}C-nmr techniques have confirmed the presence of aromatic acid residues, and established, *inter alia*, the presence of phenoxyacetic acid residues and methylene groups. Most importantly, results with ^{13}C-nmr provide strong evidence that ring cleavage fragments are present in the white-rotted lignin polymer (33,34).

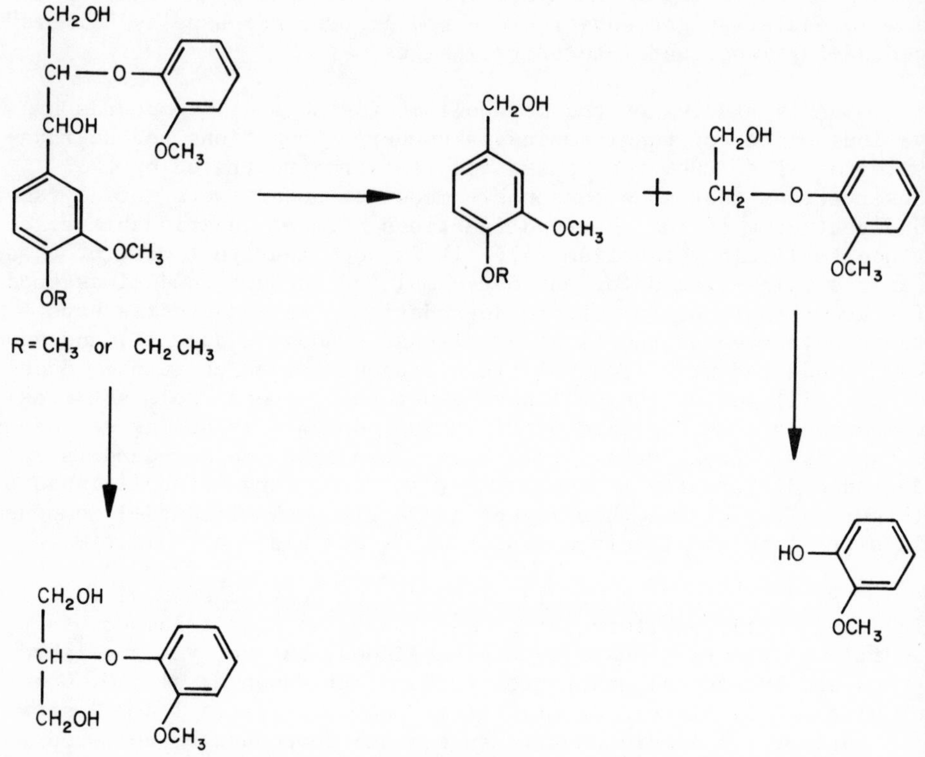

Figure 1.   Degradation of a β-aryl ether substructure (Type A, Tabl I) model compound by *Phanerochaete chrysosporium*. Reactions to righ occurred only in nitrogen-starved cultures (31).

        Identification of low molecular weight products formed during lignin degradation is also helping to elucidate the chemistry involved.   Eight low molecular weight aromatic acids have been identified in extracts of spruce wood partially decayed by *P. chrysosporium* (35).   These clearly indicate C_α-C_β cleavage and C_α-oxida tion.   More interesting than the aromatic acids are traces of a variety of compounds consisting of aliphatic residues, resulting from ring cleavage, attached to intact aromatic nuclei.   Tentative structural assignments for 14 such compounds have been made on the basis of gas chromatography/mass spectrometry (Chen et al, unpub.) Two of these structures are shown in Figure 3, along with the structures of four of the identified aromatic acids. Consideration of all of the ring-cleavage structures leads to the conclusion (which, like the structures, must be considered tentative) that aromatic ring cleavage was 2,3- or 3,4-intradiol in each case, and that the presumed o-diphenolic substrate for cleavage therefore

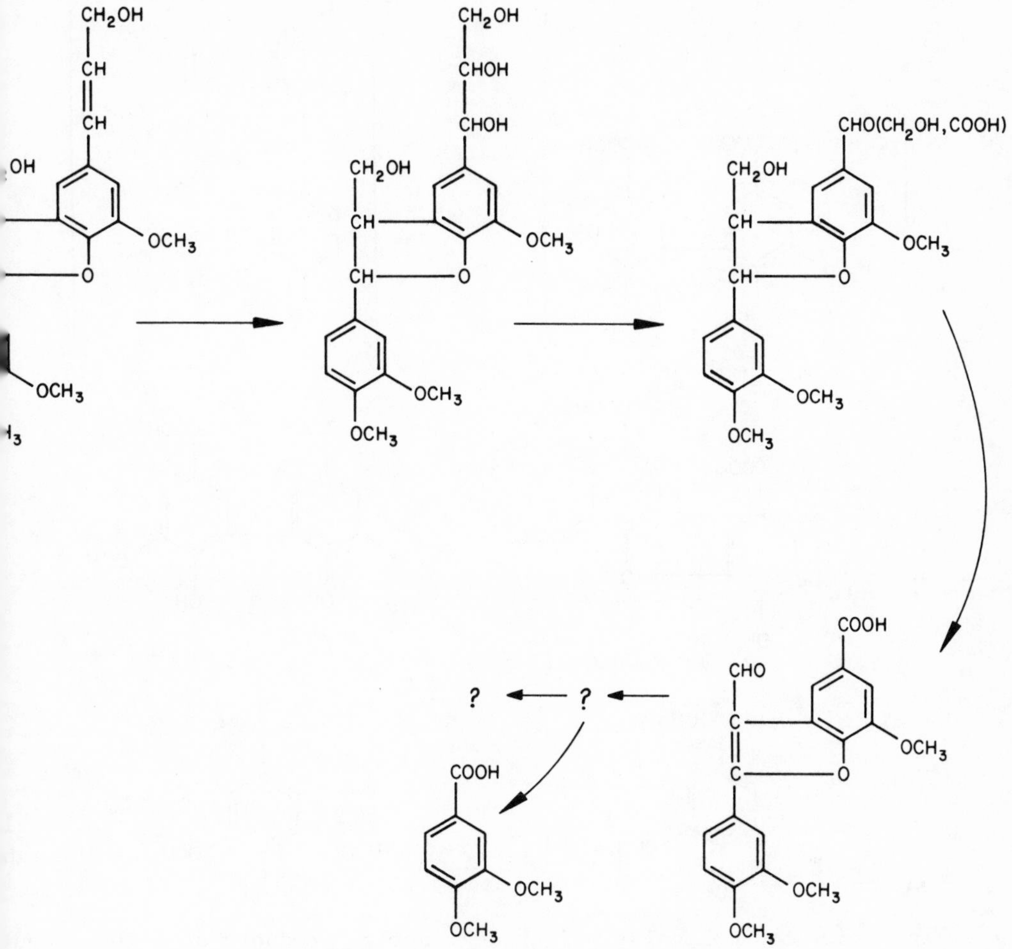

Figure 2. Degradation of a phenylcoumaran substructure (Type B, Table I) model compound in ligninolytic nitrogen-starved cultures of *Phanerochaete chrysosporium* (32).

arose via C_2-hydroxylation, and/or methoxyl demethylation. The structures of these various low molecular weight products do not establish the nature of the cleavage reaction(s) that released them from the polymer or which of the indicated reactions (C_α-oxidation, C_α-C_β cleavage, demethylation, C_2-hydroxylation, ring cleavage) occurred in the polymer.

Consideration of what another group of closely related fungi does to lignin provides some perspective here. Many brown-rot wood decay fungi belong to the same genera as white-rot fungi, from which

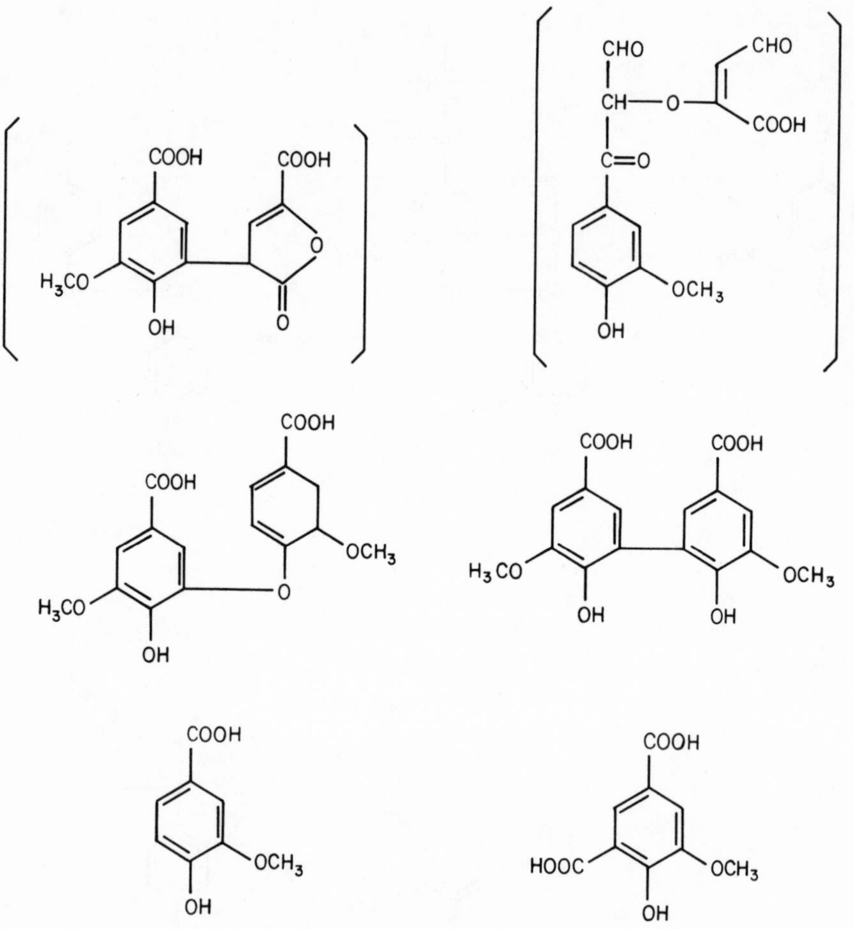

Figure 3. Low molecular weight degradation products of lignin identified or tentatively identified (brackets) in extracts of spruce wood decayed by *Phanerochaete chrysosporium* (35; C. Chen et al., unpub.).

they are not completely distinguishable taxonomically using morphological criteria, and from which they evidently evolved (36). But they decay wood quite differently. Brown-rot fungi decompose and utilize the cellulose and hemicelluloses, but cause only limited changes in lignin, leaving its polymeric nature intact (37). The changes they cause in lignin, proven by chemical means, include demethylation of methoxyl groups, aromatic hydroxylation at C_2 and limited side-chain oxidations (37,38,39). That they can cause limited aromatic ring cleavage has been shown by us (15) and by Haider and Trojanowski (40), but this clearly does not lead to extensive depletion of lignin during wood decay. The important point is that methoxyl demethylation and C_2-hydroxylation are effected in the lignin polymer by fungi very closely related to the white-rot fungi.

Degradative reactions of lignin polymer metabolism based on all the work discussed above are summarized in Table III. Figure 4 gives a schematic, hypothetical structure for a lignin polymer fragment following partial degradation by a white-rot fungus.

BIOCHEMISTRY OF LIGNIN POLYMER DEGRADATION

Both logic and experimental evidence indicate that the lignin-olytic system (polymer-degrading component) is oxidative and non-specific. That degradation is primarily oxidative is apparent from the chemical studies discussed above, and is in accord with the essential non-hydrolyzability of lignin. Non-specificity is evidenced by the facts that: (a) Lignin is degraded despite the heterogeniety of interunit linkages and the variety of neighboring groups around those linkages; (b) it is degraded despite the racemic nature of all asymmetric carbons; (c) it is degraded even after sub-stantial modification by chemical pulping and bleaching reactions (18,47,48,49,50); and (d) ligninolytic cultures metabolize a wide variety of aromatic compounds. That the degrading system is not induced by its substrate is consistent with there being only a loose connection between the structure of lignin and the activity of the degrading system.

It is difficult to rationalize these features in terms of classical enzymes. A consideration 5 years ago of the reactions known or suspected in lignin degradation, and of the types of enzymes involved in catabolism of low molecular weight aromatics, pointed to the apparent need for a variety of different enzymes (51). For some time our work has been directed at identifying specific reac-tions of lignin degradation that could be used to assay for a specific catalyst, and thereby assess its nature.

On the basis of our increasing knowledge of the chemistry discussed above, and of the recent knowledge already gained through the study of specific reactions, it seems likely that key oxidative reactions in lignin polymer degradation may not be directly mediated by enzymes. Hall (52) and Zeikus (11) in fact have speculated that active oxygen species, such as peroxide, superoxide anion, etc., might be involved instead. No direct evidence has been presented, because specific reactions involved in lignin degradation and suit-able for assays had not been identified. We now know several such reactions (as in Figures 1 and 2), which can be tied to lignin degradation on the basis of physiological characteristics. These are being examined by us and by others at present to assess the nature of the catalyst(s). There is already some experimental evidence to support non-classical biological oxidation.

TABLE III

Reactions of Lignin Polymer Degradation by White-rot Fungi

Reaction	Evidence (references), notes
Side Chains:	
C_α-C_β cleavage	Chemical (35,41,42); spectroscopic (33,42); model compound studies also show (31,32).
C_α oxidation	Spectroscopic (33,34,42); model compound studies also show (C. Chen et al., unpublished).
C_α-C_β oxidation to diol	Suspected on basis of model compound study (32).
β-aryl ether cleavage	Suspected on basis of chemical study (42); supported by model compound studies (43, C. Chen et al., unpublished).
Aromatic Rings:	
C_1-C_α cleavage	Catalyzed by phenol-oxidizing enzymes (44, 45); supported by model compound studies (31,39); importance unclear.
Methoxyl demethylation	Methoxyl content of degraded polymer (42,46); analogy with brown rot (37); model compound studies (C. Chen et al., unpublished).
C_2-hydroxylation	Suspected by analogy with brown rot (39); and on basis of structures of degradative products (C. Chen et al., unpublished).
Aromatic ring cleavage	Combined chemical, spectroscopic evidence (42); ^{13}C-nmr (33,34).

We (S. S. Bar-Lev and T. K. Kirk, unpub.) have recently demonstrated that the titer of the ligninolytic system in *P. chrysospori*ₙ depends on the concentration of culture O_2 after primary growth has occurred and during the period of synthesis of essential components of the ligninolytic system. A (functional) ligninolytic system (lignin→CO_2) is not even formed at low O_2 concentrations, which still permit rapid oxidation of glucose and good growth. The most direct interpretation of these results is that O_2 induces an enzyme system which directly or indirectly degrades lignin. Elevated oxygen concentration also enchances the rate of lignin metabolism after the system is formed.

A second kind of evidence comes from a recent study with a substructure model compound (Fig. 2). Oxidation of the cinnamyl alcohol side chain in the starting compound (2-1) to a glycerol

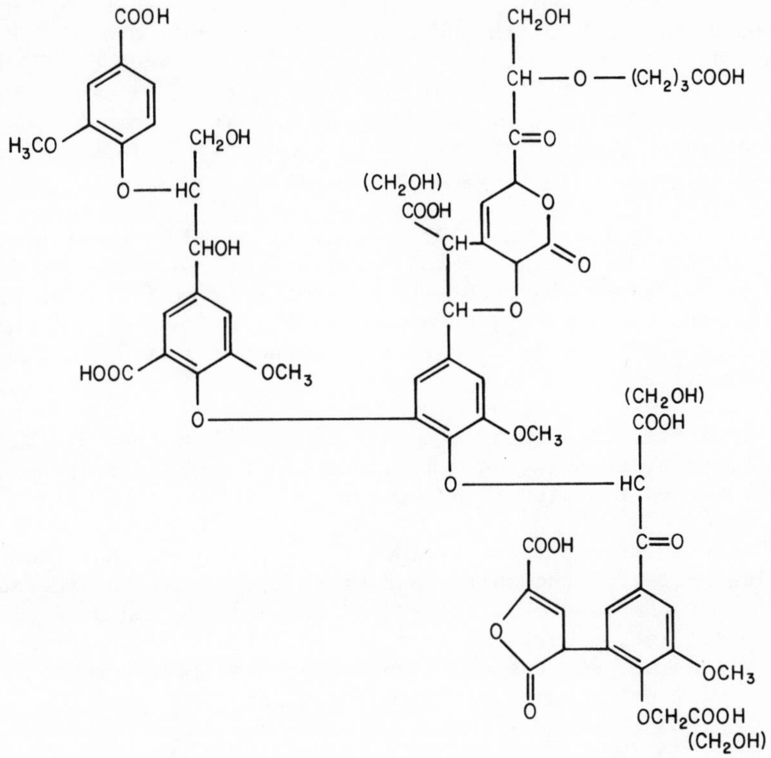

Figure 4.   Hypothetical structure for segment of spruce lignin partially degraded by a white-rot fungus.

side chain (compound 2-2) is non-stereoselective; compound (2-2) is optically inactive and is a mixture of *erythro* and *threo* forms. We have speculated that ·a non-stereoselective epoxidation, followed by non-enzymatic hydrolysis of the epoxide, occurs (32).   Non-stereoselective *enzyme*-directed conversion of (2-1) to (2-2) seem unlikely.

Brown-rot fungi can again provide useful insight. These interesting fungi rapidly depolymerize virtually all of the cellulose in intact wood (53), without removing (53) or substantially degrading (38) the lignin.   It has not been possible to isolate an enzyme from brown-rot fungi that can duplicate the effects of whole cultures on the cellulose in wood--i.e., catalyze rapid depolymerization at low weight loss (54).   Furthermore, isolated cellulases from these fungi insignificantly attack crystalline cellulose (55), and the capillaries in wood are too small anyway for enzymes to penetrate (56). Thus the evidence indicates that the depolymerization is in fact oxidative and may be non-enzymatic (55). It has been shown that Fe^{++}/H_2O_2 ("Fenton's reagent") at the pH found in brown-rotted wood (pH 3-4) mimics this depolymerization, that wood contains enough Fe^{++} for this to occur, and that the fungi produce enough extracellular H_2O_2 (57). It has been suggested that Fe^{++}/H_2O_2 is actually the cellulose-depolymerizing agent in the brown-rot fungi (57). This important question is being pursued experimentally.

Some white-rot fungi also produce enough H_2O_2 under acidic enough conditions, but white-rot fungi do not cause the depolymerization of cellulose observed with brown-rot fungi (57). To explain this apparent discrepancy, Koenigs (57) has suggested that white-rot fungi chelate the Fe^{++} so that it cannot act with the H_2O_2 to cause cellulose oxidation.

Lignin is not demethylated by the Fe^{++}/H_2O_2 reagent (T. K. Kirk and J. Koenigs, unpub.), so some other agent must be responsible for this documented reaction in brown-rot.

Taken together, these various results suggest that the lignin-oxidizing system of the white- and brown-rot fungi, and the cellulose oxidizing system of the latter group, may well be mediated directly by enzymes. Yet, a certain amount of specificity is apparently exerted, leaving open the question of what the catalyst is. This question will not remain unanswered much longer.

REFERENCES

1. Adler, E., 1977, Lignin chemistry--Past, present and future, Wood Sci. Technol., 11:169.
2. Freudenberg, K., 1968, The constitution and biosynthesis of lignin, In: "Constitution and Biosynthesis of Lignin," A.C. Neish and K. Freudenberg, eds., p. 45, Springer, New York.
3. Sarkanen, K.V. and C.H. Ludwig, eds., 1971, "Lignins: Occurrence, Formation, Structure and Reactions," Wiley-Interscience, New York, 916 p.
4. Kirk, T. K., (1981), Lignin degradation, In: "Biochemistry of Microbial Degradation," D. T. Gibson, ed., Marcel Dekker, New York.
5. Crawford, D.L. and R.L. Crawford, 1980, Microbial degradation of lignin, Enz. Microbial Technol., 2:11.
6. Crawford, D.L. and R.L. Crawford, 1976, Microbial degradation of lignocellulose: The lignin component, Appl. Environ. Microbiol. 31:714.
7. Federle, T.W. and J.R. Vestal, 1980, Lignocellulose mineralization by arctic lake sediments in response to nutrient manipulation, Appl. Environ. Microbiol. 40:32.
8. Hackett, W.F., W.J. Connors, T.K. Kirk, and J.G. Zeikus, 1977,

Microbial decomposition of synthetic ^{14}C-labeled lignins in
nature: Lignin biodegradation in a variety of natural materials,
Appl. Environ. Microbiol., 33:43.

9.   Martin, J.P. and K. Haider, 1980, Microbial degradation and
stabilization of ^{14}C-labeled lignins, phenols, and phenolic
polymers in relation to soil humus formation, In: "Lignin
Biodegradation: Microbiology, Chemistry and Potential Applications," T.K. Kirk, T. Higuchi, and H.-m. Chang, eds., CRC
Press, Boca Raton, Florida, Vol. I, p. 77.

10.   Zeikus, J.G., 1980 , Fate of lignin and related aromatic sub-
stances in anaerobic environments, In: "Lignin Biodegradation:
Microbiology, Chemistry and Potential Applications," T.K. Kirk,
T. Higuchi, and H.-m. Chang, eds., Vol. I, p. 101, CRC Press,
Boca Raton, Fla.

11.   Zeikus, J.G., 1981, Lignin metabolism and the carbon cycle:
Polymer biosynthesis, biodegradation and environmental recal-
citrance, Adv. Microbial Ecol. (in press).

12.   Ander, P., and K.-E. Eriksson, 1978, Lignin degradation and
utilization by micro-organisms, In: "Progress in Industrial
Microbiology," Vol. 14, M.J. Bull, ed., p. 1, Elsevier,
Amsterdam.

13.   Kirk, T.K. and P. Fenn, (1981), Formation and action of the
ligninolytic system in basidiomycetes, In: "Decomposition by
Basidiomycetes," J. Frankland and J. Hedger, eds., p.
Cambridge Univ. Press, Cambridge, United Kingdom.

14.   Burdsall, H.H. and W.E. Eslyn, 1974, A new *Phanerochaete* with
a *chrysosporium* imperfect state, *Mycotaxon*, 1:123.

15.   Kirk, T.K., W.J. Connors, R.D. Bleam, W.F. Hackett, and J.G.
Zeikus, 1975, Preparation and microbial decomposition of
synthetic ^{14}C] lignins, Proc. Nat. Acad. Sci., 72(7):2515-2519.

16.   Kirk, T.K., W.J. Connors, and J.G. Zeikus, 1976, Requirement
for a growth substrate during lignin decomposition by two
wood-rotting fungi, Appl. Environ. Microbiol., 32:192.

17.   Keyser, P., T.K. Kirk, and J.G. Zeikus, 1978, Ligninolytic
enzyme system of *Phanerochaete chrysosporium*: Synthesized in
the absence of lignin in response to nitrogen starvation,
J. Bacteriol., 135:790.

18.   Hiroi, T. and K.-E. Eriksson, 1976, Microbiological degradation of lignin. Part 1. Influence of cellulose on the degradation of lignins by the white-rot fungus *Pleurotus ostreatus*,
Sven. Papperstidn., Vol. 79,157.

19.   Drew, S.W. and K.L. Kadam, 1979, Lignin metabolism by *Aspergillus fumigatus* and white-rot fungi, In: "Developments in
Industrial Microbiology," Vol. 20, L.A. Underkofler, ed.,
p. 153, Soc. Ind. Microbiol., Arlington, Va.

20.   Jeffries, T.W., S. Choi, and T.K. Kirk, (1981), Nutritional
regulation of lignin degradation in *Phanerochaete chrysosporium*. Appl. Environ. Microbiol. (in press).

21.   Kirk, T.K., E. Schultz, W.J. Connors, L.F. Lorenz, and J.G.
Zeikus, 1978, Influence of culture parameters on lignin

metabolism by *Phanerochaete chrysosporium*, <u>Arch</u>. <u>Microbiol</u>.,
117:277.

22. Reid, I.D., 1979, The influence of nutrient balance on lignin
     degradation by the white-rot fungus *Phanerochaete chrysospori*
     Can. J. Bot., 57:2050.

23. Yang, H.-H., M. Effland, and T.K. Kirk, 1980, Factors influenc
     ing fungal decomposition of lignin in a representative ligno-
     cellulosic, thermomechanical pulp, <u>Biotech. Bioeng</u>. 22:65.

24. Fenn, P. and T.K. Kirk, 1979, Ligninolytic system of *Phanero-*
     chaete chrysosporium: Inhibition by *o*-phthalate, <u>Arch. Micro</u>-
     <u>biol</u>., 123 : 307.

25. Bu'Lock, J.D., 1975, Secondary metabolism in fungi and its
     relationship to growth and development, <u>In</u>: "The Filamentous
     Fungi," Vol. 1, J.E. Smith and D.R. Berry, eds., p. 33, Wiley
     New York.

26. Fenn, P. and T.K. Kirk, 1981, Relationship of nitrogen to the
     set and suppression of ligninolytic activity and secondary met
     olism in *Phanerochaete chrysosporium*. <u>Arch</u>. <u>Microbiol</u>. (in pres

27. Shimada, M., F. Nakatsubo, T. Higuchi, and T.K. Kirk, (1981),
     Biosynthesis of veratryl alcohol in relation to lignin degrada-
     tion in *Phanerochaete chrysosporium*. <u>Arch</u>. <u>Microbiol</u>. (in pres

28. Fenn, P., S. Choi, and T.K. Kirk, 1981, Ligninolytic activity
     in *Phanerochaete chrysosporium:* Physiology of transient
     suppression by NH_4^+ and L-glutamate. <u>Arch</u>. <u>Microbiol</u>. (in pre

29. Wilcox, W.W., 1968, Changes in wood microstructure through
     progressive stages of decay. <u>USDA Forest Service Research Pap</u>
     <u>FPL 70</u>, 45 p.

30. Kirk, T.K., L.F. Lorenz, and H.-m. Chang, 1975, Topochemistry
     of the fungal degradation of lignin in birch wood as related
     to the distribution of guaiacyl and syringyl lignins. <u>Wood</u>
     <u>Sci. Technol</u>., 9:81.

31. Enoki, A., G.P. Goldsby, and M.H. Gold, 1980, Metabolism of
     the lignin model compounds veratrylglycerol-β-guaiacyl ether
     and 4-ethoxy-3-methoxyphenylglycerol-β-guaiacyl ether by
     Phanerochaete chrysosporium, <u>Arch</u>. <u>Microbiol</u>. 125:277.

32. Nakatsubo, F., T.K. Kirk, M. Shimada, and T. Higuchi, (1981),
     Metabolism of a phenylcoumaran substructure model compound in
     ligninolytic cultures of *Phanerochaete chrysosporium*, <u>Arch</u>.
     <u>Microbiol</u>. (in press).

33. Chua, M.G.S., C.-L. Chen, H.-m. Chang and T.K. Kirk, (1981),
     ^{13}C-NMR characterization of spruce lignin degraded by *Phanero-*
     chaete chrysosporium, <u>Holzforschung</u> (in press).

34. Ellwardt, P.-C., K. Haider, and L. Ernst, (1981), Untersuchung
     des microbiellen Ligninabbaues durch ^{13}C-NMR-Spektroskopie an
     spezifisch ^{13}C-angereichertem DHP-Lignin aus Coniferylalkohol
     <u>Holzforschung</u> (in press).

35. Chen, C.-L., H.-m. Chang and T.K. Kirk, (1981), Low molecular
     weight aromatic acids from spruce wood decayed by *Phanero-*
     chaete chrysosporium, <u>Holzforschung</u> (in press).

36. Gilbertson, R.L., 1980, Wood-rotting fungi of North America, Mycologia, 72:1.

37. Kirk, T.K. and E. Adler, 1970, Methoxyl-deficient structural elements in lignin of sweetgum decayed by a brown-rot fungus, Acta Chem. Scand., 24:3379.

38. Kirk, T.K., 1975 , Effects of the brown-rot fungus Lenzites trabes on the lignin in spruce wood, Holzforschung, 29:99.

39. Kirk, T.K., S. Larsson, and G.E. Miksche, 1970, Aromatic hydroxylation resulting from attack of lignin by a brown-rot fungus, Acta Chem. Scand., 24:1470.

40. Haider, K. and J. Trojanowski, 1980, A comparison of the degradation of ^{14}C-labeled DHP and corn stalk lignins by micro- and macrofungi and bacteria, In: "Lignin Biodegradation: Microbiology, Chemistry and Potential Applications," T.K. Kirk, T.Higuchi, and H.-m. Chang, eds., Vol. I p. 111, CRC Press, Boca Raton, Florida.

41. Hata, K., 1966, Investigations on lignins and lignification: 33: Studies on lignins isolated from spruce wood decayed by Poria subacida Bll, Holzforschung, 20:142.

42. Kirk, T.K. and H.-m. Chang, 1975, Decomposition of lignin by white-rot fungi. II. Characterization of heavily degraded lignins from decayed spruce wood. Holzforschung, 29:56.

43. Fukuzumi, T., 1980a, Microbial metabolism of lignin-related aromatics, In: "Lignin Biodegradation: Microbiology, Chemistry and Potential Applications," T.K. Kirk, T. Higuchi, and H.-m Chang, eds., Vol. II p. 73, CRC Press, Boca Raton, Fla.

44. Freudenberg, K., J.M. Harkin, M. Riechert, and T. Fukuzumi, 1958, Die an der Verholzung beteiligten Enzyme, Die Dehydrierung des Sinapinalkohols, Chem. Ber., 91:581.

45. Ishihara, T., 1980, The role of laccase in lignin biodegradation, In: "Lignin Biodegradation: Microbiology, Chemistry and Potential Applications," T.K. Kirk, T. Higuchi and H.-m. Chang, eds., Vol. II p. 17, CRC Press, Boca Raton, Florida.

46. Ishikawa, H., W.J. Schubert, and F.F. Nord, 1963, Investigations on lignins and lignification: 27: The enzymatic degradation of softwood lignin by white-rot fungi, Arch. Biochem. Biophys., 100:140.

47. Lundquist, K., T.K. Kirk, and W.J. Connors, 1977, Fungal degradation of kraft lignin and lignin sulfonates prepared from synthetic ^{14}C-lignins, Arch. Microbiol., 112:291.

48. Fukuzumi, T., 1980b, Microbial decolorization and deforming of pulping waste liquors, In: "Lignin Biodegradation: Microbiology, Chemistry, and Potential Applications" T.K. Kirk, T. Higuchi, and H.-m. Chang, eds., Vol. II p. 161, CRC Press, Boca Raton, Florida.

49. Eaton, D., H.-m.Chang, and T.K. Kirk, 1980, Fungal decoloration of kraft bleach plant effluents, Tappi, 63:103.

50. Sundman, G., T. K. Kirk, and H.-m Chang, (1981), Fungal decolorization of kraft bleach plant effluents: Fate of the chromphores, Tappi (in press).

51.   Kirk, T.K., 1975 , Lignin-degrading enzyme system, In: "Cellu-
      lose as a Chemical and Energy Resource," C. Wilke, ed., p. 13
      Biotechnol. Bioeng. Symp. 5, John Wiley, New York.
52.   Hall, P.L., 1980, Enzymatic transformations of lignin: 2,
      Enzyme Microb. Technol., 2:170.
53.   Cowling, E.B., 1961, Comparative biochemistry of the decay of
      sweetgum sapwood by white-rot and brown-rot fungi, USDA Tech.
      Bulletin 1258, 79 p.
54.   Highley, T.L., 1977, Requirements for cellulose degradation b
      a brown-rot fungus, Mater. Org., 12:25.
55.   Highley, T.L., 1975, Properties of cellulases of two brown-ro
      fungi and two white-rot fungi, Wood Fiber, 6:275.
56.   Cowling, E.B., 1963, Structural features of cellulose that
      influence its susceptibility to enzymatic hydrolysis, In:
      "Advances in Enzymatic Hydrolysis of Cellulose and Related
      Materials," E. Reese, ed., p. 1, Pergamon, New York.
57.   Koenigs, J., 1974, Production of hydrogen peroxide by wood-
      rotting fungi in wood and its correlation with weight loss,
      depolymerization, and pH changes, Arch. Microbiol., 99:129.

DISCUSSION

Q.   WOODWARD: Is there any carbohydrate in the lignin as you
     isolate it?

A.   KIRK: From hardwoods (angiosperms), it is difficult but
     possible to isolate a carbohydrate-free lignin, but from soft
     woods (gymnosperms) it is done routinely. Our isolated
     lignins (softwoods) have been carbohydrate-free.

Q.   WOODWARD: The reason I ask is that it is commonly assumed --
     and I don't know whether there's any truth to it -- that the
     precursor for lignin is coniferyl alcohol, for which in turn
     the precursor is coniferin, which is β-glucoside. I'm really
     wondering, since the polymerization of the coniferyl alcohol
     is thought to be a non-enzymatic process, what there is about
     coniferyl alcohol as opposed to coniferin which would make it
     polymerizable whereas the coniferin itself is not?

A.   KIRK: That's an easy one. The coniferin has no phenolic
     hydroxyl -- it's tied up in the glucosydic linkage -- so it
     cannot be oxidized to a radical by peroxidase. The latest
     indications are that the coniferin is not the precursor of
     coniferal alcohol in the plant cell wall. During the poly-
     merization, the quinone methides, which are reactive inter-
     mediates, can add hemicelluloses, so that there is increasing
     evidence that there are a number of linkages, involving
     covalent bonds, between the hemicelluloses and lignin,
     particularly in angiosperm lignins.

Q.   DETROY: This is a tough question for you, I know, but a lot of these organisms degrade the labelled lignocellulosics very well, but with your particular organism, how much of the lignin from the wood chips do you degrade -- say in 20 days, using chemical analysis?

A.   KIRK: The best rate we have ever obtained (with the hardwood red alder) was between 3% and 4% a day, averaged over 14 days. One thing about these fungi is that they degrade hardwood lignins (such as red alder) much faster than softwood lignins, probably because it is less complicated chemically; there is less opportunity for condensation during the polymerization to form hardwood lignin, because of the extra methoxyl group in the precurser sinapyl alcohol.

Q.   REDDY: I'm always intriqued by the triggering of the so-called ligninolytic system by nitrogen, carbohydrate or sulfur limitation. Could you speculate as to the physiological basis for this triggering?

A.   KIRK: That's an excellent question. We have played around with it but have no answer, of course. Apparently during evolution, after lignin appeared on the earth, a second metabolic system appeared which could oxidize lignin. I don't know what its second metabolic function was, but it persisted because it gave the producing organism access to most of the world's carbohydrate. I guess there has been no selective pressure to move it out of secondary metabolism to primary metabolism. Perhaps somebody else can do a better job than I in answering your question. It is interesting to speculate as to why ligninolytic activity should have been secondary metabolic in the first place. Perhaps a secondary metabolite is converted into the lignin-oxidizing species; e.g., an acid that is converted into a peracid. Several such possibilities can be suggested.

AMYLASES: ENZYMATIC MECHANISMS

Dexter French

Department of Biochemistry and Biophysics
Iowa State University
Ames, Iowa 50011

INTRODUCTION

Starch is a major storage form for carbohydrates in nearly all green plants. Utilization of starch by the plants or by other organisms requires initial solubilization of the starch and conversion to dextrins and oligosaccharides by amylases. Various organisms have developed different strategies for starch breakdown, but all involve an initial attack by an amylase, perhaps concomitantly with another enzyme such as a dextrinase or debranching enzyme, followed by a glucosidase which converts the dextrins or oligosaccharides to glucose.

Amylases are among the most effective enzymes known. For porcine pancreatic alpha amylase and sweet potato beta amylase the turnover numbers are of the order of 1000 per second per molecule of enzyme (1).

In general, alpha amylases require calcium ions to stablilize their structure. Some bacterial alpha amylases contain essential zinc ions. Animal alpha amylases also require chloride ion, an allosteric effector (2). Other anions are less effective. Beta amylases generally are sulfhydryl enzymes and are inactivated by oxidation, SH reagents, and heavy metal ions.

Several amylases have been purified to homogeneity and crystallized. X-ray structural studies are in progress (3-5); the crystal structure of porcine pancreatic alpha amylase at 5 Å resolution is shown in Figure 1. Figures 2 and 3 show details of Taka A amylase.

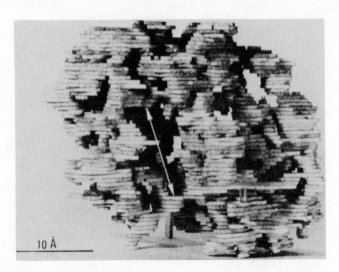

Figure 1. Balsa wood model of porcine pancreatic alpha amylase at
5 Å resolution (5). The active site is located in the crevice
indicated by the white arrow.

    Some of the enzymes exist in multimeric forms. Sweet potato
beta amylase is a tetramer (6). Porcine pancreatic alpha amylase is
apparently synthesized as a single chain, 56000 daltons, but it
undergoes some proteolysis to give smaller associated fragments with
retention of activity (7). Amylases from different tissues of a
single animal species are very similar, apparently as a consequence
of gene duplication and mutation, as well as tissue-specific regulation and expression (8). Conversely, the alpha amylases from
various bacteria, e.g. *Bacillus subtilis* (9), are surprisingly
similar in their product specificity to the alpha amylases of germinating cereals (10). Also, the animal alpha amylases give a set
of branched oligosaccharides essentially identical with those
obtained by action of the fungal alpha amylases, e.g. Taka amylase
(11-14).

    With Taka amylase and fungal glucoamylase there are isozymes
that seem to be nearly identical in their primary structures (15-17).
These isozymes have slightly different substrate specificities.

CLASSES OF AMYLASES

    Much of the early biochemistry of amylases was done in the
laboratories of breweries, where it is important to know the effec-
tiveness of malt in producing fermentable sugars from grain. It was
early recognized that there are two distinct types of activity in

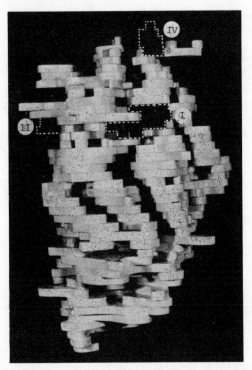

Figure 2. Model of Taka-amylase A at low resolution (3). Sites I, II, III (behind) and IV are maltotriose binding sites. Site I is the active site.

malt: an "amyloclastic" or "dextrinogenic" activity, which only appears during germination, and a "saccharogenic" activity, which is already present in the ungerminated barley but becomes several-fold more active during germination. The two activities were separated by taking advantage of the thermal stability of the amylo-clastic enzyme and the stability of the saccharogenic activity at low pH. Kuhn found that the amyloclastic enzyme gave dextrins with a downwards mutarotation, thus having an alpha anomeric configura-tion. By contrast, the saccharogenic enzyme gave beta maltose (18). Thus these enzymes were designated as alpha and beta amylases, and this classification has been retained to the present. Subsequently it has been recognized that the beta amylases attack starch or dextrins from the non-reducing ends of the molecules, thus are endwise acting or "exoases". The alpha amylases are capable of attacking long starch molecules in the interior, also, in between branch points. To contrast such interiorly acting amylases with beta amylase, they have sometimes been referred to as "randomly" acting, although this is a misleading descriptor. Reese (19,20) has proposed the generalization that the endwise acting hydrolases,

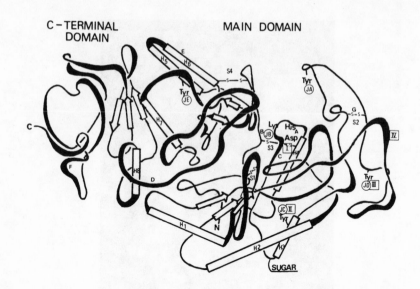

C - TERMINAL
DOMAIN   MAIN DOMAIN

Figure 3. Structure of Taka-amylase A at 3 Å resolution (4).
Possible catalytic groups (His, Asp) are located at the crevice
(I) in the upper right of the figure.

which give defined low molecular weight products, act with inversion
of configuration, whereas the interiorly acting enzymes give retention of configuration. The initial products have varying chain
length and branching pattern, and final structures are dictated by
"end effects."

There are many other ways of classifying amylases, for instance high temperature tolerant, high salt tolerant, high alkalinit
tolerant, glucose-producing (glucoamylase), maltotetraose-producing,
cyclodextrin-producing, etc. In the last analysis, each amylase
with differing structure probably has different nuances of specificity; even the same enzyme acting in different environments may
have significantly different specificities (21).

ACTION PATTERNS: SINGLE CHAIN, MULTI-CHAIN, MULTIPLE ATTACK,
PROCESSIVITY

An endwise-acting enzyme may act on a polymeric substrate in
such a way that the new chain end is essentially identical with that
of the original substrate. In this case, the same enzyme molecule
may proceed to act again. This phenomenon is called multiple or
repetitive attack, or processivity (Figure 4). The degree of
multiple attack may be expressed as the probability "f" that, having
completed one or more catalytic events at the end of a chain polymer

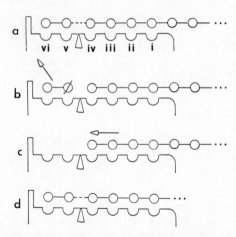

Figure 4. Multiple attack by beta amylase. The four subsites to the right constitute the "substrate-feeding" site; the two sub-sites to the left constitute the "maltose-liberating" site. (a) Productive complex. Cleavage occurs between subsites IV and V. (b) Maltose is liberated, leaving residual substrate on right-hand part of binding site. (c) Residual substrate shifts to left, giving (d) new productive complex. For repetitive attack to occur, binding by maltose in subsites V-VI must be weak in comparison with binding of residual substrate in subsites I-IV.

that the enzyme will carry out at least one more catalysis before dissociating from the substrate (22). If $f=0$, the action pattern is called multi-chain, this meaning an obligatory dissociation such that the enzyme will almost certainly attack another substrate molecule rather than return to its previous substrate. If $f=1$, the action pattern is called single chain, implying that attack is completed on a single molecule of substrate without dissociation of the E·S complex. Most amylases are somewhere between these extremes, and have a degree of multiple attack between 0 and 1.

To a first approximation, if end effects can be neglected, the kinetics of multiple attack can be formulated as in Figure 5 (22).

For such a processive reaction, the multiple attack parameter f is equal to $k_2/(k_{-1} + k_2)$. Experimental values for beta amylase (DP=35-44) or individual oligosaccharides (DP=9-13) give $f=0.75$-0.80. For potato phosphorylase acting in a synthetic mode, $f=0.3$ or less (22).

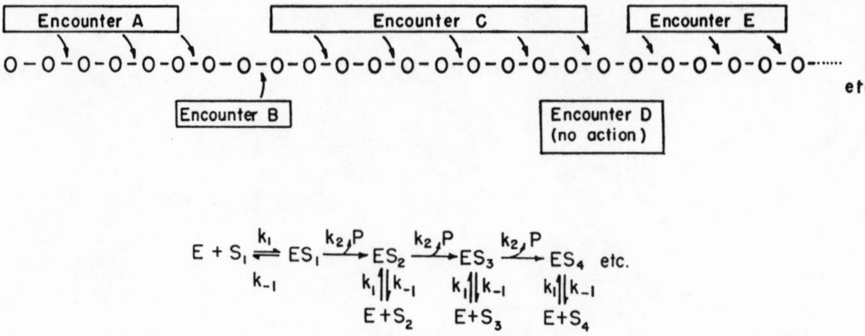

Figure 5. Kinetics of multiple attack: action of beta amylase on a starch chain (1). (a, above) Action pattern on a starch chain. Each encounter represents formation of ES, multiple attack, and dissociation. (b, below) Kinetic description of a single encounter. Following each catalytic event, a new ES complex forms, which may react (k_2 process) or dissociate (k_{-1} process).

Procine pancreatic alpha amylase also displays multiple attack following the initial "random" or interior attack on a high molecula weight substrate. Here the degree of multiple attack is about 0.88-0.92 (23).

The basic interpretation of multiple attack is simply that, once the enzyme has gone through a complete sequence of events comprising unproductive complex $\longrightarrow$ productive complex $\longrightarrow$ catalytic step (formation of $E.P_1P_2$) $\longrightarrow$ dissociation of P_2, there still remains the $E \cdot P_1$ complex which in effect is a new $E \cdot S$ (non-productive) complex. See Figure 4 (24). Rearrangement of the substrate on the enzyme active site then gives a new productive $E \cdot S$ complex and the cycle can be continued until the $E \cdot S$ complex dissociates by a k_{-1} process. On the assumption that the k_2 step is rate-limiting, the necessary condition for a high degree of multiple attack is simply a high k_2/k_{-1} ratio. It can be shown that for enzymes showing appreciable multiple attack, the Michaelis constant $K_m=k_{-1}/k_1$, (22), rather than $K_m=(k_2 + k_{-1})/k_1$ with enzymes for which there is an obligatory dissociation of all products before the catalytic event can be repeated. Moreover, if the turnover number of the enzyme k_2, the multiple attack parameter $f=k_2/(k_{-1} + k_2)$ and the Michaelis constant k_{-1}/k_1 are known, it becomes possible to calculate the absolute values for k_1 and k_{-1}. For sweet potato beta amylase, experimental values are $f=0.76$; $K_m=7.3 \times 10^{-5}$M; and $k_2=1.05 \times 10^3$ sec^{-1} per subunit (22). These values give $k_1=4.5 \times 10^6$M^{-1} sec^{-1}; $k_{-1}=3.3 \times 10^2$ sec^{-1}. The basic reasons for the high degree of multiple attack will be discussed in following sections dealing with the nature of binding sites and catalytic mechanisms.

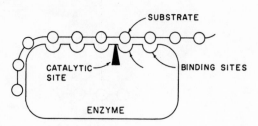

Figure 6.   Schematic representation of the active site of pancreatic
and salivary amylase. The reducing end of the substrate is to the
right.

ACTIVE CENTER, BINDING SITE AND SUBSITES

     The active center of an amylase comprises the catalytic center
the substrate binding site and subsites, and probably a water site.
No cofactors are involved. Up to now the most thoroughly studied
amylase is porcine pancreatic alpha amylase. From studies with
reducing end-labelled oligosaccharides, it can be shown that the
active center for both salivary and pancreatic amylase is as in
Figure 6. Each of the five subsites can bind one glucose unit in
a starch chain, and the catalytic site is between subsites II and
III. Evidence for this active center arrangement comes from the
cleavage patterns of reducing-end labeled oligosaccharides (Figure
7) (1,25). Maltopentaose gives only maltotriose (unlabeled) and
maltose (labeled) in a 1:1 mole ration. All other substrates give
a distribution of products. Moreover, maltotetraose and particularly
maltotriose are poor substrates relative to maltopentaose.

     The subsites I-V are of unequal binding energy (26), and
accommodate glucose units in different orientations by binding
different OH groups of the individual glucose residues. Hydroxyethyl (HE) or other substituents direct the substrates into
specific binding modes as depicted in Figure 8 (27).

     With oligosaccharide glycosides as substrates, there is a
great preference for an alpha glycosidic linkage between the glucose
unit in subsite II and the aglycone (glucose or other) in subsite
I (26). In fact, the finding attributed to subsite I may be
largely binding of the glycosidic linkage between the occupants of
subsites I and II. The effects of substituents other than hydroxyethyl (and hydroxypropyl) have not been studied systematically.
However natural branching (α-1,6-links) is permitted only at subsites I, II and V (cf. section on Action of Amylases on Branched
Substrates).

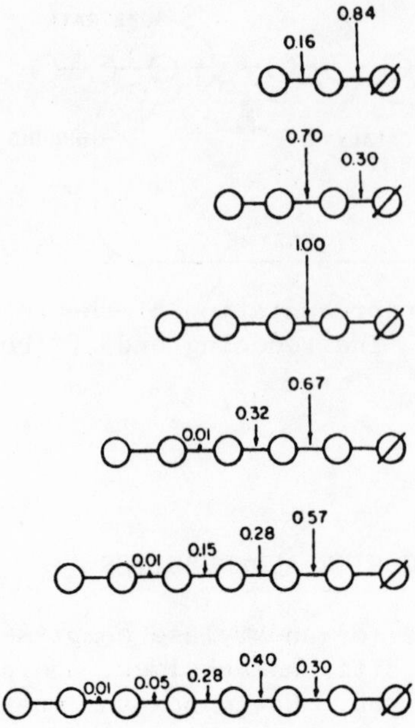

Figure 7. The frequency distribution of bond cleavage during initial action of porcine pancreatic alpha amylase on reducing end-labeled oligosaccharides. Human salivary alpha amylase gives a similar distribution (1). Relative rates of cleavage of maltotriose, malto-triose, maltotetraose and maltopentaose are about 1: 100: 1000.

For maximal k_2, all subsites must be occupied. Vacancy of subsites I or V significantly reduces k_2. Maltotriose is the minimal substrate; it occupies subsites II, III and IV. Incidentally, maltotriose can also be attacked in a termolecular process by condensing two molecules of maltotriose, forming maltohexaose. This then hydrolyzes giving maltose plus maltotetraose, which in turn gives glucose, maltose, and maltotriose (25). This termolecular process is significant only at high maltotriose concentrations. A similar termolecular reaction occurs to a small degree with malto-tetraose. With maltose, no significant termolecular reaction has been observed, possibly owing to the weak or even negative binding energy of subsite III, so that two molecules of maltose form a non-productive complex by binding at subsites I and II, and IV and V.

Details of the active site of Taka-amylase A have been worked out by Nitta et al. (28). The enzyme is reported to have a seven-subsite binding site. However the two subsites at the extreme left (Figure 9) have only weak affinity. This enzyme acts on

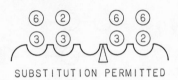

SUBSTITUTION PERMITTED

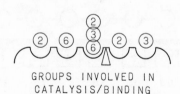

GROUPS INVOLVED IN
CATALYSIS/BINDING

Figure 8. Effect of hydroxyethyl (HE) substituents on the substrate
with porcine pancreatic alphy amylase, (above). The numbers indicate
the positions on the individual glucose units where substitution
permits formation of a productive ES complex, (below). Substitution
of OH at the indicated positions blocks formation of a productive
ES complex, (27).

the cyclodextrins and various phenyl maltosides, and shows a low
degree of multiple attack (23). The details of substrate binding to
this enzyme will probably be available soon from the x-ray structure
analysis (3,4).

Bacterial liquefying enzymes have a 9 (or 10) subsite binding
site, with the catalytic center between subsites III and IV. (Figure
10) (29). The cereal alpha amylases also have a similar extended
binding site (10).

Owing to the great expanse of the binding site, random cleavage
of only a small percentage of the total bonds in amylose gives intermediate products whose cleavage patterns are determined mainly by
end effects (10). These enzymes appear to exhibit little if any
multiple attack. With amylopectin, the major early oligosaccharide
products are from the outer chains, with a pronounced dual pattern
of product specificity, maltoheptaose and maltotriose predominating
(9). Glycogen is a poor substrate, but a branching glucose unit can
be accommodated at subsite II; this leads to products mainly in the
maltohexaose-maltooctaose range. No significant amounts of oligosaccharides are produced from the interior of the glycogen molecule.

With sweet potato beta amylase, there is an abrupt increase
in K_m and decrease in k_2 as the size of substrate is decreased from
six to five or fewer glucose units. There is no product from the
non-reducing end of the substrate except beta maltose. These facts

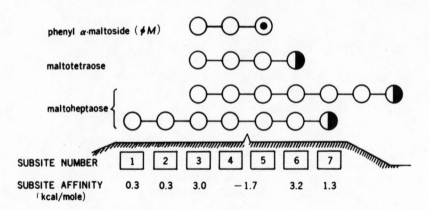

Figure 9. Active site of Taka-amylase A showing predominant productive complexes for alpha phenyl maltoside, maltotetraose and maltoheptaose (28).

suggest a six subsite active center with the catalytic group between
subsites IV and V.

The multiple attack process with beta amylase is depicted in
Figure 4. Branching at subsites I-III (30,31) does not prevent
formation of a productive complex. The branching glucose unit is
not necessarily effectively bound by the enzyme. Glucoamylase has
an active site similar to beta amylase except that there is no subsite VI (glucose being the only product from the non-reducing end),
and branching can definitely be accommodated at subsites I-IV.
Glucoamylase is also unique in that it can cleave terminal 1,6
links, although at a very slow rate relative to 1,4 links. Unlike
other amylases, it is also able to cleave maltose, though at a very
~low rate.

Recently from substrate and product specificities we have
deduced the nature of the active site of *Bacillus macerans* enzyme
(Figure 11) (33).

Possibly the first enzyme for which a multi-subsite active
center was suggested was malt alpha amylase (34). Myrbäck did not
have adequate information to establish the size of the binding site.
His drawing (Figure 12) suggests a span of about six glucose
residues for malt alpha amylase, but it is more likely that there
are about nine subsites as with the bacterial liquefying amylases
(8). It was Myrbäck's thought that branching was excluded from
the binding site, but we know now that branching can be accommodated
at certain subsites. Myrbäck also depicted the malt beta amylase

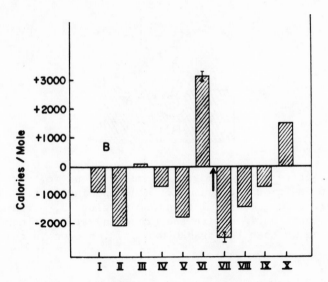

Figure 10. *Bacillus subtilis (amyloliquefaciens)* amylase binding site (29). "Subsite" X is a non-binding site (negative binding energy). Subsite interaction energies have been adjusted for substrate-induced strain to give best fit of the observed K_m and V_{max} values for various chain length oligosaccharides.

binding site in a similar fashion. French and Wild presented evidence for a five-subsite active center for potato phosphorylase (Figure 13)(35).

The minimum oligosaccharide produced in phosphorolysis is maltotetraose, which in turn is the minimum primer in the synthetic direction (35). Curiously, at least with *E. coli* maltodextrin phosphorylase, the linkage between glucose units in subsites III and IV can be α-1,6 (36).

To a first approximation, it might be thought that each subsite has its own characteristic binding energy, and that the total binding energy for a given substrate is just the sum of the binding energies for the subsites occupied. However, Thoma has shown that the K_m and k_2 values for *Bacillus* liquefying amylase are better explained if the total binding energy is less than the sum of the occupied subsite energies (29). Part of the available binding energy, about 400 cal. per subsite, is used to induce strain into the ES complex (Figure 14).

Substrate cleavage results in a net increase in binding energy. However, the individual products, especially the "right hand" product, are bound less strongly than the original substrate, so

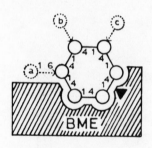

Figure 11. Active site of *Bacillus macerans* enzyme. Branching is
permitted at positions a, b and c. Ring opening at the catalytic
site (wedge), then glucanosyl transfer to glucose, gives open-chain
branched oligosaccharides with the branching at positions 4, 5 or
6 depending on whether the branch was at a, b or c in the ES complex
(33).

they can readily dissociate from the enzyme.

It seems inescapable that the single most important factor in
the great catalytic capacity of amylases lies in the extended substrate binding site, in contrast to the common glucosidases and
maltases. At the same time, the amylases have essentially zero
activity on maltose or the usual glucosides. There are a few exceptions with highly reactive glucosides such as nitrophenyl glucoside
or glucosyl fluoride, to be discussed later.

PHYSICAL STATE OF THE SUBSTATE (SOLUTION, COLLOIDAL DISPERSION,
GEL, LIPID COMPLEX, GRANULE, RETROGRADED)

The molecular conformation of starch chains in solution is
not known with certainty, but it is generally thought that they have
a flexible, somewhat extended, helical conformation (Figure 15)
(37). Short chains can rapidly transform from left to right-handed
helices. (38) Most likely the ES complex consists of a starch helix
which is stressed and distorted at the catalytic site. The cyclic
Schardinger dextrins are cleaved by some alpha amylases, particularly
by Taka amylase. However the cyclodextrins have some flexibility
and even in the crystalline state the rings may be substantially
distorted from perfect rotational symmetry (39).

Macromolecular starch is inherently insoluble in water as
evidenced by the insolubility of starch granules, and the tendency
of starch dispersions to undergo retrogradation, that is, a return
to the original insoluble state. Retrogradation includes aggregation and crystallization. The tendency of starch dispersions or

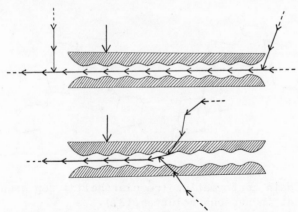

Figure 12. Binding of branched starch to malt alpha amylase as depicted by Myrbäck (34). The downward arrow represents the catalytic site of the enzyme. Branches are excluded from the binding site, or permit only poor substrate binding.

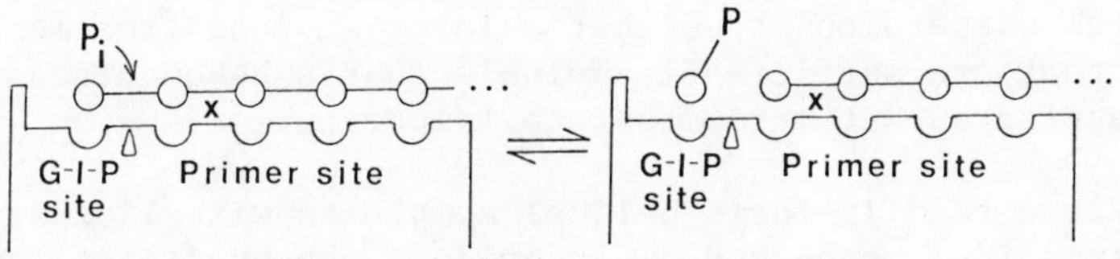

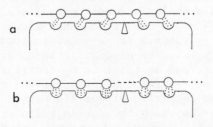

Figure 13. Active center of potato phosphorylase. The minimum acceptor ("primer") is maltotetraose (35). With *E. coli* maltodextrin phosphorylase the enzyme will permit substitution of a 1→4 linkage by a 1→6 linkage at the site marked by "x" (36).

Figure 14. Schematic representation showing tendency of enzyme to stress substrate. (a) Enzyme and substrate in relaxed conformation; poor binding, glucose residues do not match binding sites. (b) Substrate with major strain at catalytic site; glucose units in strained substrate are strongly bound by strained enzyme. Part of the binding energy is used to distort the substrate towards the **transition state** conformation.

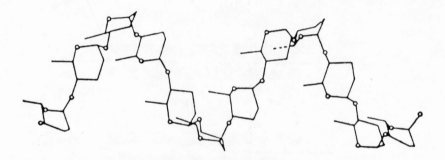

Figure 15.   Chain conformation (regular helix) representing an
amylose segment in aqueous solution (37).

pastes to form gels is dependent on the amylose content and the
molecular size or degree of degradation of the starch components.
In practical starch conversions it is usual to subject high temperature starch dispersions to either acid or amylase treatment to give
dextrins that are sufficiently soluble that subsequent enzymolysis
can be carried out at more moderate temperatures.

Amylose readily forms helical complexes with lipids, especially
with fatty acids, mono- and diglycerides, phospholipids, and synthetic detergents with linear hydrocarbon chains. Such complexes are
usually poor amylase substrates; however, in the case of *Bacillus
macerans* enzyme, the complexes are not only preferred substrates
but they also dictate the size distribution of the cyclodextrin
products (40).

Starch chains have a high tendency to form double helices, as
with native starch granules and retrograded starch (A-B type of
crystallization) (41-43). The double helix conformation of
secondary structure protects the glycosidic bonds against acidic
and enzymic hydrolysis. The glycosidic bonds are in the interior
of the double helix, and as there is no central channel, it is
impossible for water, hydrated H^+ ions, or enzyme catalytic groups
to penetrate to the sensitive glycosidic oxygen. There are two
possible exceptions in which the double helix may be the preferred
substrate, namely with Q-enzyme (branching enzyme, Fig. 16) (44)
and isoamylase (starch debranching enzyme).

With amylose, there is a critical span of molecular size
(D.P. 50-500, maximum at D.P. 80) through which retrogradation is
greatly enchanced (45). It is the author's opinion that there is
a topological problem in the formation of intermolecular double
helices from random coils. These topological constraints are

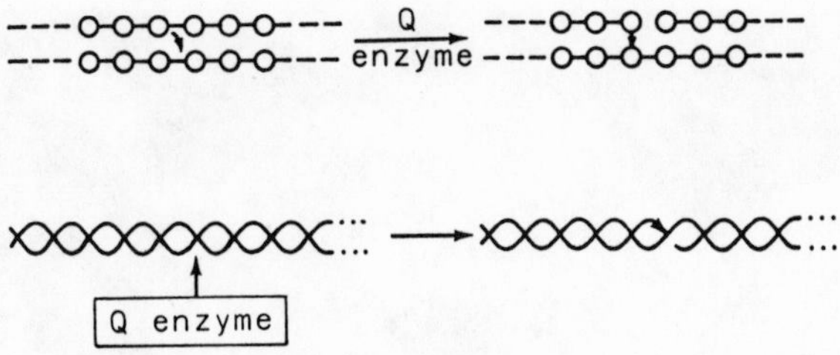

Figure 16. Action of Q enzyme (plant branching enzyme). The enzyme catalyzes an inter-chain transglycosylation. The presumed substrate conformation for the two chains is a double helix (44).

reduced by making the amylose chains shorter, so that through the critical zone of retrogradation, double helix and aggregate formation are maximized.

Raw starch granules are only slowly utilized by enzymes of mammalian digestion. Degradation of starch granules during germination of seeds is likewise a slow and incomplete process (Figure 17) (46). Bacterial digestion may be more rapid; in fact, there are some bacteria that might be classed as native starch granule-digesting (47).

ACTION OF AMYLASES ON BRANCHED SUBSTRATES

Amylases, except glucoamylases, are unable to hydrolyze α-1, 6 linkages. Therefore amylopectin, glycogen and branched dextrins are incompletely hydrolyzed, the branch linkages remaining in residual dextrins. With beta amylases, the resistant structures at the non-reducing chain ends are as in Figure 18 (30). Less rigorously treated branched substrates give quasi-limit dextrins containing one or more additional glucose units at each type of chain end (48).

With alpha amylases, the type of branched dextrin formed depends on the closeness of branch points in the substrate and the source of the enzyme. If the branch points are well separated, the animal alpha amylases (pancreatic and salivary) give a well defined set of singly branched oligosaccharides as in Figure 19 (14). When the isomaltose moieties are separated by two glucose units, the structures are cleaved as in Figure 20 (49). However, when there are fewer than two glucose units between branches, pancreatic amylase is unable to hydrolyze the structures, and multiply branched dextrins are produced, as in Figure 21 (50).

Other amylases may have different position specificity with regard to the interference by branching. Structures of residual

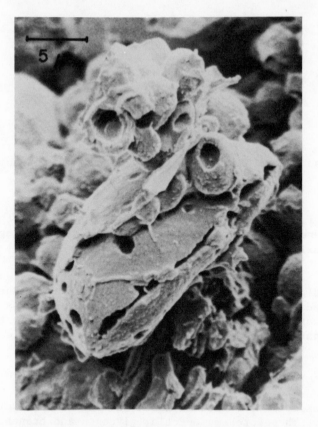

Figure 17.   Enzyme attack on starch granule during germination of
wheat (46).

branched oligosaccharides have been worked out for very few other
amylases. *Bacillus subtilis* (liquefying) amylase cleaves amylopectin with formation of branched oligosaccharides, for example
6^2-α maltosyl maltotriose (51). *Bacillus macerans* enzyme acts on
branched substrates to form branched cyclic molecules (Figure 11)
(33,50). Glucoamylases act on branched dextrins to cleave the

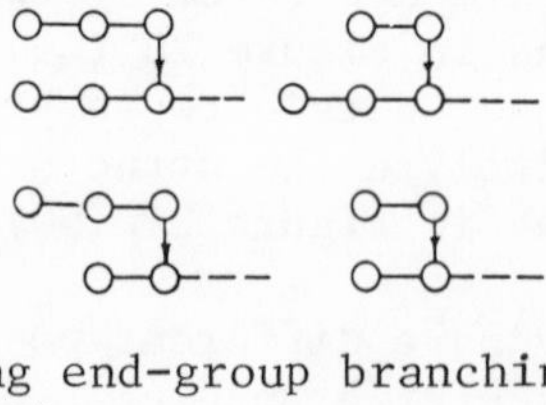

Figure 18.   Non-reducing end-group branching configurations resistant to beta amylase (30).

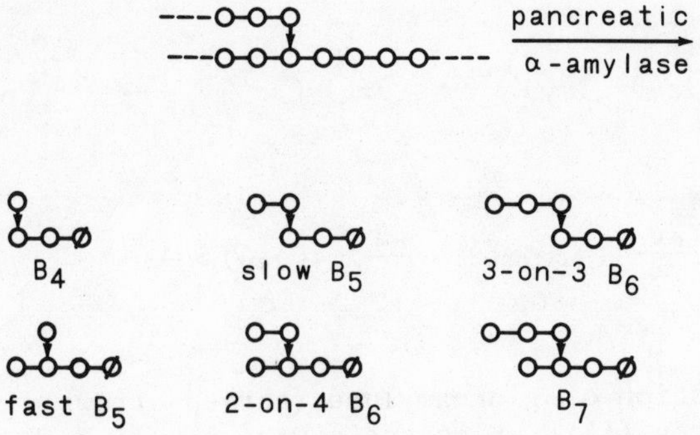

Figure 19. Singly branched oligosaccharides formed by action of pancreatic amylase on isolated branch points in amylopectin (14).

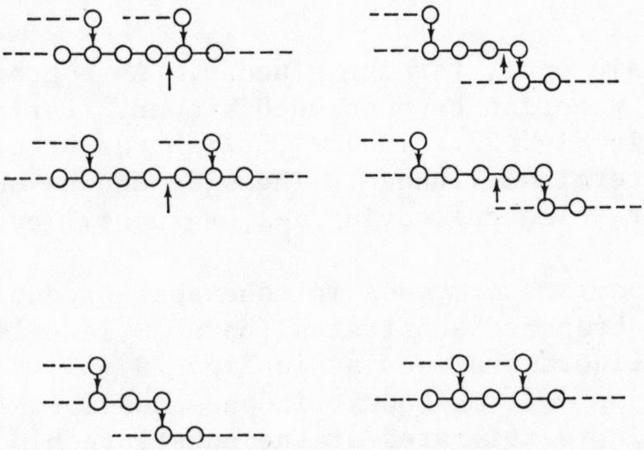

Figure 20. Action of pancreatic amylase (upward arrows) on starch configurations where branches are separated by two or three glucose units (49).

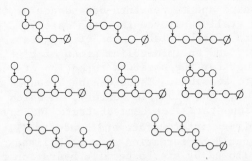

Figure 21. Doubly and triply branched oligosaccharide configurations formed by action of pancreatic amylase on amylopectin. The original oligosaccharides, which may have one or two additional glucose units on the A chains, and one additional glucose unit on the B and C chains, have been "trimmed" by glucoamylase (50).

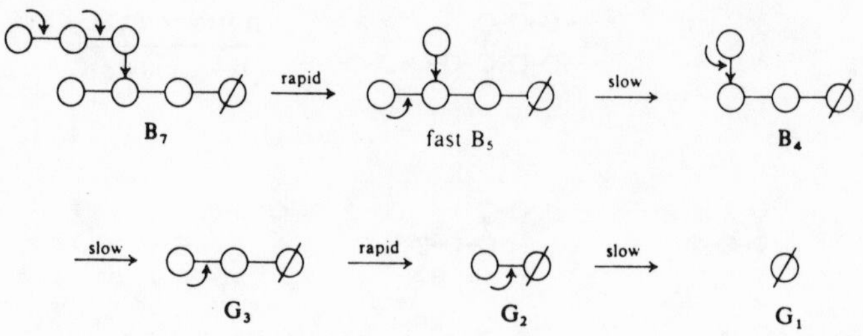

Figure 22. Action of glucoamylase (curved arrows) on singly branched oligosaccharides (14). Cleavage of the 1,6 link occurs only when the singly linked glucose (e.g., as in B_4) is in a terminal position, not when it is a single glucose side chain ("stub").

non-reducing chain ends, forming glucose. As a branch point is approached, the reaction becomes much slower. Peripheral branches are cleaved as in Fig. 22. The α-1,6 link can be cleaved only when it is the terminal linkage. The side chains on branched cyclodextrins are cleaved leaving α-1,6-glucosyl cyclodextrins (52).

With *Aerobacter aerogenes* maltohexaose-producing amylase, an exoase (53), branched substrates (beta amylase limit dextrins) give branched oligosaccharides as in Fig. 23 (53). With this enzyme, as with *E. coli* maltodextrin phosphorylase (36), a 1,6 link in the main chain is tolerated at the substrate binding site (Fig. 24).

ORGANIC REACTION MECHANISM: ROLE OF THE CATALYTIC GROUPS

From the shape and temperature-dependence of the pH-activity curves, it is generally believed that the catalytic groups in alpha amylases are a carboxylate anion of aspartate or glutamate (proton acceptor), and an imidazolium group of histidine (proton donor). To account for the observed retention of configuration, two mechanisms are feasible. There can be a double displacement (double inversion at the anomeric center), in which oxycarbonium ions are transition states between substrate and covalent intermediates, and between intermediate and products (Fig. 25). Alternatively, there could be formation of a stabilized oxycarbonium ion intermediate, followed by stereospecific hydration to yield the alpha anomeric product.

Other enzymes that act with retention of configuration e.g., *Bacillus macerans* enzyme, glucosidase, maltases, glucan phosphorylases, have similar mechanistic options.

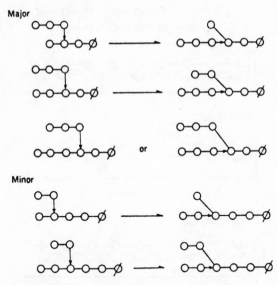

Figure 23. Branched oligosaccharides obtained by action of *Aero-bacter aerogenes* maltohexaose-producing amylase on β-limit dextrin. Left: Usual representation. Right: Alternative representation with α-1,6 linkage in hexasaccharide "main chain" (53).

        Although it was previously thought (50) that the catalytic groups in beta amylase were the same as with pancreatic (imidazolium and carboxylate), it now seems probable that they are two carboxyl groups (55). With beta amylase and other enzymes giving inversion of configuration, the initial catalytic steps are similar or identical to that with alpha amylase, up to the cleavage of the glycosidic bond and formation of an oxycarbonium ion (Figure 26).

        However, from action pattern studies it is clear that, at this point, the right-hand product (residual alpha glucan chain) does not leave the active site, but rather the reaction proceeds with the formation and liberation of beta maltose (24). The most obvious role of the COO^- group is to accept a proton from an attacking water molecule. It seems very likely that there is a significant conformational change during the catalytic process, as otherwise there would be intolerable crowding during the reaction of water with the oxycarbonium ion. Possibly the newly created reducing group goes into a reactive boat or skew form during the process. After cleavage of the glycosidic bond, the enzyme directs a stereo-specific hydration of the oxycarbonium ion. Following the catalytic steps, there is an obligatory dissociation of the left-hand product

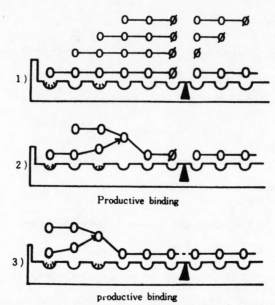

Figure 24. Schematic representation of productive complexes of *A. aerogenes* maltohexaose-producing amylase. 1) Linear substrates. 2) Outer branches of beta amylase limit dextrin; productive complex with α-1,6 link tolerated at the binding site, maltotriose A chain. 3) Same except maltose A chain (53).

(beta maltose) followed by rehydration of the enzyme and proton transfer to regenerate the catalytic groups.

ROLE OF SUBSTRATE DISTORTION

As noted in the section on the substrate binding site, part of the enzyme-substrate binding energy appears as strain at the glycosidic bond to be cleaved. Similarly, the subsite directly to the left of the catalytic center has a low or negative substrate binding energy, suggesting that, when the substrate enters this site, it is distorted by the enzyme in the direction of the transition state for catalysis. For the glucose unit occupying this one sub-site, no substitution of the OH groups is permitted. (27). This suggests that the free OH groups at carbons 2, 3 and 6 are involved in a strain or torsion as depicted in Figure 27 (27). The glucose OH groups may be involved as either hydrogen bond donors, or acceptors, or both. The hydroxyls at carbon 3 and 6, the glycosidic oxygen at carbon 4, and all the remaining glucose units to the left act to anchor the left half of the glucose unit. Tension on the OH linked to carbon 2 induces a torsion about the carbon 2-carbon-3 bond, elevating carbon 1 so that carbons 1, 2 and 6 and the ring

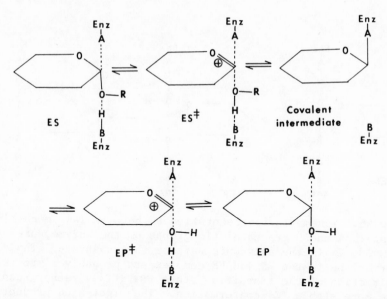

Figure 25.   Schematic representation of alpha amylase mechanism
(retention of configuration).   A and B are catalytic groups of the
enzyme, presumably carboxyl and imidazole, respectively.   OR is the
aglyconic part of the substrate.   The ring conformations in ES and
EP are probably distorted in the direction of the transition state,
rather than being in the stable $^4C_1$ conformation.   In the putative
covalent intermediate, the ring form might be more like a boat or
skew conformation.   After formation of the covalent intermediate,
the steps leading to product are mechanistically just the reverse
of the initial steps, and transfer to an acceptor other than water
might occur if the acceptor can fit appropriately into the subsites
directly to the right of the catalytic site.

oxygen are coplanar as is required for an oxycarbonium ion.   Simultaneously there is a lengthening and weakening of the C1-O1 linkage.
Following or concomitant with the rupture of the glycosidic bond,
there may be formation of a beta-linked covalent intermediate (with
alpha amylase), or beta maltose (with beta amylase).   The stereospecific hydration with alpha amylase is simply the reverse reaction,
with water taking the place of the carbon 4 OH group of the right-
hand product.

Support for the torsion concept comes from the intuitive
statement by Pauling (56) that the enzyme binds the substrate most
strongly in its transition state (highly reactive) rather than in
its ground state (unreactive), the thermodynamic argument by

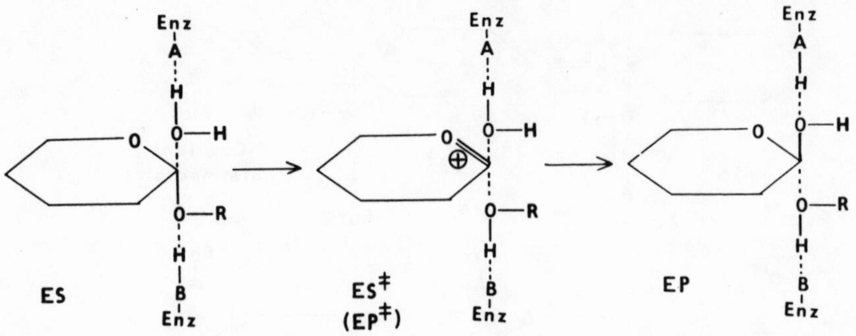

Figure 26. Schematic representation of beta amylase mechanism (inverting). A and B are catalytic groups of the enzyme, presumably carboxyl. OR is the aglyconic part of the substrate. The ring conformations in the ES and EP complex are probably distorted in the direction of the transition state $ES^{\ddagger}$ ($EP^{\ddagger}$), rather than being in the more stable ${}^4C_1$ conformation. The right-hand product, ROH, is more strongly bound to the enzyme than the left-hand product, beta maltose. There is also a specific water site. Therefore, this enzyme and other "inverting" enzymes, e.g. glucoamylase, do not normally give transglycosylation reactions.

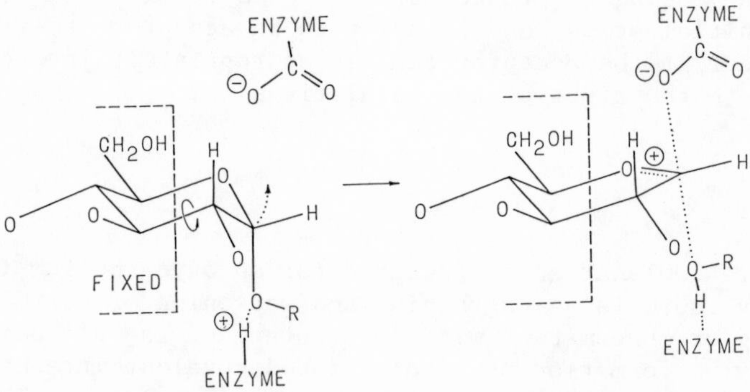

Figure 27. Substrate torsion leading to the transition state. The left-hand part of the reacting glucose unit is strongly anchored to the enzyme. Hydrogen bond formation at C2 OH exerts a torsion about the C2-C3 bond, elevating C1, lengthening the C1-O1 bond, and driving the substrate in the direction of the transition state (27).

$$\text{Non-enzymatic:} \quad S \xrightarrow{k_N} P$$

$$\text{Enzymatic:} \quad E + S \xrightleftharpoons{K_S} ES;$$

$$ES \xrightarrow{k_E} E + P$$

$$E + S \underset{\longleftarrow}{\overset{K_N^{\ddagger}}{\rightleftharpoons}} E + TX \longrightarrow E + P$$

$$K_S \updownarrow \qquad\qquad \updownarrow K_{TX}$$

$$ES \underset{\longleftarrow}{\overset{K_E^{\ddagger}}{\rightleftharpoons}} ETX \longrightarrow E + P$$

Since

$$K_S \cdot K_N^{\ddagger} = K_E^{\ddagger} \cdot K_{TX},$$

If transmission coefficients are unity,

$$\frac{1/K_{TX}}{1/K_S} = \frac{K_E^{\ddagger}}{K_N^{\ddagger}} = \frac{k_E}{k_N}$$

binding   rate
ratio   ratio

Figure 28. Wolfenden's argument that the enzyme binds the transition state much more strongly than the original substrate (57). E has been arbitrarily added in the non-enzymatic process. TX is the transition state. K_S and K_{TX} are written as dissociation constants; their reciprocals are the binding constants (57).

Wolfenden (57) which shows the energy of activation for the enzyme-catalyzed reaction must be lower than for the non-enzymic (slow) analogous reaction (Figure 28) and the fact that putative transition-state analogs, e.g. delta lactones or other compounds having an sp^2 configuration at C-1 are strong amylase inhibitors (27,58).

It is self-evident that if the enzyme exerts a stress on the substrate and therby distorts it, the enzyme itself is also subjected to an equal stress and is itself "activated". Koshland's "induced fit" concept (59) and Lumry's "rack" hypothesis (60) basically depend on this mutual stress-strain relationship. In this respect enzymes differ from lectins and antibodies; these latter may bind the ligand in its ground or undistorted state, possibly even in a lower energy state than the hydrated ligand.

AMYLASE INHIBITORS

There are many agents, such as metals, oxidizing or reducing agents, acids or alkalis, anionic polymers, which are general enzyme poisons. Here we are more interested in inhibitors that are specific for amylase or related enzymes.

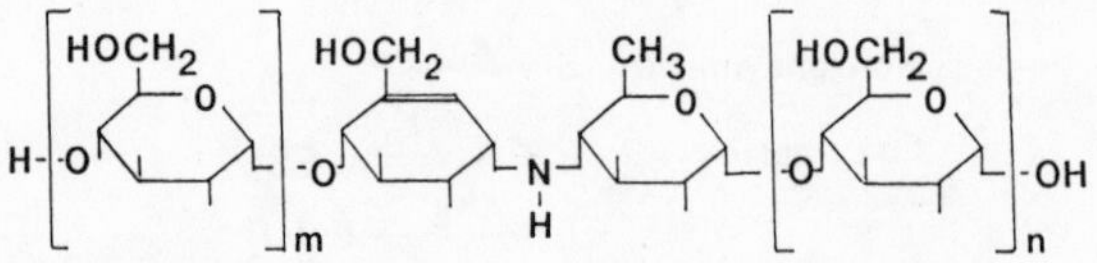

Figure 29. Structure of *Actinoplanes* pancreatic alpha amylase inhibitor. Maximal inhibition is with m=2 or 3 and n=2. Fungal alpha amylases are not inhibited. The compound with m=0 and n=2 is a strong inhibitor of intestinal sucrose, starch, and maltose digestion (67).

Product inhibition by maltose is easily demonstrated. With beta amylase, the K_I is 6mM (27). Maltose inhibits beta amylase mainly by blocking the "substrate feeding" site, that is, by binding to the right of the catalytic center. Severe inhibition by maltose does not alter the degree of multiple attack (24).

Beta amylase, potato phosphorylase and amylo-1,6-glucosidase 1,4-1,4 transferase are inhibited by the cyclic Schardinger dextrins. Although the mechanisms of inhibition are not known, probably the cyclodextrins are bound at the substrate binding site, but can not be attacked by endwise acting enzymes. By contrast, cycloheptaamylose and cyclooctaamylose (beta and gamma cyclodextrins) are substrates for pancreatic and fungal alpha amylases (61,62).

As mentioned previously, delta lactones are transition state analogs and inhibit many carbohydrases (63,64). With amylases, gluconolactone and particularly maltobionolactone are effective inhibitors (27,58). However, they are unstable in water solution, readily hydrolyzing to the corresponding aldonic acids.

Glucoamylase is non-competitively inhibited by gluconolactone (65). This result, together with ultraviolet difference and fluorescence spectra indicate that gluconolactone is bound to the left of the catalytic site (66). By contrast, mannonolactone is a competitive inhibitor and is bound to the right of the catalytic center. Similar differences in lactone binding have been found with lysozyme.

A unique type of inhibitor is produced by various Actinomycetes, especially *Actinoplanes* species (67). This inhibitor is a mixture of homologs, in which a peculiar disaccharide-like entity is linked to the right and left by α-1,4-linked glucose units. The basic structure is shown in Figure 29. Apparently, the "disaccharide" is directed to the catalytic site and blocks it.

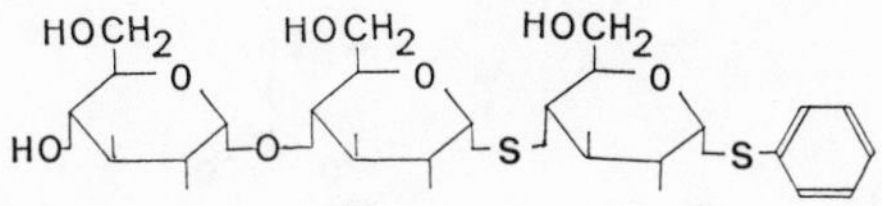

Figure 30.   Modified maltotriose, a substrate analog inhibitor for porcine pancreatic alpha amylase.   The compound binds at the active site, but the thioglycosidic bonds are not hydrolyzed by the enzyme (5).

A modified α-p-nitrophenyl maltotrioside, in which the glycosidic oxygens were replaced by sulfur, is bound at the active site of pancreatic alpha amylase, but not hydrolyzed (Figure 30) (5).

β-maltosylamine is a specific reversible inhibitor for beta amylase (68).   Polyols inhibit many carbohydrases (69), apparently by being bound in the reactive glycosyl site.

Low molecular weight proteins, found in wheat and other cereals, inhibit a variety of alpha amylases, including digestive amylases of mammals and insects (70).   These inhibitors, like antibodies or lectins, act by forming inactive complexes with amylases. Tannins found in some strains of sorghum interfere with the enzymic degradation of starch by reacting with amylase, or by forming a starch-tannin complex.

ACTION OF AMYLASES ON UNUSUAL SUBSTRATES

Hehre has studied the glycosyl fluorides as substrates or inhibitors for carbohydrases.   With pancreatic alpha amylase, alpha glucosyl fluoride is hydrolyzed and polymerized, giving oligosaccharides (71).   Alpha maltosyl fluoride gives alpha maltotetraosyl fluoride as the main product, together with other oligosaccharides (72).   With beta amylase, alpha maltosyl fluoride is directly hydrolyzed to beta maltose (73).   Beta maltosyl fluoride is inactive with alpha amylases.   With beta amylase, it requires two molecules of beta maltosyl fluoride in a termolecular reaction and gives hydrogen fluoride plus maltotetraosyl fluoride (74).   The latter, in turn, is hydrolyzed to beta maltose plus maltosyl fluoride.

D-Glucal is a substrate for both alpha and beta glucosidase, giving, respectively., alpha and beta 2-deoxyglucose (75).   When reaction is carried out in D_2O there is stereospecific labeling of C2 protons giving, with almond beta glucosidase, equatorial deuteration (R) whereas with *Candida* alpha glucosidase the product has the

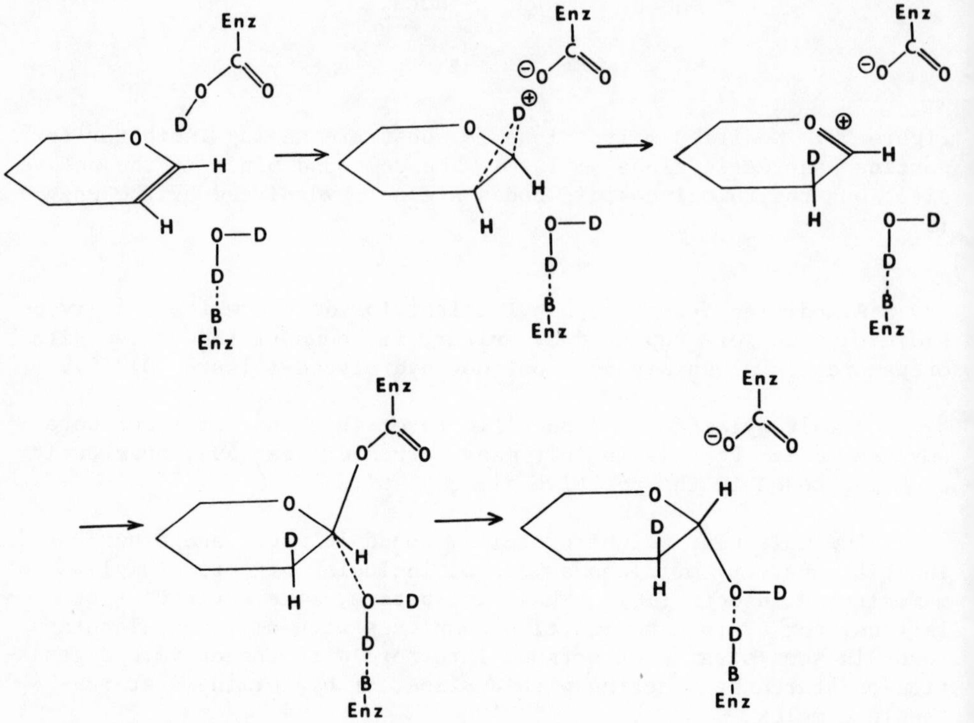

Figure 31. Mechanism of hydration of glucal by alpha glucosidase.
Reaction is carried out in D_2O to show stereo specific hydration
at C_2. Following formation of the oxycarbonium ion, the rest of
the reaction is similar to glucosidase action on glucosides (75).

deuterium in the axial (S) position (Figure 31). Presumably, similar
reactions would occur with amylases and the homologous glycals
maltal and maltotrial.

With α-maltotriosyl (1→2) β-fructofuranoside, cleavage by
pancreatic amylase gives maltotriose plus fructose (26). Analogous
reactions do not occur with the homologous maltosyl fructose or
maltotetraosyl fructose. The maltotriose moiety, being able to
completely occupy the left-hand part of the substrate binding site,
apparently directs the substrate into a non-conventional productive
ES complex.

It is generally true that amylases are specific for glycosylic
substrates in which the aglycone is a saccharide. However, Taka
amylase A (28) and *Bacillus subtilis (sacchariticus)* (21) act on
substituted and unsubstituted alpha phenyl maltosides. With the

B. subtilis enzyme, action at its optimum pH (5.4) on alpha phenyl maltoside gives phenol plus alpha maltose. However, at pH 6.18 or 6.73, a mixture of alpha and beta anomers is produced. Curiously, with various para substituted substrates (e.g. p-C$_2$H$_5$, p-Cl or p-NO$_2$) only the <u>beta</u> anomeric form of maltose is liberated. It would appear that steric factors as well as pH effects may be more important than the electronic nature of the aglycon.

SUMMARY

    Many types of amylases are found throughout the animal, vegetable and microbial kingdoms. They have evolved along different pathways to enable the organism to convert insoluble starch (or glycogen) into low molecular weight, water soluble dextrins and sugars. Alpha amylases are dextrinogenic and can attack the interior of starch molecules. The products retain the alpha anomeric configuration. Beta amylases act only at the non-reducing chain ends and liberate only beta maltose. Both alpha and beta amylases exhibit multiple (repetitive) attack, that is, after the initial catalytic cleavage, the enzyme may remain attached to the substrate and lead to several more cleavages before dissociation of the enzyme-substrate complex. Amylases have extended substrate binding sites, in the range 4-9 glucose units. This enables the enzyme to stress the substrate and lower the activation energy for hydrolysis. Similarly the enzyme exerts a torsion on the glucose unit at the catalytic site, inducing a transition state conformation (oxycarbonium ion). Alpha and beta amylases differ in the stereospecific hydration of the oxycarbonium ion, in the sequence of liberation of the right-hand <u>vs</u> the left-hand product, and the direction of motion of the retained substrate to give multiple attack.

    Substitution of individual OH groups by hydroxyethyl, etc., directs the substrate to specific positions on the enzyme, and structure analysis of the substituted products indicates how the substrate is oriented in the productive ES complex.

    The mode of inhibition by putative transition-state analogs strengthens the concept that the transition state for both alpha and beta amylases is a stabilized oxycarbonium ion.

ACKNOWLEDGEMENT

    The author is indebted to Eileen Mericle for help in the preparation of this manuscript (supported in part by Grant No. GM-08822 of the National Institutes of Health).

REFERENCES

1.   French, D., Brewers Digest 32 (1957) 50-56.
2.   Levitzki, A., and M.L. Steer, Eur. J. Biochem. 41 (1974) 171-180.
3.   Matsuura, Y., M. Kusunoki, W. Date, S. Harada, S. Bando, N. Tanaka, and M. Kakudo, J. Biochem. 86 (1979) 1773-1783.
4.   Matsuura, Y., M. Kusonoki, W. Harada, N. Tanaka, Y. Iga, N. Yasuoka, H. Toda, K. Narita, and M. Kakudo, J. Biochem. 87 (1980) 1555-1558
5.   Payan, F., R. Haser, M. Pierrot, M. Frey, J.P. Astier, B. Abadie, E. Duee, and G. Buisson, Acta Cryst. B36 (1980) 416-421.
6.   Colman, P.M. and B.W. Matthews, J. Mol. Biol. 60 (1971) 163-168.
7.   Robyt, J.F., C.G. Chittenden, and C.T. Lee, Arch. Biochem. Biophys. 144 91971) 160-167.
8.   Schibler, U., M. Tosi, A-C. Pittet, L. Fabiani, and P. K. Wellauer, J. Mol. Biol. 142 (1980) 93-116.
9.   Robyt, J.F. and D. French, Arch. Biochem. Biophys. 100 (1963) 451-467.
10.   Greenwood, C.T. and E.A. Milne, Starke 20 (1968) 139-150.
11.   French, D., and G.M. Wild, Abstracts Papers Am. Chem. Soc. 122 (1952) 5R.
12.   Nordin, P., and D. French, J. Am. Chem. Soc. 80 (1958) 1445-1447.
13.   French, D., Bull. Soc. Chim. Biol. 42 (1960) 1677-1700.
14.   French, D., in Biochemistry of Carbohydrates, Ser. 1, Vol. 5. Editor: W. J. Whelan, MTP International Review of Science (Butterworths, London, and University Park Press, Baltimore, 1975) 267-335.
15.   Yamakawa, Y., and T. Okuyama, J. Biochem. 73 (1973) 447-454.
16.   Smiley, K.L, D.E. Hensley, M. J. Smiley, and H.J. Gasdorf, Arch. Biochem. Biophys. 144 (1971) 694-699.
17.   Gasdorf, H.J., P. Atthasampunna, V. Dan, D.E. Hensley, and K.L. Smiley, Carbohydr. Res. 42 (1975) 147-156.
18.   Kuhn, R., Ber. 57 (1924) 1965-1968.
19.   Parrish, F.W., and E.T. Reese, Carbohydr. Res. 3 (1967) 424-429.
20.   Reese, E.T., A.H. Maguire, and F.W. Parrish, Can. J. Biochem. 46 (1967) 23-34.
21.   Shibaoka, T., K. Ishikura, K. Hiromi, and T. Watanabe, J. Biochem. 77 (1975) 1215-1222.
22.   Bailey, J.M. and D. French, J. Biol. Chem. 226 (1956) 1-14.
23.   Robyt, J.F. and D. French, Arch. Biochem. Biophys. 138 (1970) 662-670.
24.   French, D. and R.W. Youngquist, Stärke 12 (1963) 425-531.
25.   Robyt, J.F. and D. French, J. Biol. Chem. 245 (1970) 39197-3927.

26. Sakano, Y. and D. French, unpublished.
27. French, D., Y-C. Chan, B. England, Fed. Proc. 33 (1974) 1920.
28. Nitta, Y., K. Hiromi, and S. Ono, J. Biochem. 70 (1971) 973-979.
29. Thoma, J.A., G.V.K. Rao, C. Brothers, J. Spradlin, and L.H. Li, J. Biol. Chem. 246 (1971) 5621-5635.
30. Summer, R. and D. French, J. Biol. Chem. 222 (1956) 469-477.
31. Kainuma, K. and D. French, FEBS Letts. 6 (1970) 182-186.
32. Kainuma, K. and D. French, FEBS Letts. 5 (1969) 257-261.
33. French, D. and S. Kobayashi, Fed. Proc. 39 (1980) 1856.
34. Myrbäck, K., Arkiv. Kemi, 2 (1950) 417-422.
35. French, D. and G.M. Wild, J. Am. Chem. Soc. 75 (1953) 4490-4492.
36. Giri, N.Y. and D. French, Arch. Biochem. Biophys. 108 (1971) 505-510.
37. Rees, D.A. and W.E. Scott, J. Chem. Soc. (1971)B, 469-479.
38. Jordan, R.C., D.A. Brant, A. Cesaro, Biopolymers 17 (1978) 2617-2632.
39. Manor, P.C. and W. Saenger, J. Am. Chem. Soc. 96 (1974) 3630-3639.
40. Kobayashi, S, K. Kainuma, and S. Suzuki, Denpun Kagaku (J. Japan. Soc. Starch Sci.) 51 (1977) 691-698.
41. Kainuma, K. and D. French, Biopolymers 11 (1972) 2241-2250.
42. Wu, H-C. H. and A. Sarko, Carbohydr. Res. 61 (1978) 27-40.
43. Wu, H-C. H. and A. Sarko, Carbohydr. Res. 61 (1978) 7-25.
44. Borovsky, D., E.E. Smith, W.J. Whelan, D. French, and S. Kikumoto, Arch. Biochem. Biophys. 198 (1979) 627-631.
45. Pfannemuller, B., H. Mayerhofer and R. C. Schulz, Biopolymers 10 (1971) 243-261.
46. Dronzek, B.L., P. Hwang, and W. Bushuk, Cereal Chem. 49 (1972) 232.
47. Takaya, T., Y. Sugimoto, K. Wako, and H. Fuwa, Stärke 31 (1979) 205-28.
48. Lee, E.Y.C., Arch. Biochem. Biophys. 146 (1971) 488-492.
49. French, D., Denpun Kagaku (J. Japan. Soc. Starch Sci.)
50. Abdullah, M. and D. French, Arch. Biochem. Biophys. 137 (1970) 483-493.
51. French, D., E.E. Smith, and W.J. Whelan, Carbohydr. Res. 22 (1972) 123-134.
52. Taylor, P.M. and W.J. Whelan, Arch. Biochem. Biophys. 113 (1966) 500-502.
53. Kainuma, K., K. Wako, S. Kobayashi, A. Nogami, and S. Suzuki, Biochim. Biophys. Acta 410 (1975) 333-346.
54. Thoma, J.A. and D.E. Koshland, Jr., J. Molec. Biol. 2 (1960) 169-170.
55. Hoschke, A., E. Laszlo, and J. Hollo, Carbohydr. Res. 81 (1980) 145-156.
56. Pauling, L., Chem. Eng. News 24 (1946) 1375.
57. Wolfenden, R. Accounts Chem. Res. 5 (1972) 10-18.

58. Lazlo, E., J. Hollo, A. Hoschke, and G. Sarosi, Carbohydr. Res. 61 (1978) 387-394.

59. Koshland, D.E., Jr., Proc. Nat. Acad. Sci., U.S., 44 (1958) 98-104.

60. Lumry, R., in The Enzymes, Vol. 1, 2nd Ed. P.D. Boyer, H. Lardy and K. Myrbäck, Eds. (Academic Press, New York, 1959) 157-231.

61. Abdullah, M., D. French, and J.F. Robyt, Arch. Biochem. Biophys. 114 (1966) 595-598.

62. French, D., A.O. Pulley, J.A. Effenberger, M.A. Rougvie, and M. Abdullah, Arch. Biochem. Biophys. 111 (1965) 153-160.

63. Levvy, G.A. and S.M. Snaith, Adv. Enzymol. 36 (1972) 151-181.

64. Reese, E.T., F.W. Parrish, and M. Ettlinger, Carbohydr. Res. 18 (1971) 381-388.

65. Ohnishi, M., H. Kegal, and K. Hiromi, J. Biochem. 77 (1975) 695-703.

66. Ohnishi, M., T. Yamashita, and K. Hiromi, J. Biochem. 81 (1977) 99-105.

67. Schmidt, D.D., W. Frommer, B. Junge, L. Muller, W. Wingender, E. Truscheit, and D. Schafer, Naturwiss, 64 (1977) 535-536.

68. Walker, D.E. and B. Axelrod, Arch. Biochem. Biophys. 195 (1979) 392-395.

69. Kelemen, M.V. and W.J. Whelan, Arch. Biochem. Biophys. 117 (1966) 423-428.

70. Buonocore, V., T. Petrucci, and V. Silano, Phytochem. 16 (1977) 811-820.

71. Hehre, E.J., D.S. Genghof, and G. Okada, Arch. Biochem. Biophys. 142 (1971) 382-393.

72. Okada, G., D.S. Genghof, and E.J. Hehre, Carbohydr. Res. 71 (1979) 287-298.

73. Genghof, D.S., C.F. Brewer, and E.J. Hehre, Carbohydr. Res. 61 (1978) 291-299.

74. Hehre, E.J., C.F. Brewer, and D.S. Genghof, J. Biol. Chem. 254 (1979) 5942-5950.

75. Hehre, E.J., D.S. Genghof, H. Sternlicht, and C.F. Brewer, Biochem. 16 (1977) 1780-1787.

DISCUSSION

Q. WATKINS: I had a question about the difference in the high specific activity of amylases compared to cellulases. I was wondering if the substrate itself played a role in that?

A. FRENCH: I'm sure it does.

Q. WATKINS: If you started out with oligosaccharides of 6 glucose units, what would be the relative specific activities between cellulase and amylase?

A.   FRENCH: It depends on the particular amylase; I'll speak
      about pancreatic amylase. Substrates down to 5 glucose units
      are acted on very rapidly. Action on 4-unit chains is only
      about 10% as fast as 5, and 3 is only about 0.1% as fast as 5;
      so there is a very rapid drop off with the size. After one
      has about 5 glucose units in the substrate then increasing the
      length does not greatly increase the rate of action. The sec-
      ond factor has to do with the aggregation or state of
      dispersion of the substrate. In the case of starch, it is
      possible, not necessarily easily possible, but it is possible
      to get molecular dispersions which are acted upon much more
      rapidly than a granular starch by a ratio of perhaps 100 to
      1, or perhaps 1000 to 1; in fact some amylases are unable to
      act on granular starch, beta amylase being a specific example.
      Does that answer your question?

Q.   WATKINS: Let me state it a different way. The difference of
      specific activities was stated to be about 1000 to 1, and I
      was just wondering if you are kind of loading the dice using
      as substrates highly crystalline insoluable cellulose to
      measure cellulase activity and soluble starch to measure
      amylase activity.

A.   FRENCH: I think the ratio of activities was more like 100 to
      1 or 10 to 1, between amylase and cellulase. I don't know much
      about cellulase; the turnover number for amylase, pancreatic
      and sweet potato both, are of the order of 1000 times per
      second.

Q.   BANDURSKI: This is kind of fantasy-like, but could the amylase
      molecule move kind of agur-like down the amylase chain so that
      every time the augur turned it would successively advance two
      glucoyl units? Then the number of 4 catalytic acts would coin-
      cide with one full turn of the augur before it has to let go
      of the molecule. Somewhat related to this question, is how
      do you determine the binding affinities for the succession
      of sites along the chain?

A.   FRENCH: The answer to the first question as regards the auguring
      and whether a certain number of sucession of events represents
      one turn of the helix. That is an idea which was expressed in
      somewhat similar language by C.S. Hanes (New Phytologist 36,
      p. 101-141 and 189-239. 1937.) to account for the fact that
      maltoamylases had the ability to degrade starch into fragments
      of about 6 glucose units. He pictured that the amylose molecule
      existed in a helix with 6 glucose units per turn of the helix
      and the enzyme as coming down the helix and splitting off 6
      glucose units at a time. There isn't any truth to that although
      it was in accord with the available data, which was that the
      average size of these dextrins was about 6 glucose units. This

antedates chromotography so he had no way of knowing whether
he had a material that had precisely 6 glucose residues per
molecule or whether that was just some kind of average.

Now as regards to the other facet of the question, how do we
know that it goes down 4 times and then stops, is that it? The
answer is, the number 4 is a very statistical thing and in the
case of beta amylase, we did it by using a non-reducing end
labelled substrate and measuring the specific activity of the
maltose that is produced; we then compared that with the specific activity of maltose that is produced, when we use an interiorly labelled substrate. This is work that was done by Bailey
and French (22). Furthermore, we have taken end-labelled oligosaccharide with 13 glucose units in it, no more, no less,
subjected that to the beta amylase and looked at the products
by paper chromatography. You see, every product including
G-13 which is the original substrate un-acted on plus G-11, G-9,
G-7, G-5 and G-3, indicating that the enzyme has in some cases
taken off just one maltose unit or just 2 or just 3 or just 4,
whatever down to the end of the chain. Now we do this by using
end-labelled substrates and submitting them to paper chromatography following the intial reaction.

FERMENTATION OF PLANT POLYSACCHARIDES: ROLE OF BIOCHEMICAL GENETICS

Robert W. Detroy

Northern Regional Research Center, USDA[1]

Peoria, Illinois 61604

The application of biochemical genetics to the improvement of industrially important microorganisms has long been focused primarily on medical and agricultural products. Over the past few years, several novel ideas for genetic modification have been evoked for microbial systems. These advances in both cellular and molecular genetics and the advent of specific techniques in both *in vitro* and *in vivo* gene transfer for prokaryotic and eukaryotic organisms now give rise to applications in biotechnology for conversion of agricultural renewable resources to fuels and chemical feedstocks. These techniques include the use of directed mutasynthesis, cell and protoplast fusion, DNA transformation, and recombinant DNA technology. New and significant advances have been demonstrated in cellulosic conversions, enzymatic hydrolysis, alcohol production and tolerance, and substrate preparation relative to biological conversions. This biotechnology is now a prime candidate for transformation of fermentation genes necessary for plant polysaccharide conversions.

The efficient transformation of lignocellulosics, hemicelluloses, lignin, and starch to fermentable sugars, chemical feedstocks, and animal feedstuffs is virgin territory for the application of cell fusion and DNA cloning. Research is necessary to evaluate the transfer and regulation of genes for glycolysis and the hexose monophosphate shunt pathway.

---

[1]The mention of firm names or trade products does not imply that they are endorsed or recommended by the U. S. Department of Agriculture over other firms or similar products not mentioned.

Exploitation via molecular biology is mandated in the following areas of liquid fuels production via fermentations: alcohol from hemicelluloses, 2,3-butanediol production, high ethanol production from yeasts, alcohol tolerance, respiration-deficient yeasts, cellulase synthesis and regulation, and unexploited microbial ethanol systems.

Mutational biosynthesis is a specific technique for the generation of blocked mutants capable of producing new modified metabolite either directly or in response to some precursor analog. This technique, commonly called mutasynthesis, has been utilized effectively in the generation of new antibiotics. Gene transfer via cell fusion using intact protoplasts represents another novel approach to effect genetic transfer, especially in fungi.

The most rapidly developing area of science has been the demonstration of transformation by gene cloning or recombinant DNA technology. This technology is expanding into the industrially important yeasts and the transformation of genes into both prokaryotic and eukaryotic organisms.

The participants in the Biochemical Genetics of Fermentations session have amplified upon the need for increased gene dosage with various multi-copy plasmids for a series of sequential genes; introduction of high-level promoters for gene expression; further work on gene stability; and development of more knowledge of the genetics of microbes.

Removal of feedback controls will be a necessary component for increasing metabolite flow in the microbes evaluated. Recombinant DNA technology should also allow construction of new, possibly novel biochemical pathways.

Cloning of the glycolytic genes and their expression has been accomplished by numerous workers. Holland and Holland (1) have described the isolation and characterization of a glyceraldehyde-3-phosphate dehydrogenase (GPD) structural gene. An *Escherichia coli* transformant containing a hybrid plasmid DNA composed of vector pSF 2124 and sheared yeast DNA was cloned from a shotgun collection of transformants, using a complementary DNA probe synthesized from partially purified GPD mRNA.

Thomson and coworkers (2), using the Clarke-Carbon (3) clone bank carrying Col El-*E.coli* DNA, have identified plasmids for several of the genes of glycolysis and the hexose monophosphate shunt. Enzyme levels for the plasmid-carried genes ranged for the various plasmids from 5- to 30-fold the normal level.

The generation of suitable, stable plasmid vectors is imperative in the consideration of both gene transformation and expression.

Until recently the available yeast plasmid vectors integrated into the yeast genome, yielding low transformation values per unit DNA. The new yeast plasmid vectors display autonomous replication within a cell, yielding 5,000-20,000 transformants per unit DNA.

The availability of both *in vivo* and *in vitro* cloning methods makes it possible to consider the rational construction of various types of novel microbes--from hormone-synthesizing systems to hydrocarbon oxidation.

REFERENCES

1.   Holland, M. J. and J. P. Holland.   Isolation and characteriza-
     tion of a gene coding for glyceraldehyde-3-phosphate dehydro-
     genase from *Saccharomyces cerevisiae*.   J. Biol. Chem.   254:
     5466-5744, 1979.
2.   Thomson, J., P. D. Gerstenberger, D. E. Goldberg, E. Gociar,
     A. Orozco de Silva, and D. G. Fraenkel.   Col El hybrid plasmids
     for *Escherichia coli* genes of glycolysis and the hexose mono-
     phosphate shunt.   J. Bacteriol.   137:502-506, 1979.
3.   Clarke, L. and J. Carbon.   A colony bank containing synthetic
     Col El hybrid plasmids representative of the entire *E. coli*
     genome.   Cell 9:91-99, 1976.

MOLECULAR GENETICS AND MICROBIAL FERMENTATIONS

David A. Jackson

Genex Corporation

Rockville, Maryland

The interaction of the field of molecular genetics, especially the part of it termed recombinant DNA technology, with the business of large-scale microbial fermentations is a subject much in the news these days. From the reaction of Wall Street to the recent and prospective public offerings of genetic engineering companies, one would think these companies were in the business of synthesizing the Philosopher's Stone rather than developing methods for getting very large vats of smelly microorganisms to produce biochemicals more effectively.

In a sense, of course, microorganisms can be viewed as a modern-day equivalent of the Philsopher's Stone. Instead of transmuting lead into gold, they transmute other substances of lower value, such as molasses, into compounds of greater value, such as glutamic acid or lysine or vitamin B12 or antibiotics. Much of the current interest in the fermentation aspect of biotechnology derives from the prospect that microorganisms will, in the near future, be able to extend substantially each end of the value spectrum of compounds they act upon and produce. That is, the prospect that microorganisms will be able to economically use substrates of little present value, such as corn stover or old newspapers or various cellulosic waste streams, to make a variety of commodity chemicals and fuels has excited considerable interest. This conference attests to that interest. Similarly, the prospect that microorganisms will soon be able to produce, economically, a range of products of very high value such as interferon, a vast array of enzymes, viral coat proteins for vaccines, etc., has likewise captured the public's imagination. In order for these modern-day Philosopher's Stones to achieve a greater degree of reliability than those of the alchemists, a close collaboration must develop

between molecular geneticists, microbial physiologists, and biochemical engineers.

In this paper, I would like to consider some of the opportunities and some of the problems which will be faced in utilizing
genetically engineered microorganisms in large scale fermentations.
Throughout the discussion, unless otherwise specified the organism
will be assumed to be *E. coli* or closely related *Enterobacteriaceae*.
However, it is rapidly becoming the case that certain other species
of microorganisms, such as *Saccharomyces cerevisiae, Bacillus subtilis, Pseudomonas putida,* and several *Streptomycetes* can be
genetically engineered as well (1-4).

Figure 1 contrasts what was possible five years ago (left
side, Figure 1) with what is possible today (right side, Figure 1)
in the area of strain improvement. It shows that the nature of
both the opportunities and the problems has changed dramatically
in the past five years. Suppose, as illustrated in Figure 1, there
is a six-step pathway running from substrate S through intermediates
I_1 to I_5 to product P, and that we wish to improve the efficiency
with which a microorganism converts S to P. Until recently, the
primary techniques available for improving the wild type strain as a
production organism were first, mutagenesis and selection or screening for better producers, and second, extensive optimization of
physiological parameters affecting product yield. Given adequate
resources, these approaches can be very powerful. Obviously, a
great deal has been accomplished using them. However, they are very
labor intensive and time consuming and thus expensive. In addition,
certain desirable goals are beyond the capability of these approaches
For instance, the selection of a fundamentally new enzymatic activity (to allow utilization of a new class of substrate, for instance
in a strain which does not possess some enzymatic activity of the
desired type is essentially impossible using the mutagenesis and
selection approach.

Molecular genetics, recombinant DNA methodology in particular
now offers fundamentally new opportunities for strain improvement.
Recombinant DNA methodology in principle allows researchers to use
the whole of the genetic information in nature for strain improvement instead of just that fraction of it found within the genome of
a single species. This greatly expanded repertoire of enzymatic
activities allows strain modification of a sort essentially impossible until recently. Moreover, it allows a directed, rational
approach to strain construction using facts about known enzymes and
regulatory mechanisms where these are available. Some of the
components of such a rational approach are shown on the right hand
side of Figure 1.

One obvious approach to improving a wild type strain is to
increase the number of enzyme molecules catalyzing the conversion

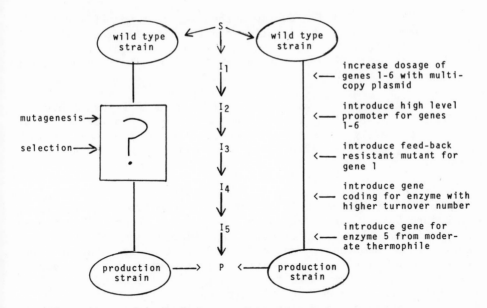

Figure 1.   Development of improved production strains.

of substrate S to product P.   Such an increase can be accomplished
by cloning the genes coding for enzymes 1 through 6 on a multicopy
plasmid.   The large increase in gene dosage is generally associated
with a significant increase in the number of molecules of enzymes
1 through 6 in the cell (5-7).   Another approach to increasing the
levels of enzyme 1 through 6 in the cell would be to put the genes
coding for these enzymes under the control of a high level pro-
motor (8).

Having achieved high levels of the enzymes for the pathway in
the cell, it does not necessarily follow that metabolite flow through
the pathway will be significantly increased.   This is because there
are other mechanisms besides enzyme limitation which can restrict
flow of metabolites through a pathway.   One common mechanism for
controlling metabolite flow is the existence of feedback inhibition
of the first enzyme in a pathway by the end product of that pathway.
Thus, a strategy for circumventing this problem would be to introduce, by recombinant DNA methods, the gene for a feedback resistant
mutant for the first enzyme in the pathway.   Another potential
problem in restricting metabolite flow may be that the turnover
number of one of the enzymes in the pathway is signifcantly lower
than that of all the others.   Should this be the case, it would be
possible to introduce into the cell the gene for an analogous
enzyme having a higher turnover number from another species of

bacteria. Finally, it is sometimes the case that one of the enzymes
in a pathway will be significantly more thermolabile than all of the
others. A strategy for dealing with this problem would be to introduce into the cell the gene for the analogous enzyme from a moderate
thermophile.

The examples of strain modification shown in Figure 1 are not
an exhaustive list. Many other specific types of genetic modification can be readily envisioned. However, each of the modifications
listed in Figure 1 has already been accomplished in at least one
instance.

For the sake of discussion, let us assume that it is possible
to introduce any biosynthetic or catabolic gene from any organism in
nature into *E. coli* or *Saccharomyces cerevisiae*. Does this unprece-
dented ability allow us to construct our microbiological Philospher's
Stone? It is important to recognize clearly that it does not. Simply
putting new genes for new enzymatic activities into a microorganism
does not insure or even make likely that it will be a successful
production strain. A number of additional problems must be dealt
with before directed molecular genetic manipulation of bacteria will
result in adequate strains for large scale fermentations.

Before considering what some of these problems are, it is
worth reviewing briefly the process by which new genetic information
can be inserted into a bacterial cell. This process is shown
schematically in Figure 2, and the important steps are listed below.

STEPS IN CLONING DNA

1.   Select enzyme whose gene is to be cloned.

2.   Select DNA containing the desired gene.

3.   Select appropriate plasmid vector.

4.   Recombine vector DNA and gene DNA.

5.   Transform appropriate cells.

6.   Identify cells containing the desired recombinant DNA.

7.   Obtain amplified DNA and characterize.

8.   Modify gene as required.

9.   Insert modified gene into compatible expression vector.

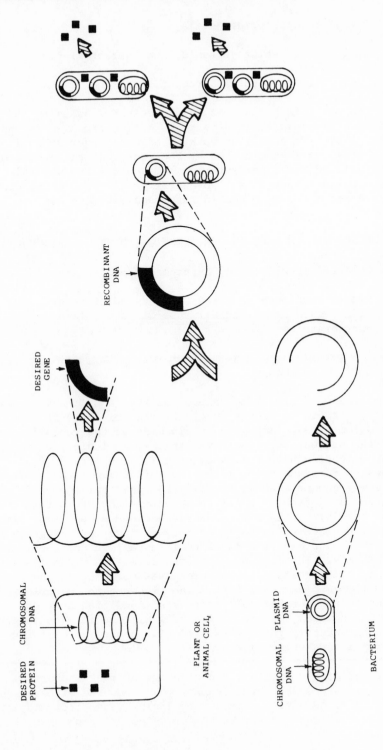

Figure 2. Scheme illustrating splicing and cloning of recombinant DNA.

10. Transform appropriate cells.

11. Grow cells, isolate plasmid, and characterize.

12. Grow cells for protein production.

The step in this process, at which decisions based on the fact that what is ultimately desired is a production organism, is the first one on this list. Moreover, at each of several other steps in this process, choices will be dictated by the fact that the organism will be used in a large scale fermentation. To understand why this is so, let us now consider some of the potential problems of using genetically engineered microorganisms in large scale fermentations.

PROBLEMS OF APPLYING MOLECULAR GENETICS TO INDUSTRIAL FERMENTATIONS

1. Genetic instability of extrachromosomal elements.

2. Poorly developed genetics for many of the most widely used or potentially useful industrial microorganisms.

3. The product may be toxic when present at high concentrations.

Each of the points listed above deserves additional comment. The genetic instability of many extrachromosomal elements is a serious problem (5,9). Recombinant plasmids or the genes inserted into them can be lost by several mechanisms, including segregation (5,9), recombination with the chromosome (10), deletion (9,11), and other types of rearrangements (11). Even if these genetic events occur at low frequency, as is usually the case, cells in which they have occurred are often at a strong selective advantage relative to those that retain the plasmid. This is because a bacterial strain which has been genetically engineered to produce very large amounts of a particular protein or metabolite is usually under considerable metabolic stress. It often has a growth rate significantly slower than that of the parental strain which does not contain the plasmid. Therefore, if the plasmid or any of the genes on the plasmid which are leading to the metabolically stressful condition are lost or otherwise inactivated, the resulting cell will be able to outgrow the cells which retain the stress-producing genes and will thus overgrow the population very quickly.

A second problem is that the genetics of many industrial microorganisms are at best rudimentary when compared with the genetics of *E. coli*. Genetic systems for cloning genes from and introducing genes into such organisms as *Corynebacteria*, obligate

anaerobes, and extreme thermophiles are essentially unknown. Unfortunately, in spite of the fact that we understand more about *E.
coli* than any other microorganism, it is not a particularly good
production organism. It remains to be seen whether genetic engineering can compensate for the current inadequacy of *E. coli*.

Product toxicity associated with product chemicals or fuels
present at high concentration in the fermentation broth is also a
potentially serious problem. Even if the genetic potential to
produce a chemical at a very high level can be introduced into a
strain, that potential may not be realizable because the product is
toxic to the cell. This is currently a problem for many of the
bacterial species proposed as ethanol producers (12), it is a
problem with butanol/acetone fermentations (13), and it is a problem
with most acidogenic fermentations and with many fermentations
involving aromatic chemicals (14).

The problems listed above are by no means necessarily insoluble
ones. A number of approaches to solving them have been and are
being tried. Some of these approaches are listed below.

POSSIBLE SOLUTIONS FOR GENETIC INSTABILITY
FOR EXTRACHROMOSOMAL ELEMENTS

1. Place an essential gene on the plasmid.

   a. antibiotic resistance gene, using sensitive cell
      as host.

   b. phage repressor gene, using a repressor defective
      phage lysogen as host.

   c. DNA synthesis function gene, using a cell mutant
      for this gene as host.

2. Regulate expression of cloned genes so that cell is
   stressed only near end of active growth phase.

3. Use as vectors replicons which are inherently more
   stable than others.

4. Avoid homology between extrachromosomal elements
   and host chromosome; use recombination defective
   host cells.

5. Avoid extrachromosomal elements carrying transposons.

Several of the points listed above deserve additional comment. The strategy of incorporating an antibiotic resistance gene on a plasmid and introducing that plasmid into a cell which is sensitive to that antibiotic is a proven method of maintaining plasmids in a viable cell population. However, for most large-scale fermentations producing products of relatively low value, this approach is un- likely to be an economically viable one. For products of very high value, such as interferon or hormones or certain enzymes, this approach may be quite acceptable. The proposal for using a plasmid carrying the repressor gene for a specific phage for which the host cell is lysogenic is an idea which has occurred independently to a number of groups. If the phage lysogen carries a repressor muta- tion, loss of the plasmid will result in induction of the phage leading to killing of the cell. Other cells in the population will be immune to attack by the phage produced so long as they retain plasmids carrying repressor genes.

A different sort of strategy for insuring that a high pro- portion of the cells in a population maintain a recombinant plasmid whose expression results in considerable metabolic stress on the cell is to regulate the expression of the cloned genes on the plas- mids so that metabolic stress occurs only near the end of the active growth phase of the population. In this way, the opportunity for overgrowth of the population by cells which have lost their recombi- nant plasmid are minimized. If the proper regulatory circuitry is built into the plasmid and/or the cell, such regulation of expression can be achieved by addition of a variety of small molecule inducers to the fermentation medium or by temperature shifts.

Point 3 listed above needs little comment. Replicons of different inherent stabilities have been isolated from bacteria and, all other things being equal, it should be advantageous to utilize the most stable replicons as the basis for vectors in production organisms.

Points 4 and 5 listed above are related. One of the signifi- cant pathways for loss of genes from a cell is by recombination leading to deletions or rearrangements (10). Avoiding nucleotide sequence homology between the DNA of the extrachromosomal element and that of the host chromosome minimizes this type of loss, as does the use of host cells which are recombination defective. Loss or rearrangement of genes has also been associated with the presence of transposons in plasmids (9). To the extent that it is possible, it would thus be wise to construct the final version of a recombi- nant plasmid to be used in a production organism so as to remove transposons.

As mentioned above, another significant problem in applying molecular genetic techniques to microorganisms of industrial importance is the fact that most of these microorganisms are poorly characterized genetically. Several promising strategies for dealing with this problem are listed below.

POSSIBLE SOLUTIONS FOR POORLY DEVELOPED GENETICS
OF INDUSTRIAL MICROORGANISMS

1. Utilize molecular genetic techniques to isolate and study genes and other genetic elements from industrial microorganisms in other microorganisms with highly developed genetic systems (e.g. *E. coli, B. subtilis*).

2. Develop systems for transferring genes into industrially useful bacteria and fungi (e.g. promiscuous plasmids, transformation or cell fusion methodologies).

3. Develop genetic systems in these organisms, using indigenous genetic elements as vectors.

Progress is being made with each of the strategies listed above. However, certain problems still remain to be solved. A common problem in trying to select for the introduction of a gene for a particular enzyme in *E. coli* is that *E. coli* may lack the transport system for the substrate of that enzyme.

A final major problem is that of product toxicity. This is a difficult problem in part because so little is known about the molecular basis of product toxicity. Potential solutions to this problem are listed below.

POSSIBLE SOLUTIONS FOR PRODUCT TOXICITY

1. Transfer genes of interest into product tolerant organisms.

2. Attempt to transfer genes leading to product tolerance into producing organisms.

3. Investigate molecular basis of product toxicity and tolerance.

Most of the solutions to the product toxicity problem are likely to be either strictly empirical or to involve a substantial amount of basic research to determine the mechanism of the toxic phenomena involved. The attempt to transfer genes of interest into organisms which already have a high level of tolerance for a particular product may be successful for one or a few genes, but it is likely to be very difficult for complex metabolic pathways. Similarly, the attempt to transfer genes leading to product tolerance into organisms which have the potential for high level production of a toxic product is likely to be quite complicated genetically. Nonetheless, this approach is worth trying since the phenotype of product tolerance can be selected incrementally and since very strong selections for the desired phenotype are generally easy to devise. Fortunately, an alternative non-genetic approach to the problem of product toxicity exists. This is the development of new chemical and biochemical engineering methods for economically removing toxic products from large scale fermentations on a continuous basis.

In conclusion, let us consider some of the more realistic opportunities offered by application of genetic engineering techniques to microorganisms, with particular emphasis on the production of chemicals and fuels.

OPPORTUNITIES IN APPLYING MOLECULAR GENETICS TO INDUSTRIAL FERMENTATIONS

1. Increase gene dosage and thus concentration of gene products; consequent increased rate of metabolite flow through pathways.

2. Increase yield of product from substrate.

3. Construct novel biochemical pathways in an organism of choice to allow:

    a. wider substrate utilization

    b. small molecule (e.g. antibiotic) modification.

4. Produce gene products not normally found in microorganisms (e.g. human proteins).

5. Put genes of interest under control of known regulatory mechanisms.

6. Utilize gene products with special physicochemical properties (e.g. thermostability).

The rationale behind point 1 above is that an increase in the gene dosage for the enzymes of a pathway has in many cases now been shown to lead to a substantial increase in the number of enzyme molecules in the pathway and a consequent increase in the rate of metabolite flow through the pathway. Control of the level of gene dosage for virtually any gene is readily achieved through the use of the appropriate multicopy plasmid. More sophisticated versions of this approach employ, in addition, high-level regulatable promoter, mutant genes coding for feedback resistant enzymes, etc. It is worth noting that removal of feedback inhibition controls is likely to be more important (and better for the cell) than producing massive amounts of a feedback inhibited enzyme in order to obtain adequate flow of metabolites.

Increased yield of product from substrates, the second of the opportunities listed above, has been a goal of fermentation microbiologists for many years. An example of the achievement of this goal through genetic engineering already exists. ICI (15,16) and Cetus (17) have both cloned the gene for the ATP-independent glutamate dehydrogenase (GDH) of *E. coli* and have introduced it on a plasmid into the obligate methylotroph *Methylophilus methylotrophus*. This organism will grow on a mixture of methanol, ammonia, and salts, but lacks the glutamate dehydrogenase pathway for assimilating ammonia. It utilizes instead the glutamine synthetase – glutamate synthetase pathway which consumes one mole of ATP for each mole of ammonia assimilated. The recombinant plasmid containing the GDH gene is both stable and expressed in *Methylophilus*. Strains containing this plasmid convert substrate carbon to biomass 4 to 7% more efficiently than the wild type organism, presumably because less ATP is reguired for ammonia assimilation because of the presence ATP independent *E. coli* GDH (15).

The ability to construct novel biochemical pathways in a microorganism so as to allow a wider range of substrates to be utilized is of considerable potential importance. An example of a novel biochemical pathway which could be constructed in *E. coli* is shown in Figure 3. *E. coli* aspartase can efficiently convert fumaric acid plus ammonia to aspartic acid. Fumaric acid costs $0.53/lb., while aspartate currently sells for approximately $3.00/lb. The *cis* isomer of fumaric acid – maleic acid – can be derived by the spontaneous hydration of maleic anhydride, which is 30% cheaper than fumaric acid. *E. coli* cannot grow on maleate but certain other organisms, including certain Pseudomonads, can (18). Introduction of a maleate isomerase gene into *E. coli* thus allows aspartate to be produced from a significantly cheaper precursor.

Another method of constructing novel biochemical pathways is currently being explored by the pharmaceutical industry for the purpose of synthesizing new types of antibiotics. The proposal here is to introduce the genes for two or more different antibiotic biosynthetic pathways into the same cell. The hope is that the action of enzymes from each pathway on the intermediates and end products of the other pathway will result in new and potentially useful species of antibiotics.

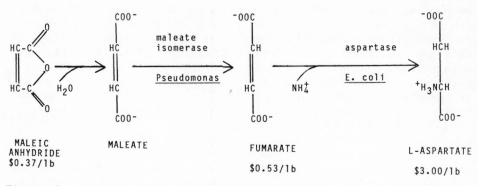

Figure 3.   Construction of a novel biochemical pathway in $E.$ $coli$
utilizing genes from different microorganisms.

The new opportunity made possible by recent advances in molecular genetics which has most attracted the interest of the public
is the possibility of using microorganisms to produce the products
of genes not normally found in microorganisms.   A number of microbia
strains producing such substances as human insulin (19), human interferon (20,21) and human growth hormone (22,23) have already been
constructed, and strains producing a much wider diversity of human,
mammalian, and viral proteins are being developed.   Another example
of a microorganism producing a novel gene product is the strain
constructed recently by Doel et al. of G.D. Searle (24).   These
workers chemically synthesized an artificial gene consisting of a
repeating nucleotide sequence which coded for the dipeptide aspartyl-
phenylalanine.   A polymer of this repeating sequence was then
inserted into a vector DNA molecule and the resulting recombinant
DNA molecule was introduced into $E.$ $coli.$ This strain of $E.$ $coli$
then produced a polymer of the dipeptide aspartyl-phenylalanine.
This polymer can be degraded enzymatically to the dipeptide which
can then be chemically methylated to yield the artificial sweeten-
ing agent aspartame.

Point 5 above, incorporating known regulatory elements which
are well-understood, may be of considerable general applicability.
Many of the problems of achieving substantial metabolite flows
through the biosynthetic pathways of diverse microorganisms involve
repression or feedback control by poorly understood or unknown
mechanisms.   It may be possible to circumvent some of these problems
by putting key genes under the control of well-understood regulatory
elements derived, for instance, from $E.$ $coli$ or $B.$ $subtilis.$

A final opportunity, also of potentially wide applicability,
is the ability to select and utilize genes coding for enzymes having

specific physicochemical characteristics. One of the most generally useful characteristics is likely to be thermostability. In cases where all except one or two of the enzymes in a pathway form a mesophile function well and are stable at 50°C for example, it may be possible to operate this pathway in an immobilized cell system at 50°C by introducing the genes from a moderate thermophile coding for enzymes analogous to those from the mesophile which are thermo-labile. The enzymes from the thermophile would be expected to be thermostable, and would thus allow the whole pathway to function at 50°C. A related strategy would be to clone genes for enzymes having particularly high turnover numbers, or which were insensitive to feedback inhibition, so as to replace enzymes which represented rate limiting steps in pathways.

In summary, while the list of applications of molecular gene-tics to large-scale fermentations presented above is not exhaustive, it does illustrate the diversity of ways in which gene cloning technology can be applied. Although it is certainly premature to conclude that genetic engineering of microorganisms for large scale fermentations will be easy or that it will be a panacea for all problems, enough has already been done to suggest that the promise of this technology is extensive and that it is realizable.

REFERENCES

1.   Hinnen, A., Hicks, J.B., Fink, G.R. (1978). Proc. Nat. Acad. Sci. USA 75: 1929-1933.
2.   Lovett, P.S., Keggins, K.M. (1979) in Methods in Enzymology (Wu, R., ed.) Vol. 68, Academic Press, New York, p342-357.
3.   Nagahari, K., Sakaguchi, K. (1978). J. Bacteriol. 133:1527-1529
4.   Bibb, M., Schottel, J.L., Cohen, S.N. (1980). Nature 283:526-531.
5.   Herschfield, V., Boyer, H.W., Yanofsky, C., Lovett, M.A., Helinski, D.R. (1974). Proc. Nat. Acad. Sci. USA 71:3455-3459.
6.   Davis, M.G., Calvo, J.M. (1977). J. Bacteriol. 131:997-1007.
7.   Panasenko, S.M., Cameron, J.R., David, R.W., Lehman, I.R. (1977). Science 196:188-191.
8.   Hallewell, R.A., Emtage, S. (1980). Gene 9:27-47.
9.   Imanaka, T. and Aiba, S. (1980). J. Gen. Microbiol. 118:253-261.
10. Hicks, J.B., Hinne, A., Fink, G.R. (1978). Cold Spring Harbor Symp. Quant. Biol. 43:1305-1313.
11. Rood, J.I., Sneddon, M.K., Morrison, J.F. (1980). J. Bacteriol 144:552-559.
12. Lee, K.J., Tribe, D.E., Rogers, P.L. (1979). Biotechnology Letters 1:421-426.
13. Walton, M.T., Martin, J.L. in Microbial Technology (Peppler,

H.J. and Perlman, D., eds.), Vol. 1, 2nd edition, Academic
Press, New York, 1979, pp. 188-209.

14. Zeikus, J.G. (1980). Ann. Rev. Microbiol. 34:423-464.

15. Windass, J.D., Worsey, M.A., Pioli, E.M., Pioli, D., Barth,
    P.T., Atherton, K.T., Dart, E.C., Byrom, D., Powell, K., Senio
    P.J. (1980). Nature 287:396-401

16. Senior, P.J., Windass, J. (1980). Biotechnology Letters 2:205
    210 (1980).

17. Gelfand, D.H. (1980). Abstracts of the Annual Meeting of The
    American Chemical Society, #60.

18. Scher, W., Jacoby, W.B. (1969). J. Biol. Chem. 244:1878-1882.

19. Geoddel, D.V., Kleid, D.G., Bolivar, F., Heynecker, H.L.,
    Yansura, D.G., Crea, R., Hirose, T., Kraszewski, A., Itakura,
    K., Riggs, A.D. (1979). Proc. Nat. Acad. Sci. USA 75:5936-5940

20. Nagata, S., Taira, H., Hall, A., Johnsrud, L., Steuli, M.,
    Ecsodi, J., Boll, W., Cantell, K., Weissmann, C. (1980).
    Nature 284:316-320.

21. Maeda, S., McCandliss, R., Gross, M., Sloma, A., Familletti,
    P.C., Tabor, J.M., Evinger, M., Levy, W.P., Pestka, S. (1980)
    in press, Proc. Nat. Acad. Sci., USA.

22. Martial, J.A., Hallewell, R.A., Baxter, J.D., Goodman, H.M.
    (1979). Science 205:602-607.

23. Geoddel, D.V., Heynecker, H.L., Hozumi, T., Arentzen, R.,
    Itakura, K., Yansura, D.G., Ross, M.J., Miozzari, G., Crea,
    R., Seeburg, Ph.H. (1979). Nature 281:544-548.

24. Doel, M.T., Eaton, M., Cook, E.A., Lewis, H., Patel, T., Carey
    N.H. (1980). Nucleic Acids Research 8:4575-4592.

THE BIOCHEMICAL GENETICS OF GLYCOLYSIS IN MICROBES

Dan G. Fraenkel

Department of Microbiology and Molecular Genetics

Harvard Medical School, Boston, MA 02115

MUTANTS AND MAPPING

Mutants for most reactions of glycolysis have been described both in *Escherichia coli* and in *Saccharomyces cerevisiae*. The pathway between glucose and pyruvate has three irreversible and seven reversible reactions (Figure 1), and most of the intermediates are needed in biosynthesis. Thus, one might expect mutants in an irreversible step to be impaired in growth on glucose but unimpaired gluconeogenically, and mutants in a reversible step to require supplementation even for gluconeogenic growth. To a first approximation this pattern is found but there are deviations (Table I). For example, *E. coli* mutants blocked between triose-P and phosphoenolpyruvate do require supplementation (e.g., by glycerol) for growth on lactate (1,2) but phosphoglucose isomerase mutants grow without supplementation by glucose (3) - probably because glucose-6-P and its products are not essential for growth of this organism. Aldolase mutants also do not require supplementation for gluconeogenic growth, and the explanation is unknown; it might relate to other aldolases (see ref. 4). The growth on glucose of a (double) pyruvate kinase mutant occurs because phosphoenolpyruvate is used by the phosphotransferase (PTS) reaction intiating glucose metabolism and such a mutant fails to grown on non-PTS sugars (5). Many of the mutants have interesting properties. The subject was reviewed in 1973 (6). Some of the more recent work is cited below; see also refs. 1-3, 5, 7-8, and 9 (the latter on glucose phosphorylation and uptake by the PTS). Other than for phosphofructokinase, characteristics of the *E. coli* glycolysis mutants will not be further considered. One common property however deserves mention; such mutants, if incubated with glucose, often accumulate metabolites before the block, and glucose may be inhibitory to growth on an otherwise permissive medium.

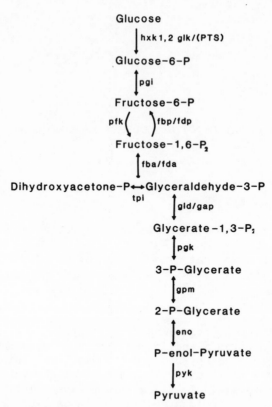

Figure 1.   Reactions between glucose and pyruvate.   Most of the gen
symbols in use or suggested are the same for *Escherichia coli* (43)
and *Saccharomyces cerevisiae* (20), but some differ, in which case
the *E. coli* symbol is given after the slash.   PTS, phosphortrans-
ferase system.

Most of the mutations are in the structural genes for the
enzyme in question.   Map positions are given in Table II, and have
been evaluated in terms of genome evolution (10).   There is no
evidence for operons, even for the two cases of very close linkage
(*pfkA* and *tpi*, and *fda* and *pgk*).

Mutants have been reported also for many of the reactions of
anaerobic pyruvate dissimilation in *E. coli* leading to the mixed
acid fermentation products: pyruvate formate lyase (*pfl*, 11), formate hydrogen lyase (*fdh*, 12, and *hyd*, 13; see also 14, 15), acetat
kinase and phosphotransacetylase (*ack* and *pta*, 16, 17), alcohol
dehydrogenase and acetaldehyde coenzyme A dehydrogenase (*adh* high
levels of both, and *acd*, deficient in the latter enzyme (18), and
fumarate reductase (*frd*, 19).

TABLE I

General Growth Phenotype of *E. coli* Glycolysis Mutants.
(The original papers should be consulted for details).

| | Minimal medium: | | |
	Glucose	Lactate	Lactate + Glycerol
wild-type	+	+	+
pgi	-/+	+	+
pfkA	-/+	+	+
fda	-	+	+
tpi	-	-	+
gap	-	-	+
pgk	-	-	+
eno	-	-	+
pykA,B	+	+	+

TABLE II

Gene Positions in *E. coli* (43, and see text).

pgi	min 91
pfkA	88
pfkB	38
fda	63
tpi	88
gap	39
pgk	63
eno	59
zwf	41
pgl	17
gnd	44
pfl	20
fdh	80
hyd	57
ack	49
pta	49
frd	94
acd	62

In *Saccharomyces*, mutant studies in glycolysis are recent
(reviewed in 20). The data in Table III indicates their growth
and again, to a first approximation, the expectations are met: blocking of the irreversible steps affects only glycolytic growth, while

TABLE III

General Growth Characteristics of Yeast Glycolysis Mutants.

	Enriched medium +		
	Glucose	Pyruvate	Pyruvate + Glycerol
wild-type	+	+	+
hxk1,2 glk	-	+	+
pgi	-	-	-
pfk1,2	-	+	+
tpi	-	-	+
pgk	-	-	+
gpm	-	-	+
pyk	-	+	+
pdc	-/+	+	+
adc	-/+	+	+

blocking the other affects both glycolytic and gluconeogenic growth. In yeast there are apparently several cases where single enzymes are responsible for the reactions, and single gene deficiency mutants are known. These include phosphoglucose isomerase (*pgi*), triose-P isomerase (*tpi*), phosphoglycerate kinase (*pgk*), phosphoglycerate mutase (*gpm*) and pyruvate kinase (*pyk*). There are several cases in yeast glycolysis where isoenzymes are known and their existence *in vivo* is to a degree confirmed by the absence of mutants for aldolase, glyceraldehyde-3-P dehydrogenase, or enolase. To prevent glucose use, three kinases must be inactivated (*hxk1, hxk2, glk; 21*).

In general, the phenotypes of yeast glycolysis mutants have not been described in detail. As with the *E. coli* mutants, incubation with glucose causes high metabolite accumulations before the block (see ref. 22), and glucose is often toxic to growth.

Many of the known yeast glycolysis mutants seem to be in the structural genes, as shown by alleles causing temperature sensitive enzymes, or by cloning. Known map positions are given in Table IV.

With respect to the yeast fermentation products themselves – mainly ethanol – there is quite detailed knowledge of the genetics of alcohol dehydrogenase (e.g., 23), and pyruvate decarboxylase mutants have been obtained (24). The pathway to glycerol has not yet been studied with mutants. Glycerol is overproduced in an alcohol dehydrogenase mutant (25).

TABLE IV

Glycolysis Gene Positions in *S. cerevisiae* (20)

HXK1	6R
HXK2	7L
GLK	3L
PGI	2R
PGK	3R
PYK	1L

CLONING OF GLYCOLYSIS GENES

In *E. coli* , cloning used to be done genetically, by construction of specialized transducing phages. *pfkA*, the gene coding for the main phosphofructokinase of *E. coli* was obtained this way (26), as was *gnd*, the gene for 6-phosphogluconate dehydrogenase (27). In such cases, the isolated phage provides the source of DNA enriched for the gene in question, whereas induction of a lysogen, or infection at high multiplicity, by increasing the number of gene copies usually increases the amount of enzyme produced. It is now often more convenient to use *in vitro* methods. Clarke and Carbon (28) cloned the *E. coli* chromosome, in pieces of average size 8×10^6 daltons, into the Col E1 plasmid, and many have screened the resulting clone bank of ca. 2000 strains, by complementation, for genes of interest. We have done so for several genes of glycolysis (Table V). In general, the amounts of gene products are substantially higher than in wild type strains. Such plasmids are a convenient source of DNA for the gene in question. For example, the hybrid plasmid carrying the gene *pfkA*, for the main phosphofructokinase of *E. coli*, Pfk-1, was used by J. Thomson to program efficient cell free synthesis of active enzyme (29).

In some cases it was not possible to find the required hybrid plasmid in the Clarke-Carbon bank. Or, one may be interested in cloning a mutant gene. Our work on *pfkB* of *E. coli* is an example. *E. coli* has a second, and very minor, phosphofructokinase, Pfk-2 of different kinetics from Pfk-1. The normal amount of Pfk-2 is low in *pfkB+* strains and inadequate for growth on sugars in the absence of Pfk-1, but a mutation, *pfkB1*, increases the amount about thirty-fold and allows growth on sugars again. To determine the nature of the *pfkB1* mutation F. Daldal has cloned both alleles, *pfkB1+* and *pfkB1*, in the vector pBR322, by selection for function in the appropriate recipient (Table VI). Subcloning to date has given both genes on ca. 2.3 kb inserts, and restriction analysis shows no differences in fragment pattern. This means that the *pfkB1* mutation is neither insertion of a large element carrying a new promoter, nor a deletion connecting the gene to another promoter.

TABLE V

E. coli Clones from the Clarke-Carbon Bank (from ref. 44)

	wild type	mutant	clone	
pfkA	0.52	0.00	13.3	(pLC16-4)
tpi	3.95	0.00	22.1	(pLC16-4)
pgi	1.67	0.00	9.2	(pLC37-5)
zwf	0.10	0.00	1.84	(pLC3-33)
pgk	2.01	0.01	9.02	(pLC15-31)
eno	0.47	0.01	3.45	(pLC10-47)

DNA sequencing should show whether it is a point mutation.

Most of the glycolysis enzymes of yeast have also been cloned
One method has been to prepare a clone bank of yeast DNA in *E. coli*
and then screen it appropriately. J. Carbon and colleagues used an
immunological technique to identify the clone for phosphoglycerate
kinase, PGK (30).   Holland and Holland (31) used a labelled probe
of DNA complementary to the mRNA for glyceraldehyde-3-P dehydrogenase, to the same purpose.   (This was possible because the yeast
glycolysis enzymes are present in high amount (Table VII), so are
their messages (32).)   This work has already shown that yeast has
three genes for glyceraldehyde-3-P dehydrogenase, and there is
knowledge of their sequence, including flanking regions (33). Such
cloning methods which do not use mutants also afford a way to obtain
mutants, by *in vitro* mutagenesis and reintroduction of the genes
into yeast.

TABLE VI
Cloning of *E. coli* Phosphofructokinase and
Fructose Diphosphatase Genes into pBR322
(F. Daldal, to be reported)

Enzyme activity

Donor	Recip.	Clone	Insert
*pfkB*1	*pfkB*⁻		
0.45	0.001	4.06	HindIII, 6.5 kb
pfkB⁺			
0.017	"	0.30	"
fdp⁺	*fdp*⁻		
0.014	0.00	1.24	EcoR1

TABLE VII

Amounts of Yeast Glycolysis Enzymes (from 20)

(% soluble protein)

Hexokinase	0.5
Phosphoglucose isomerase	1.0
Phosphofructokinase	0.3
Aldolase	4.0
Triose-P isomerase	2.0
Glycerald.-3-P DH	10.0
P-Glycerate kinase	5.0
P-Glucerate mutase	0.9
Pyruvate kinase	5.0

G. Kawasaki has cloned many of the remaining glycolysis genes by complementation in yeast. A clone bank of yeast DNA in a hybrid vector, CV13 (34), able to replicate in both yeast and *E. coli*, was used to transform the appropriate yeast mutant. In yeast, the plasmids, presumably nuclear, are carried in several copies, and protein products are in high level (Table VIII). One can also assess whether the yeast gene functions in the prokaryote. In the case of the triose-phosphate isomerase (*TPI*) it does not, but subclones which do are readily obtained by selection for function in an *E. coli tpi* mutant. In this case it seems that a deletion has joined the yeast gene to a bacterial promoter on the plasmid.

TABLE VIII

Yeast Genes Cloned by Complementation into Yeast
(G. Kawasaki, unpublished)

Vector: CV13 (pBR322 - LEU2 - 2 micron)
DNA: by Sau3A into BamH1 of CV13

	wild type	mutant	clone
Pgi	2.85	0.02	20.5, 33.8
Tpi	18.3	0.01	164, 99, 226
Pgk	1.99	0.01	15.4
Pgm	0.74	0.00	4.2, 5.6
Pyk	4.02	0.02	14.4, 19.2

TABLE IX

Glucose-6-P Dehydrogenase in *E. coli* Crude Extracts (AnO$_2$, anaerobic

			units/mg
Wild-type	Glucose		0.28
"	"	(AnO$_2$)	0.27
"	Fructose		0.22
pgi mutant	Glucose		0.23
"	Fructose		0.23

There are innumerable applications of cloning. The amino acid
sequence of yeast triose phosphate isomerase is not known but is
being obtained from the DNA (G. Kawasaki and T. Alber, in preparation). Ultimately, *in vitro* mutagenesis at specific residues should
be possible. Identification and manipulation of the high level
promoters of such genes is also being done, and may be useful for
cloning other genes in yeast.

GENE EXPRESSION

Many of the enzymes of central intermediary sugar metabolism
in *E. coli* are expressed "constitutively." This is illustrated
(Table IX) for glucose-6-P dehydrogenase in *E. coli*, whose level in
the wild type changes little whether cells are grown with glucose,
or not, aerobically or anaerobically, and, in a phosphoglucose
isomerase mutant, whether grown with glucose (so glucose-6-P is
high) or without (no glucose-6-P in the cell). Apparently, enzyme
level does not vary greatly according to need.

The absence of large induction effects in response to apparent
physiological need does not mean that enzyme levels are not regulated
at all. There are data showing significant changes in enzyme levels
according to the degree of aerobiosis (for Pfk-1 the amount is up
to three times higher anaerobically (35)), or according to carbon
source (for *pfk-1*, a level much lower on pyruvate than on glucose
(36). In general data on the effect of growth rate of glycolysis
gene expression are scarce, and it is likely that when 2-dimensional
gels are used to survey their levels various classes of control will
become apparent (F.C. Neidhardt, pers. comm.). The amount of 6-
phosphogluconate dehydrogenase varies with growth rate (37), and
as the molecular biology of this gene (*gnd*) is becoming known it may
provide a model for the understanding of expression of this type of
"constitutivity." mRNA levels have not been assessed for any such
genes.

TABLE X

Glycolysis enzyme activities in yeast wild type and *gcr* mutant grown in enriched medium containing lactate plus glycerol, with the addition of maltose as indicated. Activities are normalized for each enzyme to the activity of the wild type grown with maltose (from 45).

	GCR		gcr	
(Mal)	+	−	+	−
Hxk	100	72	100	78
Pgi	100	126	28	7
Pfk	100	109	92	58
Fda	100	183	31	5
Tpi	100	132	21	7
Gld	100	158	54	4
Pgk	100	122	45	8
Gpm	100	124	7	1
Eno	100	92	7	1
Pyk	100	124	20	7
Zwf	100	98	82	94

Yeast glycolysis enzymes also appear to be present constitutively, but the statement needs even more qualification than in the bacterial case. Oura (38) showed that the ability to perform glycolysis was similar in cells grown in glucose-limited chemostats aerobically or anaerobically. However, it should be remembered that several steps of glycolysis in yeast involve isoenzymes, so that absence of large induction effects may conceal major differences. The same qualification should not be needed for those cases where a single gene governs a particular reaction, but even then the situation is unclear. Maitra and Lobo (39) showed that the addition of glucose to acetate grown cells caused very high differential rates of synthesis of some glycolysis enzymes (particularly in one strain), and studies with mutants implicated glucose-6-P as inducer of some of the enzymes (40).

In our work we have not seen large variation in glycolysis enzyme levels in cultures fron steady state growth in several media. But there is an apparent regulatory mutation affecting the glycolysis enzymes, *gcr*. Although the original allele arose by selection for resistance to glucose toxicity in a pyruvate kinase mutant (*pyk*), its growth on glucose (in a *PYK* strain) is impaired enough that *gcr* mutants can be readily obtained by screening of glucose negative mutants (G. Kawasaki, unpub.). The enzyme pattern has two interesting characteristics (Table X): first, the levels of many glycolysis enzymes are low, ca. 5% of wild type as assayed from growth in a gluconeogenic medium; and second, in the presence of sugars, most of the affected levels are much higher (ca. 25% normal). These freatures are readily seen in 1-dimensional gels.

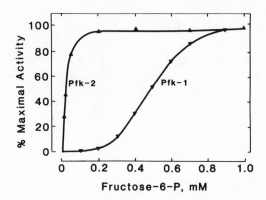

Figure 2.   Phosphofructokinase Kinetics. (Adapted from 47.)

CONTROL OF ENZYME ACTIVITY

Since so many of the enzymes of glycolysis seem to be present whether needed or not, the control of flux in the pathway might depend on activation and inhibition of key reactions, such as phosphofructokinase.   The main *E. coli* enzyme, Pfk-1, is an allosteric protein, and the minor one, Pfk-2, seems not to be (Figure 2). But the effect of loss of Pfk-1 is prevented by mutation increasing the amount of Pfk-2.   This fact implies that either the control characteristics of these enzymes are not important, or that their properties differ *in vivo* and *in vitro*.   Some data on growth (41) are in Table XI, comparing strains with wild type enzyme pattern (90) Pfk-1), with high level Pfk-2 only, or with both enzymes. Having Pfk-2 made only a small difference in growth on sugars and none on glycerol.

The lack of effect on glycerol was particularly surprising considering the kinetics (Figure 2), for one might expect that in gluconeogensis, where fructose-6-P concentration is probably low, Pfk-1 would not reform fructose-1,6-P, but Pfk-2 might.   Interestingly, although no impairment of gluconeogenic growth was seen in strains with the *pfkB1* allele (and hence high level Pfk-2) such impairment was seen in a secondary mutant derived from a *pfkB1* strain, and carrying the double mutation "*pfkB1**" (and hence a variant enzyme, Pfk-2*) (Table XII). Metabolite levels in such strains (all lacking Pfk-1) are also given in Table XII. As expected for the impaired gluconeogenic growth of the *pfkB1** strain, fructose-6-P was barely detectable, while its level was normal in the (normal) growth of the *pfkB1* strain.   In growth on glucose, on the other hand, the *pfkB1** strain (which grows well) had the expected low levels of fructose-6-P, while the strain with *pfkB1* (also growing well) had the high level of fructose-6-P characteristic of *pfkB*⁺ strains (very slow growth).   These results

TABLE XI

Growth (dt, doubling time) and yield (Y) of
E. coli strains with various *pfk* alleles
(from 46)

	$pfkA^+$ dt	$pfkB^+$ Y	$pfkA^+$ dt	$pfkB1$ Y	$pfkA^-$ dt	$pfkB1$ Y
Glucose O_2	80	4.2	80	6.0	105	4.7
" AnO_2	105	14.3	105	11.0	135	14.5
Glycerol O_2	90	7.9	95	7.9	100	7.9
" + Fum AnO_2	248	11.5	270	14.1	253	15.5

TABLE XII

Growth (dt, doubling time) and metabolite levels (mM) of *E. coli*
strains carrying various *pfkB* alleles; all strains are deleted for
pfkA (from 41).

	$pfkB^+$	$pfkB1$	$pfkB1*$
Glucose:			
dt	250	80	60
G-6-P	11.1	11.3	2.0
F-6-P	2.8	1.9	0.2
F-1,6-P_2	0.4	3.2	3.5
Glycerol:			
dt	110	95	350
G-6-P	1.2	1.0	<0.05
F-6-P	0.3	0.2	<<0.05
F-1,6-P_2	3.5	3.4	5.8

suggest that the phosphofructokinases in the two strains, Pfk-2 and Pfk-2*, differ functionally. For example, Pfk-2, might be inhibited *in vivo* by an unknown effector, so that in growth on sugars, even though there is sufficient activity for rapid flux, fructose-6-P concentration is high. The alteration in Pfk-2* might be in its control properties, so that fructose-6-P is no longer in high level during growth on glucose (which is slightly more rapid than *pfkB1* strains), but causing difficulties in gluconeogenesis. The two enzymes, Pfk-2 and Pfk-2*, have been compared and are similar in many properties, including a very high affinity for fructose-6-P as substrate. One difference is that Pfk-2 is somewhat sensitive to inhibition by fructose-6,6-P_2, and the inhibition is less in Pfk-2*. It is not known to what degree this difference accounts for growth differences (41). For example, the model may be correct but fructose-1,6-P_2 might not be the true effector. To further compli- cate matters, direct tests have shown that impaired gluconeogenic growth in *pfkB1* strains is not accompanied by futile cycling (42). Clearly, *in vivo* control of the Pfk-2 reaction in *E. coli* is not well understood.

ACKNOWLEDGEMENTS

Unpublished work from this laboratory was one by Drago Cliftor Fevzi Daldal, Glenn Kawasaki, and Dan Fraenkel, and supported by grants from the National Science Foundation (PCM-79-10682) and the National Institutes of Health (2 RO1 GM 21 098-06).

REFERENCE

1. Irani, M., and Maitra, P.K. 1974. Isolation and characteriza- tion of *Escherichia coli* mutants defective in enzymes of glycolysis. Biochem. Biophys. Res. Commun. 56, 127-133.
2. Hillman, J.D., and Fraenkel, D.G. 1975. Glyceraldehyde 3- phosphate dehydrogenase mutants of *Escherichia coli*. J. Bacteriol. 122, 1175-1179.
3. Vinopal, R.T., Hillman, J.D., Schulman, H., Reznikoff, W.S., and Fraenkel, D.G. 1975. New phosphoglucose isomerase mutants of *Escherichia coli*. J. Bacteriol. 122, 1172-1174.
4. Lengler, J. 1977. Analysis of mutations affecting the dis- similation of galactitotl (dulcitol) in *Escherichia coli* K 12. Molec. gen. Genet. 152, 83-91.
5. Pertierra, A.G., and Cooper, R.A. 1977. Pyruvate formation during the catabolism of simple hexose sugars by *Escherichia coli*: studies with pyruvate kinase-negative mutants. J. Bacteriol. 129, 1208-1214.
6. Fraenkel, D.G., and Vinopal, R.T. 1973. Carbohydrate meta- bolism in bacteria. Ann. Rev. Micro. 27, 69-100.

7. Irani, M.H., and Maitra, P.K. 1977. Properties of *Escherichia coli* mutants deficient in enzymes of glycolysis. J. Bacteriol. 132, 398-410.
8. Hillman, J.D. 1979. Mutant analysis of glyceraldehyde-3-P dehydrogenase in *Escherichia coli*. Biochem. J. 179, 99-107.
9. Roehl, R.A. and Vinopal, R.T. 1980. Genetic locus, distinct from *ptsM*, affecting enzyme IIA/11B function in *Escherichia coli* K-12. J. Bacteriol. 142, 120-130.
10. Riley, M., and Anilionis 1978. Evolution of the bacterial genome. Ann. Rev. Microbiol. 32, 519-560.
11. Varenne, S., Casse, F., Chippaux, M., and Pascal, M.C. 1975. A mutant of *Escherichia coli* deficient in pyruvate formate lyase. Molec. gen. Genet. 141, 181-184.
12. Pascal, M.C., Casse, F., Chippaux, M., and Lepelletier, M. 1973. Genetic analysis of mutants of *Salmonella typhimurium* deficient in formate dehydrogenase activity. Molec. gen. Genet. 120, 337-340.
13. Pascal, M. C., Casse, F., Chippaux, M., Lepelletier, M. 1975. Genetic analysis of mutants of *Escherichia coli* K 12 and *Salmonella typhimurium* LT2 deficient in hydrogenase activity. Molec. gen. Genet. 141, 173-179.
14. Ruiz-Herrera, J., and Alvarez, A. 1972. A physiological study of formate dehydrogenase, formate oxidase and hydrogenlyase from *Escherichia coli* K-12. Antonie van Leeuwenhoek 38, 479-491.
15. Mandrand-Berthelot, M.-A., Wee, M.Y.K., and Haddock, B.A. 1978. An improved method for the identification and characterization of mutants of *Escherichia coli* deficient in formate dehydrogenase activity. FEMS Microbiol. Lett. 4, 37-40.
16. Brown, T.D.K., Jones-Mortimer, M.C., and Kornberg, H.L. 1977. The enzymatic interconversion of acetate and acetyl-CoA in *Escherichia coli*. J. Gen. Microbiol. 102, 327-336.
17. LeVine, S.M., Ardeshir, F., and Ames, G.F.-L. 1980. Isolation and characterization of acetate kinase and phosphotransacetylase mutants of *Escherichia coli* and *Salmonella typhimurium*. J. Bacteriol. 143. 1081-1085.
18. Clark, D.P., and Cronan, J.E. Jr. 1980. Acetaldehyde coenzyme A dehydrogenase of *Escherichia coli*. J. Bacteriol 144, 179-184.
19. Guest, J.R. 1979. Anaerobic growth of *Escherichia coli* K 12 with fumarate as terminal electron acceptor. Genetic studies with menaquinone and fluoroacetate-resistant mutants. J. Gen. Microbiol.115, 259-271.
20. Fraenkel, D.G. 1981. Carbohydrate metabolism. In Molecular Genetics of Yeast. Cold Spring Harbor, in press.
21. Lobo, Z., and Maitra, P.K. 1977. Physiological role of glucose phosphorylating enzymes in *Saccharomyces cerevisiae*. Arch. Biochem. Biophys. 182, 639-645.

22. Ciriacy, M., and Breitenbach, I. 1979. Physiological effects of seven different blocks in glycolysis in *Saccharomyces cerevisiae*. J. Bacteriol. 139, 152–160.

23. Ciriacy, M. 1979. Isolation and characterization of further *cis*- and trans-acting regulatory elements involved in the synthesis of glucose repressible alcohol dehydrogenase (ADHII) in *Saccharomyces cerevisiae*. Mol. Gen. Genet. 176, 427–431.

24. Lam, K.-B., and Marmur, J. 197. Isolation and characterization of *Saccharomyces cerevisiae* glycolysis mutants. J. Bacteriol. 130, 746–749.

25. Wills, C., and Phelps, J. 1975. A technique for the isolation of yeast alcohol dehydrogenase mutants with altered substrate specificity. Arch. Biochem. Biophys. 167, 627–637.

26. Morrissey, A.T.E. 1971. Phosphofructokinase mutants of *Escherichia coli*. Ph.D. Thesis, Harvard University.

27. Wolf, R.E. Jr., and Fraenkel, D.G. 1974. Isolation of specialized transducing bacteriophages for gluconate 6-phosphate dehydrogenase (*gnd*) of *Escherichia coli*. J. Bacteriol. 117, 468–476.

28. Clarke, L., and Carbon, J. 1976. A colony bank containing synthetic Col El hybrid plasmids representative of the entire *E. coli* genome. Cell 9, 91–99.

29. Thomson, J. 1977. *E. coli* phosphofructokinase synthesized in vitro from a Col El hybrid plasmid. Gene 1, 347–356.

30. Hitzeman, R.A., Chinault, A.C., Kingsman, A.J., and Carbon, J. 1979. Detection of *E. coli* clones containing specific yeast genes by immunological screening. ICN-UCLA Symp. Molec. Cell Biol. 14, 57–68.

31. Holland, M.J., and Holland, J.P. 1979. Isolation and characterization of a gene coding for glyceraldehyde-3-phosphate dehydrogenase from *Saccharomyces cerevisiae*. J. Biol. Chem. 254, 5466–5474.

32. Holland, M.J., Hager, G.L., and Rutter, W.J. 1977. Characterization of purified poly(adenylic acid)-containing messenger ribonucleic acid from *Saccharomyces cerevisiae*. Biochemistry 16, 8–16.

33. Holland, J.P., and Holland, M.J. 1979. The primary structure of a glyceraldehyde-3-P dehydrogenase gene from *Saccharomyces cerevisiae*. J. Biol. Chem. 254, 9839–9845.

34. Broach, J.R., Strathern, J.N., and Hicks, J.B. 1979. Transformation in yeast: development of a hybrid cloning vector and isolation of the CAN1 gene. Gene 8, 121–133.

35. Reichelt, J.L., and Doelle, H.W. 1971. The influence of dissolved oxygen concentration on phosphofructokinase and the glucose metabolism of *Escherichia coli* K-12. Antonie van leeuwenhoek 37, 497–506.

36. Kotlarz, D., Garreau, H., and Buc, H. 1975. Regulation of the amount and of the activity of phosphofructokinases and pyruvat kinases in *Escherichia coli*. Biochim. Biophys. Acta 381, 257–268.

37.   Wolf, R.E., Jr., Prather, D.M. and Shea, F.M. 1979. Growth-
       rate-dependent alternation of 6-phosphogluconate dehydrogenase
       and glucose 6-phosphate dehydrogenase levels in *Escherichia
       coli* K-12. J. Bacteriol. 139, 1093-1096.
38.   Oura, E. 1974. Effect of aeration intensity on the biochemical
       composition of Baker's yeast. I. Factors affecting the type
       of metabolism. Biotech. Bioeng. XVI, 1197-1212.
39.   Maitra, P.K., and Lobo, Z. 1971a. A kinetic study of glycoly-
       tic enzyme synthesis in yeast. J. Biol. Chem. 246, 475-488.
40.   Maitra, P.K., and Lobo, Z. 1971b. Control of glycolytic
       enzyme synthesis in yeast by products of the hexokinase
       reaction. J. Biol. Chem. 246, 489-499.
41.   Daldal, F., Babul, J., Guixe, V., and Fraenkel, D.G. 1981.
       Gluconeogenic impairment in a phosphofructokinase mutant of
       Escherichia coli. To be submitted.
42.   Daldal, F., and Fraenkel, D.G. 1981. Assessment of gluconeo-
       genic futile cycling in *Escherichia coli*. To be submitted.
43.   Bachmann, B.J., and Low, K.B. 1980. Linkage map of *Escherichia
       coli* K-12, Edition 6. Microbiol. Rev. 44, 1-56.
44.   Thomson, J., Gerstenberger, P.D., Goldberg, D., Gociar, E.,
       Orozco de Silva, A., and Fraenkel, D.G. 1979. ColEl hybrid
       plasmids for *Escherichia coli* genes of glycolysis and the
       hexose monophosphate shunt. J. Bacteriol. 137, 502-506.
45.   Clifton, D., and Fraenkel, D.G. 1980. The *gcr* (glycolysis
       regulation) mutation of *Saccharomyces cerevisiae*. (To be sub-
       mitted.)
46.   Robinson, J.P., and Fraenkel, D.G. 1978. Allosteric and non-
       allosteric *E. coli* phosphofructokinases: effects on growth.
       Biochem. Biophys. Res. Commun. 81, 858-863.

MECHANISMS OF YEAST GENETICS

Helen Greer

Cellular and Developmental Biology
Harvard University
Cambridge, Massachusetts 02138

Saccharomyces cerevisiae is a lower eukaryote ideal for many
current biological studies. It shares certain properties with higher
eukaryotes: a nucleus containing multiple chromosomes packed in
chromatin structures, and specialized organelles such as vacuoles and
mitochondria. In addition, the organization of yeast structural
genes is similar to that of higher eukaryotic cells: most functionally related genes are scattered on different chromosomes rather than
linked together in operons (21). Yet, while yeast are more complex
than bacteria, they still share many of the technical advantages
which permitted rapid progress in the genetic and biochemical studies
of prokaryotic organisms. Some of the properties which make yeast
particularly amenable to study are their short generation time, the
existence of both stable haploids and diploids, and the ease of
replica plating and mutant isolation. Furthermore, the sophisticated
classical genetics of yeast allows one to fully exploit recent technological advances in genetic engineering.

To make optimal use of the yeast system for the commercial
production of certain gene products, it is clearly desirable to
understand the advantages and limitations of the organism. An overview of the general "state of the art" concerning classical and
molecular genetics in *Saccharomyces cerevisiae* is presented in this
report. Complementary reviews should also be consulted (44,51,57).

CLASSICAL GENETICS

A. Life Cycle

Saccharomyces cerevisiae is generally a heterothallic organism

217

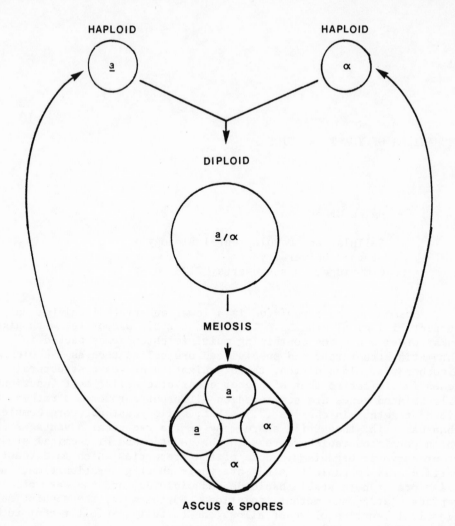

Figure 1.   The heterothallic life cycle of *Saccharomyces cerevisiae*.

with two stable haploid cell types, a and α (Figure 1).   These cells
grow vegetatively by budding, doubling about every 90 minutes (24).
The a and α cells can mate with each other, which results in zygote
formation, nuclear fusion, and the production of stable a/α diploids.
Like haploid cells, the diploids also grow vegetatively by budding.
Under appropriate starvation conditions (growth on potassium acetate
in the absence of a nitrogen source, (19)), a/α diploids are induced
to sporulate.   The process of meiosis results in the formation of a
tetrad;   four spores enclosed in an ascus sac.   Each tetrad contains two a and two α haploid spores.   Upon germination, these cells

can in turn mate to start a new cycle.

Heterothallic yeast strains can become homothallic by the introduction of the HO gene (28,67). The HO gene directs switching of
mating type in the presence of two other genes, HMR, and HML. Therefore, in homothallic strains, haploid cells are very unstable,
rapidly giving rise to a mixture of a and a cells which mate to
produce stable diploids. Because of the instability of homothallic
strains, heterothallic strains, which can be maintained as stable
haploids, are standardly used for most yeast studies.

B. Meiotic Analysis

The existence of both haploid and diploid states in yeast
greatly facilitates genetic studies, as the four progeny of meiosis
can be readily analyzed. Sporulation of diploid cells is induced
by growing the cells first on rich media, then transferring them to
starvation media (19). The resulting tetrads, which consist of
four meiotic spores enclosed in an ascus sac, are treated with snail
enzyme, glusulase, to digest the ascus sac and liberate the spores.
Genotypes of the meiotic progeny can then be determined using either
random spore or tetrad analysis.

1. Random Spore Analysis. Random spore analysis is technically easier than tetrad analysis. Average progeny ratios are
obtained from a mixed population of spores from many tetrads. After
digestion of the asci with glusulase, they are vortexed to ensure
separation of the spores from their tetrads. There are several
genetic ways to distinguish the haploid spores from the unsporulated
diploid cells that are also present in the mixture (Table I).

(a) Haploids can be identified if one of the original
parent strains carries the recessive ade2 mutation (adenine auxotrophy). This mutation confers a red color to the cells because
of the accumulation of an intermediate (18,59). If ade2 is heterozygous in a cross, all of the diploids and one half of the haploids
from meiosis will be white (wild type), while the other half of the
haploids will be red. Only the red colonies are picked and analyzed.
Unless a gene is linked to ADE2, this procedure will produce a
random sampling of haploid meiotic progeny.
(b) Diploids can be selected against if one of the parent
strains carries the can^R (canavanine resistance) marker. Canavanine, an analog of arginine, inhibits the growth of strains unless
they carry the can^R mutation. The can^R mutation is recessive to the
wildtype CAN^S (canavanine sensitive) allele. If can^R is heterozygous in the diploid, all of the diploids and one half of the haploids
will be CAN^S, and the other half of the haploids will be can^R.
Haploid progeny can therefore be selected directly on canavanine
medium (56) and
(c) If it is not convenient to use either of the above

markers in a cross, colony size can be used to distinguish haploids
from diploids. In general, haploid colonies are smaller than
diploid colonies.

The haploid progeny identified by any of the above procedures
are further analyzed to determine their phenotype by standard
replica plating procedures. Average segregation ratios for an
entire population of cells are thus obtained.

2. Tetrad Analysis: Alternatively, the four spores of individual tetrads can be analyzed as units rather than as random spores
While this procedure is technically more difficult than random spore
analysis, it yields much more genetic information. A suspension of
glusulase-treated tetrads is gently streaked onto an agar slab
placed on a glass slide so that the four spores from each tetrad
remain together (38). The slide is inverted on a microscope equippe
with a needle and a micromanipulator (55). The four spores are then
physically separated using the micromanipulator and needle, and
placed at regular intervals onto the agar slab. The slab is then
transferred to an agar petri plate, where the spores germinate to
produce colonies. These are scored by standard replica plating
procedures. A chromosomal gene which is heterozygous in the cross
will segregate 2^+ : 2^- in each tetrad. Additional information can
be obtained by simultaneously comparing segregation patterns from
two genes.

In a cross of AB x ab, the tetrads are genetically analyzed and
divided into three categories: parental ditype (PD), nonparental
ditype (NPD), or tetratype (TT) (Table II). The ratios of these
different classes indicate Mendelian versus non-Mendelian inheritance of genes A and B, centromere linkage of A and B, linkage of
A and B to each other, and actual map distance. This information
is important for classical genetic studies as well as for cloning
experiments, where it permits determination of whether a plasmid
is episomal or has integrated into the chromosome, and whether
integration has occurred at a specific locus.

An abbreviated review of tetrad analysis follows. Tetrad
analysis always compares two markers to each other. In the cross
AB x ab, in which genes A and B are unlinked, the process of meiosis
results in duplication of chromosomes, followed by their segregation
Chromosomal segregation occurs in one of two possible ways depending
upon the orientation of the chromosomes at the metaphase plate.
The chromosomes then segregate a second time. Depending upon the
orientation of the chromosomes prior to the first division, the
second division produces a PD or an NPD tetrad (Figure 2). Since
the original chromosome orientation is random, PD = NPD. Thus a
1:1 ratio of PD:NPD indicates that genes A and B are unlinked.

If one of the genes, A, is centromere linked, and a single

TABLE I
Random Spore Analysis

criterion	2n	n	n
ade2	+/ade2 *(white)*	+ *(white)*	ade2 *(red)*
can^R	+/can^R *(sensitive)*	+ *(sensitive)*	can^R *(resistant)*
size	large	small	small

TABLE II
Tetrad Types

AB x ab

Parental ditype (PD)	Non-parental ditype (NPD)	Tetratype (TT)
AB	Ab	AB
AB	Ab	Ab
ab	aB	aB
ab	aB	ab

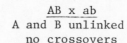

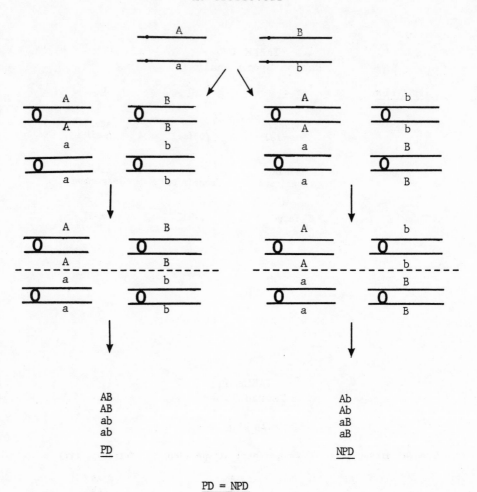

Figure 2. Tetrad pattern of a cross AB x ab in which genes A and B are unlinked and no crossovers occur. A and a are two alleles of one gene, and B and b are alleles of another gene. The chromosomes are depicted as lines and their centromeres as circles. The four chromosomes carrying either gene A, B, a, or b, duplicate and line up at the metaphase plate in one of two possible orientations. The left and right side of the figure illustrates these possibilities. The chromosomes then segregate from each other as shown by the dotted line. A second segregation then occurs to produce four haploid spores in either a PD or NPD tetrad.

crossover occurs between gene B and its centromere, a recombinant
TT tetrad is produced (Fig. 3). As the distance between B and its
centromere increases, the number of crossovers increases, producing
more TT, as well as additional PD and NPD, tetrads. When gene B is
completely unlinked to its centromere, the ratio of these tetrads can
be calculated to be 1 PD : 1 NPD : 4 TT (47). Intuitively, it is
clear that if gene B is closer to the centromere, the number of
crossovers and recombinant tetrads will diminish. Since a TT is

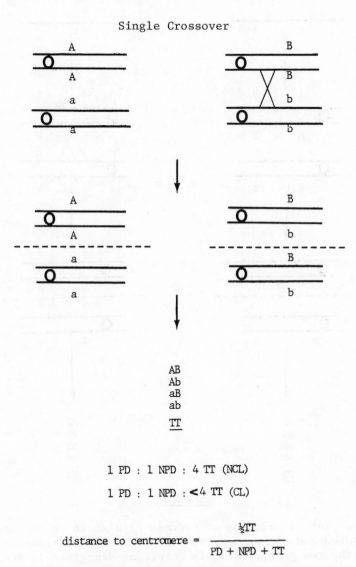

Single Crossover

AB
Ab
aB
ab

TT

1 PD : 1 NPD : 4 TT (NCL)

1 PD : 1 NPD : < 4 TT (CL)

$$\text{distance to centromere} = \frac{\frac{1}{2}TT}{PD + NPD + TT}$$

Figure 3. Tetrad pattern of a cross AB x ab in which genes A and B
are unlinked and a single crossover occurs. Meiosis occurs as described in Fig. 2 to produce a TT tetrad.

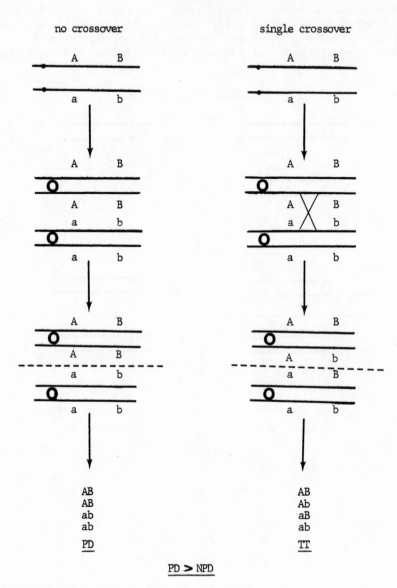

Figure 4. Tetrad patterns of a cross AB x ab in which genes A and B are linked and either no crossovers or a single crossover occurs between the two genes. Meiosis occurs as described in Fig. 2 to produce either a PD or TT tetrad.

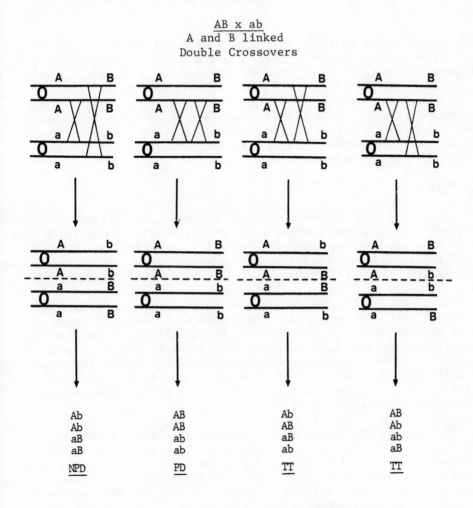

Figure 5. Tetrad patterns of a cross AB x ab in which genes A and
B are linked and a double crossover occurs between the two genes.
Different tetrads are produced depending upon which DNA strands are
involved in the crossover events. Meiosis occurs as described in
Fig. 2.

the only unique recombinant tetrad type, centromere linkage of gene B is indicated by ratios of 1 PD : 1 NPD : < 4 TT (47). The actual distance of gene B to the centromere can be calculated as ½ (TT)/ (PD + NPD + TT).

In the cross AB x ab, in which genes A and B are linked, if no crossovers occur, only PD tetrads are produced; no NPD tetrads appear (Figure 4). Therefore, if PD > NPD, it indicates linkage of genes A and B. A single crossover between A and B will generate a TT, whereas a double crossover will generate a TT, NPD, or PD tetrad, depending upon which DNA strands are involved (Figures 4 and 5). Analysis of these multiple crossover ratios permits calculation of the distance in centimorgans between two markers by the formula: (100) (TT + 6NPD)/ 2(PD + NPD + TT) (50).

C. Mapping

The results of extensive mapping studies using tetrad analysis indicate that yeast possess 17 chromosomes (46,47). About two hundred genes have already been mapped (Figure 6). As additional genes are discovered, their map positions on the yeast genome can be determined in a variety of ways (Figure 7).

1. Gene Linkage: A gene can be mapped by determining its linkage to other markers whose map positions are already known. The major problem with this approach is the high level of generalized recombination yeast cells undergo; the genome is 3500 centimorgans (46). Therefore, even physically proximal genes appear to be gene-tically unlinked. The sets of multiply marked strains that do exist for such mapping studies are difficult to use because they must carry so many mutations.

2. Centromere Linkage: If centromere linkage of the unknown gene can be established, it greatly aids the mapping process (25). Subsequent crosses to strains carrying only centromere linked muta-tions on each of the 17 chromosomes will then suffice to localize the gene. Therefore, initial mapping studies generally include a cross to a strain carrying a single centromere linked mutation to determine if the tetrad ratios are 1 PD : 1 NPD : < 4 TT, indicating centromere linkage of the unknown gene.

3. Trisomic Mapping: The principle of trisomic mapping is that extra copies of a given chromosome perturb the normal 2:2 segrega-tion ratios of markers on that chromosome (31,46,71). If a haploid strain with a mutation on a given chromosome, (-), is crossed to a strain which is disomic for that chromosome, (+/+), the resulting trisomic strain, (-/+/+), will undergo meiosis to produce tetrads with aberrant ratios of $4^+ : 0^-$, $3^+ : 1^-$, and $2^+ : 2^-$, for the mutation in question. Concomitant aberrant ratios for an unknown mutation and another known mutation indicates the chromosome on which

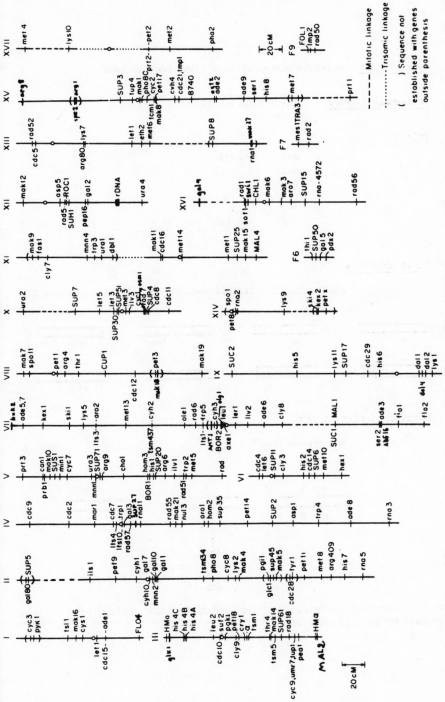

Figure 6. Genetic linkage map of *Saccharomyces cerevisiae*. From Mortimer and Hawthorne (47) with additions from the Abstracts Book of the meeting on "The Molecular Biology of Yeast", August 14 to August 19, 1979, Cold Spring Harbor Laboratory, Cold Spring Harbor, N.Y.

1. <u>Gene linkage</u>. multiply marked strains (3500 centimorgans)

2. <u>Centromere linkage</u>. 1 PD: 1 NPD: < 4 TT

3. <u>Trisomic</u>.

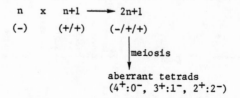

$$n \quad x \quad n{+}1 \longrightarrow 2n{+}1$$
$$(-) \qquad (+/+) \qquad (-/+/+)$$

meiosis

aberrant tetrads
$(4^+{:}0^-, \; 3^+{:}1^-, \; 2^+{:}2^-)$

4. <u>Chromosome loss</u>.

cdc6 (or cdc14) diploid $\longrightarrow 37^oC \longrightarrow 23^oC \longrightarrow$ chromosome loss

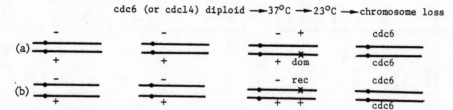

5. <u>Recombinationless strain</u>.

homozygous "rec⁻" diploid

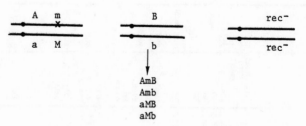

AmB
Amb
aMB
aMb

Figure 7. Mapping techniques. See text for an explanation of the
five possible procedures shown.

the unknown mutation is located. Crosses are therefore performed with strains that are each disomic for a different chromosome. Once the chromosome carrying the unmapped mutation is identified, more precise mapping studies can be undertaken to determine the linkage relationships to other genes on that particular chromosome. The major problem with trisomic mapping is the instability of strains carrying extra copies of chromosomes.

4. Chromosome Loss: The chromosome loss mapping technique depends upon the observation that diploids which are homozygous for a temperature sensitive nuclear division mutation, cdc6 or cdc14, lose chromosomes if they are grown at the non-permissive temperature and then shifted to the permissive temperature (G. Kawasaki, pers. comm.). If a set of heterozygous diploids are multiply marked with a recessive mutation on each chromosome, loss of the wild type chromosome will reveal a particular recessive mutation. The concomitant appearance of a recessive mutation with the recessive allele of the gene being mapped, indicates the chromosome map position of the unknown gene.

    (a) To map a dominant mutation, a diploid is constructed by crossing a strain carrying both the dominant mutation and cdc6 to a multiply marked strain carrying cdc6.

    (b) To map a recessive mutation, the unknown recessive mutation must first be crossed into a multiply marked haploid strain containing cdc6. The resulting strain is then crossed to a strain carrying only a cdc6 mutation. In this way, the unknown recessive allele is always on the same chromosome as one of the known recessive alleles.

The problems with this technique are: (i) not all chromosomes are lost with equal frequency during the temperature shift, and (ii) elaborate strain construction is necessary before recessive mutations can be mapped.

5. Recombinationless Strain: Basically, it is the high frequency of yeast recombination which prevents mapping of yeast genes by simple linkage studies. This problem can be circumvented by using recombinationless (rec⁻) mutants. Mapping could then be accomplished by crossing the rec⁻ mutation into the unknown mutant strain, and crossing this recombinant to another rec⁻ strain which was multiply marked with one mutation on each chromosome. The meiotic progeny of the resulting diploid would be analyzed for linkage between the unknown mutation and one of the other known recessive mutations. Although an appropriate rec⁻ yeast strain has not yet been characterized, the spoll mutation is an attractive candidate for such a mutation. This mutation greatly reduces recombination, but unfortunately also results in very poor sporulation (M. Esposito, pers. comm.).

D. Non-Mendelian Inheritance

A strain carrying a single chromosomal mutation gives a 2:2 segregation pattern when crossed to a wild type strain. However, many characteristics in yeast are not inherited from chromosomal genes. These can be identified by non-Mendelian segregation patterns of 4:0 and 0:4. However, the appearance of aberrant ratios does not, per se, indicate that a trait is carried by non-chromosomal genes. Polygenic interactions or aneuploidy can also result in aberrant tetrad ratios of 4:0, 3:1, and 2:2. These phenomena can, however, be distinguished from the non-Mendelian inheritance patterns resulting from non-chromosomal elements (e.g., mitochondria, $2u$ circles, and killer particles) by additional genetic crosses.

1. Mitochondria: Most ATP production in the yeast cell occurs via oxidative phosphorylation, localized in the mitochondria (4,60). There are approximately 20-50 mitochondria per cell (72), each containing a 75 kb genome encoding mitochondrial rRNAs, tRNAs and several cytochrome and ATPase polypeptides. Physically, the mitochondrial DNA resembles bacterial DNA in that it is circular (35). Yet, genetic and molecular studies of mitochondrial DNA have revealed the existence of a mosaic gene organization, analogous to some nuclear genes of higher eukaryotes. The mRNA from the cob-box (cytochrome b) and oxi-3 (cytochrome oxidase) are processed from larger precursors (13). Many mutations exist which block this maturation event. It has been shown that the cytochrome b intervening sequence itself codes for a trans-acting diffusible polypeptide necessary for this mRNA splicing (41).

A unique feature of yeast cells is their ability to survive without mitochondria; they can use the less efficient fermentation pathway as an alternative energy producer. Mutants which have lost part or all of their mitochondrial DNA are called p^- (42). Such mutants are easily obtained by ethidium bromide treatment of the cells (48). p^- mutants are respiratory deficient because of a loss of cytochrome function; consequently, they cannot use non-fermentable carbon sources, e.g., glycerol, ethanol, lactate, or acetate. Thus, yeast is an excellent organism for mitochondrial or fermentation studies.

2. $2u$ Circles: $2u$ circles are autonomously replicating native yeast DNA plasmids. While their function is not known, they are not essential for cell viability since certain strains have been shown to contain no $2u$ circles (43). Most strains, however, contain about 60 copies of the $2u$ circle per cell (15,35). The plasmids probably reside in the nucleus and have been shown to produce poly-A containing mRNA (7,8).

The majority of these plasmids are unit size, 6.2 kilobases, though some are found as dimers or multimers (11,52). The $2u$ circle contains two short inverted repeats separated by two large unique sequences. Both orientations of one of the unique sequences are normally generated *in vivo* by intramolecular recombination (23,36). These plasmids have been used extensively in the construction of hybrid cloning vectors for yeast transformation experiments.

3. <u>Killer</u>: Killer strains contain double stranded RNA which codes for a toxin. The toxin is secreted and is lethal to non-killer strains. Generally, killer strains are resistant to their own toxin, due to an immunity factor which is also encoded by the RNA (9,10). Killer RNA is present in the cytoplasm of killer strains in several copies per cell (5). This RNA is encapsulated in non-infectious virus-like particles and is transmitted by cytoplasmic mixing between mating cells (27,62). Many chromosomal genes, in addition to plasmid genes, appear to be essential for the expression and maintenance of the killer trait (70).

E. <u>Mutagenesis</u>

The ability to maintain yeast strains as stable haploids makes yeast far more amenable to mutant selection than other eukaryotes, because haploidy permits the isolation of recessive mutations. Many mutagens including EMS, nitrous acid, nitrosoguanidine, ICR, UV, and X-rays can be used for yeast mutagenesis (45). The treated yeast cells can then be screened for the desired mutation. By using a combination of different mutagens and selection procedures, detailed fine structure mapping can be achieved. One example is the <u>his4</u> region (which encodes the third, second, and tenth steps in the histidine biosynthetic pathway; (17)), in which hundreds of mutations, including missense, nonsense, frameshift, deletions, and insertions, have been isolated and mapped (G. Fink, pers. comm.; H. Greer, unpubl.).

In many cases, positive selection procedures can be devised to obtain desired mutants. In general, these procedures involve growing cells under conditions where wild type growth is inhibited while growth of the desired mutant is resistant to inhibition (Table III) For example, certain ura⁻ mutants are resistant to ureidosuccinic acid (2,39), cytochrome c mutants are resistant to chlorolactate (58), <u>gal1</u> and <u>gal4</u> mutations are resistant to galactose in a <u>gal10</u> background (16), <u>lys2</u> and <u>lys5</u> mutations are able to use a-amino adipate as a nitrogen source (12), and various mutations are resistant to different amino acid analogs or drugs. In addition, resistance to any one of the above substrates can be used as a selection for inactivation of a nonsense suppressor if resistance results from a suppressible nonsense mutation.

In most cases, however, a direct selection for a particular mutation is not possible. In such situations, standard screening

TABLE III
Positive Selections

phenotype	genotype

1. galactose

	gal^S	gal10	(epimerase)
	gal^R	gal10 gal1	(galactokinase)
		gal10 gal4	(positive regulator)

2. ureidosuccinic acid

	USA^S	wild type	
	USA^R	ura1	(dihydroorotate dehydrogenase)
		ura3	(OMP decarboxylase)
		ura5	(OMP pyrophosphorylase)

3. alpha-amino adipate

	aaa^S	wild type	
	aaa^R	lys2	(2-amino adipate reductase)
		lys5	(2-amino adipate reductase)

4. canavanine

| | can^S | wild type | |
| | can^R | can1 | (arginine permease) |

5. chlorolactate

| | chl^S | wild type | |
| | chl^R | cyc1 | (iso-1-cytochrome c) |

6. suppressor

| | can^S | SUP(amber) can^R(amber) auxo(amber) |
| | can^R | sup$^-$ can^R(amber) auxo(amber) |

procedures using replica plating to look for non-growth of colonies on a particular media are often used. In addition, several enrichment procedures for non-growing cells exist. These procedures resemble bacterial penicillin selections in that conditions favor survival of mutant over wild type cells. One such procedure is nystatin enrichment (Figure 8). Nystatin is an antibiotic which only kills actively growing cells (61,68). Different researchers have reported varying degrees of success with this procedure. An alternative procedure is to use the inositol selection (Figure 9). This technique takes advantage of the fact that starvation for inositol of ino$^-$ mutants (inositol auxotrophy) kills only actively growing cells (26). The disadvantage of the inositol enrichment procedure is that ino$^-$ mutations must be crossed into any strain in which mutant searches are to be undertaken. A third procedure is heat shock enrichment (Figure 10). Heat shock only kills exponentailly growing cells (69). This procedure is versatile in that no special strains are needed.

The sophisticated yeast genetic system permits standard genetic analyses, including mapping, complementation testing, and dominance

Nystatin Enrichment

Antibiotic only kills actively growing cells.

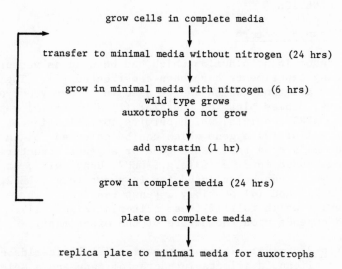

grow cells in complete media

↓

transfer to minimal media without nitrogen (24 hrs)

↓

grow in minimal media with nitrogen (6 hrs)
wild type grows
auxotrophs do not grow

↓

add nystatin (1 hr)

↓

grow in complete media (24 hrs)

↓

plate on complete media

↓

replica plate to minimal media for auxotrophs

Figure 8.   Nystatin enrichment procedure for mutants from Snow (61) and Thouvenot and Bourgeois (68).

Inositol-less Death

Inositol starvation only kills actively growing ino⁻ cells.

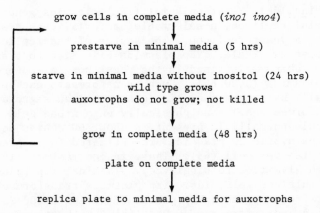

grow cells in complete media (*ino1 ino4*)

↓

prestarve in minimal media (5 hrs)

↓

starve in minimal media without inositol (24 hrs)
wild type grows
auxotrophs do not grow; not killed

↓

grow in complete media (48 hrs)

↓

plate on complete media

↓

replica plate to minimal media for auxotrophs

Figure 9.   Inositol-less death enrichment procedure for mutants from Henry et al. (26).

testing of these mutations. This property also makes yeast an ideal choice for molecular biological studies.

MOLECULAR GENETICS

A. <u>Yeast Plasmid Vectors</u>

     Many recombinant plasmids which can be used as vectors for yeast cloning experiments have been constructed (6). The most versa tile vectors are those which can be used in either yeast or bacterial host systems. These plasmids contain: (1) a bacterial replicon, such as the pBR322 origin, which permits amplification of the plasmi in <i>E. coli</i> cells; (2) a gene which can be selected for in <i>E. coli</i> cells, such as a drug resistance gene or a yeast structural gene which is expressed in <i>E. coli</i> (e.g., <u>LEU2</u>, <u>URA3</u>, <u>HIS3</u>, or <u>TRP1</u>); (3) a gene which can be selected for in yeast (e.g., <u>LEU2</u>, <u>URA3</u>, <u>HIS3</u>, or <u>TRP1</u>); and (4) possibly a yeast replicon. Three types of plasmids exist which fulfill these criteria (Figure 11). The choice of plasmid depends upon the nature of the experiment.

     1. <u>YIp Plasmids</u>: Yeast integrating (YIp) plasmids contain a bacterial replicon, a selectable bacterial gene and a selectable yeast gene, but do not contain a yeast replicon. Yeast transforma- tion occurs as a result of the integration of the entire plasmid into the yeast genome at a region of homology (29,32,65). Such integrations can be confirmed by tetrad analysis in which the trans- formed gene shows Mendelian segregation patterns of $2^+ : 2^-$. YIp plasmids transform yeast cells rather inefficiently, giving frequen- cies of about 1-10 transformant colonies per microgram of plasmid DNA (32,65). These cells contain a stable single copy of the trans- formed gene.

     2. <u>YEp Plasmids</u>: Yeast episomal (YEp) plasmids generally con- tain a bacterial replicon, a selectable bacterial gene, a selectable yeast gene, and a yeast replicon. The source of the replicon is the native yeast $2u$ circle. YEp plasmids give rise to transformants as a result of being maintained in the yeast host as autonomously replicating plasmids (3,20,65). Such transformants can be confirmed both genetically by tetrad analysis (non-Mendelian segregation ratio for the transformed gene), and physically on agarose gels. The native $2u$ circle normally is present in about 60 copies per cell (15), while the hybrid $2u$ plasmids are estimated to be present in about 5-10 copies per cell (65). Thus, in contrast to YIp transfor- mations, which give rise to single copy plasmids, YEp transformation give rise to multicopy plasmids. YEp plasmids transform cells with a much higher frequency than YIp plasmids, giving 5,000-20,000 trans formant colonies per microgram of DNA (65). Such transformants are mitotically unstable when grown under non-selective conditions.

Heat Shock

Heat shock only kills exponentially growing cells.

```
     ┌──────────►
     │      grow cells in complete media to stationary phase
     │                          │ dilute
     │                          ▼
     │              grow in minimal media (8 hrs)
     │            wild type cells enter exponential phase
     │            auxotrophs remain in stationary phase
     │                          │
     │                          ▼
     │                 heat shock (53°C, 6')
     └──────────                │
                                ▼
                    plate on complete media
                                │
                                ▼
        replica plate to minimal media for auxotrophs
```

Figure 10. Heat shock enrichment procedure for mutants from Walton et al. (69), as modified by D. Morisata and H. Greer (unpub.).

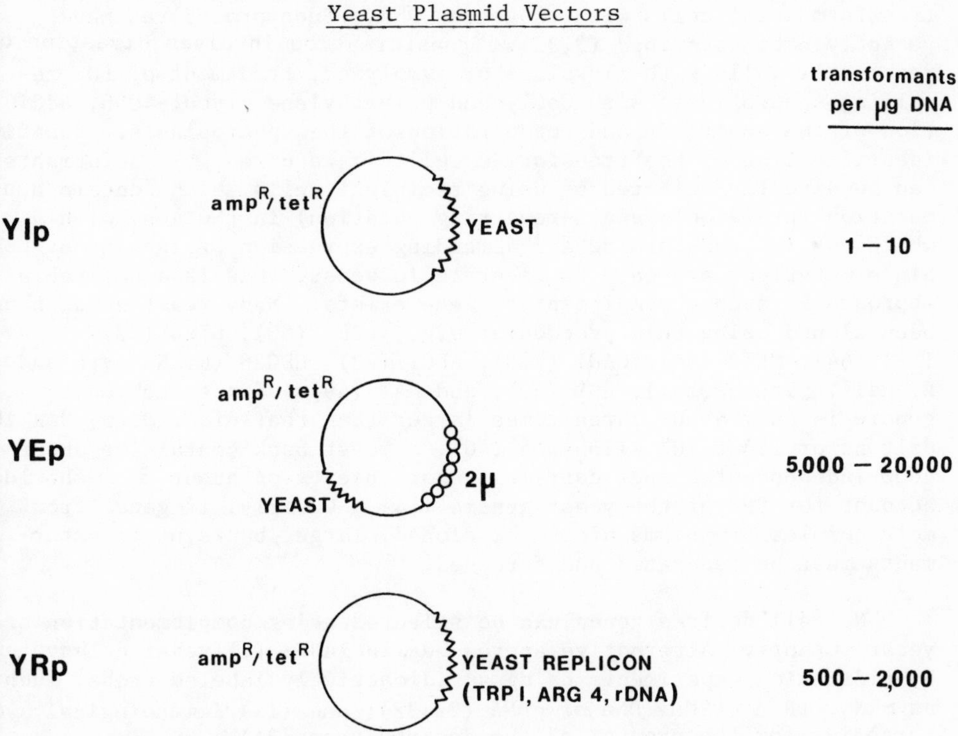

Yeast Plasmid Vectors

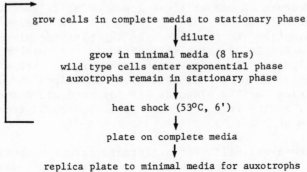

transformants
per μg DNA

YIp amp^R/tet^R YEAST   1 — 10

YEp amp^R/tet^R YEAST 2μ   5,000 — 20,000

YRp amp^R/tet^R YEAST REPLICON
(TRP I, ARG 4, rDNA)   500 — 2,000

Figure 11.   Three types of yeast plasmid vectors.

3. YRp Plasmids: Yeast replicating (YRp) plasmids contain a
bacterial replicon, a selectable bacterial gene, a selectable yeast
gene,and a chromosomal, rather than an episomal,yeast replicon. Suc
replicons are present, for example, in plasmids containing the yeast
TRP1 gene (65), ARG4 gene (37), and the ribosomal DNA genes (66).
Thus, the presence of one of these genes on a YRp vector serves the
function of simultaneously supplying both a yeast selectable marker
and replicon. Like YEp plasmids, the YRp plasmids give rise to tran
formants as a result of being maintained in the yeast host as autonomously replicating plasmids. Such transformants are mitotically
unstable when grown under non-selective conditions (63). Transforma
tion frequencies for YRp plasmids are intermediate between YIp and
YEp plasmids, giving frequencies of about 500-2,000 transformants
per microgram of DNA (65).

Given the availability of different vectors, experiments can
be designed which require either integrating or episomal, or single
or multi-copy plasmids.

B. Transformation

The use of the plasmids described above rests on the ability to
transform yeast cells with exogenous DNA. Such procedures have
recently been described (3,32). Transformation involves digestion of
yeast cell walls with glusulase or zymolyase, treatment of the resulting spheroplasts with $CaCl_2$ and polyethylene glycol-4000, addition of the donor DNA,and regeneration of the spheroplasts. Positiv
identification of the transformed cells is required. Transformants
can be directly selected by using recipient cells which contain a
mutation (preferably a non-reverting mutation) in the gene with
which one is transforming and demanding expression of that gene.
Since mutations are easy to generate in yeast, this is a desirable
approach if such a complementary gene exists. Many yeast genes have
been cloned using this procedure: e.g., LEU2 (53), HIS4 (33),
TYR1 (64), MET2 (64), CAN1 (7,8), ADC1 (73), CDC28 (K. Nasmyth and
B. Hall, pers. comm.), HML (30), and MAT (49). Since the yeast
genome is only about three times larger than that of *E. coli*, 9 x 10
daltons or 1.4 x 10^4 kilobases (40), a yeast bank containing about
4600 independent clones carrying yeast inserts of about 15 kb should
account for 99% of the yeast genome (14). Clearly, if genes from
more complex organisms are to be cloned, larger banks of transformants must be generated and screened.

Not all desired genes can be selected using complementation of
yeast mutants. Alternative approaches include: (i) yeast colony
hybridization experiments using a radioactively labeled probe, such
as mRNA, rRNA, tRNA, DNA or cDNA (22,32); and (ii) immunological
screening for the product of the desired gene (34).

C. *In vitro* Mutagenesis

Once the desired gene is cloned, it can be manipulated *in vitro* to alter the levels of production of the gene product: (i) promoter mutagenesis of the cloned gene; or (ii) fusion of the structural part of the cloned gene to a different yeast promoter. Various procedures for *in vitro* mutagenesis have been developed (1). Point mutations can be obtained using chemical mutagenesis, insertions can be created using bacterial transposable elements or other defined DNA sequences, and deletions can be generated by exonuclease or restriction enzyme digestion.

DNA which has been altered *in vitro* can be reintroduced into the yeast host by transformation (54). An example is illustrated in Figure 12. A PstI fragment containing the yeast his4 region is subcloned into a YIp plasmid containing the yeast ura3 gene. The his4ABC region (coding for three steps in the histidine biosynthetic pathway) can be deleted by subjecting the YIp plasmid to limited digestion with the restriction endonuclease EcoRI, running the digest on an agarose gel, eluting the desired fragment, and recircularizing by intra-molecular ligation. The resulting plasmid will contain the YIp sequences and some yeast sequences on either side of the his4 region at which homologous integration of the plasmid into the yeast genome can occur. This new plasmid can be used to replace the wild type chromosomal his4 region by transforming a yeast strain containing a ura3 mutation, and selecting ura$^+$ colonies (Figure 13). Duplications resulting from integration of the plasmid into the genome are unstable because of tandem regions of homology. Homologous recombination will result in the loss of vector sequences, the ura$^+$ gene, and the host his4 region. These strains can be identified by selecting ura$^-$ cells (on ureidosuccinic acid) and simultaneously screening for his$^-$ cells. The above scheme is extremely useful for introducing precisely defined deletions into yeast and of particular importance due to the difficulty of obtaining *in vivo* deletions.

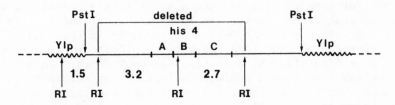

Figure 12. A YIp-his4 plasmid. The PstI fragment containing the yeast his4 region is subcloned into a YIp plasmid. The arrows indicate the PstI or EcoRI restriction endonuclease sites, and the numbers indicate the size of DNA in kilobases between EcoRI sites (M. Igo and H. Greer, unpub.). The bracket indicates the EcoRI fragment which must be deleted to remove all his4 sequences.

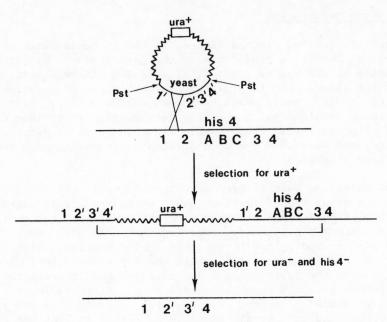

Figure 13. Insertion of the YIp-his4 deletion plasmid carrying the
URA3 gene into the yeast chromosomal genome (see Fig. 12). Integration occurs at a region of homology between the flanking his4 sequences still present on the plasmid (1',2') and the chromosome (1,2)
to produce a tandem duplication. Subsequently, the vector can recombine out using the regions of homology 3',4' and 3,4, resulting in
the stable introduction of the deleted his4 region in place of the
wild type his4 region.

    Other types of mutations, in addition to deletions, can also
be easily introduced into the yeast genome using cloned plasmids.
An example is illustrated in Fig. 14. A URA3 YIp plasmid containing
the his4 region is subjected to *in vitro* mutagenesis and used as the
donor DNA for transformations into a yeast strain containing a ura3
mutation. Ura⁺ transformants are selected, resulting in his4 duplications. Homologous recombination will result in the loss of vector
sequences, the ura⁺ gene, and the wild type host regulatory region.
These can be identified by selecting for ura⁻ cells. In addition,
it is desirable to have a positive selection for retaining in the
chromosome the *in vitro* generated regulatory mutation. For example,
a leaky temperature sensitive mutation in the his4C structural gene
requires a constitutive regulatory mutation to grow under certain
conditions. In fact, any type of *in vitro* generated mutation or
rearrangement can, in principle, be inserted into the yeast genome.

    Thus, the exploitation of the yeast transformation system has

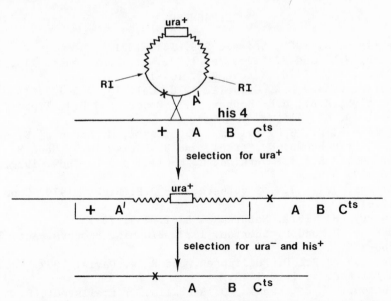

Figure 14.   Insertion of a YIp (URA3) plasmid containing part of
the his4 region (gene A) and a regulatory mutation for his4 (shown
as an "x") into the yeast chromosomal genome.   Integration and
excision occur in an analogous fashion to that described in Fig. 13.

resulted in yeast becoming the model system for recombinant DNA experiments requiring a eukaryotic host.   The development of recombinant
DNA technology, coupled with yeast genetics and transformation and
in vitro mutagenesis techniques, has precipitated a revolution in
our understanding of the molecular genetics of yeast cells.

CONCLUSION

The combination of the sophisticated nature of both classical
and molecular genetics of yeast makes it an ideal organism for both
basic gene regulation studies and also for more applied studies in
which commercial production of certain specific gene products is
desired.

ACKNOWLEDGEMENTS

I especially wish to thank Donald Morisato and Michele Igo for
help, both intellectual and technical, which was invaluable in the
writing of this manuscript. I am also grateful to Gail Mazzara for
comments on the paper and Bernard Galgoci for help with some of the
figures.

REFERENCES

1.   Abelson, J. 1980. Science 209, 1319-1321.
2.   Bach, M.L. and F. Lacroute. 1972. Mol. Gen. Genet. 115, 126-13
3.   Beggs, J.D. 1978. Nature 275, 104-109.
4.   Borst, P. and L.A. Grivell. 1978. Cell 15, 705-723.
5.   Bostian, K.A., J.E. Hopper, D.T. Roger, and D.J. Tipper. 1980.
      Cell 19, 403-414.
6.   Botstein, D., S.C. Falco, S.E. Stewart, M. Brennan, S. Scherer
      D.J. Stinchcomb, K. Struhl, and R. Davis. 1979. Gene 8, 17-24.
7.   Broach, J.R., J.F. Atkins, C. McGill, and L. Chow. 1979. Cell
      16, 827-839.
8.   Broach, J.R., J.N. Strathern, and J.B. Hicks. 1979. Gene 8,
      121-133.
9.   Bussey, H. 1972. Nature New Biol. 235, 73-75.
10.   Bussey, H. and D. Sherman. 1973. Biochim. Biophys. Acta 298,
      868-875.
11.   Cameron, J.R., P. Philippsen, and R. W. Davis. 1977. Nucleic
      Acids Res. 4, 1429-1448.
12.   Chatoo, B., F. Sherman, D. Azubalis, T. Fjellstedt, D. Mehnert
      and M. Ogur. 1979. Genetics 93:51-65.
13.   Church,G., P. Slonimski, W. Gilbert. 1979. Cell 18, 1209-1215.
14.   Clarke, L. and J. Carbon. 1976. Cell 9, 91-99.
15.   Clarke-Walker, G.D. and G. L. Miklos. 1974. Eur. J. Biochem.
      41, 263-267.
16.   Douglas, H. and D. Hawthorne. 1964. Genetics 49, 837-844.
17.   Fink, G.R. 1966. Genetics 53, 445-459.
18.   Fisher, C. 1969. Biochem. Biophys. Res. Commun. 34, 306-310.
19.   Fowell, R.R. 1969. In "The Yeasts", Vol. 1 (A.H. Rose and
      J. S. Harrison, eds.), Academic Press, N.Y.,   303-383.
20.   Gerbaud, C., P. Fournier, H. Blanc, M. Aigle, H. Heslot, and
      M. Guerineau. 1979. Gene 5, 233-253.
21.   Greer, H. and G.R. Fink. 1975. In "Methods in Cell Biology,
      Vol. XI, Yeast Cells." (D. Prescott, ed.) Academic Press, N.Y.
      247-272.
22.   Grunstein, M. and D.S. Hogness. 1975. Proc. Natl. Acad. Sci.
      USA 72, 3961-3965.
23.   Guerineau, M., C. Grandchamp, P.P. Slonimski. 1976. Proc. Natl.
      Acad. Sci. USA 73, 3030-3034.
24.   Hartwell, L.H. 1974. Bacteriol. Rev. 38, 164-198.
25.   Hawthorne, D.C. and R.K. Mortimer. 1960. Genetics 45, 1085-110
26.   Henry, S., T. Donahue, and M. Culbertson. 1975. Molec. Gen.
      Genet. 143, 5-11.
27.   Herring, A.J. and E.A. Bevan. 1974. J. Gen. Virol. 22, 387-394.
28.   Hicks, J., J. Strathern, and I. Herskowitz. 1977. In "DNA Inser
      tion Elements, Plasmids and Episomes" (A. Bukhari, J. Shapiro,
      and S. Adhya, eds.). Cold Spring Harbor Laboratory, N.Y.,
      457-462.
29.   Hicks, J.B., A. Hinnen, and G.R. Fink. 1978. Cold Spring Harbor
      Symp. Quant. Biol. 43, 1305-1313.

30.   Hicks, J., J. Strathern, and A.J. Klar. 1979. Nature 282, 478-483.

31.   Hilger, F. and R.K. Mortimer. 1980. J. Bact. 141, 270-274.

32.   Hinnen, A., J. Hicks, and G.R. Fink. 1978. Proc. Natl. Acad. Sci. USA 75, 1929-1933.

33.   Hinnen, A., P. Farabaugh, C. Ilgen, and G.R. Fink. 1979. ICN-UCLA Symp. 14, 43-50.

34.   Hitzeman, R.A., A.C. Chinault, A.J. Kingsman, and J. Carbon. 1979. INC-UCLA Symp. 14, 57-68.

35.   Hollenberg, C.P., P. Borst, E.F. Van Bruggen. 1970. Biochim. Biophys. Acta 209, 1-15.

36.   Hollenberg, C.P., A. Degelmann, B. Kustermann-Kuhn, and H.D. Royer. 1976. Proc. Natl. Acad . Sci. USA 73, 2072-2076.

37.   Hsiao, C.H. and J. Carbon. 1979. Proc. Natl. Acad. Sci. USA 76, 3829-3833.

38.   Johnston, J.R. and R.K. Mortimer. 1959. J. Bact. 78. 292.

39.   Korch, C., F. Lacroute, and F. Exinger. 1974. Mol. Gen. Genet. 133, 63-75.

40.   Lauer, G., T.M. Roberts, and L.C. Klotz. 1977. J. Mol. Biol. 114, 507-526.

41.   Lazowka, J., C. Jacq, P. Slonimski. 1980. Cell 22, 333-348.

42.   Linnane, A.W., J.M. Haslam, H.B. Lukins, and P. Nagley. 1972. Ann. Rev. Microbiol. 26, 163-198.

43.   Livingston, D.M. 1977. Genetics 86, 73-84.

44.   Mortimer, R.K. and D.C. Hawthorne. 1969. In "The Yeasts", Vol. I, (A.H. Rose and J.S. Harrison, eds.). Academic Press, N.Y. 385-460.

45.   Mortimer, R.K. and T.R. Manney. 1971. In "Chemical Mutagens" Vol. I. (A. Hollaender, ed.), Plenum Press, N.Y., p. 289-310.

46.   Mortimer, R.K. and D.C. Hawthorne 1973. Genetics 74, 33-54.

47.   Mortimer, R.K. and D.C. Hawthorne 1975. In "Methods in Cell Biology", Vol. XI (D.M. Prescott, ed.). Academic Press, N.Y. 221-233.

48.   Nagley, P. and A.W. Linnane. 1972. J. Mol. Biol. 66, 181-193.

49.   Nasmyth, K.A. and K. Tatchell. 1980. Cell 19, 753-764.

50.   Perkins, D.D. 1949. Genetics 34, 607-626.

51.   Petes, T. 1980. Ann. Rev. Biochem. 49, 845-876.

52.   Petes, T. and D.H. Williamson. 1975. Cell 4, 249-253.

53.   Ratzkin, B. and J. Carbon. 1977. Proc. Natl. Acad. Sci. USA 74, 487-491.

54.   Scherer, S. and R.W. Davis. 1979. Proc. Natl. Acad. Sci. USA 76, 4951-4955.

55.   Sherman, F. 1975. In "Methods in Cell Biology, Vol. XI. Yeast Cells." (D. Prescott, ed.). Academic Press, N.Y.,   189-199.

56.   Sherman, F. and H. Roman. 1963. Genetics 48, 255-261

57.   Sherman, F. and C. W. Lawrence. 1974. In "Handbook of Genetics" Vol. 1. (R.C. King, ed.). Plenum Publishing Corporation, N.Y. 359-393.

58.   Sherman, F., J. Stewart, M. Jackson, R. Gilmore, and J. Parker. 1974. Genetics 77, 255-284.

59. Silver, J. and N. Eaton. 1969. Biochem. Biophys. Res. Commun. 34, 301-305.
60. Sinclair, J.H., B.J. Stevens, P. Sanghavi, and M. Rabinowitz. 1967. Science 156, 1234-1237.
61. Snow, R. 1966. Nature 211, 206-207.
62. Somers, J.M. and E.A. Bevan. 1969. Genet. Res. 13, 71-83.
63. Stinchcomb, D.T., K. Struhl, and R.W. Davis. 1979. Nature 282, 39-43.
64. Storms, R.K., J.B. McNeil, P.S.Khandlkar, G. An, J. Parker, and J.D. Friesen. 1979. J. Bacteriol. 140, 73-82.
65. Struhl, K., D.T. Stinchcomb, S. Scherer, and R.W. Davis. 1979. Proc. Natl. Acad. Sci. USA 76, 1035-1039.
66. Szostak, J. and R. Wu. 1979. Plasmid 2, 536-554.
67. Takano, I. and Y. Oshima. 1970. Genetics 65, 421-427.
68. Thouvenot, D.R. and C.M. Bourgeois. 1971. Ann. Inst. Pasteur 120, 617-625.
69. Walton, E.F.,B.L. Carter, and J.R. Pringle. 1979. Molec. Gen. Genet. 171, 111-114.
70. Wickner, R. 1978. Genetics 88, 419-425.
71. Wickner,R. 1979. Genetics 92, 803-821.
72. Williamson, D.H. 1970. Symp. Soc. Exp. Biol. 24, 247-276.
73. Williamson, V.M., J. Bennetzen, E.T. Young, K. Nasmyth, and B. Hall. 1979. Nature 283, 214-216.

DISCUSSION

Q. KOHLHAW: I'm wondering with the availability of the cloned genes now, it should be possible to do trancription *in vitro*. What is the status of that, do you know?

A. GREER: The status is that currently a yeast *in vitro* transciption system does not exist. However, you can put yeast DNA into other heterologous *in vitro* systems and get message made. Several labs are trying to develop a yeast system.

PERSPECTIVES FOR GENETIC ENGINEERING OF

HYDROCARBON OXIDIZING BACTERIA

J.A. Shapiro[1], A. Charbit[2], S. Benson[1,4], M. Caruso[1,2],
R. Laux[1], R. Meyer,[3] and F. Banuett[1,5]

Department of Microbiology [1]
University of Chicago
Chicago, Illinois 60637

INTRODUCTION

　　Microbial hydrocarbon oxidation has interested biochemists and
biotechnologists associated with the petrochemical industry for
decades (34,40,55). While much of the initial interest was in the
use of hydrocarbon-oxidizing organisms in petroleum prospecting,
more recent attention has focused on the use of whole cells or
microbial enzyme systems to carry out very specific biodegradations
or bioconversions. Two developments in the past ten years have made
it a realistic possibility to envisage the rational design and construction of microorganisms for specific breakdown or interconversion of hydrocarbon substrates: (i) Rheinwald's observation that the
genes for camphor oxidation are located on a transmissible plasmid
(74,75), which quickly led to the discovery of many other transmissible plasmids in soil organisms that encode catabolic pathways
for hydrocarbon substrates, and (ii) the development of *in vitro*
and *in vivo* methods for the molecular cloning of DNA segments into
a variety of plasmid vectors.

　　In this presentation, we will evaluate where we stand with
respect to genetic engineering of hydrocarbon oxidizing bacteria for
specific applications. To do this, we will discuss the following
subjects:

　　- The nature of hydrocarbon substrates;

　　- Oxidative pathways for hydrocarbon breakdown;

[2]Unite de Genie Genetique, Institut Pasteur, 75724 Paris, France
[3]Department of Microbiology, University of Texas, Austin, TX 78712
[4]Cancer Biology Research, Frederick Cancer Res. Ctr.,Frederick, MD
[5]Institute of Molecular Biology, University of Oregon, Eugene, OR

- Degradative plasmids in *Pseudomonas* and related bacteria;
- Genetic analysis of selected hydrocarbon oxidation
  pathways;
- Genetic engineering of hydrocarbon oxidizing bacteria.

NATURE OF HYDROCARBON SUBSTRATES

Natural and synthetic hydrocarbons, including their substitute
derivatives, encompass an enormous variety of chemical structures.
In order for a microbial cell to utilize these substrates as sources
of carbon and energy, it must convert them into the normal intermediates of central metabolism, chiefly organic acids that can enter
the Krebs cycle. Although no generalization will hold for such a
diverse group of substances, there are several simplifying state-
ments which can help to understand certain characteristics of hydrocarbon degradative pathways.

(1) Unoxidized hydrocarbon substrates. Many hydrocarbon substrates have no oxidized groups. These include paraffins, aromatic
ring compounds, and more complex structures found in petroleum
deposits and elsewhere in the environment. Such substrates are
very hydrophobic and show high partition coefficients for organic
solvents. Even many hydrocarbons that are partially oxidized, such
as waxes, aliphatic alcohols, sterols, etc., also partition into
organic solvents. This thermodynamic property of many hydrocarbon
substrates influences their interaction with microbial cells. Upon
initial contact, hydrophobic substrates will partition into cellular
membranes and not into the cytoplasm where the activities of intermediary metabolism are located. Thus, in many cases, there must be
biochemical activities to oxidize membrane-bound initial substrates
to derivates that can enter the aqueous environment of the cytoplasm

(2) Linear hydrocarbon substrates. Many hydrocarbon substrate
consist of alkyl chains, sometimes attached to other structures or
with terminal substituted methyl groups (e.g., aliphatic amides).
In order to utilize the carbon in these chains, the cells need to
break them down into smaller oxidized units that are substrates for
intermediary metabolism.

(3) Cyclic hydrocarbon substrates. Both aliphatic and aromatic
hydrocarbons can have closed ring structures. The carbon in these
substrates is not available for further metabolism until the rings
have been opened to yield linear molecules that can be further
broken down.

(4) Substituted hydrocarbon substrates. Natural and synthetic
hydrocarbons often contain other atoms in place of carbon or hydroge

In natural heterocyclic compounds, sulfur or nitrogen substitutes for carbon. In synthetic derivatives of both aliphatic and aromatic hydrocarbons, various groups-but principally halogen atoms-substitute for hydrogens. In order to remove the substituent atoms and utilize the carbon in these substrates, cells must possess either (a) biochemical activities for splitting unusual covalent linkages to carbon or (b) activities that will convert the substrates to labile compounds which spontaneously release substituent atoms.

OXIDATIVE PATHWAYS

Many pathways for microbial hydrocarbon oxidation have been studied in varying detail (13,34,55). Sometimes, alternative pathways have been proposed. Rather than try to deal with all of these comprehensively, we will describe three pathways of bacterial hydrocarbon oxidation which are widely accepted as correct and for which we have information about the underlying genetic control. We will also discuss some initial studies of a pathway for breakdown of halogenated aromatic hydrocarbons.

It is useful to bear in mind that there are generally two components to each hydrocarbon oxidation pathway. As most vividly pointed out by Hans Knackmuss (personal communication) these are the throat and stomach. The throat consists of specialized activities which convert the initial hydrocarbon to a substrate for the stomach, a more generalized set of activities that digests this substrate to intermediates of central metabolism.

(1) Methyl group oxidation to carboxylic acid. One of the most common throats for unoxidized hydrocarbons is hydroxylation of a free methyl group followed by successive dehydrogenation to a carboxylic acid: $RCH_3 \rightarrow RCH_2OH \rightarrow RCHO \rightarrow RCOOH$. This initial pathway applies to the oxidation of methane, of n-alkanes, and of substituted aromatics such as toluene, xylenes, and cymene (1,14,34,85,96; Figure 1). In some cases, such as xylenols and cresol, even partially oxidized compounds are subject to initial metabolism by conversion of a methyl group to a carboxylic acid group (43,70). Typically, a multi-component mixed function mono-oxygenase catalyzes the initial hydroxylation reaction, with hydrocarbon and molecular oxygen as substrates (33,52). Thus, the pathway must be aerobic. The best characterized enzyme is the hydroxylase from alkane-oxidizing *Pseudomonas putida (P. oleovorans)*. This enzyme has three components: soluble rubredoxin, soluble rubredoxin reductase and a phospholipid-requiring membrane oxidase (initially named ω-hydroxylase; 1,33,54,69,77,78). The membrane oxidase is an inducible 40,000 dalton cytoplasmic membrane peptide (6). At least one of the soluble proteins is inducible, but these components are relatively non-specific because they are replaceable by spinach ferredoxin and ferredoxin reductase (5). A *P. aeruginosa* alkane hydroxylation

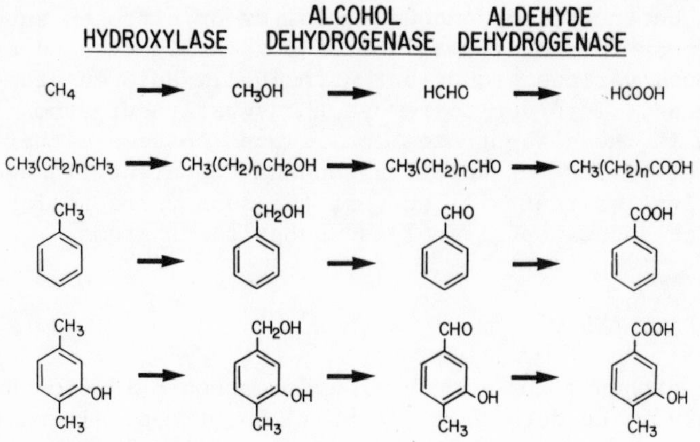

Figure 1. Methyl group oxidation to carboxylic acid. The four substrates are (top to bottom) methane (76,87), *n*-alkanes (1), toluene (96) and 2,5-xylenol (70).

complex is also separable into particulate and cytoplasmic component (86), and the methane monooxygenases from methylotrophs are also particulate activities (66,76).

Membrane proteins are also involved in subsequent alcohol and aldehyde dehydrogenation, although soluble activities may also catalyze these reactions. In the *P. putida* alkane oxidation system, there is a specifically inducible cytoplasmic membrane alcohol dehydrogenase (6,7), and inducible membrane alcohol and aldehyde dehydrogenases have also been reported in *P. aeruginosa* strains (83). Particulate preparations from methylotrophs will convert methane to formate (87).

An interesting characteristic of the initial monooxygenases is their broad substrate range. The alkane hydroxylase from *P. putida* is active on a broad series of different chain-length *n*-alkanes (54) and the enzyme from *P. aeruginosa* will catalyze the epoxidation of terminal alkenes (84). The methane monooxygenases from various methylotrophs will hydroxylate many *n*-alkanes, *n*-alkenes, ethers and cyclic compounds (40) and epoxidate C_1 to C_4 *n*-alkenes (44).

(2) β-oxidation of fatty acids. An important stomach for the breakdown of straight-chain fatty acids in β-oxidation to yield acetyl-CoA from even-numbered carbon chains and, additionally, propionyl-CoA from odd-numbered chains (Figure 2; 13). Fatty acids originate from *n*-alkanes and terminally substituted hydrocarbons such as aliphatic amides (13,64). Partial β-oxidation of internally substituted or branched molecules has also been reported (85). Studies of isocitrate lyase mutants unable to utilize acetyl-CoA as sole carbon and energy source indicated that β-oxidation is the sole

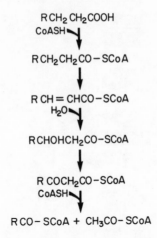

Figure 2.   Bacterial β-oxidation (13).

pathway for fatty acid utilization in *P. aeruginosa* and *P. putida* (13,64).

(3) <u>Ring fissions pathways</u>. As mentioned above, the opening of the conjugated ring structure is essential for microbial assimilation of carbon from aeromatic hydrocarbon substrates. Three kinds of stomachs have evolved to catalyze ring fission reactions (Figure 3).

(a) The *ortho* pathway for cleavage of catechol and related compounds (this is also called the β-ketoadipate pathway);
(b) The *meta* pathway for cleavage of catechol and related compounds; and
(c) The gentisate pathway.

It is not always clear why a particular aromatic substrate is utilized by one pathway or the other. For example, many throats lead to catechol or substituted catechols, which can then be further degraded by either *ortho* or *meta*- fission pathways (13). In some cases, however, a substrate requires one of the two alternative pathways because the products of the incorrect cleavage reaction are "dead-end" metabolites incapable of further catabolism or toxic to the cell (48,58). As we shall see below, this means that the choice of ring-fission pathway often determines which substrates a bacterial strain can degrade.

Preliminary studies of the chlorobenzoate-utilizing *Pseudomonas* strain B13 and its relatives indicate that the ring fission enzymes are the critical activities in catabolism of halogenated aromatic substrates (Figure 4; 15,16,17,21,49,71,72,73,80). B13 synthesizes two sets of *ortho* fission enzymes. Growth on benzoate induces a catechol 1,2-oxygenase (C12O) and muconate lactonizing enzyme (MLE) that have poor activity on chlorinated catechols and

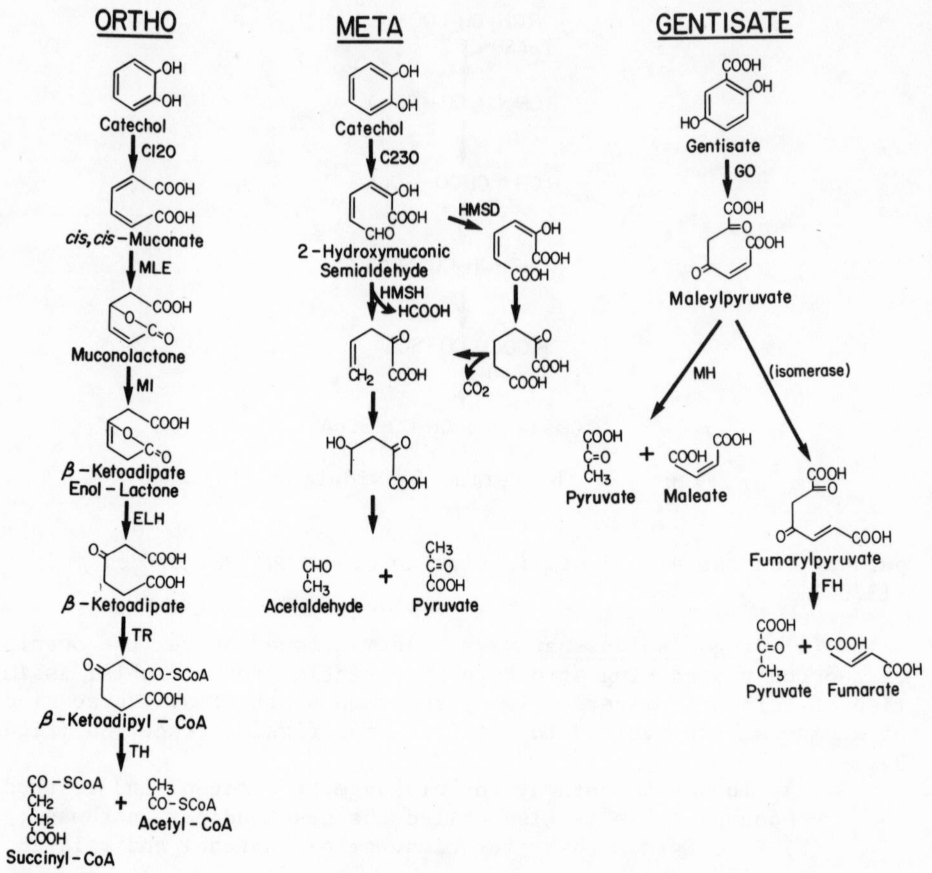

Figure 3.   Ring fission pathways.   The enzyme nomenclature follows
reference 13.   In the *ortho*-fission pathways: C120 = catechol-1,2-
oxygenase, MLE = nuconate lactonizing enzyme, MI = muconolactone
isomerase, ELH = enol-lactone hydrolase, TR = transferase, and TH =
thiolase.   In the *meta*-fission pathway: C230 = catechol-2,3-oxygen-
ase, HMSH = hydroxymuconic semialdehyde hydrolase, HMSD = hydroxymuconic semialdehyde dehydrogenase.   In the gentisate pathway: GO =
gentisate oxygenase, MH = maleylpyruvate hydrolase, FH - fumaryl
pyruvate hydrolase.

their reaction products, while growth on 3-chlorobenzoate induces
analogues of these two ortho pathway enzymes with much greater
activity on chlorinated catechols and their reaction products (16,
80).   *In vitro*, the enzymes from chlorobenzoate-grown cells will
quantitatively release Cl⁻ ions from chlorocatechol.   When *ortho*
pathway enzymes are extracted from cells grown on benzoate (or from
bacteria that cannot utilize chlorobenzoate), a low level of activit
is seen against chlorocatechol, and there is release of chloride

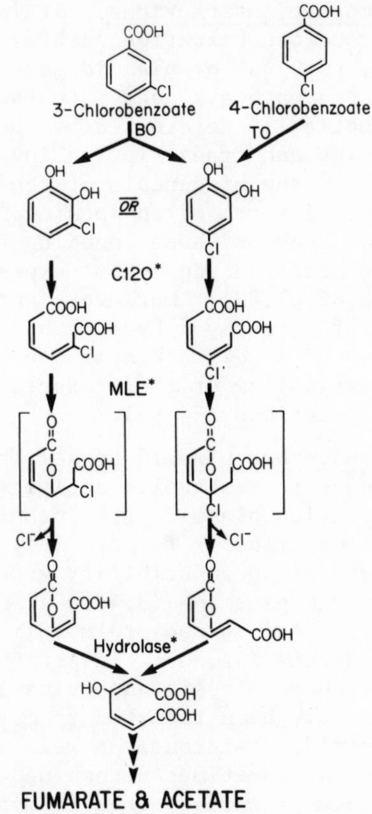

FUMARATE & ACETATE

Figure 4. Chlorobenzoate oxidation by ortho-fission (48). The starred activities are chlorobenzoate-induced in *Pseudomonas* B-13. BO = chromosomally-encoded benzoate oxidase; TO = plasmid-encoded toluate oxidase.

ions (Knackmuss, personal communication). From these results, Knackmuss (48) concluded that chloride is spontaneously released from the chlorinated muconolactone. Thus, the activities important for chlorobenzoate utilization are not specific dehalogenases but rather enzymes that will metabolize halogenated intermediates to unstable compounds that spontaneously liberate halide ions.

HYDROCARBON OXIDATION PLASMIDS

Since Rheinwald's identification of the CAM plasmid ten years ago, many other plasmids have been identified which encode all or part of various hydrocarbon oxidation pathways. These are found chiefly in Pseudomonads (9,11,12,20,31,47,50,91). We will describe several well-studied examples later. Here it may be useful to state some more general observations.

(1) <u>Plasmid-chromosome interactions</u>. It is essential to consider a particular hydrocarbon oxidation pathway as the product of a
total bacterial genome, not just of plasmid genes (24). All of the
initial plasmid-determined pathways feed into the central pathways of
cellular metabolism genetically determined by the bacterial chromosome. Plasmid replication and transcription involve the products of
chromosomal genes, as does the biogenesis of the cell membrane where
critical oxidation activities are often located. Thus, it is not
surprising that plasmids such as those encoding the catabolism of
toluene to pyruvate and acetaldehyde do not express a functional
pathway in all cells (8,46,61,88). Moreover, chromosomal mutations
can have several kinds of effects on hydrocarbon oxidation pathways.
These include inhibition of specific plasmid-encoded oxidation steps
and blocks to further catabolism of the products of initial plasmid-
determined biochemical reactions (24,94).

(2) <u>Degradative and other plasmid types</u>. There is nothing other
than the presence of genes for catabolic activities that distinguishes hydrocarbon oxidation plasmids from other kinds of plasmids,
such as drug resistance or transfer factors (81). Degradative plasmids are found among several incompatibility groups, including both
narrow and broad host-range plasmids (3,47,50). They can carry
markers for conjugal transfer, chromosome mobilization, and resistance to antibacterial agents (47,50). Insertion of drug resistance
transposons can convert them to resistance plasmids (4,8,28), and a
natural isolate has recently been reported to carry determinants for
streptomycin and sulfonamide resistance as well as toluene oxidation
(98). Degradative plasmids sometimes recombine with each other or
with antibiotic resistance plasmids, often forming hybrids carrying
catabolic genes with altered host-range, conjugal transfer or incompatibility properties (10,24,45,46,61,88). In some case, these
recombinations are independent of homologous recombination pathways
and probably involve IS elements on the plasmid molecules (45).
Because of these frequent recombination events, it is not surprising
to find determinants for a single oxidative pathway present on a
variety of different replicons (31,92).

GENETICS OF SPECIFIC OXIDATION PATHWAYS

A few hydrocarbon oxidation pathways have been subject to
genetic analysis. There is fairly detailed information about the
n-alkane and toluene oxidation pathways of *P. putida*. Rather less
is known about genetic control of other pathways. We will discuss
some preliminary work on chlorinated aromatic hydrocarbon degradation because it illustrates the need to match throats and stomachs
and to avoid the production of dead-end metabolites.

(1) <u>The alk system</u>. *P. putida* strains carrying the OCT plasmid
or recombinants of OCT and other Inc P-2 plasmids (such as CAM) can
grow at the expense of six- to ten-carbon n-alkanes (10,12,27,35).
Most of the oxidation pathway is catalyzed by apparently constitutive chromosomal gene products, but the first two steps involve

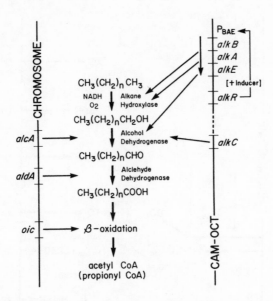

Figure 5. Genetic control of n-alkane oxidation by plasmid-bearing *P. putida* (corrected from reference 25).

inducible products of the plasmid alk (alkane utilization) loci (Figure 5; 5, 7,35). There is overlap between chromosomal and plasmid activities at the second step of the pathway, the dehydrogenation of primary alcohol to aldehyde. Studies with nitrosoguanidine-induced and transposon insertion mutations indicate the existence of both regulatory and structural genes in three different locations on these enormous Inc P-2 plasmids (>200 megadaltons; 26,36): an $alkRD$ regulatory cluster; an $alkBAE$ operon of alkane hydroxylase and alcohol dehydrogenase structural genes, located about 40 kilobase pairs from the regulatory region; and an unlinked $alkC$ alcohol dehydrogenase locus (25,27). The control of $alkBAE$ by one or more $alkR$-encoded positive regulatory proteins determines the alkane substrate range of *P. putida* (27,35). Constitutive $alkR$ mutations permit growth on undecane, which is not normally a growth substrate because it is not an inducer, while other $alkR$ mutations restrict the range of inducers (hence growth substrates) to heptane, octane and sometimes hexane or nonane (27,35). When the chromosomal $alcA$ alcohol utilization locus is mutant, the $alkR$ locus similarly determines the utilization of primary aliphatic alcohol substrates. Because of the plasmid-chromosomal overlap at the second step of the pathway, mutant bacteria only accumulate alcohol intermediates from alkane substrates when they carry at least two separate mutations ($alcA$ and $alkC$;82).

(2) <u>The tol system</u>. A variety of different plasmids enable *P. putida* and other fluorescent Pseudomonads to utilize toluene and xylenes as growth substrates (31,90,92). The best-studied of these

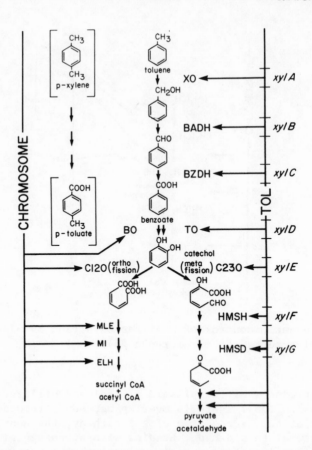

Figure 6. Genetic control of toluene and xylene oxidation by plasmid-
bearing *P. putida* (58,63,96). XO = xylene oxidase; BADH = benzyl
alcohol dehydrogenase; BZDH = benzaldehyde dehydrogenase.

plasmids is called TOL and has been the subject of intensive investigation by several laboratories. TOL encodes the oxidation pathway
outlined in Figure 6, its restriction map is known (18), and a preliminary physical map of *xyl* genes has been derived from studies of
RP4-TOL hybrid plasmids (62). The *xyl* structural genes are divided
into two distinct regulons: the genes for initial oxidation to benzoate or toulate, *xylA*, *xylB* and *xylC* are induced by toluene or
xylene but not by toluate, while the genes for the subsequent formation of catechol and the meta-fission pathway, *xylD*, *xylE*, *xylF* and
xylG are induced both by toluene or xylene and by benzoate or toluat
(30,61,62,95,96,97). Although the plasmid encodes all steps of the
oxidation pathway down to pyruvate and acetaldehyde, *E. coli* strains
carrying an RP4-TOL hybrid or a TOL::Tn401 plasmid with an inserted
resistance marker will not grow on pathway substrates (8,46,61,88);
there is, however, some inducible expression of pathway enzymes in

E. coli (61). These observations highlight the importance of having the proper host for expression of plasmid-determined catabolic phenotypes.

An important feature of the TOL-encoded pathway in Pseudomonads is the overlap with chromosomally-encoded enzymes. There are both plasmid (TO) and chromosomal (BO) gene products for the oxygenation of benzoate or toluate to catechol, and two catechol fission pathways (Figure 6). In *P. putida*, the regulation of the two ring fission pathways is different. The aromatic acid substrate induces the plasmid *meta* pathway, while the product of ring fission, *cis-, cis-* muconate, induces the chromosomal *ortho* pathway (65,95). Thus, benzoate or toluate will induce the *meta* pathway in a TOL-bearing strain, and *meta* cleavage of catechol prevents formation of the inducer for the *ortho* pathway. In certain instances, the result of this regulatory choice is paradoxical for the growth of the cell. For example, benzoate is a much better growth substrate *via* the *ortho* pathway, so that the presence of TOL leads to slower growth on benzoate (63,97). In other words, the TOL$^+$ strain has a suboptimal stomach for digesting benzoate. (Since the TOL plasmid genes may have evolved for catabolism of a substrate that requires the *meta* fission pathway and not for toluene utilization, this apparent paradox may not be relevant in nature.) This negative effect on benzoate utilization is readily corrected either by complete loss of the plasmid or by loss of a positive regulatory function (*xylS*) needed to induce the *meta* pathway. Thus TOL$^-$ or *xylS$^-$* strains outgrow TOL$^+$ strains on benzoate medium (97). We shall return to the importance of the choice of ring fission pathways in the next section on chlorobenzoate oxidation.

(3) <u>The chlorinated aromatic systems</u>. Strain B13 (15) has for alternate *ortho* fission enzymes which function on halogenated substrates (Figure 4). These genes appear to be on a plasmid because the ability to utilize 3-chlorobenzoate is readily transferred by conjugation to various *P. putida* and *P. aeruginosa* strains (72,73; W. Reineke and H.J. Knackmuss, personal communication; A.C. and J.A.S., unpublished). We shall call these genes the *clb* loci. B13 and other *clb$^+$* bacteria grown on 3-chlorobenzoate (= metachloro- benzoate or MC1) but not on 4-chlorobenzoate (= parachlorobenzoate or PC1), apparently because the chromosomal benzoate oxidase will not form parachlorocatechol (17). The analogous TOL plasmid enzyme, toluate oxidase, will form catechols from methylsubstituted sub- strates and thus, presumably, from halogenated substrates too. However, introduction of TOL into B13 (or of the *clb$^+$* loci into a TOL$^+$ strain) is not sufficient to form a bacteria that will grow on PC1, apparently because induction of the plasmid *meta*-fission path- way converts the chlorocatechol to a dead-end substrate. A secondary mutation on the TOL plasmid that blocks *meta*-pathway induction will permit growth on PC1 (72: P.A. Williams, personal communication). Thus, PC1 utilization by *clb$^+$* cells requires the introduction of a new throat, (the product of the *xylD* gene), but that throat has to

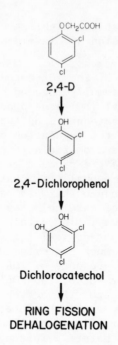

Figure 7.   Initial oxidation of 2,4-D(22).

be separated from induction of the wrong stomach in order to function
on the proper substrate (Figure 4).

B13 does not normally utilize dichlorobenzoates (DCl), but
biochemical studies on extracts and the isolation of DCl⁺ mutants
indicated that the *clb⁺* *ortho*-fission enzymes could cleave and
dehalogenate dichlorocatechols (17,37,49,72).   Other bacteria had
been isolated which could utilize dichlorinated substrates, in particular the herbicide 2,4-dichlorophenoxyacetic acid (24D or Tfd)
(Figure 7; 29,67,68).   Some of these strains, identified as *Alcali-*
genes eutrophus, carry Inc P-1 plasmids necessary for Tfd utilization (31,67). Curing experiments indicated that these plasmids only
carried genes for initial oxidation enzymes (the throat) because
the cured strain would still grown on 2,4-dichlorophenol (DCP), the
first catabolic intermediate in 24D degradation (Figure 7). In order
to investigate this pathway further, one of us (A. C.) isolated
Tfd⁺ plasmids carrying a transposable drug resistance element, Tn7,
encoding trimethoprim (Tp) resistance.   These Tfd⁺Tp plasmids could
be transferred (by virtue of their resistance markers), to *E. coli*,
where (as expected) no degradative phenotype was apparent.   Transfer
from *E. coli* to *clb⁺* and *clb⁻ Pseudomonas* strains revealed that the
Tfd⁺ plasmids encode at least two catabolic steps (Tfd → Dcp and
Dcp → dichlorocatechol.   Table I summarizes the growth characteristics of strains with different combinations of *Tfd* and *clb* genes.
Although our work on this system is not yet complete, it appears

TABLE I

Growth on Chlorinated Substrates

Bacterial genotype	Growth Substrate 3-chlorobenzoate	2,4-D	Dichlorophenol
A. eutrophus (Tfd⁺)	-	+	+
A. eutrophus (Tfd⁻)	-	-	+
A. eutrophus (Tfd⁺ clb⁺)	+	+	+
Pseudomonas	-	-	-
Pseudomonas (Tfd⁺)	-	-	-
Pseudomonas (clb⁺)	+	-	-
Pseudomonas (Tfd⁺ clb⁺)	+	+	+

We have confirmed that the Tfd⁺ plasmid pJP4 of $\underline{A}$. eutrophus JMP 134 (67) encodes two steps in 2,4-D catabolism (Figure 7) by isolating a mutant plasmid that only encodes the first step ($\underline{tfdA}^+$ $\underline{tfdB}^-$). This mutant plasmid will allow growth on 2,4-D in the $\underline{A}$. eutrophus background, where chromosomal gene products can catabolize dichlorophenol, but not in the $\underline{Pseudomonas}$ $\underline{clb}^+$ background, where a function needed for dichlorophenol utilization is lacking. $\underline{A}$. eutrophus (Tfd⁺) = JMP 134 (67), $\underline{A}$. eutrophus (Tfd⁻) = JMP 134 cured of pJP4, and $\underline{Pseudomonas}$ = $\underline{P}$. putida or $\underline{P}$. aeruginosa.

that the chromosomally-determined ring fission enzymes of these *A. eutrophus* strains may differ from those of B13. The reason is that the Dcp⁺ *A. eutrophus* is MC1⁻ unless it has received the *clb*⁺ genes from B13. Thus, there may be more than one chlorocatechol stomach in nature.

GENETIC ENGINEERING OF HYDROCARBON OXIDATING BACTERIA

Most of the sophisticated tools of recombinant DNA technology have been developed for work in *E. coli*. Some of these cannot be used directly in gram-negative hydrocarbon-oxidizing strains: colE1-derived vectors will not replicate in Pseudomonads, λ does not grown in *Pseudomonas*, and many *E. coli* promoters may not function well in *Pseudomonas*. In addition, some *in vivo* genetic engineering tools based on phage Mu will not work in hydrocarbon-oxidizing bacteria because Mu does not appear to transpose or replicate in *Pseudomonas aeruginosa* (J.A.S., unpublished). Thus, it is necessary to work out new genetic engineering methods for use in hydrocarbon-oxidizing Pseudomonads and related bacteria. (Gram-positive hydrocarbon oxidizers are yet another subject, about which less is known and which will certainly require a parallel effort).

(1) Broad host-range vectors, *Pseudomonas* plasmids include

two classes-limited host-range plasmids, which only replicate in
Pseudomonads, and broad host-range plasmids which also can replicate
in *E. coli* and in a wide variety of gram-negative species (47). In
order to take advantage of *E. coli* technology, most work on the
development of vectors for Pseudomonads has centered on this second
group of broad host-range plasmids. This includes plasmids of the
Inc P-1, P-4, and W incompatibility groups, and the characteristics
of some plasmids from these groups are summarized in Table II.

    One of the limiting steps in recombinant DNA work is trans-
formation with digested and religated DNA. In many cases, transformation of Pseudomonads is less efficient than transformation of
E. coli (4,79). One way to circumvent this problem is to transform
E. coli with fragments inserted into broad host-range vectors and
then mobilize the recombinant plasmids to the desired host. This
technique has served in two cases with methylotrophic bacteria: (a)
A methanol dehydrogenase gene was cloned by (i) shotgun cloning of
Pseudomonas AMI DNA and transformation into *E. coli* (ii) transfer of
the total recombinant plasmid population to a methanol dehydrogenase-
deficient AMI mutant, and (iii) selection of drug resistant clones
that had recovered methanol dehydrogenase activity (32). (b) The
E. coli glutamate dehydrogenase gene (*gdh$^+$*) was introduced into
Methylophilus methylotrophus by (i) *in vivo* cloning of *gdh$^+$* into
RP4 using phage Mu, (ii) subcloning in *E. coli* of a *SalI gdh$^+$* restriction fragment into the Inc P-4 vector pTB70, and (iii) conjugal
transfer of the pTB70-*gdh$^+$* hybrid into *M. methylotrophus* by selection
for drug resistance (93). Once in *M. methylotrophus* the pTB70-*gdh$^+$*
plasmid encoded expression of *E. coli* glutamate dehydrogenase at
levels about half that seen in *gdh$^+$ E. coli* strains. Since pTB70 is
present in many copies per chromosome (about 40-50 copies are seen
in other hosts with similar plasmids; 56,59,60), the level of *gdh$^+$*
expression per gene copy must be much lower in the new host cell.
Nonetheless, the expressed glutamate dehydrogenase activity permitted
a 4-7% increase in *M. methylotrophus* carbon conversion rates. The
SalI restriction site in pTB70 used for *gdh$^+$* cloning is part of the
Tn5 transposable kanamycin-resistance element, which illustrates the
utility of drug-resistance transposons for constructing broad host-
range cloning vectors (57).

    In additon to those examples of cloning in methylotrophs with
the aid of intermediate *E. coli* hosts, there is a report of successful cloning directly into a *Pseudomonas* host (59). As mentioned
above, the efficiency of transormation is generally limiting in
these experiments, but we have recently found that a particular
P. aeruginosa strain (the restriction-modification mutant PAO1161)
is highly transformable by Inc P-4 plasmids using the Lederberg and
Cohen transformation protocol (53; F.B., unpublished). Using this
strain we have been able to clone plasmid DNA fragments directly in
Pseudomonas (R. Laux, F. Banuett, T. Petes, C.J. Muster and J.A.
Shapiro, in preparation).

TABLE II

Some Broad Host-Range Cloning Vectors

Plasmid	Inc	Copy Number	Markers	Useful restriction sites	Comments	References
RP1 (= RP4, RK2, R68)	P-1	3-4	Cb Tc Km/Nm	1 EcoRI, 1 BamHI (in Tn1), 1 Bgl II, 1 Hind III (inactivates Km^r)	Tra$^+$ in all strains; poor transformation in P. aeruginosa	11, 47, 50, 56
R1162 (= R300B, RSF1010)	P-4	~50	Sm Su	1 EcoRI (sometimes inactivates Sm^r), 2 Pst (inactivate Su), 1 Hpa I, 1 Eca I, 1 Sst I	Tra$^-$ in E. coli, Tra$^+$ in P. putida and P. aeruginosa	32, 47, 50, 56, 57, 59, 60, 93, S. B. unpublished
pQSR136 (= R1162::Tn5Δ136)	P-4		Sm Su	As above plus 1 Hind III, 2 Hpa I and 2 Pst I (all in deleted Tn5)	Excellent transformation in P. aeruginosa	57, F. B. unpublished
pQSR49A (=R1162::Tn1)	P-4		Sm Su Cb	As for R1162 plus 1 Bam HI, 1 Kpn I, 3 Pst I (all in Tn1)		8, R.M., M.C. and J.A.S. unpublished
pTB70 (= R300B:: Tn5 plus extra segment)	P-4		Sm Su Km/Nm	As for R1162 plus 1 Sal I, 1 Sma I/Xma I in Tn5		93
R388	W	3-5	Tp Su	1 EcoRI, 1 SalGI, 1 Hind III, 2 Pst I	Tra$^+$ in all strains; cannot use Tp^r in P. putida due to intrinsic resistance	47, 50, J.M. Ward and J. Grinsted. 1978. Gene 3: 87-95
pUB5502	W		Tp	1 BamHI, 1 EcoRI, 1 Pst I	Tra$^-$ in E. coli; moderate transformation in P. aeruginosa	J.M. Ward and J. Grinsted, personal communication
Sa	W	3-5	Sm Km Gm Cm Su	1 Sal GI, 3 Pst I, 1 SmaI/Xma I	Tra$^+$ in all strains; resistance levels depend on host	47, 50, J. M. Ward and J. Grinsted, personal communication
pUB5578	W		Sm Km Gm	1 EcoRI (inactivates Sm^r), 1 Bam HI, 1 Pst I		J.M. Ward and J. Grinsted, personal communication

Nomenclature follows reference 47. Maps of RK2 and RP4 are in appendix B of DNA Insertion Elements, Plasmids and Episomes, 1977, A. I. Bukhari, J. A. Shapiro and S. L. Adhya (eds.), Cold Spring Harbor Laboratory, Cold Spring Harbor, New York.

(2) <u>Pitfalls in cloning in hydrocarbon oxidizers</u>. It is often useful to consider some of the possible obstacles to successful genetic engineering experiments. Some of these are apparent in the report on *M. methylotrophus* (93), and others come from unpublished work in this laboratory and elsewhere. Two points merit emphasis.

(a) Genetic manipulation of plasmids can alter their ability to replicate stably in certain hosts. Modified plasmids of the Inc P-1 and Inc P-4 groups are often stable in *E. coli* and unstable in *Pseudomonas* or methylotroph hosts. The modifications which can sometimes cause this instability are: (i) *in vitro* deletions of restriction fragments from an RP4::Tn7 plasmid (93); (ii) *in vivo* insertion of Tn5 into Inc P-4 plasmid R1162 (57; R.L. and J.A.S., unpublished); (iii) *in vitro* insertion of a 7 kb λ *lac*5 fragment into the transposon in pQSR49 (M.C. and J.A.S., unpublished); and (iv) *in vitro* recombination of Inc P-4 plasmids and col E1 derivatives (R.M., unpublished). It is not inevitable that such manipulations do cause instability, however, because Windass et al. found that pTB70, an R300B-Tn5 hybrid, was stable in *M. methylotrophus* (93), and we have isolated pBR322-Inc P-4 hybrids that are stable in *P. aeruginosa* (R.L., F.B. et al., in preparation).

(b) Certain gene products may be toxic if present in too large quantities in the cell. This is especially true of membrane proteins, as has been demonstrated for membrane-bound β-galactosidase hybrid proteins in *E. coli* (2). It is not possible to clone the *lacY* gene in high copy number plasmids because, apparently, too much of this cytoplasmic membrane protein disrupts the functional integrity of the cell envelope (M. Berman, personal communication). This same problem will almost certainly present itself with some of the membrane proteins involved in hydrocarbon oxidation. For example, the cytoplasmic membrane component of alkane hydroxylase (the *alkB* gene product) is the major membrane peptide found in alkane-grown cells (Figure 8; 6). Thus, it is likely that cloning the *alkB* gene on high copy number plasmids will prove difficult, and this has been our experience. Moreover, certain gene products like the *alkB* peptide, are already present in such high amounts that cloning for overproduction will probably not lead to a significant physiological improvement in hydrocarbon oxidation.

Thus, two conclusions come out of this rapid look at possible pitfalls in genetic engineering with hydrocarbon oxidizers. First, it is important to try several cloning vectors and be familiar with their replication behavior in different hosts. Second, it is important to know something about the details of each hydrocarbon oxidation pathway, especially about the nature of the enzymes that catalyze different steps.

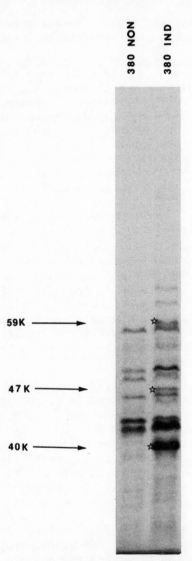

Figure 8. Total membrane peptides from an *alk*[+] *P. putida* strain (PpS 380) after growth in the presence (380IND) or absence (380NON of inducer. The alkane-induced peptides in this polyacrylamide-SDS gel are marked with a star. The 40,000 dalton peptide (40K) is the cytoplasmic membrane product of the *alkB* alkane hydroxylase structural gene (6). This inducible protein is clearly the major membrane peotide in induced cells.

PERSPECTIVES FOR GENETIC ENGINEERING OF HYDROCARBON OXIDATION PATHWAYS

   We can now discern at least four steps in the development of rational methods for modifying hydrocarbon oxidation pathways and

for constructing bacterial strains to carry out specific biodegradations or bioconversions. Some progress has been made on all of these:

(1) <u>Location of the genes for different throats and stomachs</u>.
We have seen how *in vivo* genetic techniques have made it possible to
identify groups of plasmid and chromosomal genes that encode different portions of hydrocarbon oxidation pathways. In some cases (such
as the plasmid- and chromosomally-determined oxidases that convert
substituted benzoates to substituted catechols), we see that there
can be important differences in substrate specificity between parallel enzymes that catalyze the same step. In other cases (such as
alkane hydroxylation), we see that regulation has more to do with substrate specificity than enzymatic specificity. Thus, plasmid curing
and transfer experiments, chemical and transposon mutagenesis, and
formation of conjugal hybrids between strains with different metabolic capabilities are critical to identifying genes for various
hydrocarbon oxidizing enzymes. Both biochemical studies and more
detailed genetic analysis by classical methods will be useful in dis-
tinguishing gene products which have analogous biochemical function
but different substrate specificities. It will be important to accumulate collections of mutants blocked at specific steps in hydrocarbon
oxidation pathways for two reasons: (a) to develop methods for accumulating intermediates (e.g., specific hydroxylation products), and
(b) to serve as tester strains for cloned genes.

(2) <u>Development of sophisticated cloning systems in hydrocarbon oxidizers</u>. Both *in vivo* and *in vitro* systems for cloning
specific DNA fragments are necessary.

There are preliminary steps towards *in vivo* systems with
plasmids like R68-45 which can incorporate fragments from many parts
of the bacterial genome in several species (38,41; B.W. Holloway,
personal communication). It may also be possible to develop inducible elements analogous to mini-Mu which can render any DNA segment
transposable (23). The discovery of Mu-like phages in *P. aeruginosa*
suggests that this idea is not too far-fetched (51, V.N. Krylov,
personal communication; S. Bana and J. Shapiro, unpublished). The
use of Mu cloning in the *M. methylotrophus* glutamate dehydrogenase
work shows how useful this *in vivo* technology can be (93).

In vitro cloning systems require several components, some of
which are available. These include vectors with many restriction
sites suitable for inserting foreign DNA. There are both high copy
number Inc P-4 vectors and low copy number Inc P-1 and Inc W vectors (Table II). What is lacking are <u>amplification</u> vectors and
expression vectors - that is, plasmids whose copy number can be
increased by a simple manipulation, such as a temperature shift,
and plasmids which contain high efficieny promoters whose activity
can be regulated. The study of temperate bacteriophages in *P.
aeroginosa* (42) and other hydrocarbon oxidizing bacteria

should provide a number of systems for controlled replication and transcription analogous to those derived from phage λ in *E. coli*. In addition, the cloning of well-characterized genes such as the *ami* locus from *P. aeruginosa* (19) will yield restriction fragments carrying promoters and operators functional in Pseudomonads, just as *lac* and *trp* operon fragments have done in *E. coli*.

(3) Cloning of specific throats and stomachs. Once different groups of hydrocarbon oxidation genes have been identified and mapping studies have provided an approximate idea of linkage relations between them, it will be possible to proceed to cloning individual genes or blocks of genes. The exact procedure will vary for each case. Sometimes a single cistron can be cloned into a standard strain using selection for a particular growth phenotype, but often the products of more than one locus will be necessary to express a specific activity. This is because many hydrocarbon oxidation genes appear to be under positive control so that both structural and regulatory genes are essential for expression. Frequently, these regulatory and structural genes will not be adjacent (as in the *alk* system; 25). Thus, successful cloning will require either constitutive mutant genes as donors (19) or point mutant strains as recipients. In the latter case, a single fragment will permit expression of the full phenotype because the additional needed regulatory or structural sequence(s) will be contributed by the host genome.

If several cistrons for the enzymes of a given pathway (or given throat or stomach) are adjacent, then it will probably be possible to clone a segment determining the entire set of biochemical activities. Successful experiments will require some previous genetic analysis to show that a selectable growth phenotype results from the introduction of the particular gene cluster. Take the 24D degradation pathway as an example. If the genes determining synthesis of the enzymes for conversion of 24D to dichlorocatechol are clustered, it should be possible to isolate recombinant plasmids carrying them in a clb^+ host with the B13 chlorocatechol fission activities because we already know that Tfd^+ clb^+ strains grow on 24D (Table I). The same experiment in a clb^- host would not work.

(4) Construction of strains with novel combinations of throats and stomachs. The cloning of genes for segments of hydrocarbon oxidation pathways into a variety of plasmid vectors should make it possible to extend degradative capacities by putting new throats on partial stomachs. This is essentially what Reineke and Knackmuss have done in constructing 4-chlorobenzoate degrading organisms (72, 73), and we have extended the substrate range of their strain B13 simply by introducing plasmid genes for the early steps in chlorinated phenoxyacetate degradation (Table I).

Complete degradation of hydrocarbon substrates requires the

matching of throats and stomachs to avoid the formation of non-metabolizable or toxic "dead-end" metabolites. But these so-called dead-end substances may be particularly valuable in certain applica-tions. Thus, the construction of bacteria with throats and stomachs that do not match for cell growth holds potential for the develop-ment of bioconversion systems to produce specific metabolic inter-mediates. Formation of plasmids carrying hydrocarbon oxidation genes as well as other selectable markers (such as antibiotic re-sistances) makes it possible to construct strains with defective oxidation pathways. Further sophistication can be introduced into these strain constructions once there are collections of mutants with specific pathway blocks.

To summarize, the prospects for genetic engineering of hydro-carbon oxidizing bacteria are good. What distinguishes this kind of genetic engineering from that used to produce single proteins from bacterial cells is the need to construct cells with coordinated sets of sequential biochemical activities. This will require more than wizardry with restriction endonucleases and synthetic DNA fragments, important as those tools are. Genetic engineering of hydrocarbon oxidizers will also require knowledge of the physiology of different pathways and a background of genetic analysis for each one.

ACKNOWLEDGMENTS

We thank Hans Knackmuss, George Jacoby and John Grinsted for strains and invaluable discussions. Our work on hydrocarbon oxida-tion at the University of Chicago is supported by grants from the donors of the Petroleum Research Fund, administered by the American Chemical Society, from the Louis Block Fund of the University of Chicago, and from the National Science Foundation (PCM 7903840). Work at the Institut Pasteur on 24D degradation was supported by a grant from the Union National des Caisses d'Epargne de France. Work at the University of Texas on broad host-range plasmids is supported by Public Health Service grant 5R01 GM25318. M.C. is the recipient of a fellowship from the Fondazione Cenci-Bolognetti Instituto Pasteur. R.L. is an NIH predoctoral trainee (5T32 GM07197-06).

REFERENCES

1.   Baptist, J.N., R.K. Gholson and M.J. Coon. 1963. Hydrocarbon oxidation by a bacterial enzyme system. I. Products of octane oxidation. Biochim. Biophys. Acta 69:40-47.
2.   Bassford, P., J. Beckwith, M. Berman, E. Brickman, M. Casadaba L. Guarente, I. Saint-Girons, A. Sarthy, M. Schwartz, H. Shuman and T. Silhavy. 1980. Genetic fusions of the *lac* operon A new approach to the study of biological processes. Pp 245-262, in *The Operon*, J. H. Miller and W.S. Reznikoff (eds.),

Cold Spring Harbor Laboratory, Cold Spring Harbor, New York.

3.   Bayley, S.A., D.W. Morris and P. Broda. 1979. The relationship of degradative and resistance pasmids of *Pseudomonas* belonging to the same incompatibility group. Nature 280:338-339.

4.   Benedik, M., M. Fennewald and J. Shapiro. 1977. Transposition of a β-lactamase locus from RP1 into *P. putida* degradative plasmids. J. Bacteriol. 129:809-814.

5.   Benson, S., M. Fennewald, J. Shapiro and C. Huettner. 1977. Fractionation of inducible alkane hydroxylase activity in *P. putida* and characterization of hydroxylase-negative plasmid mutations. J. Bacteriol. 132:614-621.

6.   Benson, S., M. Oppici, M. Fennewald and J. Shapiro. Regulation of membrane proteins by the *Pseudomonas* plasmid *alk* (alkane utilization) regulon. J. Bacteriol. 140:754-762.

7.   Benson, S. and J. Shapiro. 1976. Plasmid-determined alcohol dehydrogenase in alkane-utilizing strains of *Pseudomonas putida*. J. Bacteriol. 126:794-798.

8.   Benson, S. and J. Shapiro. 1978. TOL is a broad host-range plasmid. J. Bacteriol. 135:278-280.

9.   Chakrabarty, A.M. 1972. Genetic basis of the biodegradation of salicylate in *Pseudomonas*. J. Bacteriol. 112:815-823.

10.   Chakrabarty, A.M. 1973. Genetic fusion of incompatible plasmids in *Pseudomonas*. Proc. Nat. Acad. Sci., U.S.A. 70:1641-1644.

11.   Chakrabarty, A.M. 1976. Plasmids in *Pseudomonas*. Ann. Rev. Genet. 10:7-30.

12.   Chakrabarty, A.M., G. Chou and I.C. Gunsalus. 1973. Genetic regulation of octane dissimilation plasmid in *Pseudomonas*. Proc. Nat. Acad. Sci., U.S.A. 70:1137-1140.

13.   Clarke, P.H. and L.N. Ornston. 1975. Metabolic pathways and regulation: I and II. Pp. 191-340, in Genetics and Biochemistry of Pseudomonas, P.H. Clarke and M.H. Richmond (eds.), John Wiley and Sons, Ltd., London.

14.   De Frank, J.J. and D.W. Ribbons. 1977. *p*-Cymene pathway in *Pseudomonas putida*: Initial reactions. J. Bacteriol. 129:1356-1364.

15.   Dorn, E., M. Hellwig, W. Reineke and H.-J. Knackmuss. 1974. Isolation and characterization of a 3-chlorobenzoate degrading pseudomonad. Arch. Microbiol. 99:61-70.

16.   Dorn, E. and H.-J. Knackmuss. 1978. Chemical structure and biodegradability of ha-ogenated aromatic compounds: Two catechol 1,2-dioxygenases from a 3-chlorobenzoate-grown Pseudomonad. Biochem. J. 174:73-84.

17.   Dorn, E. and H.-J. Knackmuss. 1978. Chemical structure and biodegradability of halogenated aromatic compounds. Substituent effects on 1,2-dioxygenation of catechol. Biochem. J. 174:85-94.

18.   Downing, R.G. and P. Broda. 1979. A cleavage map of the TOL plasmid of *Pseudomonas putida* mt-2. Mol. Gen. Genet. 177:189-191.

19.   Drew, R.E., P.H. Clarke and W.J. Brammar. 1980. The construction *in vitro* of derivatives of bacteriophage lambda carrying the amidase genes of *Pseudomonas aeruginosa*. Molec. Gen. Genet 177:311-320.

20.   Dunn, N.W. and I.C. Gunsalus. 1973. Transmissible plasmid coding early enzymes of naphthalene oxidation in *Pseudomonas putida*. J. Bacteriol. 144:974-979.

21.   Engesser, K.-H., E. Schmidt and H.-J Knackmuss. 1980. Adaptation of *Alcaligenes eutrophus* B9 and *Pseudomonas* sp. B13 to 2-fluorobenzoate as growth substrate. Appl. Environ. Microbiol. 39:68-73.

22.   Evans, W.C., B.S.W. Smith, H.N. Fernley and J.J. Davies. 1971. Bacterial metabolism of 2,4-dichlorophenoxyacetate. Biochem. J. 122:543-551.

23.   Faelen, M., A. Resibois and A. Toussaint. 1979. Mini-mu: An insertion element derived from temperate phage Mu-1. Cold Spring Harbor Symp. Quant. Biol. 43:1169-1177.

24.   Fennewald, M., S. Benson and J. Shapiro. 1978. Plasmid-chromosome interactions in the *Pseudomonas* alkane system. Pp 170-173 in Microbiology 1978, D. Schlessinger (ed.), American Society for Microbiology, Washington, D.C.

25.   Fennewald, M., S. Benson, M. Oppici and J. Shapiro. 1979. Insertion element analysis and mapping of the *Pseudomonas* plasmid *alk* regulon. J. Bacteriol. 139:940-952.

26.   Fennewald, M., W. Prevatt, R. Meyer and J. Shapiro. 1978. Isolation of Inc P-2 plasmid DNA from *Pseudomonas aeruginosa*. Plasmid 1:164-173.

27.   Fennewald, M. and J. Shapiro. 1977. Regulatory mutations of the *Pseudomonas* plasmid *alk* regulon. J. Bacteriol. 132:622-627

28.   Fennewald, M. and J. Shapiro. 1979. Transposition of Tn7 in *P. aeruginosa* and isolation of *alk*::Tn7 mutations. J. Bacterio 139:264-269.

29.   Fisher, P.R., J. Appleton and J.M. Pemberton. 1978. Isolation and characterization of the pesticide-degrading plasmid pJP1 from *Alcaligenes paradoxus*. J. Bacteriol. 135:798-804.

30.   Franklin, F.C.H. and P.A. Williams. 1980. Construction of a partial diploid for the degradative pathway encoded by the TOL plasmid (pWWO) from *Pseudomonas putida* mt-2: Evidence for the positive nature of the regulation of *xylR* gene. Mol. Gen. Genet. 177:321-328.

31.   Friello, D.A., J.R. Mylroie, D.T. Gibson, J.E. Rogers and A.M. Chakrabarty. 1976. XYL, a non-conjugative xylene-degradative plasmid in *Pseudomonas* Pxy. J. Bacteriol. 127:1217-1224.

32.   Gautier, F. and R. Bonewald. 1980. The use of plasmid R1162 and derivatives for gene cloning in the methanol-utilizing *Pseudomonas* AM1. Molec. Gen. Genet. 178:375-386.

33.   Gholson, R.K., J.N. Baptist and M.J. Coon. 1963. Hydrocarbon oxidation by a bacterial enzyme system. II. Cofactor requirements for octanol formation from octane. Biochemistry 2:1155-1159.

34. Gibson, D.T. 1971. The microbial oxidation of aromatic hydro-carbons. Critical Review in MIcrobiology, pp. 199-223.
35. Grund, A., J. Shapiro, M. Fennewald, P. Bacha, J. Leahy, K. Markbreiter, M. Nieder and M. Toepfer. 1975. Regulation of alkane oxidation in *Pseudomonas putida*. J. Bacteriol. 123:546-556.
36. Hansen, J.B. and R.H. Olsen. 1978. Isolation of large bacterial plasmids and characterization of the P2 incompatibility group plasmids pMG1 and pMG5. J. Bacteriol. 135:227-238.
37. Hartmann, J., W. Reineke and H.-J. Knackmuss. 1979. Metabolism of 3-chloro-4-chloro-, and 3,5-dichlorobenzoate by a pseudo-monad. Appl.Environ.Microbiol. 37L421-428.
38. Hedges, R.W., A.E. Jacob and I.P. Crawford. 1977. Wide ranging plasmid bearing the *Pseudomonas aeruginosa* tryptophan synthase genes. Nature 267:283-284.
39. Heinaru, A.L., C.J. Duggleby and P.Broada. 1978. Molecular relationships of degradative plasmids determined by in situ hydridisation of their endonuclease generated fragments. Molec. Gen. Genet. 160:347-351.
40. Higgins, I.J., D.J. Best and R.C. Hammond. 1980. New findings in methane-utilizing bacteria highlight their importance in the biosphere and their commercial potential. Nature 286:561-564.
41. Holloway, B.W. 1978. Isolation and characterization of a R' plasmid in *Pseudomonas aeruginosa*. J. Bacteriol. 133:1078-1082.
42. Holloway, B. and V. Krishnapillai. 1975. Bacteriophages and bacteriocins. Pp 99-132, in Genetics and Biochemistry of Pseudomonas, P.H. Clarke and M. H. Richmond (eds.), John Wiley and Sons, London.
43. Hopper, D.J. and P.D. Kemp. 1980. Regulation of enzymes of the 3,5-xylenol degradative pathway in *Pseudomonas putida:* Evidence for a plasmid. J. Bacteriol. 142:21-26.
44. Hou, C.T., R.Patel, A.I. Laskin and N. Barnabe. 1979. Micro-oxidation of gaseous hydrocarbons: Epoxidation of C_2 to C_4 *n*-alkanes by methylotrophic bacteria. Appl.Environ.Microbiol. 38:127-134.
45. Jacoby, G.A. and A.E. Jacob. 1977. Recombination between *Pseudomonas aeruginosa* plasmids of incompatibility groups P-1 and P-2. Pp. 147-150, in DNA Insertion Elements, Plasmids and Episomes, A.I. Bukhari, J.A. Shapiro and S.L. Adhya (eds)., Cold Spring Harbor Laboratory, Cold Spring Harbor, New York.
46. Jacoby, G.A., J.E. Rogers, A.E. Jacob and R.W. Hedges. 1978. Transposition of *Pseudomonas* toluene-degrading genes and expression in *Escherichia coli*. Nature 274:179-180.
47. Jacoby, G.A. and J.A. Shapiro. 1977. Plasmids studied in *Pseudomonas aeruginosa* and other enteric bacteria. Pp. 639-656, in DNA Insertion Elements, Plasmids and Episomes, A.I. Bukhari, J.A. Shapiro and S.L. Adhya (eds.), Cold Spring Harbor Laboratory, Cold Spring Harbor, New York.

48. Knackmuss, H.-J. 1979. Halogenierte und sulfonierte Aromaten- Eine Herausforderung fur Aromaten abbauende Bakterien. Forum Mikrobiologie, June 1979:311-317.

49. Knackmuss, H.-J. and M. Hellwig. 1978. Utilization and co- oxidation of chlorinated phenols by *Pseudomonas* sp. B13. Arch Microbiol. 117:1-7.

50. Korfhagen, T.R., L. Sutton and G.A. Jacoby. 1978. Classifica- tion and physical properties of *Pseudomonas* plasmids. Pp.221- 624, in Microbiology 1978, D. Schlessinger (ed.), American Society for Microbiology, Washington, D.C.

51. Krylov, V.N., V.G. Bogush and J.A. Shapiro. 1980 *Pseudomonas aeruginosa* phages whose DNA structure is similar to Mul phage DNA. I. General description, localization of endonuclease- sensitive sites in DNA, and the structure of D3112 phages homoduplexes. Genetika 16:824-832 (in Russian).

52. Leadbetter, E.R.L. and J.W. Foster. 1959. Incorporation of molecular oxygen in bacterial cells utilizing hydrocarbons fo growth. Nature 184:1428-1429.

53. Lederberg, E.M. and S.N. Cohen. 1974. Transformation of *Sal- monella typhimurium* by plasmid deoxyribonucleic acid. J. Bacteriol. 119:1072-1074.

54. McKenna, E.J. and M.J. Coon. 1970. Enzymatic ω-oxidation of *Pseudomonas oleovorans*. J. Biol. Chem. 245:3882-3889.

55. McKenna, E.J. and R.E. Kallio. 1965. The biology of hydro- carbons. Ann.Rev.Microbiol. 19:183-208.

56. Meyer, R.J. 1979. Expression of incompatibility by derivative of the broad host-range Inc P-1 plasmid RK2. Molec.Gen.Genet. 177:155-161.

57. Meyer, R., G. Boch and J. Shapiro. 1979. Transposition of DNA inserted into deletions of the Tn5 kanamycin resistance eleme Moled.Gen.Genet. 171:7-13.

58. Murray, K., C.J. Duggleby, J.M. Sala-Trepat and P.A. Williams 1972. The metabolism of benzoate and methylbenzoates via the meta-cleavage pathway by *Pseudomonas arivilla* mt-2. Euro. J. Biochem. 28:301-310

59. Nagahari, K. and K. Sakaguchi. 1978. RSF1010 plasmid as a potentially useful vector in *Pseudomonas* species. J. Bacterio 133 1527-1529.

60. Nagahari, K., T. Tanaka, F. Hishinuma, M. Kuroda and K. Sakaguchi. 1977. Control of tryptophan synthetase amplified by varying the numbers of composite plasmids in *Escherichia coli* cells. Gene 1:141-152.

61. Nakazawa, T., E. Hayashi, T. Yokota, Y. Ebina and A. Nakazawa 1978. Isolation of TOL and RP4 recombinants by integrative suppression. J. Bacteriol. 134:270-277.

62. Nakazawa, T., S. Inouye and A. Nakazawa. 1980. Physical and functional mapping of RP4-TOL plasmid recombinants: Analysis of insertion and deletion mutants. J. Bacteriol. 144:222-231.

63. Nakazawa, T. and T. Yokota. 1973. Benzoate metabolism in *Pseudomonas putida* (*arvilla*) mt-2: Demonstration of two benzo ate pathways. J. Bacteriol. 115:262-267.

64. Nieder, M. and J. Shapiro. 1975. Physiological function of the
     Pseudomonas putida PpG6 *(Pseudomonas oleovorans)* and alkane
     hydroxylase: Monoterminal oxidation of alkanes and fatty acids.
     J. Bacteriol. 122:93–98.
65. Ornston, L.N. 1971. Regulation of catabolic pathways in
     Pseudomonas. Bacteriol. Rev. 35:87–116.
66. Patel, R.N., C.T. Hou, A.I. Laskin, A. Felix and P. Derelanko.
     1979. Microbial oxidation of gaseous hydrocarbons. II. Hydro-
     xylation of alkanes and epoxidation of alkenes by cell-free
     particulate fractions of methane-utilizing bacteria. J.
     Bacteriol. 139:675–679.
67. Pemberton, J.M., B. Corney and R.H. Don. 1979. Evolution and
     spread of pesticide degrading ability among soil microorganisms.
     Pp. 287–299, in Plasmids of Medical, Environmental and Commer-
     cial Importance, K. N. Timmis and A. Puehler (eds.), Elsevier.
68. Pemberton, J.M. and P.R. Fisher. 1977. 2,4-D plasmids and
     persistence. Nature 268:50–51.
69. Peterson, J.A., D. Basu and M.J. Coon. 1966. Enzymatic co-
     oxidation. I. Electron carriers in fatty acid and hydrocarbon
     oxidation. J. Biol.Chem. 241:5162–5164.
70. Poh, C.L. and R.C. Bayly. 1980. Evidence for isofunctional
     enzymes used in *m*-cresol and 2,5-xylenol degradation via the
     gentisate pathway in *Pseudomonas alcaligenes*. J. Bacteriol.
     143-59-69.
71. Reineke, W. and H.-J. Knackmuss. 1978. Chemical structure and
     biodegradability of halogenated aromatic compounds: Substituent
     effects on 1,2-dioxygenation of benzoic acid. Biochim. Bio-
     phys.Acta 542:412–423.
72. Reineke, W. and H.-J. Knackmuss. 1979. Construction of halo-
     aromatics utilizing bacteria. Nature 277:385–386.
73. Reineke, W. and H.-J. Knackmuss. 1980. Hybrid pathway for
     chlorobenzoate metabolism in *Pseudomonas* sp. B13 derivatives.
     J. Bacteriol. 142:467–473.
74. Rheinwald, J.G. 1970. The genetic organization of peripheral
     metabolism. A transmissible plasmid controlling camphor
     oxidation in *Pseudomonas putida*. M.S. thesis, University of
     Illinois, Urbana.
75. Rheinwald, J.G., A.M. Chakrabarty and I.C. Gunsalus. 1973.
     A transmissible plasmid controlling camphor oxidation in
     Pseudomonas putida. Proc.Nat.Acad.Sci. U.S. 70:885–889.
76. Ribbons, D.W. 1975. Oxidation of C_1 compounds by particulate
     fractions from *Methylococcus capsulatus:* Distribution and
     properties of methane-dependent reduced nicotinamide adenine
     dinucleotide oxidase (methane hydroxylase). J. Bacteriol.
     122:1351–1363.
77. Ruettinger, R.T., G.R. Griffith and M.J. Coon. 1977. Character-
     ization of the ω-hydroxylase of *Pseudomonas oleovorans* as a
     nonheme iron protein. Arch.Biochem. Biophys. 183:528–537.

78. Ruettinger, R.T., S.T. Olson, R.F. Boyer and M.J. Coon. 1974.
     Identification of the ω-hydroxylase of *Pseudomonas oleovorans*
     as a nonheme iron protein requiring phospholipid for catalytic
     activity. Biochem.Biophys.Res.Comm. 57:1011-1017.
79. Sano, Y. and M. Kageyame. 1977. Transoformation of *Pseudomonas*
     aeruginosa by plasmid DNA. J.Gen.Appl.Microbiol. 23:183-186.
80. Schreiber, A., M. Hellwig, E.Dorn, W. Reineke and H.-J. Knack-
     muss. 1980. Critical reactions in fluorobenzoic acid degrada-
     tion by *Pseudomonas* sp. B13. Appl.Enviorn.Microbiol. 39:58-67.
81. Shapiro, J.A. 1977. Bacterial plasmids. Introduction, Appendix
     B. Pp. 601-606, in DNA Insertion Elements, Plasmids and
     Episomes, A.I. Bukhari, J.A. Shapiro and S.L. Adhya (eds.),
     Cold Spring Harbor Laboratory, Cold Spring Harbor, New York.
82. Shapiro, J.A., S.Benson, M.Fennewald, A.Grund and M. Nieder.
     1976. Genetics of alkane utilization. Pp. 568-571, in
     Microbiology 1976, D. Schlessinger (ed.), American Society for
     Microbiology, Washington, D.C.
83. Tassin, J.P., C. Celier and J.P. Vandercasteele. 1973. Purifi-
     cation and properties of a membrane bound alcohol dehydrogenase
     involved in oxidation of long chain hydrocarbons by *Pseudo-*
     monas aeruginosa. Biochim.Biophys.Acta 315:220-232.
84. van der Linden, A.C. 1963. Epoxidation of α-olefins by heptane
     grown *Pseudomonas aeruginosa*. Biochim.Biophys.Acta 77:157-159.
85. van der Liden, A.C. and G.T.E. Thijse. 1965. The mechanism of
     microbial oxidation of petroleum hydrocarbons. Adv.Enzymol.
     27:469-545.
86. van Eyk, J. and T.J. Bartels. 1970. Paraffin oxidation in
     Pseudomonas aeruginosa. II. Gross fractionation of the enzyme
     system into soluble and particulate components. J. Bacteriol.
     104:1065-1073.
87. Wadzinski, A.M. and D.W. Ribbons. 1975. Oxidation of C_1 com-
     pounds by particulate fractions from *Methylococcus capsulatus:*
     Properties of methanol oxidase and methane dehydrogenase. J.
     Bacteriol. 122:1364-1374.
88. White, G.P. and N.W. Dunn. 1977. The apparent fusion of the
     TOL plasmid with the R91 drug resistance plasmid in *Pseudo-*
     monas aeruginosa. Aust. J. Biol. Sci. 30:345-355.
89. White, G.P. and N.W. Dunn. 1978. Evidence for transuctional
     shortening of the plasmid obtained by recombination between
     the TOL catabolic plasmid and the R91 R plasmid. Genet.Res.
     31:93-96.
90. Williams, P.A. 1979. Plasmids involved in the catabolism of
     aromatic hydrocarbons. Pp. 154-159, in Genetics of Industrial
     Microorganisms, O.K. Sebek and A. I. Laskin (ed.), American
     Society for Microbiology, Washington, D.C.
91. Williams, P.A. and K. Murray. 1974. Metabolism of benzoate and
     methyl benzoate by *Pseudomonas putida (arvilla)* mt-2: Evidence
     for the existence of a TOL plasmid. J. Bacteriol. 120:415-423.

92.   Williams, P.A. and M.J. Worsey. 1976. Ubiquity of plasmids in
       coding for toluene and xylene metabolism in soil bacteria:
       Evidence for the existence of new TOL plasmids. J. Bacteriol.
       125:818-828.
93.   Windass, J.D., M.J. Worsey, E.M. Pioli, D. Pioli, P.T. Barth,
       K. T. Atherton, E.C. Dart, D. Byron, K. Powell and P. J. Senin.
       1980. Improved conversion of methanol to single-cell protein
       by *Methylophilus methylotrophus*. Nature 287:396-401.
94.   Wong, C.L. and N.W. Dunn. 1976. Combined chromosomal and plasmid
       encoded control for the degradation of phenol in *Pseudomonas
       putida*. Genet.Res. 27:405-412.
95.   Worsey, M.J., F.C.H. Franklin and P.A. Williams. 1978. Regula-
       tion of the degradative pathway enzymes coded for by the TOL
       plasmid (pWWO) from *Pseudomonas putida (arvilla)* mt-2: Evidence
       for a new function of the TOL plasmid. J. Bacteriol. 124:7-13.
96.   Worsey, M.J. and P.A. Williams. 1977. Characterization of a
       spontaneously occurring mutant of the TOL20 plasmid in *Pseudo-
       monas putida* MT20: Possible regulatory implications. J.
       Bacteriol. 124:7-13.
97.   Worsey, M.J. and P.A. Williams. 1977. Characterization of a
       spontaneously occurring mutant of the TOL20 plasmid in *Pseudo-
       monas putida* MT20: Possible regulatory implications. J. Bac-
       teriol. 130:1149-1158.
98.   Yano, K. and NIshi, T. 1980. pKJ1, a naturally occurring con-
       jugative plasmid coding for toluene degradation and resistance
       to streptomycin and sulfonamides. J. Bacteriol. 143:552-560.

DISCUSSION

Q.   SCOTT: My question concerns the use of genetic engineering to
      produce a bacterium that can possibly degrade hydrocarbons.
      What types of safety precautions are being taken to make sure
      we don't produce a bacterium that possibly could be dangerous
      to the researcher?

A.   SHAPIRO: Well, I think most of these organisms are not organ-
      isms which can be pathogenic for people. You know, the guide-
      lines do get into some very strange situations. For example,
      it's exempt from the guidelines to clone these genes in
      Pseudomonas aeruginosa because *P. aeruginosa* is known to ex-
      change DNA with *E. Coli* in nature, and that's one of the
      criteria for exemption from the guidelines. However, *P. aeru-
      ginosa* is occasionally a pathogen in compromised individuals.
      The guidelines limit the use of *Pseudomonas putida*, because
      that kind of exchange has not been clearly and unequivocally
      demonstrated in nature. However, we spent a great deal of time
      researching this, and there is no single documented case where
      P. putida was a human pathogen. It is not closely related to

Pseudomonas phytopathogens either. I think there's no absolute
guarantee that one can give about this, but as far as we know
these organisms have not been signaled as pathogens. They don
like to grow at 37°, they're obligate aerobes and I think the
risks are small. But I could never say that the risks are zero

Q.   ARCURI: I have a question about the initial approach of the
     organisms to an insoluble surface. I wonder if there is any
     evidence that the cell approaches it in a specific manner?

A.   SHAPIRO: Well, we don't know about that and we really haven't
     looked into it. Normally, we grow cells on the surface of
     agar plates and we feed them vapors. If you think about what
     must be happening enzymatically in a liquid culture, it's a
     horrendously complicated system. We gave up trying to do rea
     enzyme kinetics on it because at least three phases are in-
     volved. There are the oil droplets themselves, then the cell
     membrane – which is not quite rigid but not quite a liquid
     structure – and then, there are the soluble proteins in the
     cytoplasm which are involved in the initial enzyme reaction
     as well. So, it's very complicated. For these shorter chain
     alkanes, there seems to be no evidence that special emulsifier
     or solubilizing agents are involved; for the longer alkane
     molecules, other organisms such as *P. aeruginosa*, some of
     the gram-positive bacteria, and even some *Acinetobacters*
     produce emulsifying agents. Whether those are just bits of
     the outer cell surface, or whether they are specifically
     evolved structures for doing that, isn't yet clear. In those
     cases, there may be cellular products which facilitate the
     contact between the substrate and the cell. But, I think
     very little is known about that. Obviously if large scale
     fermentations are going to be developed, it will be extremely
     useful to know more about this.

Q.   ARCURI: The reason I asked is because Marshall's group in
     Australia has found that certain bacteria approach oil drop-
     lets in an end on manner. They have a hypothesis, that this
     behavior is the result of a localization of hydrophobic sub-
     stances at the end of the cell. Now the question is how do
     cells vary if you engineer the membrane concentration of sub-
     stances to change the hydrophobic nature of this surface. How
     do cells manage to approach and stick to the oil droplets?

A.   SHAPIRO: Well, as I said, I think a lot of this is going to
     be very, very empirical, at least in the beginning until we
     know more.

Q.   DETROY: Jim, can you comment on the specificity of these
     systems for different chlorinated aromatics?

A.   SHAPIRO: Well, I'm not really an expert on that. It seems that
      the ring fission activities in Knackmuss' strain can utilize a
      wide variety of substrates, such as mono-chlorinated and di-
      chlorinated catechols. In some cases I think they can use
      fluorinated catechols. Mutants can be isolated, which will
      use substrates that the original strain won't use. So these
      enzymes seem to be able to tolerate a number of substitutions.
      In the pathway, as I understand it, the structures that are
      formed create very liabile halogen-carbon bonds which spon-
      taneously break and release halide ions. I think it's going
      to turn out that there are multiple enzyme systems for doing
      this which have different specificities. That's why I think
      it is important to go out and identify and catalog them; so
      that, if you have a substrate which proves refractory to that
      particular set of enzymes, you can look for other ring fission
      enzymes which will allow us to degrate that substrate.

Q.   JACKSON: I think the point that you make about the toxic
      effect of overproduction of membrane proteins is an important
      one. Are there data available where one can start to say how
      much overproduction does really lead to toxicity to several
      different proteins of this sort?

A.   SHAPIRO: Well, the best studied cases are with hybrid proteins
      that have been made by fusing β-galactosidase to various mem-
      brane proteins (often from the maltose transport system). Here
      it's well documented that large amounts of these hybrid pro-
      teins are toxic for the cell. You can isolate mutants which
      are no longer sensitive, either because the mutations affect
      the structure of the protein or its attachment to the membrane
      or, perhaps, the level of synthesis of some of these hybrids.
      Apparently it is difficult to clone lactose permease on a high
      copy number plasmid. This is persumably because of the same
      kind of problem related to this toxicity effect.

Q.   JACKSON: But, as I understand it, most of those studies have
      been done, as you say, with hybrid proteins. Here, according
      to one hypothesis, the toxicity is due to the non-membrane
      protein partner which cannot be properly transported through
      the membrane and clogs up the transport pores. Are there
      studies on strains that are overproducing normal membrane
      proteins?

A.   SHAPIRO: Well, that's certainly the case with the lactose
      permease, which is a normal membrane protein. When and if we
      have the hydroxylase gene on high copy number plasmids, we can
      make more of it. Of course, it may be that there are regulatory
      mechanisms which monitor the amount of protein that is made
      independently of gene dose. This problem is just one possible
      pitfall that I think it is important to signal right now.

Especially in these systems where there are alot of membrane proteins involved. Apparently, some of the catechol oxygenase are particulate enzymes, too. So hydrocarbon oxidation is not like the simple world of soluble biochemistry.

HYDROGEN FORMATION BY THE BIOPHOTOLYSIS
OF WATER VIA GLYCOLATE AND FORMATE

Lester O. Krampitz

Case Western Reserve University

Cleveland, Ohio 44106

I am substituting for Professor H. G. Wood who was scheduled to chair this session but because of last minute commitments was unable to attend this meeting. Knowing his interests in the theme of this symposium I am sure he would have opened the session with a few remarks about some of the interesting research he is doing in the field of microbial metabolism. With your permission I will utilize some of his time to report some results we have obtained on the biophotolysis of water with the formation of hydrogen.

The photosynthetic apparatus which splits water to yield oxygen and electrons is capable of forming hydrogen if proper catalysis of the reduction of protons by the electrons is available. Hydrogen formation has been accomplished in several laboratories employing the above concept. The efficiency of such systems is low and suffers from two main complications: (1) hydrogenase, the enzyme employed for the reduction of protons by the photosynthetically formed electrons, is very labile to the effects of photosynthetically evolved oxygen, and (2) the simultaneous evolution of oxygen and hydrogen would require a large area collecting device, which is apparently impractical.

An alternative concept is to employ the electrons for the reduction of CO_2 to a stable reduced product which would serve as an electron donor for the reduction of protons with the formation of hydrogen in a <u>dark</u> reaction. Such a product would be photosynthetic fuel crop.

Remarks at opening of session on Modification of Fermentation Pathways.

The photosynthetic reduction of CO_2 to formate would be an ideal product which could form hydrogen and CO_2 in a dark reaction by the formic hydrogenlyase complex present in some bacteria. The photosynthetic reduction of CO_2 to formate does not occur in quantitative proportions. The photosynthetic reduction of CO_2 to glycolat by green algae has been known for some time (1,2,3). Higher plants possess an enzyme, glycolic oxidase (4), which is a flavo protein capabile of oxidizing glycolate to glyoxylate and hydrogen peroxide. In the absence of catalase the hydrogen peroxide oxidizes the glycolate to formate and CO_2. We have employed these concepts to bring about the indirect biophotolysis of water to oxygen and hydrogen which are summarized in the following generalized equations:

$$\text{(1)} \quad 2CO_2 + 2H_2O \xrightarrow[\textit{Chlorella pyrenoidosa}]{h\nu} \quad \begin{matrix} H \\ HC - COOH + 1.5\ O_2 \\ OH \end{matrix}$$

$$\text{(2)} \quad \begin{matrix} H \\ HC-COOH + O_2 \\ OH \end{matrix} \xrightarrow[\text{oxidase}]{\text{glycolic}} \quad \begin{matrix} H \\ O = C-COOH + H_2O_2 \end{matrix}$$

$$\text{(3)} \quad O=C-COOH + H_2O_2 \xrightarrow{\text{nonenzymatic}} HCOOH + CO_2 + H_2O$$

$$\text{(4)} \quad HCOOH \xrightarrow[\text{hydrogenlyase}]{\text{formic}} H_2 + CO_2$$

$$\text{Sum 1 thru 4:}\ H_2O \xrightarrow{h\nu} H_2 + 0.5\ O_2$$

It should be noted that all reactions with the exception of equation 1 are dark reactions.

Experimental conditions for the photosynthetic formation of glycolate have been studied with several photosynthetic systems. These conditions include low partial pressure of CO_2, high partial pressure of oxygen, and high light intensities. Most of the experiments concerned with glycolate formation reported here were performed with *Chlorella pyrenoidosa* strain 1230.

The organism was grown on a chemically defined medium as described by Watt and Fogg (5) with the exception that 660 mg/liter of urea were employed as the nitrogen source. CO_2 was the carbon source. They were propagated in a 4 liter flask containing 3 liters of medium. The flasks contained a magnetic stirring bar. Incubation was at 30° in an incubator containing 3.0% CO_2, balance air. Illumination was with banks of fluorescent lights at an intensity of 10,000 lux. Time of harvest by centrifugation ranged from two to three days. The cell paste was washed once with water and finally suspended in the growth medium minus urea, adjusted usually to pH8.4,

at a concentration of 100 mg wet weight of cells per ml. Usually 4 ml
of the suspension were placed in manometric flasks (20 ml volume).
The flasks were attached to manometers and were incubated at 30°
with shaking in a Warburg apparatus equipped for illumination. The
light intensity was 10,000 lux with incandescent lamps. A manifold
was attached to the manometers and a flow of air (99.8%) and CO_2
(0.2%) was constantly passed through the flasks at a positive
pressure of 20 mm of Brodie solution. When additions to the flasks
were made (as indicated in the result section) appropriate correc-
tions were made to keep the cell concentration constant. Time of
incubation varied as indicated below. Glycolate was determined by
the method of Calkins (6).

RESULTS

Most investigators concerned with photosynthetic formation
of glycolate have employed low partial pressure of CO_2 with the
balance of the atmosphere oxygen. We were concerned with finding
optimum conditions for prolonged glycolate formation in an atmosphere of air supplemented with low partial pressure of CO_2, i.e.,
0.1 to 0.2%.

Data in Table I represent glycolate formation by resting cells
suspended in buffer, gassed with 0.2% CO_2 and balance air and
illuminated. At the conclusion of one hour 3.2 mM had accumulated.
The production of glycolate did not continue at the same rate
during the second hour. If, however, the contents of the flasks
were centrifuged and the algal pellet suspended in fresh buffer the
accumulation of glycolate during an hour interval was similar to
the first incubation period. Repeated centrifugation and resuspen-
sion in fresh medium could be performed repeatedly, as much as eight
times.

TABLE I

Main compartment 10% suspension	Gas phase 0.2% CO_2 balance air
Chlorella pyrenoidosa in Hepes buffer pH 8.4	
Time: 1 hr Temp: 30° Light: 10,000 lux	Glycolate formed 3.2 mM
Time 2 hr	3.4 mM

End product inhibition was not the cause of the lack of glycolate accumulation, since a suspension of cells in 5.0 mM glycolate
produced an additional amount of glycolate as in experiments with no
initial glycolate concentration. The supernatant fluid from an
incubation mixture that had ceased to form additional glycolate did
inhibit glycolate formation when illuminated with fresh cells.

Isolation of inhibitory substances from such a supernatant
fluid indicated that intermediates of the urea cycle were responsib
for the inhibitory effect. Analysis of the system further established that ammonium ion derived from the urea cycle intermedia
was inhibitory. We have not discovered the mode in which ammonium
ion inhibits glycolate formation. In experiments performed as outlined in Table I but with one micromole/ml of ammonium ion added,
glycolate formation was inhibited by 50 to 60%. Two micromoles/ml
totally inhibited its formation.

Pritchard and co-workers (2) had found that isoniazide stimulated glycolate formation. The effect of isoniazide is shown in
Table II. Preliminary results indicate that isoniazide somehow
relieves the inhibition by ammonium ion.

TABLE II

Main compartment	Gas phase
10% suspension	0.2% CO_2

Chlorella pyrenoidosa
in Hepes buffer pH 8.4
plus 30 mM isoniazide

Time:	1 hr	Glycolate formed
Temp:	30°	4.8 mM
Light:	10,000 lux	

Time 2 hr	5.2 mM

In order to convert the photosynthetically formed glycolate
to formate, reactions 2 and 3 above, glycolic oxidase was immobilized onto alkylamine glass by diazotization. The alkylamine glas
was prepared by treating the glass with γ-aminopropyltriethoxysilan
Five ml of a glycolate solution (10 mM) in 0.05M potassium phosphat
pH 7.5 was passed slowly through a column of the immobilized enzyme
(2 cm x 20 cm). The columm was washed with 20 ml of 0.05M phosphat
buffer. The combined eluates demonstrated that the glycolate had
been 98% converted to formate. Formate was determined by formic
dehydrogenase and NAD reduction.

The formate was converted to hydrogen and CO_2 (equation 4 above) by passing 25 ml of a 1.5 mM solution of formate through a column (2 cm x 200 cm) containing *Escherichia coli,* Crookes strain, immobilized on porous alkylamine glass. Hydrogen was determined by gas chromatography. Recovery of hydrogen was 70% of theory.

REFERENCES

1. Tolbert, N.E., and L.P. Zill, J. Biol. Chem. <u>222</u>, 895 (1956)
2. Pritchard, G.G., W.S. Griffin, and C.P. Wittingham. J. Exptl. Botany <u>13</u>, 1977 (1962)
3. Warburg, O., and G. Krippal, Z. Naturforschung 15b, 197 (1960).
4. Zelitch, I., and S. Ochoa, J. Biol. Chem. <u>201</u>, 707 (1953).
5. Watt, W.D., and G.E. Fogg, J. Exptl. Botany <u>17</u>, 117 (1966).
6. Calking, V.P., Ind. and Eng. Chem. Anal. Eds. <u>15</u>, 762 (1943).

HYDROGENASE GENES

R.C. Tait, K. Andersen, G. Cangelosi, and K.T. Shanmugam*

Plant Growth Laboratory, Dept. of Agronomy & Range
Science, University of California
Davis, California 95616

INTRODUCTION

Molecular hydrogen (H_2) plays a key role in the metabolism of
many microorganisms. H_2 can function as an electron donor or can be
the product of reduction of protons during energy-yielding processes.
The function of the protein hydrogenase plays a fundamental role in
H_2 metabolism. Hydrogenase has been found in a large number of
bacteria and algae. A number of reviews concerning the occurrence of
hydrogenase in microorganisms and its role in metabolism are available (1-4). For the purpose of this discussion, we shall consider
three basic categories of organisms containing hydrogenase. Organisms
possessing the ability to oxidize H_2 can be regarded as hydrogen uptake positive (hup^+), while those able to evolve H_2 can be divided
into two groups. In the first group, H_2 production is the result of
anaerobic fermentation reactions, while in the second group H_2 production is a result of the processes involved in biological nitrogen
fixation. Depending on the nature of the hydrogenase present, an
organism may belong to more than one of these three groups. Certain
strains of the nitrogen-fixing bacterium *Rhizobium japonicum*, for
example, are able to utilize H_2 as an energy source but also evolve
H_2 as an aspect of nitrogen fixation (5-9). The function of hydrogenase in each of these three groups is outlined below.

Group I. Hydrogen Uptake Positive

Although organisms capable of autotrophic growth in the
presence of H_2 and O_2 might be considered the prototype in this
group, a variety of bacteria are able to take up H_2, utilizing

---

* Department of Microbiology & Cell Science, IFAS, University of
Florida, Gainesville, Florida 32611

inorganic compounds other than O_2 as the terminal electron acceptor
The hydrogen bacterium *Alcaligenes eutrophus* obtains energy during
autotrophic growth by the oxidation of H_2 with O_2 as the electron
acceptor: $2H_2 + O_2 \rightarrow 2H_2O$ (10-12). In contrast, oxidation of H_2
by *Desulfovibrio vulgaris* involves utilization of sulfate as the
terminal electron acceptor: $4H_2 + SO_4^= \rightarrow S^= + 4H_2O$ (4). In utilization of H_2 during methanogenesis by *Methanobacterium* CO_2 serves as
the terminal electron acceptor: $4H_2 + CO_2 \rightarrow CH_4 + 2H_2O$ (13, 14).
During the process of photoreduction, H_2 is used in the generation
of reducing power for CO_2 assimilation: $2H_2 + CO_2 \xrightarrow{\text{(light)}} CH_2O$
$+ H_2O$ (15). The common feature of the utilization of H_2 by hydrogenase in this group of organisms is that $H_2\downarrow$ serves as a primary
source of reducing power in cellular metabolism.

Group II.   Fermentation H_2 Evolution

The evolution of H_2 during the fermentative metabolism of
organic compounds has been examined in some detail in the saccharolytic Clostridia and in the facultative anaerobe *Escherichia coli*
(for reviews see 1, 2). It has been suggested that the role of H_2
production in these organisms involves the disposal of electrons
produced during energy-yielding oxidation reactions, the promotion
of these energy-yielding reactions through removal of end products,
and the regulation of reducing power and energy pools (1).

Group III. H_2 Evolution by Nitrogen Fixing Organisms

Nitrogen fixing photosynthetic bacteria such as *Rhodospirillum*
rubrum have been found to produce H_2 from organic substrates (16,17)
The inhibition of this anaerobic photoevolution of H_2 by ammonia and
N_2 suggested that this activity is linked to N_2 metabolism (16-19).
Investigation of the phenomenon generated evidence for the existence
of an anaerobic citric acid cycle in which H_2 evolution is the resul
of the regeneration of reduced pyridine nucleotides (1, 17, 18). It
has been suggested by Gray and Gest that the terminal steps of the
photoevolution of H_2 can be represented by the relationship:

$$\text{light}$$
$$\downarrow$$
$$X{\sim}P$$
$$\downarrow$$
$$PNH + H^+ \rightarrow PN^+ + H_2 \qquad \text{(modified from 1)}$$

in which PNH = reduced pyridine nucleotides generated by the functi
of the anaerobic citric acid cycle, PN^+ = oxidized pyridine nucleotides, and $X{\sim}P$ = energy rich intermediates associated with photophos
phorylation. The function of this form of H_2 evolution may be

associated with the maintenance of reduced pyridines and phosphorylated compounds such as ATP at concentrations consistent with the
overall rate of biosynthetic activity and may constitute a regulatory
mechanism of the energy metabolism of the cell (1,18,19).

Nitrogenase preparations isolated from a variety of nitrogen
fixing organisms have been found to catalyze an ATP-dependent H_2
evolution (20,21). Schubert and Evans suggested that only 40-60%
of the electron flow through nitrogenase in *Rhizobium* species is
transferred to N_2, with the remainder lost through H_2 evolution (5).
Results obtained with *Klebsiella pneumoniae* suggest that about one-
third of the metabolic energy involved in nitrogen fixation is lost
via nitrogenase mediated H_2 evolution (22). The evolution of substantial quantities of H_2 during biological nitrogen fixation is
apparently an energy-consuming reaction mediated by the nitrogenease
complex.

Examination of the hydrogenases that have been purified and
characterized reveals that although the hydrogenases are all iron-
sulfur proteins, there exists a great diversity of structural, catalytic, and physiochemical properties among these enzymes (4). This
is illustrated by a comparison of the characteristics of hydrogenases
purified from *Clostridium pasteurianum, Desulfovibrio vulgaris* and
Alcaligenes eutrophus, shown in Table I. In view of the variation
in the physical properties of hydrogenases, the soluble hydrogenase
purified from *A. eutrophus* appears unique among the characterized
hydrogenases. This enzyme is insensitive to oxygen under reaction
conditions, contains FMN as a coenzyme and is able to react directly
with NAD.

Because of the fundamental role of hydrogenase in the metabolism of many organisms and its postulated activity in the regulation
of the overall energy state of the cell, we believe that a detailed
analysis of hydrogenase genes can be justified solely by the potential increase in information pertaining to the control of energy-
yielding processes. In addition, we are concened with five areas
of research in which the application of isolated hydrogenase genes
might provide not only significant scientific results, but also of
hydrogenase. These areas of interest are described below:

1. Manipulation of the efficiency of symbiotic nitrogen fixation. Because of the inherent H_2 production activity of nitrogenase,
it has been suggested that nitrogen fixation is relatively ineffi-
cient and that the efficiency might be improved by the recovery of
the H_2 produced by nitrogenase (5,6,8). It has been suggested that
strains of *R. japonicum* containing an uptake hydrogenase are more
energy-efficient during nitrogen fixation (6,13). The isolation and
characterization of hydrogenase genes might allow the construction
of energy-efficient strains of *Rhizobium* containing an active H_2
uptake system that would allow recovery of much of the energy lost
via nitrogenase-mediated H_2 evolution.

TABLE I

	Clostridium pasteurianum	Desulfovibrio vulgaris	Alcaligenes eutrophus	Alcaligenes eutrophus
Localization	Cytoplasm	Periplasm	Membranes	Cytoplasm
Natural electron donor/acceptor	Ferredoxin	Cytochrome C_3	?	NAD
Oxygen sensitivity	Very sensitive	Relatively stable	Stable	Stable
Molecular weight	60,000	50,000	100,000	200,000
Subunits	1 × 60,000	1 × 50,000	1 × 67,000 1 × 31,000	1 × 68,000 1 × 60,000 2 × 29,000
Fe/mol labile S^{2-}/mol	12, 12	12, 12	6, 6	12, 12 2 FMN
References	23, 24	25, 26	27	28, 29

2. Regeneration of NADH during *in vitro* enzymatic reactions.
Because of the unique properties of the soluble hydrogenase of *A. eutrophus* (soluble, insensitive to oxygen during reaction conditions, able to directly reduce NAD without other protein involvement), this protein might be utilized to regenerate NADH from NAD and H_2 in commercially important *in vitro* enzymatic reactions in which NADH is required. The construction of bacteria that overproduce this hydrogenase would be important to the purification of commercially relevant quantities of the protein.

3. Bioenergy production. In this era of decreasing energy supply and increasing energy consumption, the development of alternative energy sources is a topic of increasing importance. A detailed analysis of the regulation of hydrogenase may allow the manipulation of the fermentative and photosynthetic pathways of microorganisms to optimize the production of H_2 from organic and inorganic compounds.

4. Ruminant physiology and methanogenesis. Carbohydrate fermentation in the rumen is the result of coupled culture of methanogenic and non-methanogenic bacteria. It has been suggested that interspecies H_2 transfer from the non-methanogens to the methanogens and the subsequent use of the H_2 in the production of methane is able to alter the fermentative process. Interspecies transfer of H_2 may result in increased substrate utilization, greater amounts of ATP synthesized by the non-methanogens, increased growth of both organisms, and changes in the proportions of the reduced end products (32). An understanding of the role of hydrogenase in this process may suggest methods for increasing the production of fermentative products utilizable by the ruminant animal, thereby increasing the relative efficiency of the ruminant physiology. In addition, the analysis of the role of hydrogenase in interspecies H_2 transfer may allow the development of the methodology for the fermentative production of methane from plant materials in the absence of the currently required fermentation appartus (a cow).

5. Production of chemicals from CO_2 as a carbon source with H_2 as an energy source. Autotrophic organisms are able to provide for their total carbon requirement by the assimilation of CO_2. In the case of *A. eutrophus*, energy is provided by the oxidation of H_2. If the mechanisms involved in the control of hydrogenase function in the presence of organic substrates can be determined, one might imagine the construction of strains in which the utilization of H_2 as an energy source has been uncoupled from the availability of organic carbon sources. The anabolic pathways of these strains might then be manipulated to produce a desired end product, for example ethanol. The net result would then be a strain able to grow using H_2 as an energy source and CO_2 as a carbon source and producing a desired organic compound in the process.

It is our belief that a rational approach to the involvement
of hydrogenase in these problems involves the analysis of the molecular mechanisms involved in the control of expression of hydrogenase. We hope to accomplish this in part by the isolation and
in vitro analysis of hydrogenase genes. We are involved in a four-
part program, outlined below, the ultimate goal of which is the
development of the ability to manipulate hydrogenase genes.

1. Analysis of the physiology of hydrogenase.

2. Construction and characterization of hydrogenase
    mutants.

3. Isolation of hydrogenase genes by complementation
    of hydrogenase mutants.

4. Analysis of the structure and control of hydrogenase
    genes.

We are currently applying this approach to the hydrogenase genes of
A. eutrophus and *E. coli*. Our current state of progress shall be
described in the following sections.

Physiology of Hydrogenase

During autotrophic growth, a small group of reactions in the
Calvin cycle consume a large portion of the available energy.
Because of this, it has been suggested that the control mechanisms
of the intermediary metabolism of autotrophs will be focused on
CO_2 fixation rather than on exogenous substrate, as is the case in
most bacteria (3). Results obtained with hydrogen bacteria suggest
that there is a complex relationship between hydrogenase and intermediary metabolism. Adaptation of *A. eutrophus* H16 to growth on
fructose is blocked in the presence of H_2, and enzymes normally
induced by fructose in air are not induced by fructose in H_2 (33,
34). Repression of enzyme systems can be partially removed by the
addition of CO_2 (33) which presumably results in the removal of the
NADH and ATP produced by hydrogenase activity *via* the reactions
involved in CO_2 assimilation. Exposure of heterotrophically growing
cells to H_2 can result in the increased expression of the ribulose-1,
5-bisphosphate carboxylase gene(s)(35). In strains of *R. japonicum*
which can be grown autotrophically as hydrogen bacteria, there is
an interrelationship between the regulation of hydrogenase synthesis, CO_2 fixation, and the presence of organic carbon sources (36).
Although the mechanisms have not been elucidated, results obtained
in hydrogen bacteria suggest that biochemical and genetic controls
are involved in the interaction of hydrogenase with cellular metabolism (10).

Utilization of organic carbon sources in the absence of H_2 affects the expression of hydrogenase in *A. eutrophus* H1. Hydrogenase activity in cultures growing exponentially in the presence of succinate reaches 2-3 µM/hr/mg protein, 8-9 µM/hr/mg protein in the presence of lactate, 15-16 µM/hr/mg protein in the presence of fructose, and 35 µM/hr/mg protein under autotrophic conditions, shown in Table II. In the presence of isoleucine or pyruvate, hydrogenase levels have been observed to exceed levels found during autotrophic growth (37). In general, carbon sources that allowed rapid growth (succinate) repressed hydrogenase activity and carbon sources that allowed slower growth (fructose, isoleucine) allowed higher levels of hydrogenase activity. These observations suggest that hydrogenase is subject to a regulatory mechanism that is affected by the nature of the carbon source available to the cell.

Because of the role of cyclic AMP (cAMP) as a regulator molecule in the enteric bacteria (38-42), the effects of cAMP on hydrogenase were examined. The intracellular concentration of cAMP was greatly affected by the growth phase of a culture and the availability of an organic carbon source, as shown in Table II. The presence of 2 mM cAMP during the adaptation of stationary phase, autotrophically grown cultures to growth in the presence of organic carbon sources increased the rate of accumulation of hydrogenase activity. However, once the culture entered the exponential phase of growth, this stimulatory effect was no longer observed. Although the presence of exogenous cAMP can result in the increased rate of appearance of hydrogenase activity, the ultimate level of activity is determined not by the level of cAMP, but rather by the carbon source under utilization.

To determine whether the stimulatory effect of cAMP was the result of a biochemical stimulation of hydrogenase or the increased expression of genes involved in hydrogenase activity, the sensitivity of the stimulation to transcriptional and translational inhibitors was examined. As shown in Figure 1, the cAMP-mediated stimulation of hydrogenase activity was prevented by inhibition of either transcription or translation. Hydrogenase is apparently affected by cAMP at the level of the control of genetic expression.

The relationship of hydrogenase to organic carbon source utilization is illustrated in Figure 2. Organic carbon source utilization affects a regulatory system "R" which in turn controls the maximum level of expression of hydrogenase. Carbon utilization also affects the intracellular level of cAMP, which in turn modulates the efficiency of expression of genes required for hydrogenase function. Although data are not available concerning the nature of "R", one might suspect that this will be found to involve a repressor-operator or inducer-operator interaction and that the effects of cAMP are exerted through control of the transcriptional efficiency of the hydrogenase genes.

TABLE II

Carbon Source	Lag Phase		Logarithmic Phase	
	H_2ase Activity	[cAMP]	H_2ase Activity	[cAMP]
10% CO_2:10% O_2: 80% H_2	23.5	10.3	34.4	64.0
Lactate	4.8	37.5	8.8	19.3
+ 2 mM cAMP	9.9		7.8	
Succinate	1.4	137.0	2.5	20.6
+ 2 mM cAMP	2.3		3.4	
Fructose	5.9	34.4	15.6	15.1
+ 2 mM cAMP	12.8		14.5	

H_2ase activity in μM H_2/hr/mg protein.

[cAMP] in pM cAMP/mg protein.

Working on this assumption, we have examined *A. eutrophus* H1 for the presence of a cAMP binding protein analogous to the cAMP receptor protein (CRP) found in *E. coli*. The method described for the purification of CRP from *E. coli* (43) was applied to *A. eutrophus* H1. A cAMP binding protein was purified to apparent homogeneity as determined by polyacrylamide gel electrophoresis under native and denaturing conditions. This putative CRP protein has a subunit molecular weight of approximately 14 kilodaltons (Kd), a native molecular weight of 30-35 Kd, and binds cAMP with an apparent dissocation constant of 2.5×10^{-6} M. In comparison, CRP purified from *E. coli* has a subunit molecular weight of 22 Kd, a native molecular weight of 45 Kd, and binds cAMP with an apparent dissocation constant of $1-2 \times 10^{-6}$ M (44,45). The potential role of this cAMP binding protein in the transcription of hydrogenase genes should be clarified by the construction of mutants in which the function of this protein is altered and by the *in vitro* examination of the interaction of this protein with the isolated hydrogenase genes.

Construction and Characterization of Hydrogenase Mutants

Alcaligenes eutrophus. Experiments by Reh and Schlegel (46) and Pootjes (47) support the suggestion that plasmids may be involved in H_2 uptake in hydrogen bacteria. Evidence suggests that plasmids may determine H_2 utilization in *R. leguminosarum* (48). During the construction and characterization of mutants of *A. eutrophus* blocked in CO_2 metabolism (35), we obtained evidence for the involvement of large plasmids in the H_2 metabolism of hydrogen bacteria (49). These plasmids have been utilized in the construction of hydrogenase mutants of *A. eutrophus* H1.

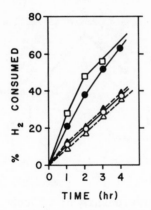

Figure 1.   Stimulation of hydrogenase activity by cAMP.

A culture of *A. eutrophus* H1 was grown in fructose minimal
medium to the stationary phase of growth, then washed, resuspended
in fresh fructose minimal medium, and incubated for 15 min under
air (in the presence of inhibitors where indicated), cAMP was added
to 2 mM, samples were evacuated and placed under N_2, and an aliquot
of H_2 injected. Hydrogenase activity was followed over a period of
3 hr by monitoring disappearance of H_2 with gas chromatography. 5 mM
methylene blue was present as the terminal electron acceptor. H_2
uptake activity of autotrophically grown cells, □ —— □. H_2 uptake
activity of cells grown in the presence of fructose, 0-0; and
fructose with the following additions: 2 mM cAMP, ●-●; 100 µg/ml
rifampicin + 2 mM cAMP, △--△; 100 µg/ml tetracycline + 2 µg/ml
cAMP, ▲--▲.

In the presence of mitomycin C, and agent which interferes with
plasmid DNA replication, *A. eutrophus* H1 was converted at a high
frequency from a hup⁺ to a hup⁻ phenotype. Two types of hup⁻ derivatives were obtained: cells unable to grow with H_2 as the energy
source, and cells capable of growth at a greatly reduced rate with
H_2 as the energy source. When examined by agarose gel electrophoresis, DNA isolated from hup⁺ strains contained a covalently
closed circular DNA of approximately 200 megadaltons (Md). Cells
which had been converted to the complete hup⁻ phenotype no longer
contained this plasmid, while the partially hup⁻ derivatives all
contained large plasmids. Co-electrophoresis of plasmids present
in hup⁺ and hup⁻ cells suggested that many of the plasmids present
in the partially hup⁻ cells contained deletions of 5-20 Md. When
the hup⁺ phenotype was conjugally transferred to a hup⁻ strain, the
hup⁺ derivative acquired the large plasmid. These observations
indicate that the large plasmid contains information necessary for
the expression of the hup⁺ phenotype. The deletions present in this

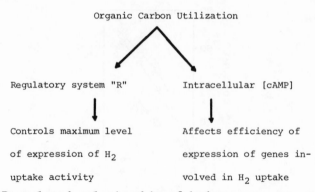

Figure 2. Postulated relationship of hydrogenase expression with organic carbon source utilization in *A. eutrophus*.

plasmid that inactivate the hup[+] phenotype represent non-reverting hup mutants which, after characterization, may be useful in the isolation of hup genes.

        In order to determine which of the two hydrogenases of *A. eutrophus* was affected by the deletions of the large plasmid, six independently derived hup[-] mutants were chosen for further characterization. Total hydrogenase activity was determined using methylene blue as an electron acceptor (50), and activity of the soluble hydrogenase was determined with NAD as the electron acceptor in cell-free extracts (29). The results are summarized in Table III. The mutants H1-3 and H1-6 contained no large plasmids and were completely lacking in both hydrogenase activities, suggesting that neither the soluble nor the membrane bound hydrogenase is present in cells cured of the large plasmid. The slow-growing mutants H1-2, H1-4, and H1-5 contain undetectable levels of the soluble hydrogenase although they contain significant levels of the membrane bound activity. The deletions present in these plasmids appear to prevent the function of the soluble hydrogenase but allow the function of the membrane bound activity. The potentially interesting H1-1 has normal H_2 uptake with methylene blue but only 10% of the normal level of NAD-reducing H_2 uptake activity. The deletion present in the plasmid in this strain may cause the synthesis of an altered soluble hydrogenase of reduced activity, may cause a reduction in the level of expression of the normal hydrogenase, or may affect a component necessary for the optimal function of the soluble enzyme. The non-reverting nature of these mutants and the inactivation of either the soluble or both hydrogenase activities makes these strains useful in the isolation of genes involved in H_2 uptake. Although the most probable situation is that the deletions directly affect the hydrogenase genes themselves, it is possible that the deletions in the plasmid affect genes whose function is necessary for the

TABLE III

Properties of *A. eutrophus* H1 derivatives
defective in H_2 utilization

| | Generation time (hr) | Plasmid size | Hup activity (μmol/hr/mg protein) e^- acceptor | |
	$H_2/O_2/CO_2$	(mdaltons)	methylene blue	NAD
A. eutrophus	2.7	$\sim$200	83	114
H1-1	7.5	$\sim$180	30	11
H1-2	8.5	$\sim$200	30	<0.2
H1-3	-	-	<1	<0.2
H1-4	10.5	$\sim$180	29	<0.2
H1-5	10.5	$\sim$180	29	<0.2
H1-6	-	-	1	<0.2

Stationary-phase cells grown in isoleucine minimal medium under
air were used. Hup activity with 5 mM methylene blue as electron acceptor was determined by following the disappearnace of
H_2 by gas chromatography. Activity using NAD as electron acceptor was determined by following the reduction of NAD spec-
trophotometrically.

expression of hydrogenase genes. In such a situation, complementation of these mutants may provide not the hydrogenase genes, but
other genes involved in H_2 uptake.

Escherichia coli. *E. Coli* is a facultative anaerobic organism
that produces H_2, a potential fuel source, during normal anaerobic
growth as a metabolic end product. In this organism formate, a
metabolic product of the enzyme pyruvate-formate lyase, is further
metabolized to H_2 and CO_2 by the enzymes formate dehydrogenase and
hydrogenase. *E. coli* is also capable of utilizing H_2 as an electron
donor during anaerobic growth in which either fumarate or malate is
used as an electron receptor (51). The presence of two enzyme
systems capable of metabolizing H_2 raises questions about the number
of hydrogenase genes coding for hydrogenase in the cell, although
purified hydrogenase is known to catalyze a reversible reaction
(52). Hydrogenase activity was detectable in both soluble and
membrane fractions of *E. coli* (53-55). Mower and his colleagues
(53) and Yamamoto and Ishimoto (54) identified multiple protein
bands with hydrogenase activity in polyacrylamide gels (native)
after electrophoresis of *E. coli* extracts (both soluble and

solubilized membrane fractions). These results suggest the possible presence of more than one hydrogenase enzyme complex in the cell although upon purification the enzyme from membrane fractions yields only one band in the polyacrylamide gels. However, it is possible that one hydrogenase catalyzes both hydrogen evolution and hydrogen uptake in association with different electron transport proteins, depending on the availability of substrates and growth conditions.

In order to better understand the role of hydrogenase in the cell, Pascal and her co-workers isolated a mutant strain of *E. coli* lacking hydrogenase activity and mapped the mutation at 57 min of the *E. coli* genetic linkage map (56,57). This mutant as well as the mutant strains described by Graham et al. (58) lacked formate de-hydrogenase activity (formate to benzyl viologen) also. These strains were isolated after nitrosoguanidine mutagenesis as colonies that are defective in H_2- dependent benzyl biologen (BV) reduction, viologen being added in an agar overlay. We have recently developed a positive and direct selection procedure for isolation of hydro-genase defective mutants of *E. coli*. Analysis of the properties of these mutants show that the hydrogenase in hydrogen evolution and hydrogen uptake is coded by one hydrogenase gene in *E. coli*.

E. coli strain Puig 446 (CGSC #4444) was mutagenized using transposon Tn10 (T^R) insertion, as described by Csonka and Clark (59). An aliquot of the mutagenized tetracycline resistant culture was spread on the surface of an agar medium containing Luria broth (60) and BV (0.5 mM). These plates were incubated under H_2 in a dessicator at room temperature. The bactericidal effect of par-tially reduced viologen dyes (51) was used to advantage in this selection procedure to obtain mutant strains that are incapable of reducing benzyl viologen from H_2. Colonies appearing after 3-5 days of incubation were picked and tested further for the presence of hydrogenase activity using tritium exchange assay (TT + $H_2O \rightleftharpoons$ HTO + HT)(50,52). Seven of the 48 clones tested produced no detectable hydrogenase activity. When the tetracycline resistance (Tn 10) was transduced from the hyd^- strains into a hyd^+, T^S strain (strain CHS26), all the T^R transductants were found to be hyd^+ indicating that the transposon Tn 10 is not in the hydrogenase gene. It is likely that the hydrogenase mutations arose spontaneously.

Strains SE-1 through SE-7 produced less than 1% of the hydro-genase activity (compared to the parent strain, Puig 446) as determined by the tritium exchange assay (Table IV). These strains also produced less than 1% of the H_2 evolved by the parent strain from glucose during fermentation. All the strains were found to be defective in the reduction of benzyl viologen (BV) from H_2 but reduced BV when formate was the electron donor. These hydrogenase minus mutants also failed to grow at the expense of H_2 and fumarate anaerobically.

TABLE IV

Properties of hydrogenase negative mutants of *E. coli*.

strain	Hydrogenase activity* (% of the parent)	H_2 production** (% of the parent)	Reduction of venzyl viologen[+] from formate	Reduction of venzyl viologen[+] from H_2	H_2 and fumarate dependent growth[++]	Reversion Frequency***
Puig 426 (CGSC #4444; parent)	100	100	+	+	+	
SE-1	0.3	0.2	+	−	−	$<10^{-9}$
SE-2	0.1	0.1	+	−	−	1×10^{-5}
SE-3	0.0	0.0	+	−	−	$<10^{-9}$
SE-4	0.1	0.0	+	−	−	2×10^{-5}
SE-5	0.8	0.6	+	−	−	$<10^{-9}$
SE-6	0.6	0.0	+	−	−	$<10^{-9}$
SE-7	0.8	0.4	+	−	−	$<10^{-9}$

* For determination of hydrogenase activity, 0.5 ml of an anaerobic, Luria broth culture was transferred to a 12x75 mm test tube and sealed with serum stopper. The gas phase in the tube was replaced with helium. Twenty-five ml of $^3H_2$ gas (1.6 mCi/ml; New England Nuclear) was added to each tube and incubated at 37°C. After 1 hr incubation the serum stopper was removed and the tube was vented in the hood for 10 min. An aliquot (50 µl) of the culture was removed, mixed with 5.0 ml Aquasol (New England Nuclear) and counted in a scintillation counter. Hydrogenase activity of the parent strain, Puig 446, was 9.0x10^5 cpm/mg cell protein.

** Hydrogen production was determined as the total amount of H_2 produced during anaerobic growth at 37°C in a medium containing Luria broth and 0.15% glucose, using a gas chromatograph as described before (63). Total H_2 produced by the parent was 27.5 µmoles/mg cell protein.

[+] Ability to reduce benzyl viologen was determined using whole cells as described before (64).

[++] Hydrogen and fumarate dependent growth was monitored using the medium described by Macy *et al*. (51).

*** Reversion frequency was determined as the number of cells in a population capable of H_2-fumarate dependent growth.

Except strains SE-2 and SE-4, all the other hyd^- strains had reversion frequencies that are less than 10^{-9}. The reversion frequencies for strains SE-2 and SE-4 were 1×10^{-5} and 2×10^{-5}, respectively. The inability of the hyd^- mutants to grow at the expense of H_2 and fumarate was utilized to genetically map the mutation. Strain SE-1 was used in these experiments and the results are presented below.

As shown in Figure 3, the hydrogenase gene was mapped at 55.5 min in the *E. coli* linkage map based on Hfr (strain KL-164; origin of transfer--61 min), mediated conjugation. The hydrogenase-plus exconjugants were selected in a medium containing H_2 as the electron donor and fumarate as electron acceptor. These hyd^+ exconjugants also produced H_2 from glucose during anaerobic fermentation. Based on bacteriophage P_1 mediated transductional analysis, the hydrogenase gene was found to cotransduce with *srl* (44%) genes. Pascal et al. (56) found that the hydrogenase and formate dehydrogenase mutations described by them cotransduced with *cys* C at 10.4% although Graham et al. (58) reported that the mutation in their mutant strains lacking both hydrogenase and formate dehydrogenase (BV) activities cotransduced with *cys* at 92%. Additional experiments involving three-factor crosses are in progress to map the *hyd* gene in strain SE-1.

The results described above show that *E. coli* has only one hydrogenase capable of reversible activity in whole cells depending on the availability of electron donors and acceptors.

Isolation of Hydrogenase Genes

The development of the methodology that allows the *in vitro* manipulation of DNA has greatly simplified the problem of the isolation of genes from bacteria like *E. coli*. In order to isolate the hydrogenase genes of *E. coli*, we have chosen to utilize the well characterized cloning vector pBR322 (65). Using the approach illustrated in Figure 4, pBR322 is digested with the restriction enzyme *Sal*I. This enzyme cleaves the DNA once at a position that is in the tetracycline resistance gene (Tc^r) present on the plasmid. *E. coli* chromosomal DNA is partially restricted with *Sal*I, and partial digestion products 12-15 kilo base pairs (kbp) in size are purified by agarose gel electrophoresis. T-4 DNA ligase is used to ligate these DNA fragments to the digested pBR322 DNA. Ligation of fragments into the *Sal*I cleavage site of pBR322 generates a recombinant plasmid in which the Tc resistance gene is interrupted by a cloned DNA fragment, inactivating tetracycline resistance. An ampicillin (Ap) resistance gene also present on pBR322 is left intact. Transformation of bacteria with this ligated DNA mixture will give rise to Ap^r Tc^r colonies containing pBR322 and Ap^r Tc^s

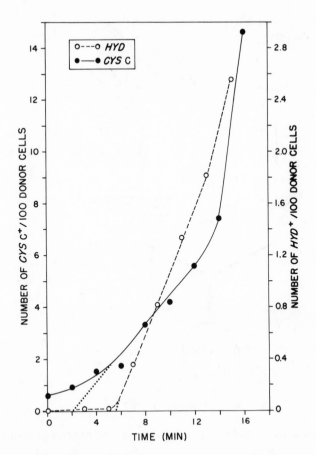

Figure 3. Results of an interrupted mating experiment using Hfr (strain KL-164) and *hyd⁻* strain SE-1. The experimental procedure was essentially as described by Miller (10).

colonies containing the recombinant plasmids. Selection of a sufficient number of the Ap[r] Tc[s] colonies will generate a gene bank in which the probability that a particular gene is present approached 100% (67). This gene bank can then be used to transform hup⁻ mutants to select for recombinant plasmids that complement the hup⁻ mutations.

Because we have been unable to directly transform *A. eutrophus* with plasmid DNA, a modification of the *E. coli* procedure must be used in the isolation of recombinant plasmids that complement *A. eutrophus* hup⁻ mutants. The plasmid cloning vector to be used is pRK290, a derivation of RK2 constructed in the laboratory of Dr. Helinski (66). This plasmid has a broader host range than does pBR322 and, although it cannot transfer itself from one

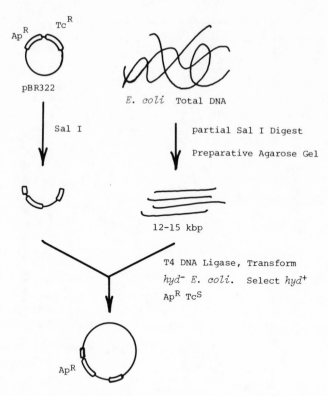

ApR TcS *hyd*+ recombinant pBR322

Figure 4.   Isolation of *E. coli* hydrogenase genes.

bacterial strain to another, in the presence of the appropriate
transfer genes, this plasmid can be made to mobilize and transfer
between bacterial strains. The procedure we are using for the
isolation of the *A. eutrophus* hydrogenase genes is outlined in
Figures 5 and 6. Unlike pBR322, there is no easy method of dis-
tinguishing pRK290 from recombinant pRK290 plasmids, so it is
desirable to form as high a proportion of recombinant plasmids as
possible during ligation. After digestion of the PRK290 with *Eco*RI
endonuclease, the DNA is treated with β-alkaline phosphatase. This
prevents the digested ends of the plasmid DNA from ligating to
themselves and eliminates the formation of circular pRK290 and
multimeric forms of pRK290 during ligation. Chromosomal DNA from
A. eutrophus can be ligated to the treated pRK290 DNA to form
recombinant plasmids, and these plasmids transformed into a strain
of *E. coli* to generate a Tc resistant recombinant pRK290 gene bank.
The procedure for the complementation of hup⁻ mutants is illustrated
in Figure 6. An aliquot of the *E. coli* strain containing the gene
bank is mixed with an aliquot of the *A. eutrophus* H1 hup⁻ mutant

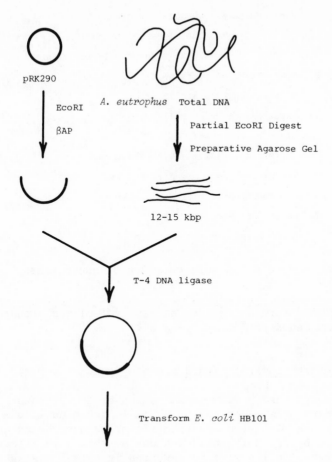

Figure 5.   pRK290 gene bank construction.

and an aliquot of an *E. coli* strain containing the plasmid pRK2013,
the plasmid used to mobilize and effect transfer of pRK290. After
allowing time for exchange to occur, cultures are plated on selective
media to determine frequency of transfer of the recombinant plasmids
and to select for *A. eutrophus* strains containing plasmids that
allow rapid autotrophic growth. In preliminary experiments we have
observed typical mobilization frequencies of 10-90%, a frequency
that is several orders of magnitude greater than the normal transfer
of P group R factors similar to RK2 from *E. coli* to *A. eutrophus*.
We have obtained several Tc^r colonies capable of normal rates of
autotrophic growth. We are currently in the process of complement-
ing the mutants described in Table V. Further analysis will be

1. Mix 3 cultures: HB101/pRK290:gene bank

                     HB101/pRK2013 (mobilizing plasmid)

                     AEH1-2 (Hup⁻ deletion mutant)

2. Concentrate on membrane filter.

    Incubate on LB plate 12 hr.

3. Resuspend and wash cells.

    Plate aliquots on:

        Minimal medium + 0.3% fructose

        Minimal medium + 0.3% fructose + 20 μg/ml Tc

        Autotrophic medium + $H_2/O_2/CO_2$ + 20 μg/ml Tc

4. Select colonies Aut⁺, Tc^R.

    Examine for plasmid presence.

Figure 6. Complementation of hup mutants.

necessary to determine whether we have yet cloned either of the
hydrogenase genes of *A. eutrophus* H1.

Analysis of the Control of Hydrogenase Genes

Although the *in vitro* examination of the structure and control
of the hydrogenase genes cannot begin in depth until the hydrogenase
genes have been isolated and identified, we have begun an *in vivo*
examination of the polypeptides whose synthesis is affected by cAMP.
Because these studies will be reported in detail elsewhere, a summary
of the observations will be presented here. Cultures growing under
different conditions were incubated in the presence of ^{35}S-methionine
and the radioactive polypeptides examined by SDS-polyacrylamide gel
electrophoresis and autoradiography. There are approximately 30
polypeptide bands, some of which are membrane-associated, that are
synthesized preferentially under autotrophic conditions. The
presence of cAMP stimulated the synthesis of six of these polypeptides and caused the synthesis of three additional bands. The
presence of H_2 during heterotrophic growth caused the increased
synthesis of certain polypeptide bands. Although the stimulatory
effects of cAMP and H_2 were not identical, there are several polypeptide bands whose synthesis is stimulated in the presence of cAMP
or H_2. The presence of both cAMP and H_2 resulted in further alterations in synthesis.

Because of the observations that the presence of H_2 during
heterotrophic growth can cause the accumulation of carboxylase (35),
radioactively labelled cell extracts were reacted with antiserum

against purified *A. eutrophus* carboxylase. The immunoprecipitates were collected and examined. The results suggest that cAMP causes the increased synthesis of carboxylase, but in the absence of H_2, either the translation of the polypeptides is incomplete or the large subunit of carboxylase is rapidly degraded to generate discrete polypeptides of low molecular weight. In the presence of both cAMP and H_2, although the level of synthesis of carboxylase may be reduced relative to the rate of synthesis in the presence of cAMP alone, the resulting large subunit of carboxylase is more stable. H_2 and cAMP appear to interact in a manner that allows complete translation of the carboxylase or that decreases the rate of proteolytic degradation of carboxylase.

Because of the apparent stimulation of both hydrogenase activity and the synthesis of carboxylase protein by cAMP, it is possible that the regulation of hydrogenases may be coupled in *A. eutrophus* to the regulation of carboxylase. In view of this possibility, in the course of the isolation of the hydrogenase genes, we shall use the appropriate mutants for the isolation of the carboxylase genes. We hope to investigate *in vitro* the details of the control of both hydrogenase and carboxylase genes and determine whether there is some form of co-ordinate regulation occurring.

Summary

For a variety of reasons, including the potential industrial applications of hydrogenase, we are interested in the isolation and analysis of hydrogenase genes. In a program focusing on the hydrogen bacterium *A. eutrophus* H1 and *E. coli*, we have developed a preliminary concept of the interaction of hydrogenase in cellular metabolism, constructed mutants deficient in hydrogenase activity, and begun the isolation of hydrogenase genes utilizing the technology allowing the *in vitro* manipulation of DNA. We hope to pursue this project to its ultimate goal: the analysis of the molecular mechanisms involved in the control of expression of these genes and the development of the ability to manipulate the production of hydrogenase.

ACKNOWLEDGEMENTS

We would like to thank Dr. B. J. Bachmann, *E. coli* Genetic Stock Center, for providing the *E. coli* strains used in this study. This work was supported by a subcontract from Solar Energy Research Institute (XR-9-8936-1) to KTS and a research grant from the National Science Foundation (PFR 77-07301). Any opinions, findings, and conclusions or recommendations expressed in the publication are those of the authors and do not necessarily reflect the view of the granting agencies. Thanks is also due to R. C. Valentine for his support and advice.

REFERENCES

1. Gray, C.T., and Gest, H. 1965. Biological formation of molecular hydrogen. Science 148, 186-192.
2. Mortenson, L.E. and Chen, J. 1974. Hydrogenase. In: Microbial Iron Metabolism (J.B. Neilands, ed.). New York, Academic Press, pp. 231-282.
3. Peck, H.D. 1968. Energy-coupling mechanisms in chemolithotrophic bacteria. Ann. Rev. Microbiol. 22, 489-518.
4. Schlegel, H.G. and Schneider, K. 1978. Distribution and physiological role of hydrogenases in microorganisms. In: Hydrogenases: Their Catalytic Activity, Structure, and Function (H.G. Schlegel and K. Schneider, eds.). Gottingen, Erich Goltze KG, pp. 15-44.
5. Schubert, K.R. and Evans, H.J. 1976. Hydrogen evolution: a major factor affecting the efficiency of nitrogen fixation in nodulated symbionts. Proc. Natl. Acad. Sci. USA 73, 1207-1211.
6. Evans, H.J., Ruiz-Argueso, T., Jennings, N., and Hanus, J. 1977. Energy coupling efficiency of symbiotic nitrogen fixation. In: Genetic Engineering for Nitrogen Fixation (A. Hollaender, ed.), New York, Plenum Publishing Corp., pp. 333-354.
7. Maier, R.J., Campbell, N.E.R., Hanus, F.J., Simpson, F.B., Russell, S.A., and Evans, H.J. 1978. Expression of hydrogenase activity in free-living *Rhizobium japonicum*. Proc. Natl. Acad. Sci. USA 75, 3258-3262.
8. Carter, K.R., Jennings, N.T., Hanus, F.J., and Evans, H.J. 1978. Hydrogen evolution and uptake by nodules of soybeans inoculated with different strains of *Rhizobium japonicum*. Can. J. Microbiol. 24, 307-311.
9. Hanus, F.J., Maier, R.J. and Evans, H.J. 1979. Autotrophic growth of H_2-uptake-positive strains of *Rhizobium japonicum* in an atmosphere supplied with H_2 gas. Proc. Natl. Acad. Sci. USA 76, 1788-1792.
10. Schlegel, H.G. and Eberhardt, U. 1972. Regulatory phenomena in the metabolism of Knallgasbacteria. Adv. Microbial. Physio. 7, 205-242.
11. Schegel, H.G. 1976. Regulatory phenomenon in the metabolism of Knallgasbacteria. Antonie van Leeuwenhoek 42, 181-201.
12. McFadden, B.A. 1978. Assimilation of one-carbon compounds. In: The Bacteria, Vol. 6 (L.N. Orston and J.R. Sokatch, eds.), New York, Academic Press, pp. 219-304.
13. Stadtman, T. C. 1967. Methane formation. Ann. Rev. Microbiol. 21, 121-142.

14. Thayer, R.K., Jungermann, K. and Decker, K. 1977. Energy
     conservation in anaerobic bacteria. Bacteriol. Rev. 41, 100-
     180.
15. Gaffron, H. 1940. Carbon dioxide reduction with molecular
     hydrogen in green algae. Amer. J. Bot. 27, 273-283.
16. Gest, H. and Kamen, M.D., 1949. Studies on the metabolism
     of photosynthetic bacteria. J. Bacteriol. 58, 239-245.
17. Gest, H. and Kamen, M.D. 1949. Photoproduction of molecular
     hydrogen by *Rhodospirillum rubrum*. Science 108, 558-559.
18. Ormerod, J.G., Ormerod, K.S. and Gest H. 1961. Light-dependent
     utilization of organic compounds and photoproduction of molecu-
     lar hydrogen by photosynthetic bacteria; relationships with
     nitrogen metabolism. Arch. Biochem. Biophys. 94, 449-463.
19. Gest, H., Ormerod, J.G. and Ormerod, K.S. 1962. Photometabolism
     of *Rhodospirillum rubrum*: light-dependent dissimilation of
     organic compounds to carbon dioxide and molecular hydrogen by
     an anaerobic citric acid cycle. Arch. Biochem. Biophys. 97,
     21-33.
20. Burns, R.C. and Hardy, R.W.F. 1975. In: Nitrogen Fixation
     in Bacteria and Higher Plants. New York, Springer Verlag.
     pp. 65-73.
21. Zumft, W.G., and Mortenson, L.E. 1975. The nitrogen-fixing
     complex of bacteria. Biochim. Biophys. Acta 416, 1-52.
22. Shanmugam, K.T., O'Gara, F., Andersen, K., and Valentine, R.C.,
     1978. Biological nitrogen fixation. Ann. Rev. Plant Physiol.
     29, 263-276.
23. Nakos, G. and Mortenson, L. 1971. Purification and properties
     of hydrogenase, an iron sulfur protein, from *Clostridium
     pasteurianum* W5. Biochim. Biophys. Acta 227, 576-583.
24. Chen, J.S. and Mortenson, L.E. 1974. Purification and pro-
     perties of hydrogenase from *Clostridium pasteurianum* W5. Bio-
     chim. Biophys. Acta 371, 283-298.
25. LeGall, J., Dervartanian, D.V., Spilker, E., Lee, J.P., and
     Peck, H.D. 1971. Evidence for the involvement of non-heme
     iron in the active site of hydrogenase from *Desulfovibrio
     vulgaris*. Biochim. Biophys. Acta 234, 525-530.
26. van der Westen, H.M., Mayhew, S.G., and Veeger, C. 1978.
     Separation of hydrogenase from intact cells of *Desulfovibiro
     vulgaris*. FEBS Letters 86, 122-126.
27. Schink, B. and Schlegel, H.G. 1979. The membrane-bound hydro-
     genase of *Alcaligenes eutrophus*. I. Solubilization, purifica-
     tion, and biochemical properties. Biochim. Biophys. Acta 567,
     315-324.
28. Schneider, K. and Schlegel, H.G. 1976. Purification and
     properties of soluble hydrogenase from *Alcaligenes eutrophus*
     H16. Biochim. Biophys. Acta 452, 66-80.
29. Schneider, K. and Schlegel, H.G. 1977. Localization and
     stability of hydrogenases from aerobic hydrogen bacteria. Arch.
     Microbiol. 112, 229-238.

30.   Schneider, K., Cammack, R., Schlegel, H.G., and Hall, D.O.
       1979. The iron-sulphur centres of soluble hydrogenase from
       Alcaligenes eutrophus. Biochim. Biophys. Acta 578, 445-461.
31.   Emerich, D.W., Ruiz-Arueso, T., Ching, T.M., and Evans, H.J.
       1979. Hydrogen-dependent nitrogenase activity and ATP forma-
       tion in *Rhizobium japonicum* bacteroids. J. Bacteriol. 137,
       153-160.
32.   Zeikus, J.G. 1977. The biology of methanogenic bacteria.
       Bacteriol. Rev. 41, 514-541.
33.   Gottschalk, G. 1965. Die Verwertung organische substrate
       durch Hydrogenomonas in Gegenwart von molekularem Wasserstoff
       Biochemische Zeitschrift 341, 260-270.
34.   Blackkolb, F. and Schlegel, H.G. 1968. Catabolite repression
       and enzyme inhibition by molecular hydrogen in hydrogenomonas
       Arch. Microbiol. 62, 129-143.
35.   Andersen, K. 1979. Mutations altering the catalytic activity
       of a plant-type ribulose bisphosphate carboxylase/oxygenase
       in *Alcaligenes eutrophus*. Biochim. Biophys. Acta 585, 1-11.
36.   Maier, R.J., Hanus, F.J. and Evans, H.J. 1979. Regulation
       of hydrogenase in *Rhizobium japonicum*. J. Bacteriol. 137,
       824-829.
37.   Tait, R.C., Andersen, K., Cangelosi, G., and Lim, S.T. 1981
       Hydrogen uptake (Hup) plasmids: characterization of mutants
       and regulation of the expression of hydrogenase. In: Genetic
       Engineering of Symbiotic Nitrogen Fixation and Conservation
       of Fixed Nitrogen (D.W. Rains and R.C. Valentine, eds.). New
       York, Plenum Press. In press.
38.   Ogden, S., Haggerty, D., Stoner, C.M., Kolodrubetz, D., and
       Schleif, R. 1980. The *Escherichia coli* L-arabionose operon:
       binding sites of the regulatory proteins and a mechanism of
       positive and negative regulation. Proc. Natl. Acad. Sci.
       USA 77, 3346-3350.
39.   deCrombrugghe, B., Chen, B., Gottesman, M., Pastan, I.,
       Varmus, H.E., Emmer, M., and Perlman, R.L. 1971. Regulation
       of *lac* mRNA synthesis in a soluble cell-free system. Nature
       New Biol. 230, 37-40.
40.   deCrombrugghe, B., Chen, B., Anderson, W., Nissley, P.,
       Gottesman, M., and Pastan, I. 1971. *Lac* DNA, RNA polymerase
       and cyclic AMP receptor protein, cyclip AMP, repressor and
       inducer are the essential elements for controlled *Lac* Trans-
       cription. Nature New Biol. 231, 139-142.
41.   Eron, L., Arditt, R., Zubay, G., Connaway, S., and Beckwith,
       J.R. 1971. An adenosine 3',5'-cyclic monophosphate-binding
       protein that acts on the transcription process. Proc. Natl.
       Acad. Sci. USA 68, 215-218.
42.   Nissley, S.P., Anderson, W. B., Gottesman, M.E., Perlman,
       R.L., and Pastan, I. 1971. *In vitro* transcription of the gal
       operon requires cyclic adenosine monophosphate and cyclic
       adenosine monophosphate receptor protein. J. Biol. Chem.
       246, 4671-4678.

43.   Boone, T. and Wilcox, G. 1978.   A rapid high-yield purification
       procedure for the cyclic adenosine 3',5'-monophosphate receptor
       protein from *Escherichia coli*.   Biochim. Biophys. Acta 541,
       528-534.

44.   Emmer, M., deCrombrugghe, B., Pastan, I., and Perlman, R. 1970.
       Cyclic AMP receptor protein of *E. coli*: its role in the synthe-
       sis of inducible enzymes.   Proc. Natl. Acad. Sci. USA 66, 480-
       487.

45.   Anderson, W.B., Schneider, A.B., Emmer, M., Perlman, R.L., and
       Pastan, I. 1971. Purification and properties of the cyclic
       adenosine 3',5'-monophosphate receptor protein which mediates
       cyclic adenosine 3',5'-monophosphate-dependent gene transcrip-
       tion in *Escherichia coli*. J. Biol. Chem. 246, 5929-5937.

46.   Reh, M. and Schlegel, H.G. 1975.   Chemolithoautotrophicals
       eine übertragbare, autonome Eigenschaft von *Nacardia opaca*
       1b. Nachr. Akad. Wiss. Göttingen.   II. Math.-Phys. Kl 12,
       207-216.

47.   Pootjes, C.F. 1977.   Evidence for plasmid coding of the ability
       to utilize hydrogen gas by *Pseudomonas facilis*.   Biochem.
       Biophys. Res. Comm. 76, 1002-1006.

48.   Brewin, N.J., Beynon, J.L., and Johnston, A.W.B. 1981. The
       role of *Rhizobium* plasmids in host specificity.   In: Genetic
       Engineering of Symbiotic Nitrogen Fixation and Conservation
       of Fixed Nitrogen (D.W. Rains and R.C. Valentine, eds.), New
       York Plenum Press. In press.

49.   Andersen, K., Tait, R.C., and King, W.R. 1980.   Plasmids re-
       quired for utilization of molecular hydrogen.   Submitted to
       Proc. Natl. Acad. Sci. USA.

50.   Lim., S.T. 1978.   Determination of hydrogenase in free-living
       cultures of *Rhizobium japonicum* and energy efficiency of soy-
       bean nodules.   Plant Physiol. 62, 609-611.

51.   Macy, J., Kulla, H., and Gottschalk, G. 1976. H_2- dependent
       anaerobic growth of *Escherichia coli* on L-malate: succinate
       formation.   J. Bacteriol. 125, 423-428.

52.   Adams, M.W.W. and Hall, D.O. 1979.   Purification of the mem-
       brane-bound hydrogenase of *Escherichia coli*.   Biochem. J.
       183, 11-22.

53.   Ackrell, B.A.C., Asato, R.N. and Mower, H. F. 1966.   Multiple
       forms of bacterial hydrogenases.   J. Bacteriol. 92, 828-838.

54.   Yamamoto, I. and Ishimoto, M. 1978.   Hydrogen-dependent growth
       of *Escherichia coli* in anaerobic respiration and the presence
       of hydrogenases with different functions.   J. Biochem. (Tokyo)
       84, 673-679.

55.   Glick, B.R. Wang, P.Y., Schneider, H., and Martin, W.G. 1980.
       Identification and partial characterization of *Escherichia
       coli* mutant with altered hydrogenase activity.   Can. J. Bio-
       chem. 58, 361-367.

56.   Pascal, M.C., Casse, F., Chippaux, M., and LePelletier, M.
       1975. Genetic analysis of mutants of *Escherichia coli* K-12

and *Salmonella typhimurium* LT2 deficient in hydrogenase
activity. Mol. Gen. Genet. 141, 173-179.

57. Bachman, B.J. and Low, K.B. 1980. Linkage map of *Escherichia coli* K-12. Edition 6. Bacteriol. Revs. 44, 1-56.

58. Graham, A., Boxer, D.H., Haddock, B.A., Mandrand-Berthelot,
M.A., and Jones, R.W. 1980. Immunochemical analysis of the
membrane-bound hydrogenase of *Escherichia coli*. FEBS Letters
113, 167-172.

59. Csonka, L.N. and Clark, A.J. 1979. Deletions generated by the
transposon Tn10 in the *srl recA* region of the *Escherichia coli*
K-12 chromosome. Genetics 93, 321-343.

60. Miller, J.F. 1972. Experiments in Molecular Genetics. New
York, Cold Spring Harbor Laboratory.

61. Hassan, H.M. and Fridovich, I. 1978. Superoxide radical and
the oxygen enchancement of the toxicity of paraquat in
Escherichia coli. J. Biol. Chem. 253, 8143-8148.

62. Anand, S.R. and Krasna, A.I. 1965. Catalysis of the H_2-HTO
exchange by hydrogenase. A new assay for hydrogenase. Biochemistry 4, 2747-2753.

63. Andersen, K. and Shanmugam, K.T. 1980. Energetics of biological nitrogen fixation: determination of the ratio of
formation of H_2 to NH_4^+ catalyzed by nitrogenase of *Klebsiella
pneumoniae in vivo*. J. Gen. Microbiol. 103, 107-122.

64. Hom, S.S.M., Hennecke, H. and Shanmugan, K.T. 1980. Regulation
of nitrogenase biosynthesis in *Klebsiella pneumoniae:* effect
of nitrate. J. Gen. Microbiol. 117, 169-179.

65. Bolivar, F., Rodriquez, R.L., Greene, P.J., Betlack, M.C.,
Heyneker, H.L., Boyer, H.W., Crosa, J.H., and Falkow, S. 1977.
Construction and characterization of new cloning vehicles.
II. A multipurpose cloning system. Gene 2, 95-113.

66. Ditta, G., Stanfield, S., Corbin, D., and Helinski, D.R. 1980.
Broad host range DNA cloning system for gram-negative bacteria
construction of a gene bank of *Rhizobium meliloti*. Proc. Natl
Acad. Sci. USA. In press.

67. Clarke, L. and Carbon, J. 1976. A colony bank containing
synthetic ColEl hybrid plasmids representative of the entire
E. coli genome. Cell 9, 91-99.

DISCUSSION

Q. FRAENKEL: In your introduction, when you discussed *Rhizobium
japonicum,* you talked about the hydrogenase. Is that a
soluble hydrogenase?

A. TAIT: There's been very little work done on the hydrogenase
of *R. japonicum*. From discussion with Dr. Evans, I understand
that it is a particulate or membrane-bound hydrogenase. It
may ·be that we will have to ultimately clone both the soluble

and the membrane bound hydrogenases and use both genes as hybridization probes in *R. japonicum* to check for the presence of both of these genes.

Q.   FRAENKEL: I just had one other small question. Do you have any idea what is on the rest of that large plasmid?

A.   TAIT: We worked very hard looking for other phenotypic markers on this plasmid because hydrogen uptake is not a good marker to transfer into other strains. We looked for drug resistance markers, for a number of aromatic carbon source utilization pathways, at nutritional requirements, and at just about everything you can imagine. We found no additional markers. The only thing that we can find on this plasmid is hydrogen uptake. My suspicion is that it is probably a plasmid that contains aromatic pathways or carbon source utilization pathways, but we have not been able to identify any.

Q.   WOOD: Has anybody shown that those strains of *R. japonicum* containing the hydrogenase do in fact grow faster in some kind of a controlled experiment and that hydrogenase really does make a difference?

A.   TAIT: In terms of nitrogen fixed per carbon provided, if you look at the hup$^+$ the hup$^+$ is clearly a more efficient strain. Now whether that carries over into the field is a topic of some debate. To some extent the numbers have gotten so close in terms of statistical significance that it is not yet clear if you really do get a benefit to the plant under agricultural conditions. I think it is fairly clear that hydrogenase function is beneficial under laboratory conditions.

CONVERSION OF REDUCTASES TO DEHYDROGENASES

BY REGULATORY MUTATIONS

Edmund C. C. Lin

Department of Microbiology and Molecular Genetics
Harvard Medical School
Boston, Massachusetts 02115

Nicotinamide adenine dinucleotide (NAD^+)-linked oxidoreductases catalyze reactions that are generally in favor of NAD^+ formation at neutral pH. However, *in vivo* enzymes of this kind can function as either dehydrogenases or reductases. We have a case in which an enzyme that normally acts to reduce L-lactaldehyde is converted by a series of mutations that affect gene expression to an enzyme that acts to oxidize L-1, 2-propanediol. In *Escherichia coli* both aerobic and anaerobic utilization of L-fucose requires the expression of an inducible trunk pathway mediated by fucose permease (1), fucose isomerase (2), fuculose kinase (3), and fuculose 1-phosphate aldolase (4). The aldolase cleaves the six carbon substrate into dihydroxy-acetone phosphate and lactaldehyde (Figure 1). Anaerobically, lactaldehyde is completely reduced to propanediol by L-1, 2-propanediol: NAD^+ 1-oxidoreductase (propanediol oxidoredutase), an enzyme with a molecular weight of 76,000 consisting of two electro-phoretically indistinguishable subunits (5). For each mole of fucose fermented, one mole of propanediol is secreted into the medium (6). The sacrifice of one half of the carbon skeleton of fucose in this way permits the further metabolism of dihydroxyacetone phosphate without an exogenous hydrogen acceptor. Aerobically, lactaldehyde is completely oxidized to pyruvate sequentially by L-lactaldehyde: NAD^+ 1-oxidoreductase (lactaldehyde dehydrogenase) and a lactate dehydrogenase of the flavoprotein class (6,7) thereby channeling all of the carbon atoms from fucose into central metabolic pathways. Synthesis of the two key branch enzymes in the fucose system requires not only the presence of the inducer, but also the proper respiratory condition: induction of propanediol oxidoreductase requires anaerobiosis, whereas induction of lactaldehyde dehydro-genase requires aerobiosis (Table I).

305

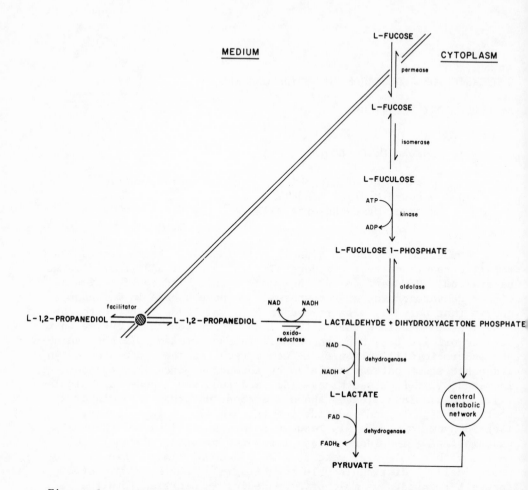

Figure 1.   Scheme for propanediol and fucose metabolism in *E. coli*.
The enzyme catalyzing the interconversion of propanediol and lactalde
hyde is referred to as propanediol oxidoreductase since the actual
role of this protein depends upon the strain in which it is found.
FAD and $FADH_2$, the oxidized and reduced forms of flavine adenine
dinucleotide; NAD and NADH, the oxidized and reduced forms of nicotinamide adenine dinucleotide.

Under aerobic conditions, wild-type *E. coli* fails to utilize propanediol as a sole source of carbon and energy by the action of the oxidoreductase because the lack of the proper inducer and the presence of molecular oxygen prevents the synthesis of the protein. Several series of mutants capable of growing aerobically on propanediol at progressively more rapid rates have been isolated and partially characterized. In every case, the capacity to use propanediol is associated with constitutive aerobic synthesis of propanediol oxidoreductase. Both this enzyme and L-lactaldehyde dehydrogenase are essential for the new growth property (1,7,8,9).

Sustained selection of the mutants on propanediol results, however, inevitably in the loss of growth ability on fucose. This growth failure can be accounted for by the disturbance of the regulatory mechanism that controls the expression of the fucose system. In particular, fucose permease, fucose isomerase, and fuculose kinase become noninducible (1). Typical changes in the regulatory pattern of gene expression of the fucose system resulting from selection on propanediol are illustrated in Table II. The cell extract of wild-type strain 1 grown aerobically on casein hydrolysate contained negligible activity of propanediol oxidoreductase. The additional presence of fucose in the growth medium resulted in a fourfold elevation of enzyme activity. Strain 413, the mutant selected for growth on propanediol, exhibited a basal level of the oxidoreductase ten times that found in wild-type cells. The addition of fucose raised the level another four times. Strain 421, a derivative of strain 413, produced the oxidoreductase at an even higher basal level. However, the permease, isomerase, and kinase can no longer be induced. The aldolase, in contrast, became constitutive. The inability to form the first three proteins in the trunk pathway explains the growth failure of strain 421 on fucose and perhaps also the inability of fucose to increase further the level of the oxidoreductase. Strain 3, a propanediol-utilizing mutant selected independently from wild-type strain 1, has properties similar to those of strain 421.

The pleiotropic changes in the levels of enzyme activities of the trunk pathway are probably mechanistically tied to the increased constitutive synthesis of the oxidoreductase and are therefore likely to be regulatory in nature. This interpretation is supported by the properties of three independent fucose-positive revertants of strain 3. These revertants, strains 54, 55, and 56, all show partial or full constitutive synthesis of the permease, isomerase, and kinase (Table III).

Mutants of strain 3 and 421 were selected by serial transfer of cells into media containing initially 12 to 20 mM L-1, 2-propanediol. Strain 430 was selected from strain 3 by culturing cells in media in which the propanediol concentration was not allowed to exceed 0.5 mM. Thus the selective pressure was for increased scavenging power rather than for a high rate of growth under sub-

TABLE I. Activities of Fucose Pathway Enzymes in Crude Extracts
of Wild-Type *E. coli* as a Function of Growth Conditions.[a]

Carbon source	O₂	Specific activity[b]					
		Fucose permease	Fucose isomerase	Fuculose kinase	Fuculose 1-phosphate aldolase	Propanediol oxidoreductase	Lactaldehyde dehydrogenase
CAA[c]	+	0	36	27	0	20	93
CAA + fucose	+	55	500	440	240	80	100
Fucose	+	58	520	420	130	42	280
Glucose	+					6	15
CAA + pyruvate	−					89	0
Fucose	−	64	750	310	270	240	32
Glucose	−					0	0

[a] Adapted from reference 1.

[b] Fucose permease activity is expressed in nanomoles per minute per milligram of dry weight at 37°C; all other activities are expressed in nanomoles per minute per milligram of protein at 25° C.

[c] Casein hydrolysate.

strate abundant conditions. Four phenotypic changes were detected
in strain 430: (i) the aldolase gene is inactivated; (ii) the constitutive oxidoreductase activity level is increased; (iii) lactaldehyde
dehydrogenase is synthesized constitutively and at an elevated level;
and (iv) at low concentrations of propanediol the rate of specific
transport (facilitator diffusion) across the cell membrane is enhanced [data not given in Tab. II, see ref. (10)]. The last three
changes appear to act together by facilitating the rate of entry of
propanediol into the cell followed by the conversion of the compound
to an ionized metabolite, L-lactate. The significance of the loss
of the aldolase activity is not yet known. It is possible that by
increasing the expression of the gene for the oxidoreductase yet
another step, the aldolase gene became nonexpressible. It is also
possible that a separate mutation abolished the aldolase activity
which became a liability to the cells growing on propanediol because
of a cul-de-sac accumulation of fucose 1-phosphate.

Strain 430, in contrast to strain 3, can no longer be reverted
to grow on fucose. Such being the situation, one might expect that
continued selection on propanediol would eventually lead to the
deletion of all the genes in the trunk pathway.

The enzymatic patterns of the wild-type, mutant, and pseudo-
revertant strains together indicate that the fucose system consists
of a regulon with probably four or more operons respectively encoding: (i) the permease (see partial constitutivity of its activity
versus full constitutivity of the isomerase and the kinase in strains
54, 55, and 56 as shown in Tab. III); (ii) the isomerase and the
kinase; (iii) the aldolase; and (iv) the oxidoreductase. The structural gene for lactaldehyde dehydrogenase is probably under the
control of an independent regulatory protein, since the enzyme can
be induced by propanediol in strain 413 without concomitant induction of enzymes of the trunk pathway.

The extraordinarily complex changes in enzymatic patterns
associated with the selection on propanediol probably reflects the
fact that high expression of the oxidoreductase operon requires the
remodeling of a common regulatory element, the function of which is
also intricately linked to the expression of the other operons in the
system. The complexity of the control reflects the need for having
two kinds of signals for gene expression: a specific inducer and an
indicator of respiratory state. The evolution of the propanediol
pathway provides a striking contrast to several previously studied
systems in which the structural gene of an enzyme mobilized for a new
function by virtue of its side specificity belongs to a system under
simpler repressor control, such as that found in the lactose system
of *E. coli*. In these cases, the constitutive synthesis of the critical
enzyme can result from a random mutation that destroys repressor
function. The synthesis of the other gene products that share the

TABLE II. Activities of Fucose Pathway Enzyme in Extracts of Various Mutants Grown Aerobically on Different Media.[a]

Strain	Carbon source	Specific activity[b]					
		Fucose permease	Fucose isomerase	Fuculose kinase	Fuculose 1-phosphate aldolase	Propanediol oxidoreductase	Lactaldehyde dehydrogenase
1	CAA[c]	0	36	27	0	20	93
	CAA + fucose	55	500	440	240	80	100
413	CAA	0	20	40	10	210	160
	CAA + fucose	50	460	420	190	990	160
	Propanediol	0	10	0	0	260	330
421	CAA	0	15	20	390	1,300	120
	CAA + fucose	0	15	20	380	1,200	130
	Propanediol	0	10	0	180	1,300	300
3	CAA	0	43	80	490	410	130
	CAA + fucose	0.08	30	46	490	390	110
	Propanediol		43	57	490	420	260
430	CAA	0	20	48	0	750	380
	CAA + fucose				0	680	420
	Propanediol				0	720	410

[a] Adapted from references 8 and 10.

[b] Fucose permease activity is expressed in nanomoles per minute per milligram of dry weight at 37°C; all other activities are expressed in nanomoles per minute per milligram of protein at 25° C.

[c] Casein hydrolysate.

TABLE III. Activities of Fucose Pathway Enzymes in Crude Extracts of Revertants of Strain 3 Grown Aerobically.[a]

Strain no.	Carbon source	Specific activity[b]				
		Fucose permease	Fucose isomerase	Fuculose kinase	Fuculose 1-phosphate aldolase
54	CAA[c]	0.3	110	110	470
	CAA + fucose	0.3	100	120	500
55	CAA	8.0	230	160	500
	CAA + fucose	7.0	240	160	440
56	CAA	15.0	600	550	370
	CAA + fucose	15.0	630	400	420

[a] Adapted from reference 1.

[b] Fucose permease activity is expressed in nanomoles per minute per milligram of dry weight; all other activities are expressed in nanomoles per minute per milligram of protein.

[c] Casein acid hydrolysate.

same control, whether or not they are necessary for the new pathway, thereby also becomes constitutive. The only price exacted from the mutant may be the gratuitous synthesis of several proteins when neither the original nor the novel substrate is present in the environment. With sufficient time, however, the situation might be remedied by gene duplication, which would then permit the reestablishment of repression for one set of genes according to the original pattern, and the development of a new set of rules for the expression of the other set of genes to fit the new environment. Thus the mutant may gain a new metabolic function without sacrificing the original pathway.

Recently another NAD^+-linked oxidoreductase was found to acquire a new role in *E. coli* under experimental conditions. From a strain genetically doubly blocked in the normal catabolic pathway mediated by glycerol kinase and glycerol 3-phosphate dehydrogenase was obtained mutants that produce greatly elevated levels of an oxidoreductase as the first enzyme for glycerol dissimilation. Although the original role of the enzyme is yet to be established, the increased basal activity in anaerobically grown wild-type cells indicates that its original role was that of a reductase (11, 12). If so, this would be another example in which the physiological direction of the reaction catalyzed by an NAD^+-linked enzyme is reversed by mutations affecting gene expression.

The physiological performance of nicotinamide adenine dinucleotide-linked oxidoreductases can be influenced by a number of factors: the pH of the environment, the levels of the oxidized and reduced forms of the coenzyme, the concentrations of the substrates undergoing oxidation or reduction, and the relative affinities of the protein for the substrates. Since pH and coenzyme concentrations in the cell can undergo only limited changes and cannot be used as signals for specific metabolic control, investigations on the function and evolution of the oxidoreductases tended to be focussed on internal substrate concentrations and the K_m's of the enzymes. The model systems presented direct attention to yet another important facet in the evolution of the oxidoreductases: the control of gene expression. It was demonstrated that the normal metabolic flow catalyzed by an oxidoreductase can be readily reversed by altering the permissive condition for enzyme synthesis and by presenting the cell with the product instead of the substrate.

ACKNOWLEDGEMENTS

We thank Sarah Monosson for editorial assistance.

This work was supported by grant PCM76-81071 A01 from the National Science Foundation and by Public Health Service grant 5 R01 GM11983 from the National Institute of General Medical Sciences.

REFERENCES

1. Hacking, A.J. and E.C.C. Lin. 1976. J. Bacteriol. 126:1166-1172.
2. Green, M. and S.S. Cohen. 1956. J. Biol. Chem. 219:557-568.
3. Heath, E.C. and M.A. Ghalambor. 1962. J. Biol. Chem. 237:2423-2426.
4. Ghalambor, M.A. and E.C. Heath. 1962. J. Biol. Chem. 237:2427-2433.
5. Boronat, A. and J. Aguilar. 1979. J. Bacteriol. 140:320-326.
6. Cocks, G.T., J. Aguilar, and E.C.C. Lin. 1974. J. Bacteriol. 118:83-88.
7. Sridhara, S. and T.T. Wu. 1969. J. Biol. Chem. 244:5233-5238.
8. Hacking, A.J. and E.C.C. Lin. 1977. J. Bacteriol. 130:832-838.
9. Sridhara, S. T.T. Wu, T.M. Chused, and E.C.C. Lin. 1969. J. Bacteriol. 98:87-95.
10. Hacking, A.J., J. Aguilar, and E.C.C. Lin. 1978. J. Bacteriol. 136:522-530.
11. St. Martin, E.J., W.B. Freedberg, and E.C.C. Lin. 1975. J. Bacteriol. 131:1026-1028.
12. Tang, C.T., F.E. Ruch, and E.C.C. Lin. 1979. J. Bacteriol. 140:182-187.

DISCUSSION

Q. KRAMPITZ: Are there any conversions of lactaldehyde by an interim molecular oxidation and reduction to acetate? Or, is there oxidation on the alpha carbon to form methylglyoxal?

A. LIN: We have not encountered any; that's another possibility.

cAMP AND REGULATION OF CARBOHYDRATE METABOLISM

James L. Botsford

Department of Biology
New Mexico State University
Las Cruces, New Mexico 88003

Cyclic nucleotides including cAMP and cGMP are found in many procaryotes. Table I provides a representative selection of bacteria from which cAMP has been identified and quantitated. With only a few exceptions, the mechanism of action of these nucleotides and the physiological consequences of variations in the intracellular levels are not known. cGMP has also been found in a variety of bacteria (Table II), it is usually present in amounts at least an order of magnitude smaller than those observed for cAMP. Intracellular concentrations of cGMP of 3-35 nM have been reported for *Escherichia coli* (3). 30 nM cGMP is equivalent to 18 molecules per cell if the volume of a cell is assumed to be 10^{-15} l. It has been proposed that cGMP in *E. coli* is an artifact of adenylate cyclase activity (70). However, a guanylate cyclase activity distinct from adenylate cyclase by several criteria has been purified and partially characterized from *E. coli* (40). In animal cells, it was originally proposed that cAMP and cGMP act in opposition, the "Yin Yang Effect." This hypothesis has received less support as more evidence has accumulated (59). In bacteria in which both cAMP and cGMP levels have been measured including *Caulobacter crescentus* (69); *E. coli* (3,17); *Streptomyces hygroscopius* (15); and *Rhizobium japonicum* (36,37), no readily apparent relationship between the levels of the two nucleotides is found.

Cyclic nucleotides other than cAMP and cGMP have been found in *Corynebacterium murisepticum* and *Micrococcus* spp. These nuceotides include cIMP, cCMP, and cyclic deoxyadenosine monophosphate (27,28,29,30). It is uncertain if these nucleotides are significant metabolites. No functions for them has been reported.

TABLE I

cAMP in Representative Bacteria Other than Enteric Coliforms*

Bacterium	Function Implicated	Reference
Anabaena variabilis	heterotrophic growth	25
Bordetella pertusis	unknown	24
Caulobacter crescentus	differentiation	69
Mycobacterium smegmatis	unknown	34
Myxococcus xanthus	differentiation	45
Pseudomonas aeruginosa	unknown	71
Rhizobium japonicum	expression of hydrogenase	37
Streptomyces hygroscopius	antibiotic production	15

*This list is not intended to be exhaustive. cAMP has been isolated and its concentration determined in each example given. See Rickenberg (56) for a more complete list.

Several bacteria do not contain detectable cAMP. These bacteria include *Bacillus licheniformis* (3), *B. magaterium* (67), *B. brevis* (65), *Bacteroides fragilis* (26), and *Lactobacillus plantarum* (60). While cAMP is not found in the genus *Bacillus*, cGMP is found. However, the concentration is quite small, 0.9 to 8 pmoles/gm dry weight equivalent to less than 1 to 8 molecules/cell (68). The significance of the nucleotide has been questioned (68). Despite the absence of cAMP, these bacteria seem to regulate the synthesis of inducible enzymes much like the enteric coliforms which do contain cAMP (74).

cAMP has been identified in *Pseudomonas aeruginosa* (71). Intracellular concentrations are comparable to those observed in the enteric coliforms. However, little is found in the culture medium. With the exception of enteric coliforms very little cAMP appears to be excreted by bacteria. Several catabolic enzymes in *P. aeruginosa* are sensitive to catabolite repression. cAMP does not appear to be involved in this effect.

It should be emphasized that with the exception of cAMP metabolism in the enteric coliforms, little is known about the metabolism of either cAMP or cGMP except that the nucleotides are present and under some conditions, the amounts vary (Tables I and II). Most reports of cyclic nucleotides in the literature are restricted to investigations in which large amounts of the nucleotide are added to the growth medium and the effect on some function noted. This approach provides only the most preliminary evidence.

TABLE II
cGMP in Representative Bacteria*

Bacterium	Function Implicated	Reference
Bacillus brevis	RNAase activity	65
Bacillus licheniformis	unknown	3
Bacillus megaterium	unknown	68
Corynebacterium murisepticum	unknown	28
Caulobacter crescentus	differentiation	69
Microbacterium spp.	unknown	28
Rhizobium japonicum	hydrogenase activity	36
Streptomyces hygroscopius	antibiotic production	15
Escherichia coli	unknown	3, 17, 70

*This list is not intended to be exhaustive. cGMP has been isolated and its concentration determined in each example given.

cAMP AND CATABOLITE REPRESSION IN *E. COLI* AND *S. TYPHIMURIUM*.

The mechanism of action for cAMP in the enteric coliforms is known in considerable detail and has been recently reviewed (46, 48a). Briefly, cAMP binds reversibly to an allosteric protein termed the cAMP receptor protein, or CRP, to form an active CRP-cAMP complex. In the *lac* operon, the regulatory element, the CRP-cAMP complex, binds in the promoter region at a site several nucleotides from the RNA polymerase binding site. This binding permits RNA polymerase to bind and transcription to be initiated. The details of the mechanisms of action for the CRP-cAMP complex are less certain in the case of the arabinose operon (35) and the galactose operon (9). The basic features appear to be the same even though these operons are regulated differently than is the *lac* operon.

The intracellular levels of cAMP have been found to vary with the carbohydrate available to the cell (13, see 46 for a review of this area). In general, intracellular levels of cAMP are inversely proportional to the growth rate afforded the cells by that carbon source. The formation of the CRP-cAMP complex necessary for induction of catabolic operons is proportional to the intracellular concentration of cAMP. When cAMP production is inhibited, as when cells grow with glucose as a carbon source, there is little active CRP-cAMP complex present. As a consequence, the cell is unable to induce for additional catabolic pathways regardless of the presence of the appropriate inducer (13,46,47). This model is supported by

very elegant biochemical studies of regulation of gene expression
of the *lac* and *gal* operons *in vitro* in systems of coupled transcription and translation and in purified systems of transcription
(46,47). Measurements of intracellular levels of cAMP correlate
well with conditions of catabolite repression (13), at least under
most conditions (18, see 77 for a discussion of this point.)

Recently, at least three different lines of evidence have been
offered that argue that catabolite repression is not simply a consequence of the intracellular concentration of cAMP. These data
argue that catabolite repression is mediated by several distinct
mechanisms.

First, several mutations suppressing deletion mutations of
adenylate cyclase (*cya*) have been isolated and described (10,72).
The mutations map in the *crp* region and result in altered CRP function. Apparently the CRP is in an active conformation in the absence
of cAMP. In some of these strains, synthesis of β-galactosidase is
still sensitive to catabolite repression (10,72; J.G. Harman and
W.J. Dobrogsz, Abst. Ann. Meet. ASM, 1980, K 95, p142; J.G. Harman,
personal communication).

A second line of evidence comes from studies of a factor found
in the culture medium of wild type *E. coli* growing in minimal glucose
medium. This factor causes catabolite repression of the *lac* and
gal operons as well as of tryptophanase. This repression is distinct from cAMP mediated effects (11,75). This factor termed the
CMF, catabolite modulator factor, has been characterized only to
the extent that it is of low molecular weight, has no net charge,
and is stable to acid, base, and heat. CMF causes catabolite
repression of the *lac* operon in strains having a *cya* deletion and
the mutation in *crp* that suppresses the *cya* deletion.

A third line of evidence comes from the work of Wanner et al.
(77). They determined the specific activity of β-galactosidase in
cells growing with different carbon sources. They found an 18 fold
variation in the specific activity of the enzyme over a 5.6 fold
range in growth rates. This variation in specific activity could
be reduced but not eliminated by the addition of 5 mM exogenous
cAMP. This "residual variation" required the *lac* promoter region
to be fully functional indicating that the control was mediated by
the initiation of transcription and was a consequence of the cata-
bolites present in the medium. The authors concluded that cAMP
alone can not account for catabolite repression.

Magasanik (41) pointed out that it is doubtful that the CRP-
cAMP complex could fully account for catabolite repression. Inducer
exclusion could also play a critical role. Subsequent investigations have borne this out. Many lines of evidence indicate that

glucose transport prevents transport of other carbohydrates (39) and that this can be distinct from any effect glucose has on cAMP levels in the cell (12,61,62). Furthermore, the results of Ullmann's group (11,75) and those of Wanner et al.(75) suggest that additional factors, apart from the CRP-cAMP complex, could affect transcription. These factors could interact with the CRP. A dialyzable factor in cell extracts from *E. coli* grown with glucose was found to inhibit the binding of cAMP to the CRP in vitro (7). This inhibition appeared to be uncompetitive. This inhibitory effect could be distinct from cAMP and could alter the conformation of the CRP.

These lines of evidence suggest that cAMP is but one regulatory element mediating catabolite repression.

REGULATION OF cAMP LEVELS IN *E. COLI* AND *S. TYPHIMURIUM*.

cAMP levels in bacterial cells, as in animal cells, can be regulated by three means. The nucleotide can be excreted into the growth medium. The nucleotide can be degraded by the enzyme cAMP phosphodiesterase. The rates of cAMP production can vary in response to growth conditions.

cAMP is excreted from washed cells of *E. coli* (43). This excretion is energy dependent (63) and has been studied in detail in membrane vessicles (16). When cells grow exponentially in steady state conditions, cAMP is excreted at a rate proportional to its synthesis (13). The significance of cAMP excretion is not certain. Excretion has been observed under conditions that do not affect the induction of β-galactosidase (18)*.

cAMP is degraded by the enzyme cAMP phosphodiesterase. The enzyme from *E. coli* has been partially purified and characterized (44). The K_m for the activity is about 0.5 mM, several orders of magnitude greater than the intracellular concentration of cAMP. The specific activity does not vary with growth conditions (4,44). The enzyme is not found in some strains of *E. coli*. These strains make somewhat more cAMP than do strains having the activity (5). The *cpd* gene in *E. coli* has not been mapped and no strains isogenic except for this allele have been constructed. However, such strains

---

* Most of the cAMP in a culture of *E. coli* is in the extracellular fraction. If a culture with 10^9 cells/ml has a total of 100 pmoles cAMP/ml, there are 100×10^{-12} moles/ml x 6.024×10^{23} molecules/ mole = 6×10^{13} molecules cAMP/ml. If the intracellular concentration of cAMP is 1 μM, then there are 10^{-6} moles/1 x 1 cell 10^{-15} $1 \times 6.04 \times 10^{23}$ molecules/mole x 10^9 cells = 6×10^{11} molecules in the cells. $(6 \times 10^{11}/6 \times 10^{13}) \times 100$ = 1% of the cAMP in the culture is intracellular. See ref. 51 for another approach.

TABLE III
Rates of cAMP Production in *S. typhimurium* LT-2 (cpd⁺)
and *S. typhimurium* 3311 (cpd⁻)

Strain	cAMP*
LT-2	12.2
3311	38.4

*Results expressed as pmoles cAMP ml^{-1} min^{-1} A_{660}^{-1} as calculated from at least squares fit plot of cAMP vrs. time. Cells were grown to mid log phase in M-9 glucose medium, washed by filtration and resuspended in M-9 medium without glucose. Samples were taken at time = 0, 5, 10, 15, and 20 min. Samples were treated and assayed for cAMP as described previously(4).

of *S. typhimurium* have been constructed (1). Rates of cAMP production in the *cpd⁻* strain are higher than in the *cpd⁺* strain (Table III) The activity does reduce the net rate of cAMP production in *S. typhimurium*. The effect of enzyme activity on intracellular levels of cAMP remains to be determined.

The study of regulation of rates of cAMP production has a serious constraint. The enzyme responsible for synthesis of cAMP, adenylate cyclase, is membrane associated in *E. coli*. When the membrane is disrupted, the specific activity of the enzyme is insufficient to account for the rates of cAMP production seen *in vivo*. Furthermore, the activity is no longer inhibited by sugars that inhibit the activity in whole cells (50). This precludes a classical biochemical characterization of the activity. Several techniques to study the regulation of adenylate cyclase activity *in vivo* have been developed. Cells can be pulsed with highly radioactive adenosine and the cAMP made in the first few minutes after the pulse can be measured (51). Cells can also be treated with toluene to make them permeable to ATP and the rate of cAMP production determined (21). Cells can be simply washed rapidly and then aerated in the presence and in the absence of a carbon source to determine the inhibition of cAMP production caused by that carbon source. Apparently cells preferentially channel resources into cAMP production as the rate remains linear for at least 20 minutes regardless of the carbon source (4,49). The first technique, the adenosine pulse method, is quite tedious and has the disadvantage that only initial rates of cAMP production can be determined. In the second technique the toluene treatment is very critical (21). The last technique, aerating washed cells, provides rates of cAMP synthesis comparable to those observed using the other techniques. However, ATP could become limiting under some conditions with this simple assay.

By all these methods of assay, adenylate cyclase is seen to be inhibited by sugars. The sugars need not be metabolized, only to be transported. The inhibitory sugars include those transported by the phosphenolypyruvate phosphotransferase system (PTS) including

TABLE IV

Rates of cAMP Production as a Function of Carbon Source in
Batch Culture and in Carbon Limited Continuous Culture[a]

	Batch Culture[b]		Continuous Culture[c]	
Carbon Source	Present	Absent	0.1 hr^{-1}	0.3 hr^{-1}
glucose	2.6	150	3.4	6.3
fructose	3.9	98	3.1	6.3
glycerol	3.5	65	3.4	6.6
ribose	3.3	54	4.7	9.1

[a]Rates of cAMP production in terms of pmoles cAMP ml^{-1} min^{-1} mg protein^{-1}.

[b]"Present" means carbon source present while rates of cAMP production were
     measured.

"Absent" means carbon source not present while rates of cAMP production were
     measured.

[c]These rates were calculated with the data presented in Figures 1 and 2 from
     regression lines fitted to the data (J. G. Harman, M.S. Thesis, NMSU, 1977).

glucose and fructose; sugars transported by facilitated diffusion
including glycerol; and sugars transported by active transport proton
motive mechanisms such as lactose (19,53,62). Mechanisms to account
for this inhibition by PTS sugars have been proposed (12,48,52,64).
Inhibition of cAMP production by the transport of lactose has been
partially characterized (49). Apparently the activity of adenylate
cyclase responds to the proton gradient established as a consequence
of lactose transport. The mechanisms involved in inhibition of
adenylate cyclase by PTS sugars are not at all certain and conflict-
ing evidence has been offered (66,79). Some of the anomolous
effects seem to be strain specific (14).

Regardless of the mechanisms involved, cAMP production is
influenced by the carbon source (13,46; see Table IV for representative data). And these differences are in part, a consequence of
transport of the carbon source available to the cell. But it has
been proposed that synthesis of adenylate cyclase is repressed (46,
53) when cells grow with some carbon sources. Genetic and physiological evidence supports this proposal (4). In these experiments,
adenylate cyclase activity was determined by measuring rates of
cAMP production in washed cells aerating without a carbon source.
This provided an estimate of the specific activity of the enzyme
in the absence of inhibition by a carbon source (4). The inhibitory
effect of carbon sources was determined by including the sugar in
the aeration medium. It was found that when cells were grown with
a carbon source such as glucose that inhibits adenylate cyclase

activity severely, adenylate cyclase activity measured in the absence
of a carbon source was very high. Conversely, when cells were grown
with a carbon source such as succinate or glycerol that inhibits
adenylate cyclase only a little, adenylate cyclase activity measured
in the absence of a carbon source was low. This inverse relationship between inhibition of adenylate cyclase and the apparent
specific activity of the enzyme in the absence of a carbon
source (that is, a measure of the absolute amount of the enzyme) is
teleologically satisfying. When cells grow with glucose, cAMP production is maximally inhibited and cells are unable to induce
alternative catabolite operons. Conditions of catabolite repression
prevail. When glucose is exhausted, adenylate cyclase is no longer
inhibited and copious amounts of cAMP are made. The cells can then
induce alternative catabolic pathways unlimited by the availability
of cAMP. On the other hand, when cells grow with carbon sources
that do not inhibit adenylate cyclase, cAMP production is already
sufficient for induction of alternative catabolic pathways (4).

   Mutations in crp affect the apparent repression of adenylate
cyclase. It has been proposed that the CRP functions as a classical
negative repressor for adenylate cyclase (4). According to this
model, the CRP-cAMP complex active in initiation of transcription
(the promoter function) also functions as a classical negative
repressor for cya expression (the repressor function). There are
about 1200 CRP molecules per haploid genome in $E.$ $coli$ (2). If the
intracellular concentration of cAMP is on the order of 1 μM in
glucose grown cells, these cells contain about 600 molecules of
cAMP per cell. Most of the CRP molecules are inactive (conditions
of catabolite repression) and adenylate cyclase would be derepressed.
Were the intracellular concentration of cAMP to increase by a factor
of 2 or 3, nearly all the CRP would be in active conformation and
adenylate cyclase would be repressed.

   This model for repression of adenylate cyclase has received
support recently (31,42, H.V. Rickenberg, personal communication).
These investigations show that in broken cell extracts, the specific
activity of adenylate cyclase varies depending upon the carbon
source. This variation requires a functional crp allele (42).

   This model for regulation of adenylate cyclase is highly
speculative. The specific activity of an enzyme, particulary a
membrane associated enzyme with complex interactions with transport
functions, is not necessarily proportional to the number of molecules of that enzyme. An alternative is that the amount of adenylate
cyclase could be invariant and the production of a component necessary for activation of adenylate cyclase could respond to the
carbon source available (55, M.H. Saier, personal communication).

   We have observed that cells with a ColE1::cya hybrid plasmid

TABLE V
cAMP Production in Strains Having ColE1::cya Hybrid Plasmids

Strain[a]	Genotype	cAMP Production[b]
JA 200	wild type	54.7
JA200/pLC23-3	ColE1::cya	85.8
JA200/pLC29-5	ColE1::cya	39.5
JA200/pLC36-14	ColE1::cya	88.0
JA200/pLC41-4	ColE1::cya	60.0
8306/pLC23-3	cya del./ColE1::cya	90.1

[a]Strains are from the Clarke-Carbon E. coli ColE1 clone bank (6). Presumably each strain carries a different hybrid plasmid.

[b]cAMP production reported as pmoles cAMP ml^{-1} min^{-1} mg $protein^{-1}$ measured in cells grown with glucose and the necessary amino acid supplements, washed, and aerated in the absence of glucose. All strains could transfer cya and ilv to appropriate auxotrophic strains indicating that the plasmid had not become integrated. cAMP production in the 8306/LC23-3 strain is typical indicating that cya on the plasmid can be expressed normally. 8306 has a deletion for cya.

(6) do not overproduce cAMP (Table V). The additional copies of the *cya* gene could be repressed since there are 1200 molecules of the putative repressor in the cell. The excess adenylate cyclase may not be fully functional because there is not a commensurate excess of a component needed to activate the enzyme. The lack of a gene dosage effect of *cya* expression could be due to a pecularity of the ColE1 plasmid; cAMP does seem to be involved in the maturation of this plasmid (32).

REGULATION OF cAMP PRODUCTION WHEN CELLS GROW IN CARBON LIMITED CHEMOSTATS

Nutrient limited chemostats provide a reproducible, steady state condition that is physiologically quite different from conventional batch cultures. In a chemostat, cell numbers are determined by the concentration of the limiting nutrient. The growth rate of the culture is determined by the flow rate of fresh medium into the culture chamber replacing the spent medium (33,73). Cells respond to the situation in a chemostat in ways that would not always be predicted from studies in batch cultures. The major outer membrane proteins are present in different proportions when cells grow in chemostats (76). The specific activity of many enzymes in cells grown in chemostats is not as would be expected when cells

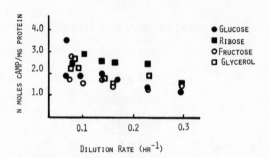

Figure 1. cAMP levels in cultures as a function of dilution rate
when cells grow in chemostats. Samples were taken after cultures
reached steady state conditions and assayed for total cAMP as
described previously (4). These data were taken from Harman (M.S.
Thesis, NMSU, 1977).

grow in batch culture (8,20). Catabolite repression of several
inducible catabolic enzymes is reduced when cells grow in carbon
limited chemostat culture (38).

From studies of regulation of cAMP production in batch cultures, we know that adenylate cyclase activity is inhibited by
transport of a carbon source. Furthermore, repression of adenylate
cyclase appears to be inversely proportional to inhibition of the
activity; that is, when the activity is inhibited, synthesis of
adenylate cyclase is derepressed. *A priori*, it would be anticipated
that as cells grow more slowly in carbon limited chemostat culture,
the rate of cAMP production should increase because the transport
systems would be unsaturated an increasing proportion of time. On
the other hand, if the activity is less inhibited as cells grow
more slowly, synthesis of adenylate cyclase should become more
repressed. The increasing repression might offset the decreasing
inhibition as cells grow more slowly.

This was tested (J.G. Harman, M.S. Thesis, NMSU, 1977; 19).
Salmonella typhimurium 3311 *cpd* was grown in chemostats with limiting glucose, fructose, glycerol or ribose. Glucose and fructose
are transported by PTS mechanisms, glycerol by facilitated diffusion, and ribose by an active transport mechanism (54,58). The
dilution rate varied from approximately 0.1 hr^{-1} (a 10 hour generation time) to 0.4 hr^{-1} (a 2.5 hour generation time). The concentrations of the sugars were adjusted so that approximately 10^9
cells/ml were present with all 4 carbon sources.

The data in Figure 1 show that the total production of cAMP
decreases as cells grow more rapidly. With the exception of ribose,

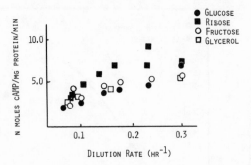

Figure 2. Rate of cAMP production as a function of dilution rate when cells grow in chemostats. This figure represents the data in Figure 1 calculated to provide the rates of cAMP synthesis. These data were taken from Harman (M.S. Thesis, NMSU, 1977) and appear in a somewhat different form in Ref. 19)

the results are quite similar. If the rate of cAMP production is calculated by multiplying the concentration of cAMP by the dilution rate, it can be seen that the rate of cAMP production increases as cells grow more rapidly (Figure 2).* In Table IV, these data are presented in another form and compared with the results obtained with conventional batch cultures. In contrast to the situation in batch culture, rates of cAMP production in carbon limited chemostat cultures are not affected much by the carbon source in *S. typhimurium*.

Somewhat similar results have been obtained with *E. coli* growing in glucose or succinate limited chemostat culture in which the intracellular and extracellular fractions of cAMP were determined (78). However, cAMP production was much lower, less than half, when cells grew with limiting succinate than when cells grew with limiting glucose.

In these experiments, the rates of cAMP production are much lower when cells grow in chemostats with limiting carbon sources

---

* In a chemostat, if cell numbers or anything produced by cells is to remain at a steady state concentration, the rate of production must equal the dilution rate of fresh medium into the culture chamber. For example: assume the culture chamber has a volume of 100 ml and cAMP at a concentration of 100 pmoles ml^{-1} is measured. If the flow rate of fresh medium into the chemostat is 33.33 ml hr^{-1}, the resulting dilution rate is 0.3 hr^{-1} and the cells must make 100 pmoles ml^{-1} cAMP x 0.3 hr^{-1} = 33 pmoles ml^{-1} cAMP hr^{-1} to maintain a steady state concentration of 100 pmoles ml^{-1}.

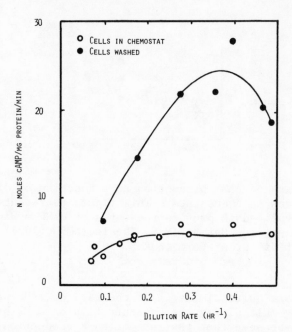

Figure 3.   Rates of cAMP production in bacteria grown in glucose
limited chemostats at various dilution rates and aerated in the
absence of a carbon source (19).

than when they grow in batch culture.   This observation leads to the
question: is cAMP production lower when cells grow in carbon limited
chemostat culture because adenylate cyclase is repressed under these
conditions or because adenylate cyclase is inhibited?   Could both
inhibition and repression be acting?   We tested this by growing cells
with limiting glucose in chemostats with dilution rates of slightly
less than 0.1 hr^{-1} to slightly greater than 0.5 hr^{-1}.   A sample was
taken for measurements of the total cAMP in the culture.   A second
sample was taken, the cells washed rapidly by filtration, and the
rates of cAMP production were determined after the cells were resuspended in medium without a carbon source.   The results of this
experiment are presented in Figure 3.

These results suggest that adenylate cyclase is both inhibited and repressed when cells grow in these conditions, since
rates of cAMP production were always higher in washed cells aerating
in the absence of a carbon source than when growing in the chemostat.
At least at the slower dilution rates this inhibition was not due
to glucose.   Glucose did not accumulate in concentrations greater
than 20 μM.   When cells grew in batch culture, cAMP production was
not inhibited by glucose until the concentration exceeded 50 μM
(19, see also 14).   Presumably some other inhibiting catabolite(s)

accumulated under these conditions. The peak in cAMP production in washed cells coincided with the dilution rate at which glucose was detectable at a concentration of 14 μM in the growth chamber. This concentration is also the K_s for growth of *E. coli* in chemostats with limiting glucose (23) and is presumably the K_s for growth of *S. typhimurium* under these conditions. This concentration is also approximately the K_m for glucose transport by the PTS system (54). The significance of this peak in the context of our experiments is not certain.

Adenylate cyclase appeared to be more repressed as cells grew more slowly if measurements of cAMP in washed cells provides a valid measure of the absolute amounts of adenylate cyclase present. Rates of production in washed cells increased as cells grew more rapidly and cAMP production was more inhibited.

The initial hypothesis was supported. When cells grew with limiting glucose in the chemostat, adenylate cyclase activity was less inhibited, that is the rate of cAMP production by washed cells was little more than the rate of cAMP production by cells in the chemostat at the slowest dilution rate. And as the inhibition to adenylate cyclase decreased, the specific activity of the enzyme also declined. Repression and inhibition combined to reduce the rates of cAMP production in carbon limited chemostat culture to much less than uninhibited rates observed in conventional batch culture (Table IV).

There are several alternative explanations for the data. The putative activator of adenylate cyclase may be limited when bacteria grow in carbon limited chemostat culture. The putative activator or perhaps adenylate cyclase per se may be much less stable under these conditions. Synthesis of adenylate cyclase may be repressed in response to longer generation times as has been shown for several enzymes in glutamate metabolism (20), superoxide dismutase (22) and the *trp* operon (57).

CONCLUDING REMARKS

At the present time it is impossible to generalize about a role for cAMP of cGMP in carbohydrate metabolism in procaryotes. In bacteria other than the enteric coliforms, very little information concerning cyclic nucleotides is available. Catabolite repression is observed in bacteria in which cAMP is not found. Catabolite repression is observed in other bacteria in which cAMP is found but the catabolite repression appears to be unaffected by the nucleotide. cGMP is found in some bacteria but in very small concentrations. Except in a few dimorphic procaryotes (e.g. *Caulobacteria* and *Strep-tomyces*), it has no apparent function.

In the enteric coliforms, cAMP is certainly a key factor in
regulation of induction of catabolic enzymes. Catabolite repression
is mediated, in part , by the intracellular concentrations of cAMP.
Induction of catabolic operons is limited by the availability of
the CRP-cAMP complex. However, regulation of cAMP production is
not at all certain even in descriptive terms. Our current understanding of cAMP metabolism in the enteric coliforms is summarized
in Figure 4.

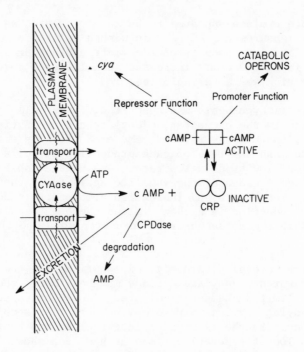

Figure 4.   cAMP metabolism in *E. coli*. This figure summarizes what
is known about cAMP metabolism in *E. coli* and presumably in other
enteric coliform bacteria.

    CYAase-adenylate cyclase. This enzyme is inhibited by trans-
port of PTS sugars and sugars such as lactose transported by poton
motive mechanisms.

    CPase-cAMP phosphodiesterase. This enzyme degrades cAMP and
reduces the net production of cAMP. Its activity does not appear
to change with culture conditions.

    CRP-cAMP receptor protein. This is an allosteric regulatory
protein that forms an active complex with cAMP. This complex is
required for initiation of transcription of several operons and
could serve as a repressor of *cya* expression.

ACKNOWLEDGEMENTS

The author's work has been supported by grants from the National Science Foundation and by participation in the NIH-MBS program (1-506-RR-08136 to NMSU). The author would like to express his appreciation to Alan Peterkofsky and Milton H. Saier for considerable correspondence resulting in valuable insights.

REFERENCES

1. Alper, M.D. and B.N. Ames. 1978. Transport of antibiotics and metabolic analogs by systems under cyclic AMP control: Positive selection of *Salmonella typhimurium cys* and *crp* mutants. J. Bacteriol. 133:149-157.
2. Anderson, W.B., A.B. Schneider, M. Emmer, R.L. Perlman, and I. Pastan. 1971. Purification and properties of the cyclic adenosine 3', 5'-monophosphate receptor proetin which mediates cyclic adenosine 3',5'-monophosphate dependent gene transcription in *Escherichia coli*. J. Biol. Chm. 245:5929-5937.
3. Bernlohr, R.W., M.K. Haddox, and N.D. Goldberg. 1974. Cyclic 3',5'-monophosphate in *Escherichia coli* and *Bacillus liceniformis*. J. Biol. Chm. 249:4329-4331.
4. Botsford, J.L. and M. Drexler. 1978. The cyclic 3',5'-adenosine monophosphate receptor protein and regulation of cyclic 3',5'-adenosine monophosphate synthesis in *Escherichia coli*. Molec. Gen. Genet. 164:47-56.
5. Buettner, M.J., E. Spitz, and H.V. Rickenberg. 1973. Cyclic adenosine monophosphate in *Escherichia coli*. J. Bacteriol. 114:1068-1075.
6. Clarke, L. and J. Carbon. 1976. A colony bank containing synthetic ColE1 hybrid plasmids representative of the entire *E. coli* genome. Cell 9:91-99.
7. Danley, D.E., M. Drexler, and J.L. Botsford. 1977. Differential binding of cyclic adenosine 3',5'-monophosphate to the cyclic adenosine 3',5'-monophosphate receptor protein in
8. Dean, A.C.R. 1972. Influence of environment on the control of enzyme synthesis. J. Appl. Chem. and Biotech. 22:245-257.
9. deCrombrugghe, B. and I. Pastan. 1978. Cyclic AMP, the cyclic AMP receptor protein and their dual control of the galactose operon. In: The Operon. Editors: J.H. Miller and W.S. Reznikoff. Cold Spring Harbor, New York. Cold Spring Harbor Laboratory. pp. 303-324.
10. Dessein, A., M. Schwartz, and A. Ullmann. 1978. Catabolite repression in *Escherichia coli* mutants lacking cyclic AMP. Molec. Gen. Genet. 162:83-91.
11. Dessein, A., G. Tillier, and A. Ullmann. 1978. Catabolite modulator factor: physiological properties and in vivo effects. Molec. Gen. Genet. 162:89-94.

12. Dills, S.S., A. Apperson, M.R. Schmidt and M.H. Saier, Jr.
     1980. Carbohydrate transport in bacteria. Microbiol. Rev.
     44:385-418.

13. Epstein, W., L.B. Rothman-Denes, and J. Hesse. 1975. cAMP
     as mediator of catabolite repression in *Escherichia coli*.
     Proc. Nat. Acad. Sci. USA 72:2300-2303.

14. Feucht, B.U. and M.H. Saier. 1980. Fine control of adenylate
     cyclase by the phosphoenolpyruvate:sugar phosphotransferase
     systems in *Escherichia coli* and *Salmonella typhimurium*. J.
     Bacteriol. 141:603-610.

15. Gersch, D., W. Romer, H. Bocker and H. Thrum. 1978. Variation
     in cAMP and cGMP in antibiotic producing strains of *Strepto-
     myces hydroscopius*. FEMS Microbiol. Lett. 3:39-46.

16. Goldenbaum, P.E. and G.A. Hall. 1979. Transport of cyclic
     adenosine 3',5'-monophosphate across *Escherichia coli* mem-
     brame vessicles. J. Bacteriol. 140:459.

17. Gonzales, J.E. and A. Peterkofsky. 1975. Diverse directional
     changes of cAMP relative to cGMP in *E. coli*. Biochem. Biophys.
     Res. Comm. 67:190-198.

18. Haggerty, D.M., and R.F. Schleif. 1975. Kinetics of the onset
     of catabolite repression in *Escherichia coli* as determined by
     lac mRNA initiations and intracellular cAMP levels. J.
     Bacteriol. 123:946-953.

19. Harman, J.G. and J.L. Botsford. 1979. Synthesis of adenosine
     3',5'-cyclic monophosphate in *Salmonella typhimurium* growing
     in continuous culture. J. Gen. Microbiol. 110:243-246.

20. Harvey, R.J. 1970. Metabolic regulation in glucose limited
     chemostat cultures of *Escherichia coli*. J. Bacteriol. 104:
     698-706.

21. Harwood, J. and A. Peterkofsky. 1975. Glucose sensitive
     adenylate cyclase in toluene treated cells of *Escherichia
     coli*. J. Biol. Chem. 250:4656-4662.

22. Hassan, H.M. and I. Fridovitch. 1977. Physiological function
     of superoxide dismutase in glucose limited chemostat cultures
     of *Escherichia coli*. J. Bacteriol. 130:805-811.

23. Herbert, D. and H.L. Kornberg. 1976. Glucose as the rate-
     limiting step in the growth of *E. coli* on glucose. Biochem.
     J. 156:449-456.

24. Hewlett, E. and J. Wolff. 1976. Soluble adenylate cyclase
     from the culture medium of *Bordetella pertusis*. Purification
     and properties. J. Bacteriol. 127:890-898.

25. Hood, E.E., S. Armour, J.D. Ownby, A.K. Hauda and R.A.
     Bressan. 1979. Effect of nitrogen starvation on the level of
     cAMP in *Anabaena variabilis*. Biochim. Biophys. ACTA 588:193-
     199.

26. Hylemon, P.B. and P.V. Phibbs, Jr. 1974. Evidence against the
     presence of cyclic AMP and related enzymes in selected strains
     of *Bacteroides fragilis*. Biochem. Biophys. Res. Comm. 60:88-
     95.

27. Ishiyama, J. 1976. Isolation of cyclic deoxyadenosine 3',5'-monophosphate from the culture fluid of *Corynebacterium murisepticum*. J. Biol. Chem. 251:438-440.

28. Ishiyama, J. 1976. Isolation of inosine 3',5'-monophosphate from bacterial culture medium. J. Cycl. Nucleo. Res. 2:21-23.

29. Ishiyama, J. 1975. Isolation of cyclic 3',5'-guanosine monophosphate from bacterial culture fluids. Amino Acid and Nucleic Acid 32:87-88.

30. Ishiyama, J. 1975. Isolation of 3',5'-pyrimidine mononucleotides from bacterial culture fluids. Biochem. Biophys. Res. Comm. 65:286-288.

31. Janecek, J., J. Naprtek, Z. Dobrova, M. Jiresova, and J. Spizek. 1979. Adenylate cyclase activity in *Escherichia coli* cultured under various conditions. FEMS Microbiol. Lett. 6:305-310.

32. Katz, L. and D.R. Helinski. 1974. Effects of inhibitors of RNA and protein synthesis on cAMP stimulation of plasmid ColE1 replication. J. Bacteriol. 119:450-460.

33. Kubitschek, H.E. 1970. Introduction to research with continuous culture. Englewood Cliffs, NJ. Prentice-Hall pp260.

34. Lee, C.H. 1977. Identification of adenosine 3',5'-monophosphate in *Mycobacterium smegmatis*. J. Bacteriol. 132:1031-1033.

35. Lee, N. 1978. Molecular aspects of *ara* regulation. In: The Operon. Editors: J. H. Miller and W.S. Reznikoff. Cold Spring Harbor, NY. Cold Spring Harbor Laboratories. pp 389-409.

36. Lim, S.T. and K.T. Shanmugam. 1979. Effect of cyclic guanosine 3',5'-monophosphate on nitrogen fixation in *Rhizobium japonicum*. J. Bacteriol. 139:256-263.

37. Lim, S.T. and K.T. Shanmugam. 1979. Regulation of hydrogen utilization in *Rhizobium japonicum* by cyclic AMP. Biochim. Biophys. ACTA 584:479-491.

38. McFall, E. and J. Mandelstam. 1963. Specific metabolic expression of three induced enzymes in *Escherichia coli*. Biochem. J. 89:391-399.

39. McGinnis, J.F. and K. Paigen. 1973. Site of catabolite inhibition of carbohydrate metabolism. J. Bacteriol. 114:885-887.

40. Macchia, V., S. Varrone, H. Weissbach, D.L. Miller and I. Pastan. 1975. Guanylate cyclase in *Escherichia coli*. J. Biol. Chem. 250:6214-6220.

41. Magasanik, B. 1970. Glucose Effects: Inducer exclusion and repression. In: The Lactose Operon. Editors: J. Beckwith and D. Zipser. Cold Spring Harbor, NY. Cold Spring Harbor Laboratory. pp 189-220.

42. Majerfeld, I.H., D. Miller, E. Spitz and H.V. Rickenberg. 198. Regulation of the synthesis of adenylate cyclase by the cAMP-cAMP receptor protein complex. Molec. Gen. Genet. In press.

43. Makman, R.S. and E.W. Sutherland. 1965. Adenosine 3',5'-phos-
     phate in *Escherichia coli*. J. Biol. Chem. 240:1309-1314.
44. Nielsen, L.D., D. Monard, and H.V. Rickenberg. 1973. Cyclic
     3',5'-adenosine monophosphate phosphodiesterase of *Escherichia
     coli*. J. Bacteriol. 116:857-866.
45. Parish, J.H., K.R. Wedgwood, and D.G. Herries. 1976. Morpho-
     genesis in *Myxococcus xanthus* and *Myxococcus virescens*. (Myxo-
     bacteriales). Arch. Microbiol. 107:343-351.
46. Pastan, I. and S. Adhya. 1976. Cyclic adenosine 3',5'-mono-
     phosphate in *Escherichia coli*. Bacteriol. Rev. 40:527-551.
47. Pastan, I. and R.L. Perlman. 1970. Cyclic adenosine mono-
     phosphate in bacteria. Science 169:339-344.
48. Peterkofsky, A. 1981. Transmembrane signaling by sugars
     regulates the activity of *Escherichia coli* adenylate cyclase.
     In: *Microbiology* 1981. Editor: D. Schlessinger. Washington
     D.C. American Society for Microbiology. In Press.
48a. Peterkofsky, A. 1976. Cyclic nucleotides in bacteria. Adv.
     Cyc. Nucleo. Res. 7:1-45.
49. Peterkofsky, A. and C. Gazdar. 1979. *Escherichia coli* adeny-
     late cyclase complex-Regulation by the proton electrochemical
     gradient. Proc. Nat. Acad. Sci. USA 76:1099-1102.
50. Peterkofsky, A. and C. Gazdar. 1973. Measurements of cAMP
     synthesis in intact *E. coli* B. Proc. Nat. Acad. Sci. USA
     70:2149-2152.
51. Peterkofsky, A. and C. Gazdar. 1971. Glucose and the metabo-
     lism of adenosine 3',5'-cyclic monophosphate in *Escherichia
     coli*. Proc. Nat. Acad. Sci. USA 68:2794-2798.
52. Peterkofsky, A., J.E. Gonzalez, and C. Gazdar. 1978. The
     Escherichia coli adenylate cyclase complex. Regulation by
     enzyme I of the phosphoenol pyruvate:sugar phosphotransferase
     system. Arch. Biochem. Biophys. 188:47-55.
53. Peterkofsky, A., J. Harwood, and C. Gazdar. 1975. Inducibility
     of sugar sensitivity of adenylate cyclase of *E. coli*. B.
     Jour. Cyc. Nucleo. Res. 1:11-20.
54. Postma, P.W. and S. Roseman. 1976. The bacterial phosphoenol
     pyruvate:sugar phosphotransferase system. Biochim. Biophys.
     ACTA 457:213-257.
55. Rephaeli, A.W. and M.H. Saier, Jr. 1976. Effects of *crp*.
     mutations on adenosine 3',5'-monophosphate metabolism in
     Salmonella typhimurium. J. Bacteriol 127:120-127.
56. Rickenberg, H.V. 1974. Cyclic AMP in Procaryotes. Ann. Rev.
     Microbiol. 28:357-394.
57. Rose, J.K. and C.Y. Yanofsky. 1972. Metabolic regulation of
     the tryptophan operon of *E. coli*. Repressor independent
     regulation of transcription initiation frequency. Jour. Molec.
     Biol. 69:103-110.
58. Roseman, S. 1977. Transport of sugars across bacterial
     membranes. In: *Biochemistry of Membrane Transport*. Editors:
     G. Semenza and E. Carafoli. Berlin. Springer-Verlag. pp. 582-
     597.

59. Ross, E.M. and A.G. Gilman. 1980. Biochemical properties of hormone sensitive adenylate cyclase. Ann. Rev. Biochem. 49:533-564.

60. Sahyoun, N. and I.F. Durr. 1972. Evidence against the presence of 3',5'-cyclic adenosine monophosphate and relevant enzymes in *Lactobacillus plantarum*. J. Bacteriol. 112:421-426.

61. Saier, M.H. 1979. The role of the cell surface in regulating the internal environment. In: The Bacteria. Vol. VII. Editors: J.R. Sobatch and L.N. Orston. New York: Academic Press pp168-267.

62. Saier, M.H. 1977. Bacterial phosphoenolpyruvate:sugar phosphotransferase systems: Structural, functional and evolutionary interrelationships. Bacteriol. Rev. 41:856-871.

63. Saier, M.H., B.U. Feucht, and M.F. McCamman. 1975. Regulation of intracellular cyclic AMP levels in *Escherichia coli* and *Salmonella typhimurium*. Evidence for energy dependent excretion of the cyclic nucleotide. Jour. Biol. Chem. 250:7593.

64. Saier, M.H. and E.G. Moczydlowski. 1978. The regulation of carbohydrate transport in *Escherichia coli* and *Salmonella typhimurium*. In: Bacterial Transport. Editors: Barry P. Rosen. New York: Marcel Dekker, Inc. pp103-122.

65. Sarkar, N. and H. Palus. 1975. A guanosine 3',5'-monophosphate sensitive nuclease from *Bacillus brevis*. J. Biol. Chem. 250:684-690.

66. Scholte, B.J. and P.W. Postma. 1980. Mutation in the *cyp* gene of *Salmonella typhimurium* which interferes with inducer exclusion. J. Bacteriol. 141:751-757.

67. Setlow, P. 1973. Inability to detect cAMP in vegetative or sporulating cells or dormant spores of *B. megaterium*. Biochem. Biophys. Res. Comm. 52:365-372.

68. Setlow, B. and P. Setlow. 1978. Levels of cGMP in dormant, germinating and outgrowing spores and growing a sporulating cells of *Bacillus megaterium*. J. Bacteriol. 136:433-436.

69. Shapiro, L. 1976. Differentiation in the *Caulobacter* cell cycle. Ann. Rev. Microbiol. 30:377-407.

70. Shibuya, M., Y. Takabe, and Y. Kaziro. 1977. A possible involvement of *cya* gene in the synthesis of cyclic guanosine 3':5'-monophosphate in *E. coli*. Cell 12:521-528.

71. Siegel, L.S., P.B. Hylemon, and P.V. Phibbs, Jr. 1977. Cyclic adenosine 3',5'-monophosphate and activities of adenylate cyclase and cyclic adenosine 3',5'-monophosphate phosphodiesterase in *Pseudomonas aeruginosa* and *Bacteriodies*. J. Bacteriol. 129:87-96.

72. Takebe, Y., M. Shibuya, and Y. Kaziro. 1978. A new extragenic suppressor of *cya* mutations. J. Biochem. 83:1615-1623.

73. Tempest, D.W. 1970. The place of continuous culture in microbiological research. Adv. Microb. Phys. 4:223-249.

74. Ullmann, A. 1974. Are cyclic AMP effects related to real physiological phenomena? Biochem. Biophys. Res. Comm. 57:348-355.

75.   Ullmann, A., F. Tillier, and J. Monod. 1976. Catabolite modu-
      lator factor: A possible mediator of catabolite repression in
      bacteria. Proc. Nat. Acad. Sci. USA 73:3476-3479.
76.   Villarejo, M., J. Stanovich, K. Young, and G. Edlin. 1979.
      Differences in membrane proteins, cAMP levels and glucose
      transport between batch and chemostat cultures of *Escherichia
      coli*. Curr. Microbiol. 1:345-349.
77.   Wanner, B.L., R, Kodaira, and F.C. Neidhardt. 1978. Regulation
      of *lac* operon expression: Reappraisal of the theory of cata-
      bolite repression. J. Bacteriol. 136:947-954.
78.   Wright, L.F., D.P. Milne, and C. J. Knowles. 1979. The regula-
      tory effects of growth rate and cyclic AMP levels on carbon
      catabolism and respiration in *E. coli* K-12.   Biochim. Biophys.
      ACTA   483:73-80.
79.   Yang, J.K., R.W. Bloom, and W. Epstein. 1979. Catabolite and
      transient repression in *Escherichia coli* do not require enzyme
      I of the phosphotransferase system. J. Bacteriol. 138:275-279.

METABOLIC COMPROMISES INVOLVED IN THE GROWTH OF MICROORGANISMS IN NUTRIENT-LIMITED (CHEMOSTAT) ENVIRONMENTS

David W. Tempest and Oense M. Neijssel

Laboratorium voor Microbiologie, Universiteit van
Amsterdam, Nieuwe Achtergracht 127, 1018 WS
Amsterdam, The Netherlands

INTRODUCTION

Biochemical research, particularly over the past 50 years or so, has revealed ever more clearly the underlying unity of living processes. And this possibly has obscured to some extent the fact that there are nevertheless important physiological differences between microbial cells and, say, the cells of higher animals. One of the most fundamental of these, and one which undoubtedly has considerable evolutionary significance, is evident in the ways in which the different cells accommodate to environmental change. Clearly, the cells of higher animals have evolved to spend the whole of their existence in a closely regulated environment, and this is a condition of life for them. But microbial cells are markedly different. They generally are exposed to environments that fluctuate extensively (and often rapidly) and, being free-living creatures, they do not possess the capacity to regulate their surroundings. Instead, they respond to environmental change by changing themselves - structurally and functionally - and seemingly have acquired in the course of evolution a whole armoury of sophisticated control mechanisms whereby to effect such change. As most people realize, it is this enormous versatility of microbial cells (their structural and functional plasticity) that makes them economically, as well as ecologically, of considerable importance; it also makes them fascinating objects for study.

One serious problem, however, faces persons attempting to study this so-called phenotypic variation; that is, that microorganisms interact with their environment in a way that causes it to change continuously. Consequently, if one grows microorganisms in a closed system (that is, the classical batch culture method) one cannot obtain prolonged steady state environmental conditions; and

335

one then must recognize that inevitably one will be dealing with
populations whose properties are changing continuously with time.
There is only one practical way around this problem and that is to
grow organisms in an open system – that is, a continuous-flow culture
system. Moreover, if one employs the chemostat mode of continuous
culture then further benefits accrue in that not only can one obtain
a wide range of controlled environments, but also a range of unique
environments in which organisms may express properties that are not
otherwise expressed, or expressed only transiently. And by relating
these properties to the precise conditions provoking their expression
insight frequently may be gained into their functional significance.
It is the purpose of this article to detail some of these properties
and to place them in a rational physiological context.

Before proceeding to a detailed description of microbial response to nutrient-limited environments, however, it is useful to
consider in a little more detail the question of cell-environment
interaction as it may relate to the behaviour of organisms in natural
ecosystems. For, as already indicated, it is logical to suppose that
the physiological plasticity of microorganisms is related to their
need to cope with the vicissitudes of life outside the laboratory
culture. In this connection, it is relevant to draw attention to the
enormous growth rate potential of most microorganisms which we study
routinely. For example, in broth culture, *Escherichia coli* is able
to double in mass within 20 min. Thus, if one *E. coli* organism
(weighing about 0.2 pg) and its progeny were to grow at an unrestricted rate for as little as 3 days, then there would be produced
a mass of organisms equal to about 1000-times the mass of the Earth.
So why is it, one might reasonably ask, that the surface of this
planet is not deep with *E. coli*? The simple answer must be that, in
natural ecosystems, organisms rarely grow at their potentially maximum rate. Hence it is important to consider why this is so: or, to
put it another way, to consider what may constrain the growth of
organisms in natural ecosystems. Many factors, of course, may play
a part; microorganisms may be limited in their growth by extremes
of temperature, pH,salinity and/or water activity, as well as by the
presence of noxious substances, predators and parasites. But over
and above these, one factor that will consistently constrain the rate
at which these populations grow must be the availability of nutrient
substances. For what we know with certainly is that heterotrophic
organisms require to consume at least 2 g of some carbon substrate
(such as glucose) to synthesize 1 g of biomass. Consequently,
irrespective of other considerations, the availability of nutrient
substances always would ultimately limit the extent to which any
population could grow – be it in the laboratory culture or in some
natural ecosystem. On the basis of this argument, then, it is
reasonable to conclude that nutrient insufficiency will be the most
common environmental extreme to which microorganisms are routinely
exposed and that, in consequence, such conditions will have exerted

a potent selective force in the evolution of microbial species. One may anticipate, therefore, that a substantial part of the microbe's metabolic machinery will be directed to coping with this ubiquitous condition.

Nutrient-limited growth conditions are, of course, precisely those that are extant in a chemostat culture, and the very fact that organisms grow readily in chemostat environments attests to the ability of these creatures to cope with this putatively common environmental extreme. Not surprisingly, however, in so doing they often express a physiology that is very different from that expressed in batch culture. And since the bulk of our knowledge of microbial physiology has derived from studies of organisms grown in batch culture, this seemingly has led a number of microbial physiologists to believe that batch cultures are essentially "normal" and that organisms growing in chemostat culture are "aberrant". But there are no good grounds for so believing, and it is more prudent simply to accept that organisms growing in chemostat culture necessarily are different, physiologically, from those growing in batch culture, and that these differences can be both rationalized and exploited.

PHYSIOLOGICAL ASPECTS OF NUTRIENT-LIMITED GROWTH

If, as argued above, nutrient-limited growth conditions have exerted a strong selective pressure in the course of evolution, then one might predict that microorganisms would possess the capacity to modulate their physiology in at least four aspects to accommodate to such restrictive conditions. Thus, (1.) it is reasonable to assume that they would either possess constitutively, or else be able to induce (or derepress) the synthesis of high-affinity uptake systems for all the potentially growth-limiting nutrients. Failing this, one would expect them, under appropriate conditions, to be able to over-produce some lower-affinity uptake system so as to increase the V_{max} of the primary substrate uptake mechanism. In this way, organisms would enhance their capacity to compete with other species normally present in natural ecosystems for the limiting supply of nutrient (17,47,48,51). At the same time, (2.) it would be necessary for them to regulate the uptake of all the other (non-limiting) nutrients – particularly the carbon and energy source – so as to prevent intermediary metabolites accumulating to potentially traumatic levels (6,7). Clearly (3.) some rearrangement of metabolism would be desirable in order to circumvent, as far as was physiologically possible, those bottlenecks imposed by the specific nutrient limitation. Finally, (4.) organisms would need to modulate coordinately the rates of synthesis of all their macromolecular components in order to allow balanced growth to proceed at a grossly submaximal rate. Much evidence has accumulated that accords with these predicted responses, and selected examples are specified below.

Modulation of Substrate Uptake Mechanisms

High- and low-affinity uptake systems for a wide variety of substrates have been reported to be present in a number of different organisms; for example, in *E. coli* these include uptake systems for glucose (30), gluconate (15), magnesium (37), potassium (41) and phosphate (52,53). However, with batch cultures it is not always easy to derive a clear understanding of the relevance of these different uptake systems to the growing cell since, in general, one is not able to culture organisms for prolonged periods of time in the presence of low, enzyme-subsaturating, concentrations of the appropriate nutrient. With chemostat cultures, however, one can routinely establish and maintain steady state nutrient-limiting growth conditions. And by judiciously varying a number of environmental parameters, and determining quantitatively their effect on the appropriate enzyme activities, the functional significance of these enzymes (and enzyme systems) can be more readily assessed.

For example, *Klebsiella aerogenes* possesses two mechanisms for the uptake and assimilation of glycerol (Fig. 1). Now studies with batch cultures revealed that organisms synthesized glycerol kinase when growing aerobically, on glycerol, but glycerol dehydrogenase when growing anaerobically (32). The rationale underlying this switch in the pathway of glycerol assimilation was sought in the fact that glycerol phosphate dehydrogenase was a flavoprotein and hence would not be able to function anaerobically in the absence of an electron acceptor such as fumarate or nitrate. Glycerol dehydrogenase, on the other hand, circumvents this bottleneck by being linked to NAD. So the reason for dual pathways of glycerol assimilation seemed quite clear: one was the strictly aerobic pathway and the other, the strictly anaerobic pathway; and this conclusion was strengthened by the finding that glycerol dehydrogenase was rapidly

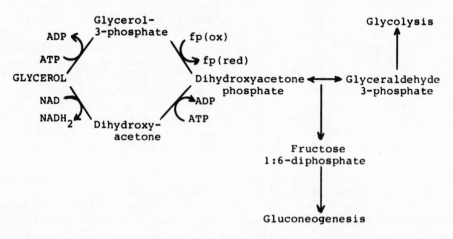

Figure 1. Pathways of glycerol assimilation in *Klebsiella aerogenes*.

destroyed in the intact cell engaged in aerobic metabolism. But it
is relevant to point out here that the affinity for glycerol of
glycerol kinase and glycerol dehydrogenase are widely different, the
reported apparent K_m values being, respectively, $1-2 \times 10^{-6}M$ (19)
and $2-4 \times 10^{-2}M$ (36). And the picture revealed by chemostat studies
is markedly different from that obtained with batch cultures, as
can be adduced from the data shown in Figure 2. This shows the
influence of glycerol concentration on the rate of respiration of
washed suspensions of *K. aerogenes* that were grown, respectively,
in glycerol-limited and ammonia-limited <u>aerobic</u> chemostat culture.
Clearly, the glycerol-limited cells possessed a high-affinity
glycerol uptake system (characteristic of glycerol kinase) but the
glycerol sufficient (ammonia-limited) cells possessed a low affinity
glycerol uptake system that was more characteristic of glycerol dehydrogenase. And analysis of extracts of these glycerol-sufficient
cells failed to reveal the presence of glycerol kinase whereas they
possessed significant levels of glycerol dehydrogenase (Table I).
Further consideration of Table I shows (1.) that no glycerol kinase
activity could be detected in anaerobic cultures, (2.) no glycerol

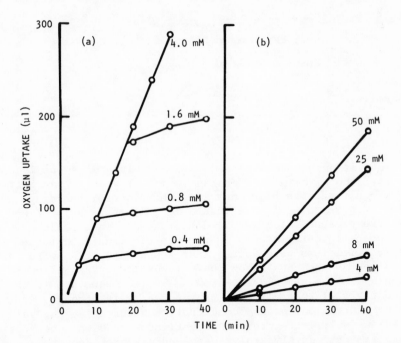

Figure 2.   Oxidation of glycerol by *Klebsiella aerogenes* washed suspensions that had been grown (a) glycerol-limited and (b) ammonia-
limited in aerobic chemostat culture (D = 0.17 h^{-1}; 35°C; pH 6.8).
The washed bacteria were incubated in a Gilson respirometer in a
50 mM phosphate buffer, pH 7.0, at 35°C. The concentration of
organisms was about 0.8 mg/ml and the concentration of glycerol
varied as indicated on the plots. (From ref. 36)

TABLE I

Glycerol Kinase and Glycerol Dehydrogenase Activities of Variously-
limited *Klebsiella aerogenes* Organisms that had been Grown in
Chemostat Culture at a Dilution Rate of 0.17 h^{-1} (35°C; pH 6.8)(36).

Growth-limitation	Carbon source	Other conditions	Specific activity (nmol substrate used/min / mg cell protein)	
			Glycerol kinase	Glycerol dehydrogenase
Carbon + Energy	Glycerol	Aerobic	122	<1
	Glucose	Aerobic	106	<1
	Glycerol	Anaerobic	<1	282
	Glucose	Anaerobic	<1	101
Sulphate	Glycerol	Aerobic	<1	11
	Glucose	Aerobic	<1	<1
	Glycerol	Anaerobic	<1	50
	Glucose	Anaerobic	<1	22
Ammonia	Glycerol	Aerobic	<1	9

kinase activity could be detected in other glycerol-sufficient cultures, (3.) the glycerol dehydrogenase activity of glycerol-limited
anaerobic cultures was high, but (4.) the glycerol dehydrogenase
activity of glycerol-sufficient aerobic cultures was low. And
whereas the presence of glycerol dehydrogenase in aerobic glycerol-
sufficient cells correlated with the kinetic studies detailed in
Figure 2, criticisms were voiced that these activities were far too
low to allow for the conclusion that glycerol dehydrogenase was
functioning in the aerobically-growing cells. However, it was shown
subsequently (21) that glycerol dehydrogenase is strongly activated
by low concentrations of Mn^{2+} and that, consequently, the values
reported in Table I are gross underestimates. So we interpret our
findings in terms of glycerol kinase and glycerol dehydrogenase
representing alternative high- and low-affinity uptake systems for
glycerol. And the advantage to the organism in synthesizing glycerol
dehydrogenase under aerobic glycerol-sufficient conditions resides
in the fact that it affords a greater measure of control over the
uptake of excess glycerol (under glycerol-sufficient conditions)
since it is linked directly to the pyridine nucleotide pool and
therefore sensitive to the redox state extant within the growing cell

Anaerobically, of course, glycerol kinase cannot function (as already mentioned) and under glycerol-limiting conditions the organisms are obliged to utilize the low-affinity uptake system. Hence, entirely predictably, under these anaerobic low-glycerol conditions the organisms must synthesize vast amounts of glycerol dehydrogenase in order to scavenge glycerol from their environment.

As suggested previously, it is reasonable to suppose that when growing in nutrient-limited environments, at a grossly submaximal rate, organisms would need to regulate the uptake of all other (non-limiting) nutrients. Indeed, that an overconsumption of glycerol can have deleterious effects has been elegantly demonstrated both with mutants of $E. coli$ that were constitutive for glycerol kinase and lacked feedback control of this enzyme (55), and with $K. aerogenes$ organisms that were induced to synthesize high levels of glycerol kinase and then exposed to glycerol in environments that would not fully support cell synthesis (40). In both cases, glycerol added in concentrations greater than 1 mM caused a rapid loss of viability. One might expect, then, that when organisms lack a low-affinity system for the uptake of some nutrient, then other mechanisms will operate to regulate the rate of penetration of excess nutrient into the cell.

Regulation of Uptake of Excess (Non-limiting) Nutrients

With organisms like $E. coli$ and $K. aerogenes$ there are known to exist dual, or even multiple, uptake systems for glucose (28), though the majority of these are linked to the phosphotransferase system (31) and have a relatively high affinity for glucose. Hence, one might anticipate that such cells will possess coarse and fine control mechanisms that serve to regulate the flow of glucose into the cell to a rate sufficient to meet the biosynthetic and bioenergetic demands of cell synthesis. Much evidence from batch culture studies of wild-type and mutant organisms broadly accords with this supposition (27); but again, data obtained with chemostat cultures are fascinatingly different.

With cultures of $K. aerogenes$ growing in a glucose-simple salts medium in a chemostat at a relatively low rate ($0.17 \ h^{-1}$) it was found that the rate of glucose uptake and metabolism varied markedly with the nature of the growth limitation (Table II).

Thus, at this fixed growth rate the glucose-limited culture took up glucose at a substantially lower rate than did any of the other glucose-sufficient cultures, but assimilated it into cell substance with a greater efficiency - the sole products formed being cells and CO_2. Under all other conditions, the rate of glucose uptake was more than double that expressed by the glucose-limited culture and a variety of intermediary metabolites were excreted in

TABLE II

Glucose Utilization Rates, and Rates of Product Formation, in Variously-limited Chemostat Cultures of *Klebsiella aerogenes* (D = 0.17 h⁻¹; 35°C; pH 6.8).

Limitation	Glucose	Glucose (+ DNP)	Ammonia	Ammonia* (+ DNP)	Sulfate	Phosphate	Magnesium	Potassium
Glucose used	36 8	65.8	107.4	253	98.7	112.8	124.6	175
Products formed:								
Cells	20	20	20	20	20	20	20	20
CO_2	15.6	43.2	20.2	17.4	20.8	20.4	31.4	56.3
Pyruvate	–	–	5.2	28.1	21.9	–	9.6	10.1
2-Oxoglutarate	–	–	22.5	17.2	1.8	–	9.6	3.0
Acetate	–	1.2	4.0	8.1	9.6	4.5	17.7	13.3
Gluconate	–	–	–	11.2	–	9.5	0.1	31.9
2-Ketogluconate	–	–	–	143	–	39.9	11.9	20.5
Succinate	–	–	–	–	2.3	–	–	–
D-Lactate	–	–	–	–	–	–	10.9	–
Polysacc. (Exocell.)	–	–	36.0	–	7.0	15.1	–	–
Protein (Exocell.)	–	–	–	–	1.8	–	2.5	8.0
Carbon recovery	97	98	100	97	86	97	91	93

*Dilution rate = 0.11 h⁻¹

All values are expressed as matoms carbon per hour and are normalized to a cell production rate of 20 matoms carbon per hour. Data of ref. 34 and 35.

substantial amounts. Almost all these "overflow" products were more
highly oxidized than glucose; these were, of course, highly aerated
cultures, and it is clear that excess reducing equivalents released
as a consequence of excess glucose catabolism were oxidized through
to water. Thus, there was no accumulation of typical fermentation
products that are characteristic of oxygen-limited growth, or of
the growth of Crabtree-positive yeasts in aerobic glucose-sufficient
media.

The range of overflow products formed differed both quantitatively with the nature of the growth limitation. For example,
ammonia-limited cultures produced much 2-oxoglutarate, phosphate-
limited cells much 2-ketogluconate and potassium-limited cells
much gluconic acid. All glucose-sufficient cultures, however,
produced acetate and substantial amounts of CO_2.

What, then, is the possible physiological significance of
this overflow metabolism? What advantages accrue to the organism
in not regulating the rate of glucose uptake and metabolism to that
rate extant in glucose-limited cultures? Perhaps the significance
of overflow metabolism can be best assessed by considering the
special metabolic requirements of the primary uptake system for
the growth-limiting nutrient. Thus, when growing under conditions
of ammonia limitation, *K. aerogenes* derepresses the synthesis of a
high-affinity ammonia uptake system that involves two enzymes –
glutamine synthetase and glutamate synthase (50). Both enzymes
effect reactions that require three substrates; ammonia, glutamate
and ATP, and glutamine, 2-oxoglutarate and NADPH, respectively.
Hence, in order to function effectively in the assimilation of low
concentrations of ammonia, these two enzymes require an unrestricted
supply of glutamate, 2-oxoglutarate, ATP and NADPH. These conditions
could not be met fully if, under ammonia limitation, the uptake of
glucose was highly constrained; and clearly it is not. It is not
difficult to appreciate, therefore, the physiological significance
of an overflow of 2-oxoglutarate under conditions of ammonia limitation; nor similarly, the overflow of much pyruvate by sulphate-
limited cultures. In the case of phosphate limitation, it is
obvious that since phosphate is assimilated primarily via ATP synthesis (from ADP), and the latter occurs primarily by way of respiratory chain activity, that a sufficiency of ADP and reducing
equivalents must be maintained for the cells to scavenge phosphate
from their environment. The excess reducing equivalents are generated with a minimum participation of phosphate by the cells converting glucose to gluconic acid and ketogluconic acid, and excreting
these into the medium. It should be pointed out, however, that there
is no evidence of a glucose dehydrogenase operating in these *K. aerogenes* organisms and it seems most probable that gluconic acid arises
from a phosphorylated precursor.

One of the most intriguing growth limitations is that imposed

by the availability of potassium. Potassium is unique among the
major nutrients that are essential for microbial growth in that it
is contained within the cell in an unmodified and largely unbound
state. Moreover, the concentration extant in the cytoplasm is
surprisingly high (that is, about 50-100 mM for Gram-negative bacteria like *K. aerogenes*), and this often may be substantially in
excess of that concentration present in the growth medium (14). It
follows, therefore, that under many conditions organisms will need
to maintain a sizeable transmembrane K^+ gradient, and that this may
be energetically expensive - though difficult to quantify. Again,
this is the kind of situation that is particularly amenable to
analysis by continuous culture methods since, by such means, it is
possible to expose organisms to a range of steady state conditions
in which the transmembrane K^+ gradient is caused to vary progressively. Thus, in a simple experiment (Fig. 3), *K. aerogenes* was
grown aerobically in a glucose-limited chemostat culture (at a fixed
dilution rate, termperature and pH value) and the input K^+ concentration progressively lowered from a value that provided a 10-fold
excess (10 mM) to 1 mM, which was just sufficient to meet the cells'
K^+ requirement. The culture population density, and the cellular
potassium content, did not change markedly, but the extracellular
K^+ concentration decreased from a value of about 9 mM to less than

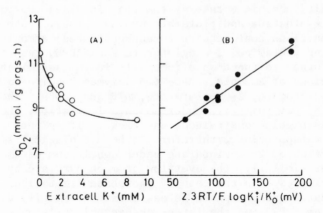

Figure 3. (a) Relationship between the specific rate of oxygen
uptake and the extracellular concentration of potassium extant in
a glucose-limited culture of *Klebsiella aerogenes* growing at a
dilution rate of 0.4 h^{-1} (35°C; pH 6.8). At the lowest potassium
input concentration (1 mM) the extracellular K^+ concentration was
at the limit of detection by flame photometry. (b) Plot of the
specific respiration rate as a function of the electrochemical
potential of the K^+ gradient. A glucose-limited chemostat culture
of *Klebsiella aerogenes* was grown in the presence of a graded excess
of potassium from less than 0.05 mM to about 9 mM. (Data of ref. 22)

0.005 mM. Thus, the transmembrane K^+ gradient (K_i^+/K_o^+) increased from about 10, at the higher input K^+ concentration, to a value in excess of 2,000 at the lowest K^+ input concentration. It is clear (Fig. 3A) that associated with this progressive increase in the transmembrane K^+ gradient was a corresponding increase in the steady state respiration rate. Hence it can be concluded that, in order to maintain such a gradient, organisms need to expend energy which, presumably, is related quantitatively to the value of its electro-chemical potential. The latter can be calculated from the Nernst equation:

$$\Delta\tilde{\mu}_K+ = 2.303 \log (K_i^+/K_o^+).RT/F$$

where K_i^+ and K_o^+ are the concentrations of K^+ inside and outside the cell, respectively, and the constants R, T and F have their usual meaning (activity coefficients are ignored). And significantly, plotting the specific respiration rate as a function of this calcu-lated electrochemical potential of the K^+ gradient revealed a straight-line relationship (Fig. 3B). One can thus begin to appre-ciate the nature of the physiological problems generated by a potassium limitation. The more potassium the organisms scavenge from their environment, the greater will be the transmembrane K^+ gradient, and hence the greater the amount of respiratory energy required to support it. Indeed, at least in principle, this trans-membrane K^+ gradient may form an infinite energy sink, and the ulti-mate constraint to scavenging potassium from a potassium-limited environment well may be the limit to which organisms can increase their respiration rate (22).

With this background information, it is not surprising to find in Table II that a potassium limitation provoked the highest rate of glucose catabolism. Moreover, it is logical that the main overflow products (gluconic acid and 2-ketogluconic acid) should be similar to those found with a phosphate-limited culture since, in both cases, the primary requirement seemingly is for a high rate of flux of respiratory energy. Consistent with this conclusion is the further finding that addition of the uncoupler 2,4-dinitrophenol (DNP) to aerobic chemostat cultures of *K. aerogenes* provoked a marked increase in the steady state respiration rate with, of course, an accompanying increase in the rate of glucose uptake. In the case of a glucose-limited culture, almost all the extra glucose taken into the cell was catabolized to CO_2, whereas with an ammonia-limited culture the extra glucose was converted almost quantitatively to 2-ketogluconic acid (Table II).

Physiological compromises such as those indicated above require that microorganisms possess the capacity to take up carbon substrate at a high rate, relative to the rate of cell synthesis, and to partially dissociate catabolism from anabolism; and this they clearly can do.

Regulation of Synthesis of Cellular Polymeric Constituents

When organisms are cultured in the presence of growth rate-limiting concentrations of some essential nutrient, other than the carbon and energy source, then one might expect synthesis of the cells' polymeric constituents to be influenced in two ways: (i) formation of those polymers that contain substantial amounts of the specific growth-limiting nutrient will be highly constrained, whereas (ii) formation of those polymers that do not contain any of the growth-limiting nutrient will be promoted.

Such a pattern of regulation is evident in the synthesis of polysaccharides by organisms growing in carbon substrate sufficient environments (Table III). But not all carbon substrate sufficient cultures behaved similarly; polysaccharide (mainly glycogen) accumulated to the highest level in slowly-growing ammonia-limited cells, and to a lesser extent in phosphate- and sulfate-limited cells. But the polysaccharide content of slowly-growing Mg^{2+}- or K^+-limited cells was even less than the basal (structural) polysaccharide level of glycerol-limited cells. However, it is known that some of the enzymes of glycogen synthesis are strongly activated by Mg^{2+} (9) which could account for the inability of Mg^{2+}-limited cultures to synthesize glycogen; and glycogen synthesis is also promoted by a high energy charge which, as already stated, is unlikely to be generated within the K^+-limited cell. In general, then, the above findings (Table III) accord with those which one might broadly predict.

In this connection, more surprising was the finding that cells of Gram-positive species (like *Bacillus subtilis* and *Staphylococcus aureus*) were able to modulate the rates of synthesis of their major

TABLE III

Influence of Growth Rate and the Nature of the Growth Limitation on the Total Carbohydrate Content of *Klebsiella aerogenes* Growing in Chemostat Culture. Data of ref. 11.

Dilution rate (h^{-1})	g. carbohydrate per 100 g dry bacterial cells					
	Glycerol-	Ammonia-	Phosphate-	Sulphate-	Mg^{2+}	K^+-limitation
0.1	4	22	18	13	2	2
0.2	3	16	13	8	2	3
0.4	3	10	8	6	3	4
0.8	3	4	4	3	4	5

anionic wall polymers in response to specific growth limitations
(49). Thus, under phosphate-sufficient growth conditions (either
carbon-, nitrogen-, sulfur-, potassium- or magnesium-limitation)
organisms possessed walls that were rich in teichoic acid - a polyol
phosphate polymer (4). Under phosphate limiting growth conditions,
however, synthesis of this wall-bound polymer was completely suppressed and instead an anionic polymer devoid of phosphate (teichuronic acid) was synthesized (Table IV). It is important to stress
here that teichoic acid is an integral part of the wall structure
(as is teichuronic acid, when it is formed), and that it generally
accounts for 50% or more of the wall dry weight. Yet this polymer
can be completely deleted from the wall and replaced (no doubt functionally) by teichuronic acid following a relatively minor change
in the growth environment; that is a lowering in the phosphate supply
relative to that of other essential nutrients. Accompanying this
phenotypic change in wall composition is a dramatic change in the
ability of the cells to bind a specific bacteriophage (SP50) as
seen in Figure 4. The specificity of this phage for teichoic acid,
along with the ability of *B. subtilis* cells to modulate synthesis of
teichoic acid in response to changes in the supply of phosphate,
have been extensively exploited by Archibald and his colleagues to
study processes of bacterial wall growth and turnover (see, for
example, refs. 1,3,44). But it is not yet clear what the value is
to the cell in being able to coordinately regulate the syntheses
of teichoic acid and teichuronic acid though, by so doing, they
markedly diminish their quantitative requirement for phosphate (from
about 3.2 to 1.7 g/100 g equivalent dry weight of cells; see ref.
49).

TABLE IV

Effect of Different Growth Limitations on the Cell-wall Composition
of *Bacillus subtilis* var *niger*. Grown in Chemostat Culture at a
Dilution Rate of 0.3 h^{-1} (35°C; pH 7.0). Data of ref. 13.

Growth-limiting nutrient	Content (in g/100 g dry weight isolated cell walls) of					
	Protein	Phosphorus	Teichoic acid	Hexose	Glucuronic acid	Galactos-amine
Glucose	10.0	3.9	35-42	20	<3	<3
Ammonia	11.5	4.8	45-52	23	<3	<3
Sulfate	12.5	4.9	45-53	23	<3	<3
Potassium	10.5	4.3	39-46	20	<3	<3
Magnesium	12.5	6.9	62-74	32	<3	<3
Phosphate	10.0	0.5	<3	<2	25	17

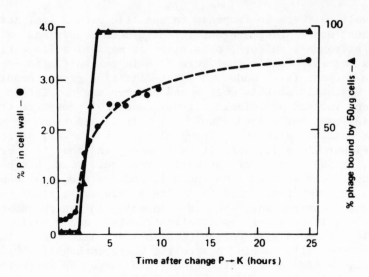

Figure 4.   Increase in wall-bound teichoic acid (●) and phage-binding
activity (▲) of *Bacillus subtilis* harvested during the transition
phase between a phosphate limitation and a potassium limitation
(D = 0.18 h⁻¹; 37°C; pH 7.0).   Wall teichoic acid content was determined by measurement of the phosphorus content (percent dry weight
of wall) of isolated walls.   From ref. 3.

        Some consistency also is apparent in the patterns of synthesis
and excretion of proteins and enzymes by nutrient-limited bacterial
cultures.   This is particularly the case with organisms like *Bacillus
licheniformis* 749/C that are known to synthesize some exocellular
enzymes (like penicillinase) constitutively (39).   Thus, when growing
under conditions of phosphate limitation, this organism produced
exocellular ribonuclease and alkaline phosphatase, as well as penicillinase (54), and when limited in its growth by the availability
of a suitable nitrogen source (in this case glutamate) the organism
produced substantial amounts of protease (Table V).   The excretion
of protein by cells that were nitrogen-limited, as well as when they
were either sulfur- or carbon-limited, is rather surprising; nevertheless, it is clear (Table V) that the amounts of protein excreted
were generally substantially less than when the culture was phosphate
limited.   And the value to the cell of diverting 1-5% of its protein
synthesis to the formation of exocellular enzymes like protease,
under conditions of nitrogen limitation, is obvious.

        Seemingly, then, microorganisms possess the ability to modu-
late extensively their structure and functioning so as to optimize
and/or maximize their utilization of the growth-limiting nutrient.
Moreover, it is clear that this optimization process may require
compromises in the efficiency with which non-limiting nutrients

TABLE V
Influence of Growth Rate and the Nature of the Growth Limitation on
the Secretion of Proteins by *Bacillus licheniformis* 749/C.
Also, the Secretion of Protease by Nitrogen-limited Cultures.
Data of ref. 54 and unpublished data of J.T.M. Wouters (pers comm.)

Dilution rate (h^{-1})	Exocellular protein ($\mu g/mg$ dry wt. cells)					Exocellular protease of N-limited cells (units/mg exocellular protein)
	*Carbon-	Sulfur-	PO_4^{3-}-	Mg^{2+}-	N-limitation	
0.1	–	–	43.2	16.6	6.3	704
0.2	10.0	16.6	31.1	26.5	7.3	638
0.3	19.3	11.9	26.9	19.3	18.3	296
0.4	18.8	12.6	25.7	13.0	28.8	142
0.5	24.5	12.6	25.1	18.9	18.3	169
0.6	–	12.2	20.0	22.1	17.6	18

*The carbon and nitrogen source was Na-(L)-glutamate. When carbon substrate
was in excess of the growth requirement, then the medium was supplemented
with glucose (6.0 g/l).

(particularly the carbon and energy source) are utilized. But
irrespective of the extent to which metabolic compromises are invoked, it is reasonable to assume that the end-product still must
be a viable functional cell. Hence it is appropriate to consider
finally, and very briefly, the mechanisms by which organisms are
able to coordinately regulate the rates of synthesis of all their
components so as to allow growth to proceed at a low, submaximal,
rate.

Regulation of Cell Synthesis

It follows from the fact that steady state populations of
microorganisms can be maintained for prolonged periods of time in
chemostat cultures, operated at grossly submaximal rates, that
organisms must possess effective mechanisms for coordinately regulating the rates of synthesis of all their macromolecular components.
But whether there exists some well-defined lower limit to the rate
at which cell synthesis can proceed is by no means certain. What
is clear, however, is that the macromolecular composition of organisms varies substantially and progressively with changes in either

the specific growth rate (20) or, at a constant growth rate, with
changes in the incubation temperature (46). In particular, the
cellular ribosome and RNA contents vary in a manner that suggests
a fixed rate of protein synthesis per ribosomal unit, irrespective
of the growth rate (25). And along with these changes in ribosome
content are changes in cell size such that the ribosome content per
cell varies even more markedly. Indeed, to such an extent does
cell composition vary with the growth condition that Herbert (20)
was moved to remark that "...it is virtually meaningless to speak
of the chemical composition of a microorganism without at the same
time specifying the environmental conditions that produced it. Such
a statement as 'the RNA content of *Bacillus subtilis* is 16.2%' is by
itself as incomplete and misleading as the statement 'the boiling
point of water is 70°C'. While the latter statement might be true
(on the summit of Mount Everest, for example), it is incomplete
and misleading because it says nothing of the effect of pressure
on boiling point. The former statement is likewise true but misleading, since the RNA content of *B. cereus* can vary from 3-30%,
depending on the environment in which the organisms are growing".

Marked changes in cell size involve corresponding changes in
the surface area/volume ratio; and if the cell envelope is of a
constant thickness, then one might expect that the wall content
(as a proportion of the total cell mass) would increase with a
decrease in the mean cell size. This is clearly evident with cultures of both Gram-positive and Gram-negative bacteria (Table VI).

TABLE VI

Influence of Growth Rate and Growth-limiting Component of the
Medium on the Average Wall Content of *Bacillus subtilis* var *niger*
and *Klebsiella aerogenes*, Grown in Chemostat Culture. From ref. 13.

Dilution rate (h^{-1})	Bacterial wall content (%, w/w)			
	Bacillus subtilis		Klebsiella aerogenes	
	Mg^{2+}-limited	PO_4^{3-}-limited	Mg^{2+}-limited	PO_4^{3-}-limited
0.05	–	37.3	–	–
0.1	26.9	23.0	19.8	20.5
0.2	23.5	21.0	–	–
0.3	18.5	17.3	15.0	14.6
0.7	–	–	13.0	11.0

Hence, not only must control mechanisms operate to match the rate
of rRNA synthesis to the demands of protein synthesis, but other
mechanisms must be invoked to modulate differentially the rates of
synthesis of cell wall polymers (mucopeptide, protein, lipid, lipo-
polysaccharide, teichoic acid, etc.) to a level appropriate to the
specific rate of cell synthesis. Although a considerable amount
is known regarding the biosynthesis and assembly of bacterial cell
walls (see, for example, refs. 16,38,42), the nature of those control mechanisms that coordinately regulate cell wall synthesis
remain largely obscure. This latter topic is obviously one to which
studies using the chemostat culture technique is particularly appropriate and, one might expect, will be increasingly applied in the
coming years.

CONCLUSIONS

        Central to studies of microbial behaviour in low-nutrient
(chemostat) environments is the presumption that most natural ecosystems will be essentially nutrient-limited. This being so, then
the enormous metabolic flexibility of microorganisms might reasonably be considered to reflect in part properties necessarily acquired
in the course of evolution to cope with these particular, ubiquitous,
extreme natural conditions. And thus, this metabolic flexibility
will be expressed in full range in chemostat environments. In this
respect, the chemostat possesses four special properties that can
be readily exploited; these are:

(1.) They allow one to impose upon microorganisms a wide range of
unique (nutrient-limited) environments; environments in which organisms may express properties that might not ever be expressed in
batch culture - or expressed only transiently.
(2.) They allow one to vary environmental parameters independent of
each other, and without invoking changes in growth rate. Thus,
changes in cell physiology following a change in the incubation
temperature, for example, can be dissociated from changes that
accompany variations in growth rate - which, in batch culture, always
follows a change in the incubation temperature.
(3.) They allow one to establish and maintain steady state conditions, thereby facilitating quantitatively meaningful analyses of
cell structure and functioning. Such a "quantitatively meaningful
analysis" is evident in studies of ribosomes and protein synthesis
(26), synthesis of cell wall components (13), substrate uptake mechanisms (5,10,24), and the energetics of cell synthesis (23,33,43,
45), among many other topics.
(4.) Finally, chemostat environments impose a high selective pressure on microbial populations, thereby facilitating selection of
mutants with specialized properties (8,18,29).

        The few examples presented in this brief review of metabolic compromises associated with the growth of microorganisms in nutrient-limited environments serve, we hope, to illustrate the enormous research potential of chemostat culture. And adding to this, the obvious utility of this technique in industrial processes, such as those of single cell protein production, it is abundantly obvious that considerably more attention ought to be paid to the study of microbial behaviour in chemostat environments than has been the case hitherto.

REFERENCES

1.   Anderson, A.J., Green, R.S. and Archibald, A. R. (1978). Wall composition and phage-binding properties of *Bacillus subtilis* W23 grown in chemostat culture in media containing varied concentrations of phosphate. FEMS Microbiol. Lett., 4, 129-132.
2.   Archibald, A.R. (1976). The use of bacteriophages to detect alterations in the cell surface of *Bacillus subtilis*. In: Continuous Culture 6 (A.C.R. Dean, D.C. Ellwood, C.G.T. Evans and J. Melling, eds.) pp 262-269. Ellis Horwood Ltd., Chichester
3.   Archibald, A.R. and Coapes, H.E. (1976). Bacteriophage SP50 as a marker for cell wall growth in *Bacillus subtilis*. J. Bacteriol 125, 1195-1206.
4.   Baddiley, J. (1972). Teichoic acids in cell walls and membranes of bacteria. Essays in Biochem. 8, 35-77.
5.   Brown, C.M. (1976). Nitrogen metabolism in bacteria and fungi. In: Continuous Culture 6 (A.C.R. Dean, D.C. Ellwood, C.G.T. Evans and J. Melling, Eds.) pp 170-183. Ellis Horwood Ltd., Chichester.
6.   Calcott, P.H. and Postgate, J.R. (1972). On substrate-accelerated death in *Klebsiella aerogenes*. J. Gen. Microbiol. 70, 115-122.
7.   Calcott, P.H. and Postgate, J.R. (1974). The effects of β-galactosidase activity and cyclic AMP on lactose-accelerated death. J. Gen. Microbiol. 85, 85-90.
8.   Clarke, P.H. (1974). The evolution of enzymes for the utilisation of novel substrates. Symp. Soc. Gen. Microbiol. 24, 183-217.
9.   Dawes, E.A. and Senior, P.J. (1973). The role and regulation of energy reserve polymers in micro-organisms. Adv. Microbial Physiol. 10, 135-266.
10.   Dawes, E.A., Midgley, M. and Whiting, P.H. (1976). Control of transport systems for glucose, gluconate and 2-oxo-gluconate, and of glucose metabolism in *Pseudomonas aeruginosa*. In: Continuous Culture 6 (A.C.R. Dean, D.C. Ellwood, C.G.T. Evans and J. Melling, eds.) pp 195-207. Ellis Horwood Ltd., Chichester.
11.   Dicks, J.W. and Tempest, D.W. (1967). Potassium-ammonium antagonism in polysaccharide synthesis by *Aerobacter aerogenes*. Biochim. biophys. Acta 136, 176-179.
12.   Ellwood, D.C. and Tempest, D.W. (1969). Control of teichoic

acid and teichuronic acid biosynthesis in chemostat cultures
of *Bacillus subtilis* var *niger*. Biochem. J. 111, 1-5.

13. Ellwood, D.C. and Tempest, D.W. (1972). Effects of environ-
     ment on bacterial wall content and compostion. Adv. Microbial
     Physiol. 7, 83-117.

14. Evans, C.G.T., Herbert, D. and Tempest, D.W. (1970). The
     continuous cultivation of micro-organisms 2. Construction of
     a chemostat. In: Methods in Microbiology (J.R. Norris and D.
     W. Ribbons, eds.) pp 277-327. Academic Press, London.

15. Faik P. and Kornberg, H.L. (1973). Isolation and properties
     of *E. coli* mutants affected in gluconate uptake. FEBS Lett. 32,
     260-264.

16. Ghuysen, J.M. (1977). Biosynthesis and assembly of bacterial
     walls. Cell Surface Reviews, 4, 463-569.

17. Harder, W. and Veldkamp, H. (1971). Competition of marine
     psychrophilic bacteria at low temperatures. Antonie van Leeuwen-
     hoek, 37, 51-63.

18. Hartley, B.S., Burleigh, B.D., Midwinter, G.G. Moore, C.H.
     Morris, H.R.,Rigby, P.J.W., Smith, M.J. and Taylor, S.S. (1972)
     Where do new enzymes come from? In: Enzymes: Structure and
     Function, 8th FEBS Meeting, vol 29 (J. Drenth, R.A. Oosterbaan
     and C. Veeger, eds.) pp 151-176. North-Holland, Amsterdam.

19. Hayashi, S. and Lin, E.C.C. (1965). Capture of glycerol by
     cells of *Escherichia coli*. Biochim. biophys. Acta 94, 479-487.

20. Herbert, D. (1961). The chemical composition of micro-organisms
     as a function of their environment. Symp. Soc. gen. Microbiol.
     11, 391-416.

21. Hueting, S., de Lange, T. and Tempest, D.W. (1978). Properties
     and regulation of synthesis of the glycerol dehydrogenase
     present in *Klebsiella aerogenes* NCTC 418 growing in chemostat
     culture. FEMS Microbiol. Lett 4, 185-189.

22. Hueting, S., de Lange, T. and Tempest, D.W. (1979). Energy
     requirement for maintenance of the transmembrane potassium
     gradient in *Klebsiella aerogenes* NCTC 418: A continuous culture
     study. Arch. Microbiol. 123, 183-188.

23. Jones, C. W. (1977). Aerobic respiratory systems in bacteria.
     Symp. Soc. gen. Microbiol. 27, 23-59.

24. Kavanaugh, B.M. and Cole, J.A. (1976). The regulation of nitro-
     gen metabolism in *Escherichia coli*. In: Continuous Culture 6
     (A.C.R. Dean, D.C. Ellwood, C.G.T. Evans and J. Melling, eds.)
     pp 184-194. Ellis Horwood Ltd., Chichester.

25. Kjeldgaard, N.O. and Kurland, C.G. (1963). The distribution
     of soluble and ribosomal RNA as a function of the growth rate
     J. molec. Biol. 6, 341-351.

26. Koch, A.L. (1971). The adaptive responses of *Escherichia coli*
     to a feast and famine existence. Adv. Microbial Physiol. 6,
     147-217.

27. Kornberg, H.L. (1973). Fine control of sugar uptake by
     Escherichia coli. In: Rate Control of Biological Processes.
     17th Symp. Soc. exptl. Biol. (D.D. Davies, ed.) pp 175-193.

University Press, Cambridge.

28. Kornberg, H.L. (1976). Genetics in the study of carbohydrate transport by bacteria. J. gen. Microbiol. 96, 1-16.

29. Kubitschek, H.E. (1974). Operation of selection pressure on microbial populations. Symp. Soc. gen. Microbiol. 24, 105-130.

30. Kundig, W. (1974). Molecular interactions in the bacterial phosphoenolpyruvate phosphotransferase system (PTS). J. Supramol Structure. 2, 695-714.

31. Kundig, W., Ghosh, S. and Roseman, S. (1964). Phosphate bound to histidine in a protein as an intermediate in a novel phosphotransferase system. Proc. Nat. Acad. Sci. U.S.A., 52, 1967-2074.

32. Lin, E.C.C., Levin, A.P. and Magasanik, B. (1960). The effect of aerobic metabolism on the inducible glycerol dehydrogenase of *Aerobacter aerogenes*. J. biol. Chem. 235, 1824-1829.

33. Neijssel, O.M. (1976). The significance of overflow metabolism in the physiology and growth of *Klebsiella aerogenes*. Thesis: University of Amsterdam.

34. Neijssel, O.M. (1977). The effect of 2,4-dinitrophenol on the growth of *Klebsiella aerogenes* NCTC 418 in aerobic chemostat cultures. FEMS Microbiol. Lett. 1, 47-50.

35. Neijssel, O.M. and Tempest, D.W. (1975). The regulation of carbohydrate metabolism in *Klebsiella aerogenes* NCTC 418 organisms, growing in chemostat culture. Arch. Microbiol. 106, 251-258.

36. Neijssel, O.M., Hueting, S., Crabbendam, K.J. and Tempest, D.W. (1975). Dual pathways of glycerol assimilation in *Klebsiella aerogenes* NCIB 418. Their role and possible functional significance. Arch. Microbiol. 104, 83-87.

37. Nelson, D.L. and Kennedy, E.P. (1972). Transport of magnesium by a repressible and a nonrepressible system in *Escherichia coli*. Proc. Nat. Acad. Sci. U.S.A. 69, 1091-1093.

38. Osborn, M.J., Rick, P.D., Lehmann, V., Rupprecht, E. and Singh, M. (1974). Structure and biogenesis of the cell envelope of Gram-negative bacteria. Ann. N.Y. Acad. Sci. 235, 52-65.

39. Pollock, M.R. (1961). The measurements of the liberation of penicillinase from *Bacillus subtilis*. J. gen. Microbiol. 26, 239-253.

40. Postgate, J.R. and Hunter, J.R. (1964). Accelerated death of *Aerobacter aerogenes* starved in the presence of growth-limiting substrates. J. gen. Microbiol. 34, 459-473.

41. Rhoads, D.B. and Epstein, W. (1977). Energy coupling to net K^+ transport in *Escherichia coli* . J. Biol. Chem. 252, 1394-1401.

42. Rogers, H.J. and Perkins, H.R. (1968). Cell Walls and Membranes. E. F. and N. Spon Ltd., London.

43. Stouthamer, A.H. (1977). Energetic aspects of the growth of micro-organisms. Symp. Soc. gen. Microbiol. 27, 285-315.

44. Sturman, A.J. and Archibald, A.R. (1978). Conservation of phage receptor material at the polar caps of *Bacillus subtilis* W23.

FEMS Microbiol. Lett. 4, 255–259.

45.   Tempest, D.W. (1978). The biochemical significance of microb-
      ial growth yields: A reassessment. Trends in Biochem. Sci.
      3, 180–184.
46.   Tempest, D.W. and Hunter, J.R. (1965). The influence of tem-
      perature and pH value on the macromolecular composition of
      magnesium-limited and glycerol-limited *Aerobacter aerogenes*
      growing in a chemostat. J. gen. Microbil. 41, 267–273.
47.   Tempest, D.W. and Neijssel, O.M. (1978). Eco-physiological
      aspects of microbial growth in aerobic nutrient-limited
      environments. Adv. Microbial Ecol. 2, 105–153.
48.   Tempest, D.W., Dicks, J.W. and Meers, J.L. (1967). Magnesium-
      limited growth of *Bacillus subtilis*, in pure and mixed cultures
      in a chemostat. J. gen. Microbiol. 49, 139=147.
49.   Tempest, D.W., Hicks. J.W. and Ellwood, D.C. (1968). Influence
      of growth condition on the concentration of potassium in
      Bacillus subtilis var. *niger* and its possible relationship
      to cellular ribonucleic acid, teichoic acid and teichuronic
      acid. Biochem. J. 106, 237–243.
50.   Tempest, D.W., Meers, J.L. and Brown, C.M. (1970). Synthesis
      of glutamate in *Aerobacter aerogenes* by a hitherto unknown
      route. Biochem. J. 117, 405–407.
51.   Veldkamp, H. and Jannasch, H.W. (1972). Mixed culture studies
      with the chemostat. J. appl. Chem. Biotechnol. 22, 105–123.
52.   Willsky, G.R. and Malamy, M.H. (1974). The loss of phoS
      periplasmic protein leads to a change in the specificity of
      a constitutive inorganic phosphate transport system in
      Escherichia coli. Biochem. Biophys. Res. Commun. 60, 226–233.
53.   Willsky, G.R. and Malamy, M.H. (1976). Control of the synthesis
      of alkaline phosphatase and the phosphate binding protein in
      Escherichia coli. J. Bacteriol. 127, 595–609.
54.   Wouters, J.T.M. and Buysman, P.J. (1977). Production of some
      exocellular enzymes by *Bacillus licheniformis* 749/C in
      chemostat cultures. FEMS Microbiol. Lett. 1, 109–112.
55.   Zwaig, N., Kistler, W.S. and Lin, E.C.C. (1970). Glycerol-
      kinase, the pacemaker for the dissimilation of glycerol in
      Escherichia coli. J. Bacteriol. 102, 753–759.

DISCUSSION

Q.   WOOD: It strikes me that in your dinitrophenol experiment,
      which was very striking, this *Aerobacter* was converted to
      a *Pseudomonas aeruginosa* or *P. fluorescenes* or *Citrobacter*.
A.   TEMPEST: Yes, but we were quite certain that we were growing
      Aerobacter aerogenes; we checked it very frequently. What is
      rather difficult to understand is how 2-ketogluconate arises.
      If you have any suggestions, I'd like to know of them because
      we have been completely unable to find a glucose dehydrogenase.

It seems most probably that the glucose is metabolized through glucose-6 phosphate and 6-phosphogluconate, but then there seems to be no known reaction that will yield a 2-ketogluconat

WOOD: Well, you may not have found the dehydrogenases, but I think it would be reasonable to predict that those are membrane-bound cytochrome-linked dehydrogenases such as you find in *Pseudomonas* and they were not easy to find in the membranes of other organisms.

TEMPEST: Yes, that could be.

Q.   TSUCHIYA: Do you have any idea of what the different holding times or dilution rates might have done to your results?

A.   TEMPEST: Yes, this was a comparative study at a single dilution rate and the data on that one slide was a year of work. What you can say is that the rate of glucose consumption doesn't increase with growth rates under these excess conditions. So, you might expect to get even more of these products formed. However, we haven't examined this systematically.

THE METHANOGENIC BACTERIA, THEIR ECOLOGY AND PHYSIOLOGY

Robert A. Mah

Division of Environmental and Nutritional Sciences
School of Public Health
University of California
Los Angeles, California   90024

A study of the methane fermentation is unavoidably concerned with a study of microbial ecology because of the obligatory inter-actions between two major physiological participants, the chemo-heterotrophic non-methanogenic bacteria and the methanogenic bacteria. In natural anaerobic habitats containing complex organic compounds and where light, sulfate, and nitrate are limited, these two groups of bacteria are linked in the degradation of organic substrates. The ultimate formation of methane and CO_2 marks the last step in a series of dissimilatory reactions by which organic compounds are completely degraded. CH_4 is the most reduced form of carbon and CO_2 the most oxidized form of carbon.

Figure 1 gives an example of the types of bacterial partici-pants and the intermediate products formed during a hypothetical digester fermentation of a complex polysaccharide. The actual spe-cies of bacteria may differ from one habitat to another depending on physical/chemical conditions of temperature, pH, osmotic pressure and substrate composition (macromolecules of polysaccharides, pro-teins, nucleic acids, lipids, etc. and/or their oligomers). The fermentation is initiated (Figure 1) when the complex polysaccharide (e.g., starch, cellulose) is hydrolyzed by cellulolytic or amylolytic bacteria to free sugars. These unit constituents are freely avail-able as fermentative substrates to a wide variety of chemohetero-trophic non-methanogenic bacteria. *Clostridium propionicum*, *Clos-tridium acetobutylicum*, *Eubacterium limosum*, and members of the coli-form group are examples of organisms whose known metabolic pathways lead to the formation of the end products chiefly found in the diges-ter fermentation, namely butyrate, propionate and acetate. Other products include H_2, CO_2 and formate. Formate is rapidly converted via the formic hydrogenlyase reaction to H_2 and CO_2 and may not be

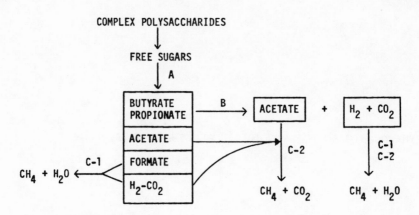

I. Nonmethanogens   II. Methanogens

   A. Clostridium acetobutyricum   C-1. H_2-oxidizing methanogens
      Eubacterium limosum
      Clostridium propionicum   C-2. Aceticlastic methanogens
      Coliforms

   B. Volatile fatty acid oxidizers
      Syntrophomonas wolfeii
      Syntrophobacter wolinii

Figure 1. Methanogenic fermentation of complex polysaccharides.

detectable. Likewise, H_2 may not be detectable because it, too, is rapidly metabolized.

The complete decomposition of the starting organic substrates depends on their conversion to acetate and then to CH_4 and CO_2. For example, the final stoichiometric conversion of 1 mole glucose to 3 moles CH_4 and 3 moles CO_2 takes place via the intermediate formation of 2 moles acetate. In order to oxidize the intermediates of glucose metabolism (e.g., butyrate or propionate) to the level of acetate, the electrons generated from the oxidation reactions must be removed. This is accomplished by proton reduction to form H_2 and ultimately by oxidation of the H_2 and reduction of CO_2 to form CH_4. The resulting acetate is also converted to methane by a unique aceticlastic reaction which splits the acetate into CH_4 and CO_2 (see Table I). The methane comes from the methyl group and the CO_2 from the carboxyl group (4).

The oxidation of butyrate and propionate is accomplished by some unusual anaerobic organisms only recently co-cultured by Bryant and his co-workers (3,8,9). Metabolic evidence for the existence of these volatile acid oxidizers came from the work of Smith and his collaborators (11) who demonstrated the formation of H_2 during oxidation of butyrate and propionate by digesting sludge. The oxidation of these volatile acids to acetate depended upon removal of electrons by an obligate proton reduction reaction to form H_2. This oxidation reaction is thermodynamically possible only when H_2 is maintained at a vanishingly low concentration. This is normally accomplished during the sludge fermentation by rapid oxidation of H_2 coupled to the reduction of CO_2 to methane. Identification of the obligate proton-reducing (H_2-producing) acetogenic organisms was accomplished by co-culturing them on a lawn of sulfate-reducing bacteria which acted as an efficient electron sink for removal of H_2 (8). Two new species and genera were described. *Syntrophomonas wolfeii* oxidized butyrate (in addition to valerate, caproate, heptanoate, and octanoate) to acetate and H_2; *Syntrophobacter wolinii* oxidized propionate to acetate, H_2, and CO_2. *S. wolfeii* is a gram-negative curved rod with rounded ends; it has 2-8 laterally inserted flagella along the concave side of the cell (9).

The volatile acid oxidation carried out by these acetogenic, H_2-forming bacteria is an important reaction in the methane fermentation. Smith (11) estimated that 80% or more of the acetate formed in sludge digesters may be accounted for by propionate oxidation. In cases of digester failure, propionate may be the chief acid to accumulate.

Two main types of methanogenic reactions occur in the methane fermentation; the oxidation of H_2 and reduction of CO_2 to methane and the splitting of acetate to methane and CO_2. H_2 oxidation-CO_2 reduction may be ascribed chiefly to members of the non-aceticlastic genera such as *Methanobacterium*, *Methanobrevibacter*, and *Methanospirillum*. The methanogenic reaction carried out by these types of organisms effectively maintains the H_2 at concentrations sufficiently low enough to make the oxidation of propionate and butyrate thermodynamically possible. The resulting acetate product is, in turn, converted by the aceticlastic methanogens, primarily in the genus *Methanosarcina*, to form 67% or more of the methane generated.

There are three main physiological groups of bacteria which are interlinked in the overall conversion of organic compounds to CH_4 and CO_2:

1.) The chemoheterotrophs (Fig. 1, reaction A organisms) initiate the fermentation by hydrolyzing macromolecules into their unit constituents, making them available for fermentation by a wide variety of fermentative organisms. The chief products of this initial stage of fermentation are butyrate, propionate, acetate, formate, H_2, and CO_2. The formation of these and not other reduced products is probably aided by H_2 removal due to action of the methanogens. In the absence of H_2 removal in pure cultures, an increase in reduced products occurs. Thus, a shift in the proportion of these products with more acetate and less butyrate and propionate might be predicted in the methane fermentation.

2.) The acetogenic obligate proton reducers (Fig. 1, reaction B organisms) are syntrophic partners with the H_2-oxidizing methanogens. Since these volatile acid oxidizers may dispose of their electrons only by proton reduction, this demands a mechanism for H_2 removal by the methanogens in order to make the reaction thermodynamically feasible. The net result is the oxidation of volatile acids to the level of acetate.

3.) The methanogens (Fig. 1, reactions C-1, C-2 organisms) serve not only as an electron sink by way of their H_2-oxidizing reactions, they also serve to remove the end product, acetate, from solution by converting it into two gases, CH_4 and CO_2, which may leave the system.

Thus, the methane fermentation appears to be mediated by a complex interaction of many types of bacteria in which physiological inter-dependencies are expressed in terms of product-substrate feeding relationships as well as in cross-nutrient vitamin relationships. Control reactions involving regulatory products such as H_2 are still poorly understood both in terms of the overall mixed culture fermentation as well as at the pure culture level.

The methanogenic bacteria are physiologically united by their requirement to form methane as a final product of energy metabolism (Figure 2). Most species oxidize H_2 and reduce CO_2 to form methane as their preferred pathway of methanogenesis. Carbon monoxide may be converted to methane, but it is not known as an important methano-genic substrate. Except for the aceticlastic methanogens, most species which use H_2-CO_2 will also use formate. Some aceticlastic isolates are incapable of oxidizing H_2 and some prefer acetate or methanol over H_2-CO_2 as methanogenic substrates (see later). How-ever, the aceticlastic organisms, especially those in the genus *Methanosarcina*, are the most diverse metabolically; in addition to acetate and H_2, they also use methanol and methylamines. The methanogenic reactions are summarized in Table I.

The taxonomy of the methanogenic bacteria has been extensively revised because of new information based on comparative studies of their distinctive 16S rRNA oligonucleotide sequences, lack of pep-tidoglycan in their cell walls, unique lipid composition and cofac-tors such as coenzyme M, F_{420}, F_{343} (1). The methanogenic bacteria appear to comprise a separate phylogenetic and physiological group of procaryotes called archaebacteria. Seven genera containing 15 species have been described (See Table II). In addition to the three original genera, *Methanobacterium*, *Methanosarcina*, and *Methano-coccus*, four new genera have been added: *Methanobrevibacter*, *Methano-microbium*, *Methanogenium*, and *Methanospirillum*. As a group, they are morphologically diverse, including short, long, or bent rods, filaments, cocci, irregular coccoid elements, and aggregates of pseudosarcina.

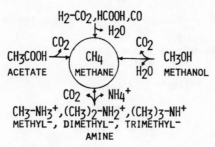

Figure 2.   Formation of methane from various methanogenic substrates.

The nutrient requirements for the methanogens range from simple to complex. For example, both *Methanobacterium formicicum* and *Methanobacterium thermoautotrophicum* may grow chemoautotrophically on H_2-CO_2. Others, like *Methanobrevibacter ruminantium*, require complex growth factors. In addition to selecting any one of the limited substrates shown in Fig. 2, methanogenic media should also include the following (4):

1. Inorganic salts such as KH_2PO_4, $NaCl_2$, Na_2CO_3
2. NH_4^+ or perhaps an organic nitrogen source
3. Specific or complex growth requirements such as acetate, yeast extract, trypticase, coenzyme M, KCl, NaCl, and trace metals
4. An appropriate pH (usually near pH 7.0)
5. An appropriate temperature (mesophilic range, 35-37°C for most)

TABLE I

Methanogenic Reactions

	$\Delta G^{O'}$ (kcal)
1. Acetate	
$^O CH_3^\triangle COO^- + H_2O \longrightarrow {}^O CH_4 + H^\triangle CO_3^-$	-7.4
2. Methanol	
$4CH_3OH \longrightarrow 3CH_4 + HCO_3^- + H^+ + H_2O$	-75.2
3. H_2-CO_2	
$4H_2 + H^+ + HCO_3^- \longrightarrow CH_4 + 3H_2O$	-32.4
4. Amines	
$4CH_3NH_3^+ + 3H_2O \longrightarrow 3CH_4 + HCO_3^- + 4NH_4^+ + H^+$	-53.8
$2(CH_3)_2NH_2^+ + 3H_2O \longrightarrow 3CH_4 + HCO_3^- + 2NH_4^+ + H^+$	-52.5
$4(CH_3)_3NH^+ + 9H_2O \longrightarrow 9CH_4 + 3HCO_3^- + 4NH_4^+ + 3H^+$	-159.8
5. Formate	
$4HCOOH + H_2O \longrightarrow CH_4 + 3HCO_3^- + 3H^+$	-31.1

TABLE II
Medium for Aceticlastic Methanogens

1. Liquid V/V
   33% culture supernatant
      (from inoculum source)

   67% Barker's salt solution:

      100 ml tap water

         0.1 g NH_4Cl

         0.04 g $K_2HPO_4 \cdot 3H_2O$

         0.01 g $MgCl_2 \cdot 6H_2O$

2. Nutrients W/V

         0.2%   Trypticase BBL

         0.2%   Yeast Extract Difco

         0.0001%   Resazurin

         0.15% $NaHCO_3$

         0.05%   Cysteine

         0.02% $Na_2S \cdot 6H_2O$

         1.0%   Calcium acetate

3. Atmosphere
         100% N_2 gas

A typical growth medium for isolating and culturing aceticlastic methanogens is given in Table II. This medium has the advantage
of permitting visual detection of aceticlastic colonies from among
a mixture of non-aceticlastic colonies because of the precipitation
of $CaCO_3$ in and around colonies after the acetate is metabolized
and removed from the medium by its conversion to CH_4 and CO_2 (5).

Methanogenic bacteria have been isolated from many anaerobic
habitats starting comparatively recently in 1947 when Schnellen isolated the first pure cultures of *Methanosarcina barkeri* and *Methanobacterium formicicum* from aquatic sediments. Methanogens have since
been isolated from such diverse environments as the Cariaco Trench;
hot springs; intestinal tracts of man and animals, especially rumi-
nants; digesters; lagoons; trees; and soil (1,4). The selected
characteristics of the methanogens given in Table III show that all
genera contain species capable of metabolizing H_2-CO_2. Only one
genus, *Methanosarcina*, characteristically also metabolizes methanol,
acetate, and the methylamines. Two exceptions to this general

behavior are *Methanobacterium soehngenii* which only utilizes acetate and no other substrate (16) and *Methanococcus mazei* which utilizes the same substrates as *M. barkeri* and is apparently more closely related to *Methanosarcina* than to *Methanococcus* (6).

Phase contrast photomicrographs and electron micrographs of some of these organisms are shown in Figures 3,4,5,6,7 and 8. *Methanobrevibacter ruminantium* (Fig. 3A) was isolated from the rumen of cattle by Smith and Hungate (13). It is the most numerous methanogen in the rumen. This short, non-motile gram positive rod requires coenzyme M and 2 methyl-butyrate as growth factors and utilizes H_2-CO_2 and formate as methanogenic substrates. *Methanomicrobium mobile* (Fig. 3B) was also isolated from the rumen of cattle (10). This short rod is motile by means of a single polar flagellum; it grows on H_2-CO_2 or formate and requires rumen fluid to provide a growth factor. *Methanobacterium formicicum* (Fig. 3C) is a long rod which may be grown chemoautotrophically on H_2-CO_2 but may also use formate. *Methanobacterium bryantii* (Fig. 3D), another long rod, uses H_2-CO_2 but not formate. This organism is the methanogenic "MOH" partner of the ethanol-oxidizing rod which formed the co-culture known as *Methanobacterium omelianskii* (2). *Methanobrevibacter arboriphilus* (Fig. 3E), a non-motile short slender rod also grows on H_2-CO_2 and not formate. This organism was isolated from a living tree (17). *Methanobacterium thermoautotrophicum* (Fig. 3F) grows chemoautotrophically at 65-70°C and uses only H_2-CO_2 as a methanogenic substrate.

Methanococcus voltae (1), a motile irregular coccoid organism is shown in Fig. 4A; this organism uses both H_2-CO_2 and formate and requires 1.2-4.8% NaCl for growth. *Methanospirillum hungatei*, a long motile spirillum, also uses H_2-CO_2 and formate (Fig. 4B).

Methanobacterium soehngenii is a long filamentous rod, sometimes punctuated with empty areas within a lengthy cell filament. The organism shown in Fig. 5 was present in the acetate enrichments of Toenniessen (15); these enrichment cultures had an infinite hydraulic and cell retention time because of the continual addition of glacial acetic acid and withdrawal of gas but not liquid from the culture vessel. *M. soehngenii* was recently cultured by Zehnder et al. (16).

Four strains of *Methanosarcina barkeri* are shown in Fig. 6. A variety of cell aggregates and cell sizes can be seen. *M. barkeri* strain 227 is shown in Fig. 6A; a gas vacuolated strain is shown in Fig. 6B; the newly designated type species (1) isolated by M.P. Bryant is shown in Fig. 6C, and a large cell type isolated by P.H. Smith is shown in Fig. 6D. A transmission electron micrograph taken by Jack Pangborn of thin sections of the gas vacuolated strain is shown in Fig. 7. Note the amorphous cell wall and random distribution of the gas vesicles.

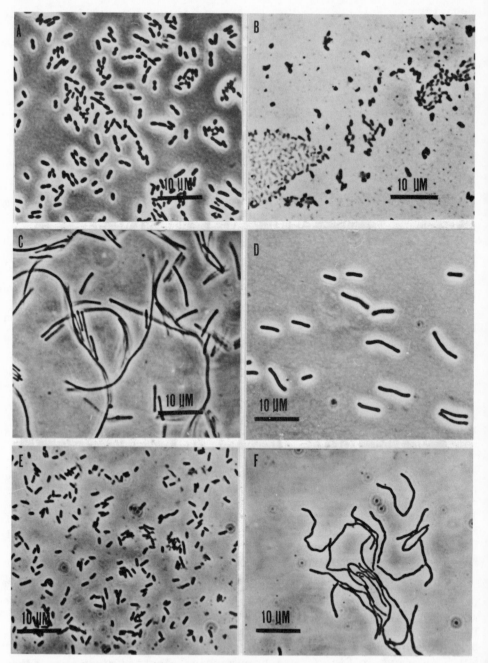

Figure 3. Phase contrast photomicrographs of wet mounts, Zeiss GFL, 43X objective, unless otherwise indicated. Approximate size as indicated. (*caption continued on next page*)

M. mazei undergoes a life cycle (6) in which an individual element forms an aggregate pseudosarcina shape comprised of a multitude of irregular elements which are freed at maturity by the slightest physical pressure. Fig. 8 shows a series of scanning electron micrographs of *M. mazei* taken by Jack Pangborn. A young culture is seen in Fig. 8A, an older culture is shown in Fig. 8B, and a specimen which was physically abraded on the surface (Fig. 8C) discloses the individual irregular units of which the mature cell aggregates are composed.

Thus far, only three aceticlastic methanogenic species have been isolated in pure culture. They are *Methanosarcina barkeri*, *Methanococcus mazei*, and *Methanobacterium soehngenii*. *M. soehngenii* has a generation time of 9 days or more; it exhibits a low K_m for acetate and therefore competes effectively for acetate at low concentrations. Nevertheless, it may not be a numerically important organism in continuously stirred tank reactors (CSTR's) because of its slow growth rates. *M. barkeri* and the related *M. mazei* are more ubiquitous in these types of digester systems. Future culture research on CSTR and fixed bed systems should lead to new isolations of other aceticlastic organisms.

Of the three aceticlastic isolates, most of the physiological studies have been done on isolates of *Methanosarcina*. H_2 exerts a regulatory effect on the aceticlastic reaction and prevents all strains of *Methanosarcina* (and the related *M. mazei*) from metabolizing acetate. This inhibitory effect is exerted in varying degrees depending on strain differences (7). For example, since *Methanosarcina* strain TM-1 cannot metabolize added H_2 (18), it is unable to use acetate as long as H_2 remains in the gas atmosphere. Once H_2 is flushed out, acetate metabolism resumes. Strain SMC metabolizes H_2 more slowly than acetate (7). Consequently, if H_2 is added to a culture of SMC on acetate, the aceticlastic reaction is inhibited while the H_2 is gradually oxidized and CO_2 reduced to form CH_4. Strain 227 metabolizes H_2 more rapidly than acetate. In this case, when H_2 is added to strain 227 on acetate, H_2 is rapidly metabolized, and the aceticlastic reaction is inhibited for the shorter duration of the H_2 in the gas atmosphere.

Cultures grown for several transfers on methanol are unable to use acetate without a lag (13). However, cultures grown on acetate use methanol and acetate simultaneously. Under these conditions, methanol apparently serves as a preferred electron acceptor to produce methane at the expense of increased oxidation of the

---

A. *Methanobrevibacter ruminantium*; B. *Methanomicrobium mobile*; photograph by M.J.B. Paynter (stained preparation); C. *Methanobacterium formicicum*; D. *Methanobacterium bryantii*; E. *Methanobrevibacter arboriphilus*; F. *Methanobacterium thermoautotrophicum*.

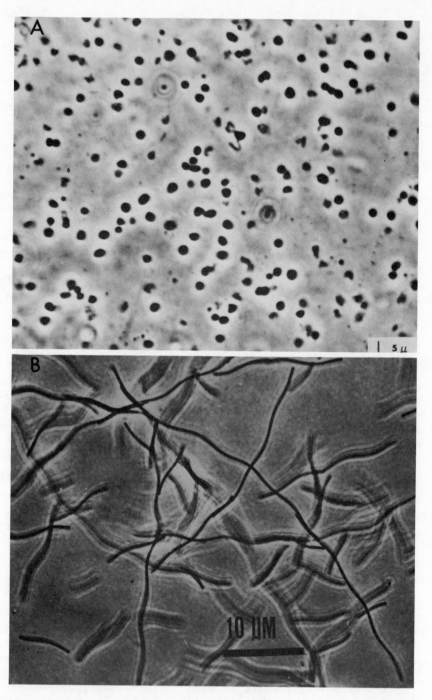

Figure 4. Approximate sizes as shown. A. *Methanococcus voltae;*
phase contrast photomicrograph by Janice Ward and P.H. Smith; B.
Methanospirillum hungatei.

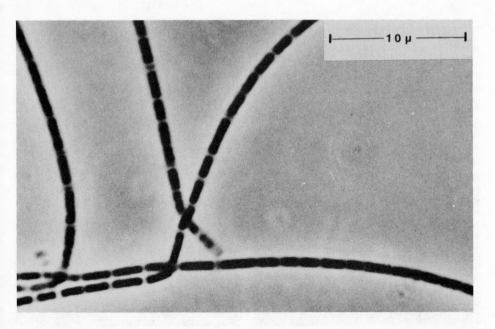

Figure 5. *Methanobacterium soehngenii;* photomicrograph by G. Toenniessen.

methyl group of acetate (7). Little or no oxidation of methanol may take place. When H_2 was added to a methanol-using culture, methanol still serves as the preferred electron acceptor to produce methane with little or no oxidation of methanol occurring. Even in the case of strain TM-1 (which normally cannot use H_2), methanol is reduced to methane by H_2 with virtually no oxidation of methanol. In this latter case, some H_2 oxidation may also be coupled to limited CO_2 reduction as long as methanol is present in the medium.

Much additional research is needed on pure culture isolation of methanogens (especially aceticlastic methanogens) and obligate proton-reducing acetogenic organisms. A better understanding of the overall methane fermentation is only beginning to emerge because of basic findings on the physiology of and interactions among the microbes involved. Knowledge of the metabolism and biochemistry of pure cultures coupled to studies on known mixtures of pure cultures are essential for future applications of this fermentation.

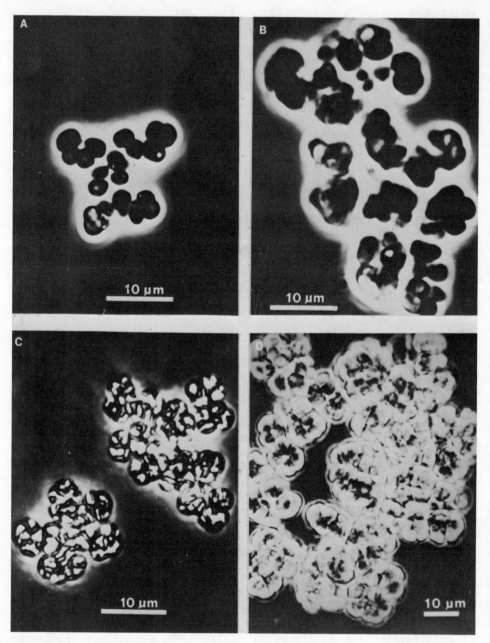

Figure 6.   A.   *Methanosarcina barkeri* strain 227; B.   *M. barkeri*
strain, isolated by M.P. Bryant; C.   *M. barkeri* strain W, gas vacuolated; D.   *M. barkeri* strain, isolated by P.H. Smith.

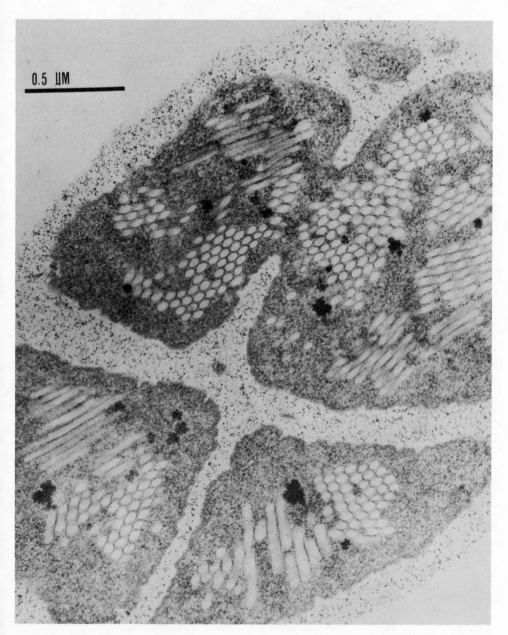

Figure 7. Thin section of *M. barkeri* strain W, transmission electron micrograph by Jack Pangborn.

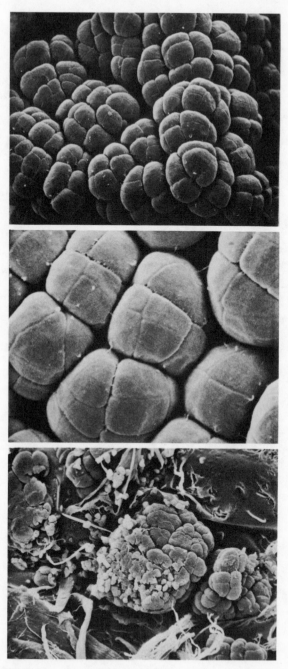

Figure 8. *Methanococcus mazei*. Scanning electron micrographs (SEM) by Jack Pangborn. Upper picture shows SEM (50X) of young culture. Middle picture shows an older cluster. Bottom picture, clump was physically abraded to show irregular components within.

TABLE III
Characteristics of Methanogenic Species in Pure Culture

Species	Morphology	Growth Substrates
Methanobacterium		
formicicum	Long rod to filament	H_2-CO_2, formate
bryantii	Long rod	H_2-CO_2
thermoautotrophicum	Long rod to filament	H_2-CO_2
soehngenii	Long filaments	Acetate
Methanobrevibacter		
ruminantium	Lancet-shaped cocci	H_2-CO_2, formate
smithii	Lancet-shaped cocci	H_2-CO_2, formate
arboriphilus	Short rods	H_2-CO_2
Methanomicrobium		
mobile	Short rods	H_2-CO_2, formate
Methanogenium		
cariaci	Irregular small cocci	H_2-CO_2, formate
marisnigri	Irregular small cocci	H_2-CO_2, formate
Methanospirillum		
hungatei	Short to long wavy spirillum	H_2-CO_2, formate
Methanosarcina		
barkeri	Pseudosarcina	H_2-CO_2, methanol methylamines, acetate
Methanococcus		
vannielii	Irregular small cocci	H_2-CO_2, formate
voltae	Irregular small cocci	H_2-CO_2, formate
mazei	Pseudosarcina to irregular coccoid elements	H_2-CO_2, methanol methylamines, acetate

REFERENCES

1. Balch, W.E., G.E. Fox, L.J. Magrum, C.R. Woese, and R.S. Wolfe 1979. Methanogens: reevaluation of a unique biological group. Microbiol. Revs. 43:260-296.

2. Barker, H.A. 1940. Studies upon the methane fermentations. VI. The isolation and culture of *Methanobacterium omelianskii*. Ant. v. Leeuwenhoek 6:201-220.

3. Boone, D.R. and M.P. Bryant. 1980. Propionate degrading bacterium *Syntrophomonas wolinii* (sp. nov., gen. nov.) from methanogenic ecosystems. Abst.Ann.Meeting, Amer.Soc. Microbiol p. 203.

4. Mah, R.A. and M.R. Smith. 1981. The methanogenic bacteria. In The Prokaryotes. Springer Verlag. ed., H.G. Schlegel. In press

5. Mah, R.A., M.R. Smith and L. Baresi. 1978. Studies on an ace-tate-fermentating strain *Methanoscarcina*. Appl. Environ. Microbiol.   1174-1184.

6. Mah, R.A., 1980. Isolation and characterization of *Methano-coccus mazei*. Current Microbiol. 3:321-326.

7. Mah, R.A., M.R. Smith, T. Ferguson, and S.H. Zinder. 1980. Methanogenesis from H_2-CO_2, methanol, and acetate by *Methano-sarcina*. In Proc. of the C-1 Symposium Sheffield, England. In press.

8. McInerney, M.J., M.P. Bryant, and N. Pfennig. 1979. Anaerobic bacterium that degrades fatty acids in syntrophic association with methanogens. Arch. Microbiol. 122:129-135.

9. McInerney, M.J. and M.P. Bryant. 1980. Isolation and character ization of *Syntrophomonas wolfei* (sp. nov., gen. nov.) a new anaerobic syntrophic, fatty acid-degrading bacterium. Abst. Ann. Meeting, Amer. Soc. Microbiol., p. 94.

10. Paynter, M.J.B. and R.E. Hungate. 1968. Characterization of *Methanobacterium mobilis*, sp. n., isolated from the bovine rumen. J. Bacteriol. 95:1943-1951.

11. Smith, P.H. 1980. EPA Report. 600-2-80-093. "Studies of metha-nogeric bacteria in sludge."

12. Smith, P.H. and R.E. Hungate. 1958. Isolation and characteri-zation of *Methanobacterium ruminantium*, n. sp. J. Bacteriol. 75:713-718.

13. Smith, M.R. and R.A. Mah. 1978. Growth and methanogenesis by *Methanosarcina* strain 227 on acetate and methanol. Appl. Env. Microbiol. 36:870-879.

14. Smith, M.R., S.H. Zinder, and R.A. Mah. April/May 1980. Micro-bial methanogenesis from acetate. Process Biochem.

15. Toenniessen, G. 1971. Studies on acetate and methanol ferment-ing methanogenic enrichments. Ph.D. Thesis.UNC,Chapel Hill,N.C

16. Zehnder, A.J.B., B.A. Huser, T.D. Brock, and K. Wuhrmann. 1980 Characterization of an acetate-decarboxylating non-hydrogen-oxidizing methane bacterium. Arch. Microbiol. 124:1-11.

17. Zeikus, J.G. and D.L. Henning. 1975. *Methanobacterium arbop-hilicum*. sp.nov., an obligate anaerobe isolated from wetwood o

living trees. Ant. v. Leeuwenhoek. J. Microbiol. Serol. 41:543-552.

18. Zinder, S.H. and R.A. Mah. 1979. Isolation and characterization of a thermoph8lic strain of *Methanosarcina* unable to use H_2-CO_2 for methanogenesis. Appl. Env. Microbiol. 38:996-1008.

DISCUSSION

Q. OLSEN: You were mentioning the cell-wall chemistry of the methanogens and also the Gram stain reactions, and I was just wondering if there is any meaning to the Gram stain reactions of these bacteria?

A. MAH: I think mainly to satisfy the usual laboratory characteri-zation reactions that one puts organisms through, I don't think it has the same kind of reference as with other procaryotic organisms.

Q. LEADBETTER: Is anything known about the nature of the carbon-nitrogen bond cleavage mechanism in the amine utilization under these anaerobic conditions?

A. MAH: I'm not familiar with that. Perhaps Dr. Gottschalk can make a comment on that.

GOTTSCHALK: Well, we are certain that oxidase reactions are not involved in just utilizing the methyl groups in trimethyl-amine. It seems that trimethylamine is hydrolyzed to yield methanol, and methanol is then utilized in the usual way.

Q. WOOD: I'm kind of curious about the biosynthetic reactions that lead to all of the cell material that must be formed from these simple substrates. Can you comment on that?

A. MAH: We haven't done any work on the assimilatory reactions at all in our lab. The organisms appear to use both acetate as well as CO_2 as starting compounds. I believe Dr. Zeikus' group has done much of the work on this aspect of the metabolism of the methanogens.

WOLFE: I'd like to make one comment as an extension of Dr. Mah's talk. I think the first 75 to 80 years of anaerobic waste treatment in this country has been misguided. The process was not designed around the needs of the methanogens. That is, the sanitary engineer in the past wanted to stir everything homo-geneously and the biocatalysts were discarded along with the treated sludge. New processes are now being designed that use

fixed beds or films where the generation time of the methanogens is separated from the retention time of the fermentor.
When this is done the slow growing catalysts are retained, and
generation time does not limit the process. The future lies
in this direction. Would you agree with that, Bob?

A.   MAH: Yes, very much. The continuously stirred tank reactor,
      I think, is an engineering concept. In order for methanogens
      to be operative in these CSTR systems, their generation times
      must be shorter than the retention times of the reactors. Thus
      slower growing methanogens will wash out. In fixed bed
      systems, a dense population of organisms remains attached to
      the substratum, and even slower growing methanogens may be
      important.

ANAEROBIC FERMENTATIONS OF CELLULOSE TO METHANE

H.D. Peck, Jr. and M. Odom

Department of Biochemistry
University of Georgia
Athens, Georgia 30602

The microbial populations responsible for the anaerobic degradation of cellulosic biopolymers appear to be taxonomically diverse and
variable, but the basic pattern of these complex fermentations is
similar wherever they occur. This in turn suggests that the common
denominator of these microbial populations is overall physiology
rather than taxonomy. For example, if one compares the microorganisms
found in mesophilic and thermophilic fermentations of cellulose to
CO_2 and CH_4, individual isolates from these fermentations will, by
and large, be taxonomically distinct, but physiologic counterparts
in terms of the overall reactions catalyzed can be readily identified
in each fermentation. This is perhaps implicit in the general concept
of a "food chain"; however, within this single constraint, it allows
for extensive diversity in terms of pH, temperature, products, product
composition, substrates, inhibitors, product and substrate tolerance
and nutrition. This diversity is currently the object of a considerable research effort which should define the environmental parameters for the degradation of complex cellulosic biopolymers and lead
to the isolation of new types of bacteria.

A second basic property of cellulose fermentation is the highly
interactive relationships among the involved microorganisms (1). In
the mature cellulose-CH_4 fermentation, all the substrate is converted
to CH_4, CO_2 and cell mass without the accumulation of any intermediates. These interactions stem largely from the fact that the
fermentation is a complete food chain in which one organism's product
is another organism's substrate. Thus, bacteria are present in these
fermentations which convert the different fermentation products
originating from the initial fermentation of cellulose, namely,
propionate, butyrate, lactate, ethanol, etc., to substrates for the
methanogenic bacteria, H_2, CO_2 and acetate. The formation and

utilization of H_2 produced in these bioconversions is of major
importance for understanding this particular food chain. H_2 is
clearly a major product/substrate in the food chain but its concentration is maintained at a low level (1 µM) by the H_2-utilizing
methanogenic bacteria for the reduction of CO_2 to methane and in high
sulfate environments by the sulfate reducing bacteria (2). The
existence of this H_2-sink has an extensive impact on the composition
of the intermediate fermentation products and in fact allows reactions to provide energy for growth which would not be possible
under conditions where molecular H_2 accumulates. This penomenon was
first clearly recognized by the Urbana group (3, 4) and termed
"interspecies H_2 transfer". It is a basic concept for any understanding of the ecology of anaerobic microbes as exemplified by those
involved in the anaerobic fermentations of cellulose to CH_4 and
CO_2. Specific interactions clearly exist at other levels but these
have not been fully documented and analyzed. Extensive nutritional
interactions can be anticipated and Allison et al (5) have shown
growth requirements of fatty acids produced in the fermentation for
cellulolytic bacteria from the rumen. There also appear to be
types of inhibitions by intermediates formed during the fermentation, but whether these effects represent true regulatory phenomena
or the results of cultivation in the laboratory under artifical
conditions has not been resolved (6). It is clear that one can not
yet generalize concerning the effects of inhibitory products and
substrates on the growth of isolated bacteria involved in the
cellulose-CH_4 fermentation. Hungate (7) reported that the growth
of pure cultures of cellulase producing bacteria on cellulose was
much slower than expected from the rate of cellulose degradation in
mixed cultures, others have isolated cellulase producing strains
which grow well in pure culture (8-10). The growth of the slow
strains can be dramatically increased and the composition of product
altered by establishing co-cultures with cellobiose-fermenting
strains (11) but co-cultures appear to have little effect on the
growth or products formed by the faster growing isolates. Similarly,
there is not yet a pattern to be found in the inhibitions of growth
observed by fermentation products on the growth of organisms
involved in the cellulose-CH_4 food chain. Again, these inhibitions
may be entirely artificial in that the microorganism never encounter
the high product levels in nature that are produced on laboratory
media; nevertheless these inhibitions must be understood before
these bacteria can be used for the commercial production of fuels
and chemicals.

CELLULOSE DEGRADATION IN THE PRESENCE OF HIGH SULFATE

There are three different patterns for the degradation of
cellulose which can presently be identified in nature. The first
of these patterns is the conversion of cellulose to CO_2 in the
presence of excess sulfate. This pattern is largely restricted

to the mesophilic marine environments with excess sulfate but one might expect that a similar pattern might be found in sulfate springs both at high and low temperature (12). The major unique feature of this pattern is the involvement of the sulfate reducing bacteria both in the oxidation of the products resulting from the fermentation of cellulose and the removal of H_2 by interspecies H_2 transfer as shown in Scheme 1.

Scheme 1. The Anaerobic Degradation of Cellulose to CO_2 in the Presence of Sulfate

Stage 1. Primary and Ancillary Bacteria

$$\text{Cellulose} \longrightarrow \begin{matrix}\text{Cellobiose}\\ + \\ \text{Glucose}\end{matrix} \longrightarrow \begin{matrix}\text{Lactate}\\ \text{Alcohols}\\ \text{Fatty acids}\end{matrix} + \begin{matrix}\text{Acetate}\\ H_2\\ CO_2\end{matrix}$$

Stage 2. Secondary Bacteria (sulfate reducers)

$$\begin{matrix}\text{Lactate}\\ \text{Alcohol}\\ \text{Fatty acids}\end{matrix} + SO_4^{-2} \longrightarrow \text{Acetate} + CO_2 + S^{-2}$$

Stage 3. Acetate and H_2 Oxidizing Bacteria

$$4H_2 + SO_4^{-2} \longrightarrow S^{-2} + 4H_2O$$

$$\text{Acetate} + SO_4^{-2} \longrightarrow 2CO_2 + S^{-2}$$

$$\text{Acetate} + 4S^{o} \longrightarrow 2CO_2 + 4S^{-2}$$

Substrates and Final Products

$$\text{Cellulose} + SO_4^{-2} \longrightarrow CO_2 + S^{-2}$$

The methanogenic bacteria, although possibly present, do not appear to play a role in this bioconversion. This is indicated by the fact that, in marine sediments, there is no significant methane formation until the supply of sulfate is exhausted (13). Stage 1 of the conversion involves the fermentation of cellulose to CO_2, H_2 and classic fermentation products such as lactate, acetate, alcohols and fatty acids, both odd and even numbered (1). Cellobiose and/or glucose are often accumulated by isolated cellulase-producing bacteria (8, 9) and may be inhibitory for the degradation of cellulose. These inhibitory sugars can be removed by non-cellulase-producing bacteria and have been indicated in the scheme as ancillary bacteria. The additional complexity of Stage 1 will in nature be dependent on the types of cellulosic substrates available and the environment. Stage 2 involves the conversion of fermentation products from Stage 1, other than acetate, CO_2 and H_2, to acetate with the reduction of sulfate to sulfide. The complex of bacteria required for these conversions has been termed the "acetogenic bacteria"; however, the term "aceto-genic" should be reserved for microorganisms capable of catalyzing the reduction of CO_2 to acetate and, as suggested by Boone and Bryant (14), they have been referred to as secondary bacteria. It should be emphasized that these secondary conversions in the presence of sulfate do not involve the production of significant amounts of H_2 or interspecies H_2 transfer, only the formation of acetate and CO_2 with the concomitant reduction of sulfate to sulfide. Lactate, formate and ethanol are usual substrates for the growth of both recognized genera of the sulfate reducing bacteria, *Desulfovibrio* and *Desulfotomaculum* (15), and recently several new isolates of the sulfate reducing bacteria have been studied (Widdel and Pfennig, pers. comm.) which are capable of converting either odd or even numbered fatty acids and alcohols to acetate and CO_2 in the presence of sulfate. Thus, sufficient physiological types of sulfate reducing bacteria have now been described to account for the utilizing of most fermentation products of cellulose in this anaerobic bioconversion.

In the third stage, acetate and H_2 are oxidized to CO_2 and H_2O with the reduction of SO_4^{-2} to sulfide. Gaseous CO_2 probably diffuses rapidly from its site of formation or is incorporated into cell materials. H_2S either reacts with metals in the immediate environment or diffuses into the overlying water where it is oxidized to S^O and sulfate by chemosynthetic and photosynthetic bacteria or oxidized to S^O by oxygen. All *Desulfovibrio* reduce sulfate with H_2 and some species can grow mixotrophically on H_2, CO_2, SO_4^{-2} and acetate (16). *Desulfovibrio* has also been used in the presence of sulfate as a "H_2-sink" instead of the H_2-utilizing methanogenic bacteria for the growth of H_2 producing bacteria in co-culture (14). By means of interspecies H_2 transfer, their presence probably tends to shift the cellulose fermentation in Stage 1 away from lactate and ethanol formation and towards acetate and fatty acid formation thus allowing the production of more ATP per glucose unit fermented (4). Acetate can be oxidized to CO_2 and H_2O by at least two different physiological types of bacteria found in these environments. *Desul-fotomaculum acetoxidans* oxidizes acetate (also ethanol, butanol and butyrate) to CO_2 in the presence of sulfate as its electron acceptor (17). A second bacterium, *Desulfuromonas acetoxidans,* oxidizes acetate (also ethanol, butanol and propanol) to CO_2 and H_2O in the presence of elemental sulfur and other electron acceptors such as malate (18). The elemental sulfur used for this oxidation probably arises from the chemical and biological oxidation of sulfide as it diffuses from the anaerobic environment. The bacterium was originally isolated from a stable association with a *Chlorobium* sp. (known as *Chloropseudomonas ethylica*) and represents the first demonstration of a "sulfur cycle". Both organisms have been isolated from marine environments and it is highly likely that they play an important essential role in the removal of acetate in high sulfate environments.

Acetogenic bacteria such as *Acetobacterium woodii* (19), which catalyze the formation of acetate from CO_2 and H_2, may also play a role in these bioconversions by utilizing H_2 formed in Stage 1, however, these microorganisms have not yet been isolated from marine environments (20). Thus, the various metabolic types of bacteria have been isolated and described to account for the complete bio-conversion of cellulose to CO_2 in the presence of sulfate. Almost certainly additional types of anaerobic bacteria will be isolated and considerable effort will be required to evaluate the significance of each organism in this important biological process.

INTERSPECIES HYDROGEN TRANSFER

Interspecies H_2 transfer can be simply viewed as the transfer of molecular hydrogen from a H_2-producing microorganism to a H_2-utilizing microorganism in mixed or co-cultures with the maintenance of a low partial pressure of H_2 (4). The phenomenon was first described in the classical studies of the Urbana group (3) on *Methanobacillus omelianskii* and extended to many types of micro-organisms (4). The H_2-utilizing methanogens, the sulfate reducing bacteria (*Desulfovibrio*) and a fumarate-reducing bacterium, *Vibrio succinogenes*, have been utilized as H_2-oxidizing organisms and, in effect, CH_4 formation, sulfate respiration or fumarate respiration are essentially added to the metabolic potential of the H_2 producing microorganism in the mixed culture. From the nutritional point of view, the relationships of H_2 producing organisms to interspecies H_2 transfer can be regarded as simple, facultative and obligatory. In simple interspecies H_2 transfer, any hydrogen produced is consumed by the H_2-utilizing bacteria and there may or not be a change in fermentation products and increase in growth; however, the H_2 pro-ducing organism does not require interspecies H_2 transfer for growth on the particular substrate. An example of this type of inter-species H_2 transfer is the co-culture of *Ruminococcus albus* with an H_2 utilizing bacterium, *V. succinogenes* (21). When grown by itself, *R. albus* produces ethanol, acetate, H_2 and CO_2 but when grown in co-culture, it forms only acetate, CO_2 and H_2, which is utilized by *V. succinogenes* to reduce fumarate to succinate. *R. albus* gains additional ATP by not having to reduce acetyl CoA to ethanol but its growth is not dependent on the removal of H_2.

Similar co-cultures have been described for *R. flavefaciens* and
Methanobacterium rumminantium (22) and the *M. omelianskii* association of an ethanol oxidizing bacterium and a methanogen (23). It is
interesting as pointed out by Wolin (4) that the hydrogenases of
the H_2-producing organism are all pyridine nucleotide linked. Simple
interspecies H_2 transfer is thus similar to nitrate reduction in the
clostridia which alters fermentation products and increases ATP yield
but is not essential for growth (24).

In facultative interspecies H_2 transfer, growth on certain
substrates requires interspecies H_2 transfer, but growth with other
substrates does not. This situation has been extensively studied
by Bryant et al (25) for the growth of several species of *Desulfovibrio* with H_2-utilizing methanogens. Most *Desulfovibrio* grow well
on pyruvate, fumarate, lactate plus sulfate, ethanol plus sulfate
but not on lactate or ethanol alone. However, in the presence of
the methanogen, the *Desulfovibrio* can grow as well on lactate or
ethanol as in the presence of sulfate as shown in Scheme 2.

Scheme 2.   Sulfate Reduction and Interspecies H_2 Transfer

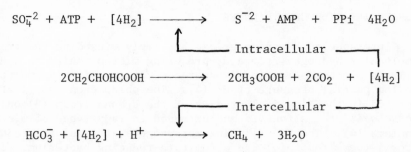

$$SO_4^{-2} + ATP + [4H_2] \longrightarrow S^{-2} + AMP + PPi \quad 4H_2O$$

Intracellular

$$2CH_2CHOHCOOH \longrightarrow 2CH_3COOH + 2CO_2 + [4H_2]$$

Intercellular

$$HCO_3^- + [4H_2] + H^+ \longrightarrow CH_4 + 3H_2O$$

Lactate is oxidized to acetate, CO_2 and eight reducing equivalents,
represented here as $4H_2$, with the formation of two high energy
phosphates at the substrate level. In the presence of sulfate, the
four reducing equivalents are utilized intracellularly for the
reduction of sulfate to sulfide. In the absence of sulfate, the
four reducing equivalents are transferred intercellularly as molecular H_2, and utilized by the methanogen for the reduction of CO_2
to methane. The resulting low partial pressure of H_2 essentially
thermodynamically "pulls" the oxidation of lactate with the production of high energy phosphate at the substate level as acetyl
phosphate. The other genus of the sulfate reducing bacteria,
Desulfotomaculum, has also been reported to grow on lactate in the
presence of a methanogen and absence of substrate amounts of
sulfate 96). Neither of the two genera of sulfate reducing bacteria
have been shown to have pyridine nucleotide coupled hydrogenases,
but the significance of this observation is unknown. Interspecies
H_2 transfer represents a new mode of growth for the sulfate-reducing
bacteria and may account for their widespread occurrence in low
sulfate environments.

The bioenergetics of sulfate reduction in *Desulfovibrio* and *Desulfotomaculum* have been shown to be quite different with regard to the metabolism of inorganic pyrophosphate (PPi) produced during the formation of adenylyl sulfate (APS) by ATP sulfurylase (Reaction 1; 26).

(1) $ATP + SO_4^{-2}$ ──────────────→ $APS + PPi$

In *Desulfovibrio*, the PPi is hydrolyzed to 2 orthophosphate (Pi) by inorganic pyrophosphatase (Reaction 2),

(2) $PPi + H_2O$ ──────────────→ $2Pi$

and these microorganisms must carry out electron transfer coupled phosphorylation in order to produce ATP for growth (27). Extracts of *Desulfotomaculum* exhibit only low levels of pyrophosphatase but contain high levels of PPi: acetate kinase (Reaction 3).

(3) $PPi + acetate$ ──────────────→ $Acetyl-P + Pi$

By means of this reaction, *Desulfotomaculum* is able to conserve the energy of the pyrophosphate bond and obtain one ATP from substrate level phosphorylation during growth on lactate plus sulfate. Relative growth yields of *Desulfovibrio* and *Desulfotomaculum* indicate that the latter does not carry out "significant" electron transfer coupled phosphorylation in this mode of growth and that *Desulfovibrio* generates three times as much ATP per sulfate reduced as *Desulfotomaculum*. Thus, *Desulfovibrio* has a bioenergetic advantage in a sulfate rich environment, and this may account for the observation that marine species of *Desulfotomaculum* are rare (15). When growing by interspecies H_2 transfer, and in the absence of sulfate, both genera of sulfate reducing bacteria are bioenergetically equivalent in that they obtain ATP only from substrate phosphorylation, 2 ATP's per CH_4 produced. In this mode of growth, the two types of organisms will be bioenergetically more competitive and this may account for the widespread distribution of both *Desulfotomaculum* and *Desulfovibrio* in fresh water environments.

Obligatory H_2-transfer applies to the situation of microorganisms whose only mode of growth is in co-culture with H_2 utilizing organisms. Bryant and his coworkers have recently isolated two bacteria of this type from primary anaerobic digestor sludge; *Syntrophobacter wolinii* which degrades proprionate to acetate, CO_2 and presumably H_2 (14) and an unnamed isolate that degrades even numbered fatty acids, butyrate, caproate and caprylate, to acetate and H_2 and odd numbered fatty acids, valerate and heptanoate, to acetate, propionate and H_2 (28). Growth was only obtained in co-culture with an H_2-utilizing methanogen or an H_2-utilizing sulfate reducing bacterium plus sulfate. Both microorganisms are gram-negative rods and strict anaerobes. The basic rationale for the obligatory nature of interspecies H_2 transfer lies in the free energy changes associated with the oxidation of these fatty acids and formation of H_2. The conversion of butyrate, for example, to acetate and H_2 (Reaction 4) has a substantial positive change in free energy ($\Delta G^{o\prime} = + 48$ KJ/reaction),

(4) butyrate + $2H_2O \longrightarrow$ 2 acetate $2H_2 + H^+ (\Delta G^{o\prime} = + 48$ KJ/reaction)

while the reduction of CO_2 to CH_4 by H_2 (Reaction 5) exhibits a negative change in free energy ($\Delta G^{o\prime} = 135$ KJ/reaction).

(5) $4H_2 + HCO_3^- + H^+ \longrightarrow CH_4 + 3H_2O$ ($\Delta G^{o\prime} = -135$ KJ/reaction)

The reaction catalyzed by the co-culture (Reaction 6) has a net negative change in free energy ($\Delta G^{o\prime} = -39$ KJ/reaction) which is sufficient to allow the growth of both physiological types of bacteria.

(6) 2 butyrate + $HCO_3^{-1} + H_2O \longrightarrow$ 4 acetate + H^+ CH_4
    ($\Delta G^{o\prime} = -39$ KJ/reaction)

Saturated fatty acids are important products of cellulose degradation but are not converted directly to CH_4 by methanogens and these observations of Bryant and coworkers clearly establish the microbiology and physiology of their conversion to substrates for the methane bacteria and effectively establish the vital importance of interspecies H_2 transfer in these complex anaerobic fermentations.

CELLULOSE FERMENTATION TO CH_4 AND CO_2

Numerous observations have suggested that a special relationship exists between the H_2-utilizing methanogens and the sulfate reducing bacteria (13, 29). These bacteria were demonstrated to be spatially associated in fresh water (30) and marine (31) sediments and it has been suggested that the sulfate reducing bacteria help to maintain the anaerobic conditions required for the growth of methanogens. The addition of sulfate inhibits methanogenesis in anaerobic digestors and in marine environments; methanogenesis only commences upon exhaustion of the supply of sulfate. The conversion of the cellulose-sulfate fermentation to the cellulose-methane fermentation is complex and little information is available concerning the mechanism of this change in fermentation pattern to that shown in Scheme 3.

Scheme 3. Cellulose Fermentation to Methane and CO_2

Stage 1. Primary and Ancillary Bacteria

$$\text{Cellulose} \longrightarrow \begin{array}{c} \text{Cellobiose} \\ + \\ \text{glucose} \end{array} \longrightarrow \begin{array}{c} \text{Lactate} \\ \text{Alcohols} \\ \text{Fatty acids} \end{array} + \begin{array}{c} \text{Acetate} \\ H_2 \\ CO_2 \end{array}$$

Stage 2. Secondary Bacteria

$$\begin{array}{c} \text{Lactate} \\ \text{Alcohols} \\ \text{Fatty acids} \end{array} \longrightarrow \text{Acetate} + CO_2 + H_2$$

Stage 3. Removal of Acetate and H_2

$$4H_2 + HCO_3^{-1} + H^+ \longrightarrow CH_4 + 3H_2O$$

$$CH_3 COO^- + H^+ \longrightarrow CH_4 + CO_2$$

$$4H_2 + 2CO_2 \longrightarrow CH_3COOH + 2H_2O$$

Substrate and Final Products

$$\text{Cellulose} \longrightarrow CO_2 + CH_4$$

In all probability, there occur both short and longer term changes in both the microbiology and physiology when fermentation is shifted to CH_4 formation. The overall fermentation becomes more dependent on interspecies H_2-transfer both for the removal of H_2 formed by the primary and ancillary microorganisms in Stage 1 and for the oxidation of fermentation products in Stage 2 by the secondary bacteria discussed in the previous section. Longer term changes probably involve increased numbers of H_2-utilizing methanogenic bacteria, growth of acetate-utilizing methanogenic bacteria which appear to be largely absent in marine environments and changes in the secondary bacteria from sulfate reducing bacteria capable of oxidizing fatty acids to fatty acid oxidizers which are completely dependent on interspecies H_2 transfer. The role of the acetogenic bacteria forming acetate from H_2 and CO_2 is not known, but they may be capable of participating in interspecies H_2 transfer and it is possible to devise a series of reactions whereby cellulose can be converted to CO_2 and CH_4 without relying on the H_2 utilizing methanogens.

The basic fermentation of cellulose to CH_4 and CO_2 shown in Scheme 3 occurs mainly in environments low in sulfate such as anaerobic digestors, fresh water sediments in lakes and swamps and marine environments where sulfate concentrations are low (32). It is characterized by the complete conversion of cellulose to CO_2 and CH_4 and the fact that acetate rather than CO_2 is the major source of CH_4 up to 70% (33).

CELLULOSE FERMENTATION IN THE RUMEN

The fermentation of cellulose as it occurs in the rumen has been the most extensively studied of these fermentations and provided much of the basic information available concerning the microbiology and physiology of cellulose degradation (1, 34). The basic pattern of the rumen fermentation of cellulose to CO_2, CH_4 and fatty acids is shown in Scheme 4.

Scheme 4.   Cellulose Fermentation to Methane, $CO2$ and Fatty Acids
            (Rumen)

Stage 1.   Primary and Ancillary Bacteria

                         Cellobiose   Acetate H_2

Cellulose ⎯⎯⎯→   +   ⎯⎯⎯→   +   +

                         glucose   Higher CO_2
                                              Fatty Acids

Stage 3. H_2-Utilizing Methanogenic Bacteria

        $4H_2 + HCO_3^{-1} + H^+$ ⎯⎯⎯⎯⎯⎯→ $CH_4 + 3H_2O$

Substrates and Final Products

Cellulose   ⎯⎯⎯→ $CH_4 + CO_2$ + Acetate + Fatty Acids

Fatty acids, mainly acetic, propionic and butyric, serve as energy sources for the ruminant and the secondary microorganisms of Stage 2 are usually absent from the rumen. CO_2 is the sole precursor of methane and the acetate utilizing methanogens are also not found in the rumen. Hungate (35) has suggested that the reason for the lack of conversion of these volatile fatty acids to CO_2 and CH_4 lies with the difference in net growth rates found in anaerobic digestors (0.1/day) and the rumen (0.1/hr). Thus, a bacterium with a net growth rate less than that of the rumen will be rapidly diluted out. The slow growth rate exhibited by the secondary bacteria, the fatty acid isolate of Bryant (54-84 hr) and S. Wolinii (87 hr) suggest that this may indeed be the case (28, 14). This may also be the reason for the absence of the acetate-utilizing methanogens which

are also known to have long generation times (36,37), and the acetogenic bacteria which theoretically should be of value in the rumen
(20).

INTERACTIONS BETWEEN PRIMARY AND ANCILLARY MICROORGANISMS

The classic work of Hungate (7) established that mesophilic
cellulolytic bacteria can be isolated from soils and established
criteria for the purity of cultures. He also reported that pure
cultures of the mesophilic cellulolytic bacteria grow much slower on
cellulose than mixed cultures and do not completely hydrolyze the
substrate, cellulose. Hungate suggested that associated contami-
nating bacteria in some manner stimulate the degradation of cellulose; similar results were later reported by Enebo (38) working with
thermophilic cellulose fermenters. On the other hand, mesophilic
and thermophilic cellulose fermentors have been isolated in pure
culture which ferment cellulose at reasonable rates (8-10). Cellobiose and/or glucose often accumulate in these cultures and the
degradation of cellulose commonly is incomplete suggesting end-product
inhibition (39). The inconsistencies in these observations probably
reflect the taxonomic and physiological diversities of the primary
cellulase-producing microorganisms isolated from different environments. We have recently observed stimulation of mesophilic and thermophilic cellulose fermentations in co-cultures of primary cellulase
producing microorganisms and ancillary non-cellulase producing microorganisms and resulting changes in fermentation patterns (11).
Stable anaerobic, mesophilic and thermophilic cellulose/methane
enrichment cultures have been established from soil and maintained
in the laboratory for the isolation of anaerobes capable of fermenting cellulose and cellobiose. Four cultures of mesophilic
cellulose fermenters have been isolated in pure culture which are
all gram negative curved rods but seem to differ in their abilities
to produce molecular H_2 and in their fermentation products. Due to
their slow growth, it has not been possible to obtain reliable fermentation balances but they all form mixtures of acetate, ethanol,
propionate, lactate and succinate. Sixteen cultures of ancillary
bacteria were isolated which have the ability to ferment cellobiose
and usually glucose but not cellulose. The effect on growth and
fermentation patterns of co-cultures of primary and ancillary microorganisms was investigated and typical results are shown in Table I.

The cultures were incubated for 25 days at $37^{\circ}C$ with an amount
of cellulose equivalent to 35 μmoles of glucose/ml. No methane was
formed by any of the cultures. Over the course of the experiment,
neither the primary nor ancillary bacteria in pure culture exhibited
significant growth on cellulose; however, co-cultures degraded 50%
of the cellulose to products: H_2, CO_2, ethanol and acetate in Expt.1
and H_2, CO_2, ethanol, acetate and lactate in Expt. 2. Not all,
but a majority of isolates which ferment cellobiose, will form

TABLE I

Stimulation of Cellulose Degradation by Reconstituted Cultures (25 days).

Microbial Type	H_2	CO_2	Products (μmoles/ml) Ethanol	Acetate	Propionate	Butyrate	Lactate	Cellulose utilized (μmoles/glucose/ml)
Expt. 1								
Cellulose fermentor (A)	0	3.0	0.09	0.16	.1	0.07	.09	4.0
Cellobiose degrader (2)	0	0	0	0	0	0	0	0
Cellulose fermentor (A) plus cellobiose degrader (2)	49.3	30.36	5.13	33.0	0.7	0.24	.12	16.89
Expt. 2								
Cellulose fermentor (B)	0	0	1.47	.62	0	0	0	1.0
Cellobiose degrader (2)	0	0	0	0	0	0	0	0
Cellulose fermentor (B) plus cellobiose degrader (2)	32	20.02	4.6	14.8	+	0	5.77	16.78

(Note)

The two strains of cellulose fermentors are indicated as A & B and the different strains of cellobiose fermentors as 2, 3 and 4.

successful associations and bacteria which ferment glucose but not
cellobiose do not form successful associations. It should be pointed
out that primary organisms will grow under these conditions, but it
requires 4-6 weeks to obtain significant levels of products. As it
was not possible to obtain more rapid growth of the primary bacteria
either using spent media, vitamin supplements or fatty acids, we have
interpreted the stimulation of growth to be due to the removal by
the ancillary bacteria of cellobiose and possibly other reducing
sugars, which are known to inhibit both the biosynthesis and catalytic activity of cellulase. This conclusion is strongly supported by
the data in Table II which shows the effect of the ancillary bacterium
on the fermentation products of a successful association. The data
clearly demonstrate again the requirement for a primary and ancillary
organism to obtain significant utilization of cellulose in the time
period of the experiment. In addition, the products formed by the
primary bacterium on glucose and the ancillary bacterium on cellobiose are indicated. If one assumes that the fermentation products
of the primary bacteria are the same on cellulose as glucose, one can
conclude that the pattern of fermentations observed in successful
associations more closely resembles that of the ancillary bacterium
than the primary microorganism. Thus, the primary organism forms
ethanol and acetate in a ratio of about 1:5 on glucose and the
secondary bacterium exhibits an ethanol/acetate ratio of 2:1 on
cellobiose; the ratio in mixed cultures of these two organisms is
2:1, almost identical to the ethanol/acetate ratio produced by the
ancillary bacterium fermenting cellobiose. The higher yield of H_2
by the mixed culture appears to be due to the conversion of formate
to H_2 and CO_2.

     In the second experiment, the same cellulose fermentor was
grown with an ancillary bacterium, which is a homoacetate fermentor.
The formation of H_2 and ethanol are essentially eliminated in the co-
culture and the major product is acetate as was observed with the
secondary bacterium growing on cellobiose. As the results can not
be explained by interspecies H_2 transfer, we have made the following conclusions regarding the microbiology of successful associations.
First, most of the products of cellulase activity are utilized by
the secondary bacterium with the result that the inhibition of the
activity and/or biosynthesis of cellulase by cellobiose and reducing sugars is prevented. Second, the fermentation patterns suggest
that the presence of the ancillary microorganism does not greatly
enhance the actual growth of the primary bacterium, indicating that
the stimulation of the degradation of cellulose is not due to a
nutritional synergism in co-culture. Third, the fermentation of
cellulose can be catalyzed by different co-cultures resulting in
the formation of different products. Fourth, the fact that the
fermentation pattern is largely determined by secondary microorganisms greatly simplified the selection of mixed cultures to
produce a single desired product. It should therefore be entirely

TABLE II

The Effect of The Ancillary Bacteria on the Fermentation Products
of Successful Associations

Bacterial Types	Substrate	Products μmoles/ml			
		H_2	Ethanol	Acetate	Formate
Cellulose fermentor (B)	Cellulose*	0	0	0	0
Cellulose fermentor (B)	Glucose	58.5	9.6	54.2	0
Cellobiose fermentor (3)	Cellobiose	12.0	41.0	21.4	10.0
Cellulose plus	Cellulose	29.0	37.8	18.7	1.0
Cellobiose (3) fermentor					
Cellobiose fermentor (4)	Cellobiose	1.0	1.1	68	0
Cellulose plus	Cellulose	3.2	0.4	65.6	0
Cellobiose (4) fermentor					

*
Significant growth of the cellulose fermentor was not observed.

(Note)
The two strains of cellulose fermentors are indicated as A & B and
the different strains of cellobiose fermentors as 2, 3 and 4.

possible to "design" cellulose-fermentations to desired single products under desired conditions when enough cellobiose-fermenting
isolates or mutants are available.

We have also been interested in the anerobic conversion of
cellulose to methane both from the aspect of the microbiology of the
process and its applicability to the practical formation of methane.
The presence of the primary and ancillary bacteria are required for
the degradation of cellulose and the inclusion of an H_2-utilizing
methane bacterium only marginally stimulated the extent of the
fermentation. H_2 and CO_2 were converted to CH_4 indicating that the
methane bacteria grew; however, a small amount of H_2 did accumulate
in the culture. In general, the accumulation of small amounts of
H_2 does not appear to effect the course of the fermentation. Similar
results with mixtures of thermophilic cellulytic and methanogenic
bacteria have been presented by Weimer and Zeikus (39). It should

be noted that the presence of a methane bacterium did not prevent
the accumulation of significant amounts of reduced products. On
occasion, H_2-utilizing methanogenic bacteria have been observed to
markedly stimulate a cellulose fermentation; however, most of our
evidence indicates that the methane bacteria, although forming
methane in mixed cultures do not "pull" the breakdown of cellulose.

These results suggest that there can be extensive interactions
other than interspecies H_2 transfer in the degradation of cellulose
to products (Stage 1); however, these interactions may be quite
artificial as the levels of intermediates or products which the
organism encounter under laboratory conditions are probably considerably higher than the bacteria encounter during the complete conversion of cellulose to methane. Nevertheless, studies with this type
of co-culture should provide basic information concerning the microorganisms involved, the breakdown of cellulose and a simple and
direct technique for modifying the cellulose fermentation for the
production of fuels and chemicals. Similar observations have been
made utilizing thermophilic microorganisms with both increased reaction rates and changes in fermentation patterns. Again the critical feature appears to be the capability of fermenting cellobiose.

HYDROGEN METABOLISM IN *DESULFOVIBRIO*

The metabolism of molecular H_2 has figured centrally in the
development of our present concepts concerning the biochemistry and
physiology of respiratory sulfate reduction and hydrogenase has been
extensively studied. Most species of *Desulfovibrio* contain a hydrogenase with high specific activity (40) which is soluble and largely
localized in the periplasmic space (41); however, in at least one
instance, the enzyme is membrane-bound (42). The soluble hydrogenase is a non-heme iron protein containing three $[Fe_4S_4]$* clusters
per molecular weight of 50,000 (43) and requires cytochrome c_3
(Mr = 13,000) for activity with naturally occurring electron
acceptors (44). Hydrogenase is produced whether these bacteria are
grown on H_2 plus sulfate or organic substrates plus sulfate. In the
later case, H_2 was not believed to be formed as a major fermentation
product and the role of hydrogenase, if any, in this mode of growth
has been problematical (15).

Desulfovibrio is the only group of bacteria which can clearly
participate in interspecies H_2 transfer as the H_2-producing or the
H_2-utilizing microorganism and there has been considerable interest
in the bioenergetics and physiology of H_2 metabolism in these
bacteria. Hatchikian et al (45) first reported the accumulation of
hydrogen during growth on lactate plus sulfate, but there was no
stoichiometry between the amount of H_2 produced and the sulfate
reduced. More recently, Tsuji and Yagi (46) have reported a burst

of H_2 production during the early stages of growth and a reutilization of the H_2 during later stages of the growth cycle. These investigators also reported the presence of two hydrogenases, one of
molecular weight 70,000 and another of 180,000. They suggested that
the lower molecular weight hydrogenase was involved in hydrogen
utilization and the higher molecular weight hydrogenase in H_2 production. The physiological role of the low molecular weight
hydrogenase was viewed as similar to the role of hydrogenase in
nitrogen-fixation where it scavenges hydrogen produced during
N_2-fixation, thereby conserving ATP (47).

    We have been investigating the localization of various elec-
tron transfer proteins, dehydrogenases and reductases, in cell
fractions from *Desulfovibrio*. APS reductase, bisulfite reductase
and pyruvate dehydrogenase have been localized in the cytoplasm and
fumarate reductase found to be bound to the internal aspect of the
cytoplasmic membrane. Some additional data is presented in Table III
for lactate dehydrogenase, formate dehydrogenase and hydrogenase.
The basic approach is to assay intact cells and extracts for the
enzyme activity with a non-permeant electron donor or acceptor such as
a viologen dye (44). Similar activities with whole cells and extracts indicate the enzyme is external to the cell membrane. An
increase in activity in broken cell preparations relative to intact
cells indicates that the activity is localized in the cytoplasm or
on the inner aspect of the cytoplasmic membrane. The data in
Table III have been normalized to the activities found in crude
broken cell preparations. In French press cell fractions of *D-
desulfuricans*, lactate dehydrogenase appears to be bound to the
inner aspect of the cytoplasmic membrane and a portion of the hydrogenase localized in the cytoplasm (Steenkamp, D. J. and H. D. Peck,
Jr., unpublished results). Formate dehydrogenase exhibited slightly
greater activity with intact cells than in extracts suggesting that
it is localized on the exterior aspect of the cytoplasmic membrane.
Lysozyme spheroplasts of *D. gigas* were examined for the same enzymatic activities; however, it was not possible to find lactate dehydrogenase. A significant fraction of the hydrogenase was localized in
the cytoplasm and formate dehydrogenase again appears to be on the
external surface of the cytoplasmic membrane. Spheroplasts were
utilized to reduce the external concentration of the lower molecular
weight hydrogenase in order that the stimulation of activity could
be observed upon lysis. The hydrogenase of *Dt. ruminis* was exclusively localized on the interior surface of the cytoplasmic
membrane and these bacteria lack an external periplasmic hydrogenase (Liu, C.L. and H.D. Peck, Jr., unpublished results). In
contrast to *Desulfovibrio* the H_2 metabolism of *Desulfotomaculum* has
been less well studied but seems to be quite limited in terms of
H_2 utilization. There is no report of the reduction of sulfate with
H_2 by *Dt. nigrificans* and *Dt. orientis* and although *Dt. ruminis*
has been reported to reduce sulfate with H_2, the cells required the

TABLE III
Localization of Hydrogenase, Formate Dehydrogenase and Lactate
Dehydrogenase in Cell Fractions from the Sulfate Reducing Bacteria

% Activity

Enzymatic Activity	Intact Cells or Spheroplasts	Crude Preparations	Membranes	Supernatant
D. desulfuricans				
(French Press)				
lactate dehydrogenase	Trace	100	79	Trace
hydrogenase	53	100	10	95
Formate dehydrogenase	137	100	Trace	84
D. gigas				
(spheroplasts)				
lactate dehydrogenase	-	NF	-	-
hydrogenase	33	100	-	-
Formate dehydrogenase	126	100	24	70
Dt. ruminis				
(French Press)				
hydrogenase	Trace	100	93	Trace

presence of 2% yeast extract (49). The reduction of other sulfur
compounds is slow compared to the rates observed with *Desulfovibrio*
but *Dt. nigrificans* is able to grow in association with methanogens
(6) and these results together indicate that it is the internal
hydrogenase which is important for interspecies H_2 transfer, the
external hydrogenase being largely responsible for H_2 utilization.

In order to investigate the role of the internal hydrogenase
in *Desulfovibrio* the amount of internal hydrogenase relative to
intact cells was determined with *D. gigas* under conditions of
sulfate limitation in a chemostat. The results that are shown in
Figure 1, indicate over a two-fold increase in internal hydrogenase
at the lower dilution rates. Using selective lysis of the sulfate
reducing bacteria by lysozyme, it has been possible to demonstrate
similar ratios of external and internal hydrogenase in mixed cultures of *D. vulgaris* and a methanogen. In contrast to these results,
Badziong and Thauer (50) have reported that *D. vulgaris*, grown on
H_2 and sulfate, does not contain any cytoplasmic hydrogenase. These
observations suggest that the internal hydrogenase may be involved
with the metabolism of organic substrates such as lactate and ethanol.

The sulfate reducing bacteria, members of the genus *Desulfo-*
vibrio, were the first nonphotosynthetic anaerobic microorganisms

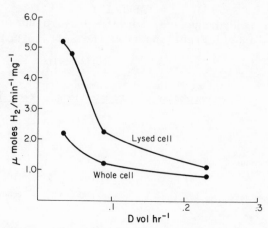

Figure 1.   The effect of sulfate limitations on the external and
internal hydrogenases of *D. vulgaris*.   (Dilution volume per hour.)

in which an electron transfer coupled phosphorylation was demonstrated. This phosphorylation was shown first with whole cells (51),
and subsequently with cell-free extracts, utilizing hydrogen as the
electron donor and fumarate (52) or sulfite (53) as the electron
acceptor.

        Due to the requirement of ATP for sulfate reduction, growth
with sulfate as electron acceptor and most organic substrates requires electron transfer coupled phosphorylation in order to obtain
a net yield of ATP for growth (27).   From the results of enzyme
localization studies with *D. vulgaris* (Marburg) grown on H_2 and
sulfate, Badziong and Thauer (50) have proposed a scheme for energy
coupling in *Desulfovibrio* which involves vectorial electron transfer
across the membrane with a proton gradient being produced by the
scalar production of protons from the oxidation of H_2 on the membrane
surface and the consumption of protons in the cytoplasm by the
reduction of sulfate.   The protons produced would of course be
utilized for the production of ATP via ATPase.   This mechanism is
quite different from the chemiosmotic model for respiratory sulfate
reduction proposed by Wood (54) in that it does not involve a typical
Mitchell loop.   A rapid proton production coupled to the oxidation
of H_2 and reduction of sulfite has been studied in our laboratory
and can best be explained by vectorial electron transfer (Liu, C.L.
and H.D. Peck, Jr., unpublished results).   The gradient is collapsed
by uncoupling agents and shows an $H^+/2e$ ratio of 1.9 - 2.1.   From
these results we propose that vectorial electron transfer is the
major mechanism for energy coupling in the sulfate reducing bacteria
when growing on both organic and inorganic substrates.   The scheme,
shown in Figure 2, involves the oxidation of lactate and pyruvate
to acetate, CO_2 and H_2, which, as a permeant molecule, can diffuse

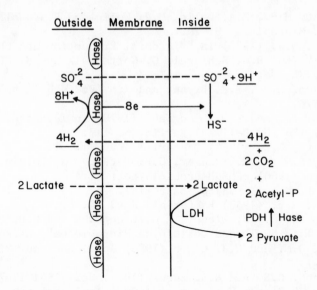

Figure 2 . Proposed bioenergetics of hydrogen metabolism in *Desulfoviobrio*.

across the cytoplasmic membrane can be utilized by the periplasmic hydrogenase for the reduction of sulfate and formation of a proton gradient. It is very similar to interspecies H_2 transfer and explains the unique property of *Desulfovibrio* in being both an efficient hydrogen-producing and H_2-utilizing bacterium. Consistent with this observation we have found that the protein composition of the membranes is quite simple containing only 4-6 major protein bands depending on growth conditions and a requirement for external hydrogenase to obtain lactate oxidation with sulfate reduction in spheroplasts. The proposed scheme is supported by enzyme localization studies and offers an explanation for many of the observations regarding H_2 metabolism in these bacteria. A major problem with this scheme involves the production of H_2 by hydrogenase E'_o = -414 mv) from the oxidation of lactate to pyruvate E'_o = -190 mv. However, the periplasmic hydrogenase may maintain the intracellular concentration of H_2 low enough to "pull" the oxidation in the direction of H_2 formation as occurs during interspecies H_2 transfer.

ACKNOWLEDGEMENT

These studies were supported in part by a grant from the U.S. Department of Energy under Contract No. DEAS-09-97 ER-10499.

REFERENCES

1. Bryant, M.P. (1979) J. Anim. Sci. 48: 193.
2. Hungate, R.E. (1967) Arch. Mikrobiol. 59: 158.

3.   Bryant, M.P., E.A. Wolin, M.J. Wolin and R.S. Wolfe (1967)
      Arch. Microbiol. 59: 20.
4.   Wolin, M.J. (1975) in "Microbial Production and Utilization of
      Gases" (Ed. H.G. Schlegel, G. Gottschalk and N. Pfennig) E.
      Goltz KG, Gottingen, p. 141.
5.   Allison, M.J., M.P. Bryant and R.N. Doetsch (1958) Sci. 128:
      474-475.
6.   Wiegel, J. and L.G. Ljungdahl (1979) in Technische Mikrobio-
      logie (Ed. H. Dellweg) Berlin, p. 117.
7.   Hungate, R.E. (1950) Bacteriol. Rev. 14: 1.
8.   Khan, A.W., J.H. Saddler, G.B. Petel, J.R. Colvin and S.M.
      Martin (1980) FEMS Microbiol. Lett. 1:47.
9.   Bryant, M.P. (1958) J. Bacteriol. 76: 529.
10.   McBee, R.H. (1950) Bacteriol. Rev. 14: 51.
11.   Dilworth, G., J. Wiegel, L.G. Ljungdahl and H.D. Peck, Jr.
      (1980) in "Colloque Celluloyse Microbienne", Marseille, p. 111
12.   Ward, D.M. and G.J. Olson (1980) Appl. Environ. Microbiol.
      40: 67.
13.   Martens, C.S. and R.A. Berne (1974) Sci. 185: 1167.
14.   Boone, D.R. and M.P. Bryant (1980) Appl. Environ. Microbiol.
      40: 626.
15.   Postgate, J.R. (1978) "The Sulphate Reducing Bacteria",
      Cambridge Univ. Press.
16.   Badziong, W., R.K. Thauer, and J.G. Zeikus (1978) Arch. Micro-
      biol. 116: 41.
17.   Widdel, F. and N. Pfenning (1977) Arch. Microbiol. 112: 119.
18.   Pfenning, N. and H. Bibel (1976) Arch. Microbiol. 110: 3.
19.   Batch, W., E.S. Schoberth, R.S. Tanner and R.S. Wolfe (1977)
      Ent. J. Syst. Bacteriol. 27: 355.
20.   Braun, M., S. Schoberth and G. Gottschalk (1979) Arch. Micro-
      biol. 120: 201.
21.   Iannotti, E.L., D. Kafkewitz, M.J. Wolin and M.P. Bryant (1973
      J. Bacteriol. 114: 1231.
22.   Wolin, M.J. (1975) Am. J. Clin. Nutr. 27: 1320.
23.   Reddy, C.A., M.P. Bryant and M.J. Wolin (1972) J. Bacteriol.
      109: 539.
24.   Hasan, M. and J.B. Hall (1975) J. Gen Microbiol. 87: 120.
25.   Bryant, M.P., L.L. Campbell, C.A. Reddy and M.R. Crabill (1977
      J. Bacteriol. 33: 1162.
26.   Liu, C.L. and H.D. Peck, Jr. (1981) J. Bacteriol (in press).
27.   Peck, H.D., Jr. (1962) Bacteriol. Rev. 26: 67.
28.   McInerney, M.J., M.P. Bryant and N. Pfenning (197) Arch.
      Microbiol. 122:129.
29.   Abram, J.W. and D.B. Nedwell (1978) Arch. Microbiol. 117: 93.
30.   Cappenberg, T.E. (1974) Antonie Van Leeuwenhuck. J. Microbiol.
      Serol. 40:285.
31.   Jurgensen, B.B. (1978) Geomicrobiol. 1: 49.
32.   Mah, R.A., D.M. Ward, L. Baresi and T.L. Glass (1977) Ann.
      Rev. Microbiol. 31: 309.

33.   Smith, P.H. and R.A. Mah (1966) Appl. Microbiol. 14: 368.
34.   Hungate, R.E. (1966) "The Rumen and Its Microbes." Academic
      Press.
35.   Hungate, R.E. (1976) in Microbial Production and Utilization
      of Gases (Ed. H.G. Schlegel, G. Gottschalk and N. Pfenning)
      P. 119.
36.   Smith, M.R. and R.A. Mah (1978) Appl. Environ, Microbiol. 36:
      870.
37.   Zehnder, A.J.B., B.A. Huser, T.D. Brock and K. Wuhrmann (1980)
      Arch. Microbiol. 124: 1.
38.   Enebo, L. (1954) Dissertation, Royal Inst. Technology,
      Stockholm.
39.   Weimar, P.J. and J.G. Zeikus (1977) Appl. Environ. Microbiol.
      33: 289.
40.   Sadana, J.C. and V. Jagannathan (1956) Biochim. Biophys. Acta
      19: 440.
41.   Bell, G.R., J. LeGall and H.D. Peck, Jr. (1974) J. Bacteriol.
      120: 994.
42.   Yagi, T., K. Kimura, H. Daidogi, F. Sakai, S. Tumura and H.
      Inokuchi (1976) J. Biochem. (Tokyo) 79: 661.
43.   Van der Westen, H.M., S.G. Mayhew and C. Veeger (1978) FEBS
      Lett. 86: 122.
44.   Bell, G.R., J.P. Lee, H.D. Peck, Jr. and J. LeGall (1978)
      Biochemie 60: 315.
45.   Hatchikian, E.C., M. Chaigneau and J. LeGall (1976) in
      Microbial Production and Utilization of Gases (Ed. H. G.
      Schlegel, G. Gottschalk and N. Pfennig) E. Goltze KG, Gottin-
      gen, p. 109.
46.   Tsuji, K. and T. Yagi (1980) Arch. Microbiol. 125: 35.
47.   Dixon, R.O.D. (1976) Nature 262: 173.
48.   Jones, R.W. and P.B. Garland (1977) Biochem. J. 164: 199.
49.   Coleman, G.S. (1960) J. Gen. MIcrobiol. 22: 423.
50.   Badziong, W. and R.K. Thauer (1980) Arch. Microbiol 125: 167.
51.   Peck, H.D. Jr. (1960) J. Biol. Chem. 235: 2734.
52.   Barton, L.L., J. LeGall and H.D. Peck, Jr. (1970) Biochem.
      Biophys. Res. Commun. 41: 1036.
53.   Peck, H.D. Jr. (1966) Biochem. Biophys. Res. Commun. 22: 112.
54.   Wood, P.M. (1978) FEBS Lett. 95: 12.

SOME ASPECTS OF THERMOPHILIC AND EXTREME

THERMOPHILIC ANAEROBIC MICROORGANISMS

L.G. Ljungdahl, F. Bryant, L. Carreira, T. Saiki,* and
J. Wiegel**

Department of Biochemistry
University of Georgia
Athens, Georgia 30602

An interest for industrial use of thermophilic, anaerobic
bacteria has clearly emerged since the 1973 oil shortages. Such
bacteria are capable of converting biomass, mostly cellulose, hemicellulose and starch to desirable industrial feedstock chemicals such
as acetate, ethanol, acetone, butanol, etc. (1). The thermophilic
bacteria are also convenient sources of enzymes, which are more
thermostable and more resistant toward denaturation when compared
with corresponding enzymes from mesophilic microorganisms (2).
Clearly, enzymes from thermophiles have properties which are desirable when considering industrial applications. The idea of using
thermophilic microorganisms industrially is not new. For instance,
several British patents since 1920 deal with fermentations of
cellulose using thermophilic, aerobic, as well as anaerobic, microorganisms (3). Curiously, these efforts were to produce ethanol
from renewable resources to be used as liquid fuel for combustion
engines. This idea has now been rediscovered some sixty or more
years after it was formulated. The cycle is complete. The problem
for today is not whether we can or can not ferment biomass to
desirable products but rather which are the best microorganisms to
use, how can we improve them, and what is the best technology.

In our laboratory, where we have had a longstanding interest
in anaerobic, thermophilic bacteria (4), we have been especially

---

*Present address: Department of Agricultural Chemistry, University
           of Tokyo, Bunkyo-ku, Tokyo 113, Japan

**Present address: Department of Microbiology, Universitat Gottingen
           · D-3400 Gottingen, West Germany

interested in the physiology of *Clostridium thermoaceticum* (5,6).
However, our studies also include the more extreme thermophilic
anaerobes, *Clostridium thermohydrosulfuricum* (7), and the recently
isolated *Thermoanaerobacter ethanolicus* (8). *C. thermoaceticum* may
be of use in the production of acetate, whereas the other two
bacteria appear suitable for fermentations leading to ethanol. In
this presentation, we will first deal with some properties of the
three thermophilic bacteria obtained from Icelandic hot springs with
temperatures from 55°C to 97°C and with pH-values from 3 to 9.

CLOSTRIDIUM THERMOACETICUM

  C. thermoaceticum was first described by Fontaine et al. (9).
It grows between 45°C and 65°C with the optimum temperature at 60°C.
Out of over forty carbohydrates including the most common disaccharides and polysaccharides that have been tested (9,10,11), *C. thermoaceticum* ferments only D-glucose, D-fructose, D-xylose, and pyruvate.
Acetate is the only product with the sugars; pyruvate, in addition,
yields CO_2. Theoretical fermentation balances are as follows:

$$C_6H_{12}O_6 \longrightarrow 3\ CH_3COOH$$

$$2C_5H_{10}O_5 \longrightarrow 5\ CH_3COOH$$

$$4CH_3COCOOH + 2H_2O \longrightarrow 5\ CH_3COOH + 2\ CO_2$$

In actual fermentations, between 85 to 90% of the theoretical yield
of acetate is obtained. This lower yield is partly due to the
incorporation of the substrates (about 5%) into cell carbon (9) and
to loss of sugars due to caramelizing which occurs at thermophilic
temperatures (7,9).

  Fermentations with *C. thermoaceticum* have been performed with
mixtures of xylose, fructose and glucose in equal concentrations
(10). Xylose is fermented faster than either of the two hexoses; the
fermentation of the latter starts when about half of the xylose is
fermented. In mixtures of glucose and fructose, the utilization of
glucose does not start until the fructose is almost completely
fermented. Clearly, fructose prevents the fermentation of glucose
by *C. thermoaceticum*. The mechanism of the inhibition by fructose
of the glucose utilization is not known. However, preliminary
results indicate that fructose represses the formation of an enzyme
needed for the fermentation of glucose. The apparent "diauxie" type
of fermentation exhibited by *C. thermoaceticum* may affect its use
in continual fermentations of mixtures of xylose, fructose and
glucose.

  It is indeed remarkable, that *C. thermoaceticum* has the
capacity to ferment one mol of glucose or fructose to three mol

of acetate, one of which is apparently synthesized from carbon dioxide (12). Several laboratories including those of H. A. Barker, E. R. Stadtman, ours, and especially that of H. G. Wood have been involved in elucidating this fermentation. Since an earlier review (5) exists and a new one (6) is soon to be published we will not discuss details of the fermentations, but merely summarize them.

The fermentative pathway of glucose by *C. thermoaceticum* is outlined in Figure 1. It is well established, although on the enzyme level much remains to be elucidated and that work, as we will see, often leads to exciting findings. Glucose is metabolized via the glycolytic pathway to form pyruvate with the generation of ATP and NADH. Half of the pyruvate is used in a transcarboxylation reaction also involving a methylcorrinoid. The other half of the pyruvate is assumed to be metabolized in the pyruvate-ferredoxin oxido-reductase reaction, which yields acetyl-CoA, CO_2 and reduced ferredoxin. Acetyl-CoA is converted to acetate in reactions that are catalyzed by phosphate acetyltransferase and acetate kinase. The latter enzyme has sigmoidal kinetics with regard to ATP, which suggests a regulatory mechanism (13).

C. thermoaceticum lacks hydrogenase and is unable to evolve hydrogen. Instead carbon dioxide serves as the acceptor of electrons generated during glycolysis and in the oxidation of pyruvate. The reduction of carbon dioxide ultimately leads to the formation of acetate. Tracer studies (12) indicate that acetate was totally synthesized from CO_2. However, this is not correct. The methyl group of the acetate is formed from CO_2 which in a series of reductive steps with formate and tetrahydrofolate derivatives as intermediates, yields a methylcorrinoid, the methyl group of which combines with the carboxyl group of pyruvate to form acetate (14). The carboxyl group of pyruvate is in isotope equilibrium with CO_2 and, consequently, isotopically labeled CO_2 is incorporated into the carboxyl group of acetate via pyruvate with the result of an apparent direct fixation of CO_2.

Recently, Diekert and Thauer (15) discovered that *C. thermoceticum* and *Clostridium formicoaceticum* (*C. formicoaceticum* like *C. thermoaceticum* ferments fructose to three mol of acetate (16, 17)) contain a carbon monoxide dehydrogenase which catalyze the reaction:

$$CO + H_2O \rightleftharpoons CO_2 + 2H^+ + 2e$$

The formation of this enzyme is dependent on the presence of nickel in the growth medium (18) and Drake et al. (19) found that the purified enzyme contains nickel.

Drake et al. (20), studying the enzyme system which converts methyltetrahydrofolate and pyruvate to acetate, found that five

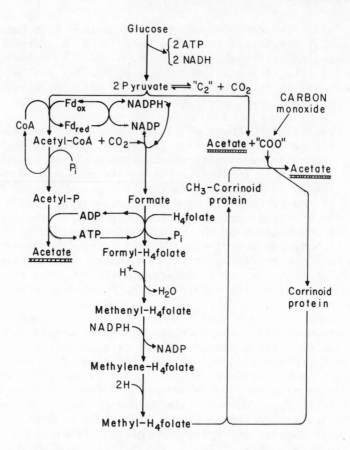

Figure 1.   Pathway of fermentation of glucose to three mol of acetate by *C. thermoaceticum*.

protein fractions, F_1, F_2, F_3, F_4 and ferrdoxin are required. Interestingly, fraction F_3 contains nickel and catalyzes the carbon monoxide dehydrogenase reaction. Moreover, it was found that a synthesis of acetate from carbon monoxide and methyltetrahydrofolate is catalyzed by the nickel enzyme (Fraction F_3) in combination with the protein fraction F_2. Pyruvate was not involved. Therefore, one may speculate that carbon monoxide and the carboxyl group of pyruvate may both yield a hypothetical "C_1" unit, which, with methyltetrahydrofolate, yields acetate. This is shown in Figure 2.

The first enzyme in the synthesis of acetate from CO_2 is formate dehydrogenase (Figure 1). In *C. thermoaceticum*, this enzyme is NADP-dependent and the reaction is as follows:

$$CO_2 + NADPH \rightleftarrows HCOO^- + NADP^+$$

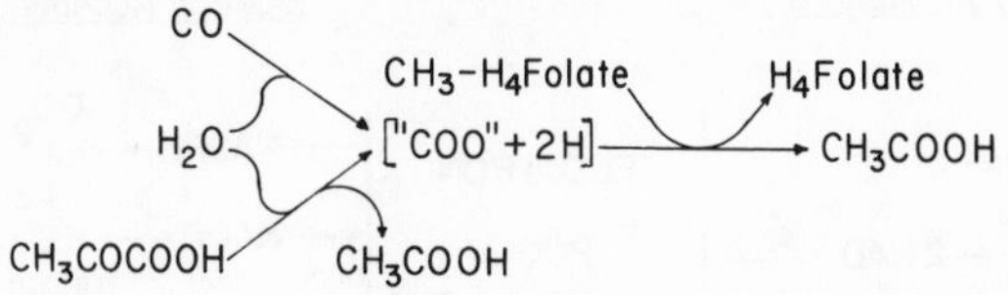

Figure 2. Hypothetical "COO"-unit formed from CO or the carboxyl group of pyruvate in the synthesis of acetate by *C. thermoaceticum*.

The formation of this enzyme is dependent on the presence of selenite and tungstate or molybdate in the growth medium (21). Selenium is required, however, tungsten and molybdenum may substitute for each other. In competition experiments using ^{185}W-tungstate and molybdate, it was shown that tungsten was incorporated into the active enzyme although the molybdate concentration in the medium was 100 times that of tungstate (22). Recently, we suggested (23) that the *C. thermoaceticum* formate dehydrogenase is a selenium-tungsten protein, which also contains non-heme iron and inorganic sulfur. On of us (T. Saiki) has now purified the enzyme to a specific activity of about 700 µmol min^{-1} mg^{-1}. The enzyme, having a M_r of 300,000, appears to consist of three different subunits and to contain one g-at of W, 2 g-at of Se and 30 - 47 g-at of Fe and of inorganic sulfur, respectively. A small amount, 0.15 g-at, of molybdenum was also present.

The exciting reports from H. G. Wood's and R. K. Thauer's laboratories regarding the involvement of a nickel enzyme in the synthesis of acetate from CO_2 and our finding of a selenium-tungsten non-heme iron formate dehydrogenase in *C. thermoaceticum* point out the importance of trace elements in this bacterium.

Perhaps the most fundamental characteristic of the fermentation of glucose to three mol of acetate by *C. thermoaceticum* is the fact that CO_2 functions as the electron acceptor. In Figure 3 are listed the electron-generating and the electron-accepting reactions. As is shown, electrons generated in the glyceraldehyde dehydrogenase reaction are accepted by NAD, whereas those generated by oxidation of pyruvate are accepted by ferredoxin. In contrast, NADPH serves as the electron donor in the formate dehydrogenase and in the methylene-H_4folate dehydrogenase reactions, whereas $FADH_2$ is the likely donor with methylene-H_4folate reductase. It is obvious that some kind of electron transport must occur to couple the electron-generating reactions forming NADH and reduced ferredoxin with the electron-accepting reactions using NADPH and a reduced flavin. There exists the possibility that this electron transport may be coupled to the production of ATP. Exceptionally high growth yields are obtained with *C. thermoaceticum* (10) and this seems to indicate that more energy (ATP) is available for growth than what can be predicted to be formed by substrate phosphorylation.

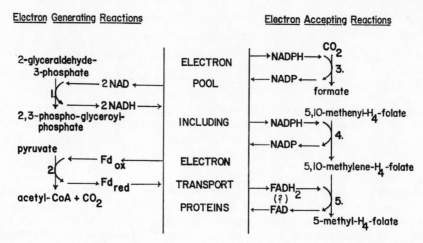

Figure 3. Electron generating and accepting reactions in fermentations by *C. thermoaceticum*. The enzymes are: 1, glyceraldehyde 3-
phosphate dehydrogenase; 2, pyruvate-ferredoxin oxidoreductase; 3,
formate dehydrogenase; 4, methylene-H_4folate dehydrogenase; 5,
methylene-H_4folate reductase.

All our attempts to demonstrate a direct transhydrogenation
between NADH and NADP have failed, and the electron transfer between
the electron-generating and electron-accepting reactions remains to
be fully explained. However, our studies have led to the isolation
of a ferredoxin (24), two rubredoxins (25), a FMN-containing rubredoxin reductase (26) and to the demonstration of a cytochrome b and
menaquinone (27) in *C. thermoaceticum*.

Ferredoxin is involved in the final steps of acetate synthesis
from CO_2, in which methyltetrahydrofolate or a methylcorrinoid
together with the carboxyl group of pyruvate form acetate (20, 28).
The role of ferredoxin in these steps is not clear, however, its
role may be connected with the function of pyruvate. A pyruvate-
ferredoxin oxido-reductase has been demonstrated in *C. thermoaceticum* (24,29) and extracts from this bacterium catalyze the transfer
of electrons from reduced ferredoxin to NADP. Ferredoxin is also
an acceptor of electrons in the oxidation of carbon monoxide (19).
Interestingly, in this reaction, cytochrome b also serves as an
electron acceptor.

A role for the rubredoxins in the metabolism of *C. thermoaceticum* is yet to be found. However, both rubredoxins are irreversibly
reduced by NAPH or NADPH in a reaction which is catalyzed by a FMN-
containing protein (26). This protein, which we refer to as

rubredoxin reductase, catalyzes the following reactions:

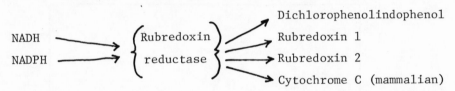

The rubredoxin reductase has been purified to homogeneity. It has a M_r of 30,000 and contains 1 mol of FMN. The FMN of the enzyme in the presence of NADH or NADPH is completely reduced. This reduction appears irreversible and the enzyme does not function as a NADH-NADP transhydrogenase.

It is evident from the above discussion that electron transfer reactions are playing an important role in *C. thermoaceticum*. It is predicted that these reactions will be found to be important in the regulation of the rates of fermentations of glucose, fructose and xylose by this bacterium. Thus, further studies of these reactions are warranted, especially if one considers using *C. thermoaceticum* for industrial applications.

CLOSTRIDIUM THERMOHYDROSULFURICUM

Extreme thermophilic bacteria are those that grow and reproduce at temperatures about 70°C (2). Tansey and Brock (30) have compiled an extensive list of thermophilic microorganisms. This list contains a rather large number of aerobic, but only few anaerobic, extreme thermophiles. In our laboratory, we have for a number of years been searching for anaerobic, extreme thermophiles in natural environments (31). It is evident that the list of these microorganisms will greatly increase in the future. So far, our studies have led to the isolation of *Clostridium thermohydrosulfuricum* (7) from many soil and mud samples and to the discovery of *Thermoanaerobacter ethanolicus* (8), which will be discussed later in this presentation.

Klaushofer and Parkkinen (32) first isolated *C. thermohydro-sulfuricum* from juices in an Austrian sugar factory. Hollaus and Sleytr (33) studied its taxonomy and cell wall fine structure. Our finding (7) that this microorganism occurs in many different natural habitats has been confirmed by Zeikus (1).

C. thermohydrosulfuricum grows between 38°C to 78°C. Optimal growth occurs around 70°C, at which temperature the doubling time is about 70 min. The pH-optimum is rather narrow (between 6.9 - 7.5) although it grows from pH 5.5 to pH 9.3. It has a wide substrate spectrum and grows on glucose, galactose, mannose, fructose, xylose, ribose, cellobiose, sucrose, maltose, raffinose, starch and

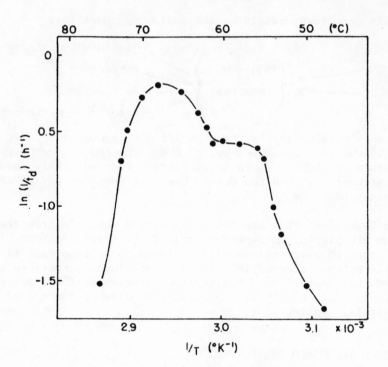

Figure 4. Arrhenius plot. Natural log of growth rate of *C. thermo-hydrosulfuricum* versus the reciprocal of temperature (°K) (7).

pectin. The stoichiometry of the fermentation of glucose may be expressed as follows:

$$C_6H_{12}O_6 + 0.5 \ H_2O \longrightarrow$$
$$\underline{\hspace{1cm}} C_2H_5OH + 0.5 \ CH_3COOH + 0.5 \ CH_3CHOHCOOH + 1.5 \ CO_2 + H_2$$

However, variations in this stoichiometry are often observed and we have obtained ethanol yields as high as 1.5 mol per mol of glucose. Thus, this organism may be useful for the production of ethanol. Thi will undoubtedly be discussed by Dr. Zeikus (34) during this sympo-sium.

During our studies of the rate of growth of *C. thermohydro-sulfuricum* as a function of temperature, we found that the increase in the growth rate did not follow a straight line in an Arrhenius plot as has been found for many microorganisms. Instead, the line in the Arrhenius plot exhibited a plateau between 55°C and 62°C (7) (Figure 4). Thus, the growth rate of *C. thermohydrosulfuricum* is the same at 62°C as it is at 55°C. We do not know the reason for this critical temperature interval, but it is conceivable that it reflects a transition temperature above which new proteins have to be synthesized for the microorganism to function. Evidence for such a concept has been presented by Haberstich and Zuber (35). To obtain an indication of such a possibility, we have studied the protein composition of *C. thermohydrosulfuricum* grown at 50°C and 70°C using the method of O'Farrell (36). In this technique, the proteins are separated by two-dimensional polyacrylamide gel electrophoresis. In the first dimension, the separation is based on isoelectric points, whereas, in the second dimension, it is based on molecular weights of the proteins. The results are shown in Figure 5.

The first impression is that the protein "maps" of the 50°C- and the 70°C-grown bacteria are much alike. This indicates that the maps are from the same bacterium, which rules out the possibility that the culture consists of two different bacteria -- one which grows below the critical temperature and a second which grows above that temperature. However, differences exist between the two maps. There are fewer proteins in the 70°C-grown cells in comparison with those grown at 50°C. This is especially evident in the middle region where proteins of Mr 60,000 and with pI between 5.5 and 6.5 appear. Clearly, cells grown at 70°C synthesize fewer proteins than cells grown at 50°C. More interestingly, however, is the fact that a few proteins marked by arrows are more noticeable in 70°C-grown cells than in those grown at 50°C. These proteins may be of importance for the bacterium's ability to grow at the higher temperature. Although our results are preliminary and should be interpreted with caution, they seem to indicate that in *C. thermohydrosulfuricum* the synthesis of some proteins is turned off at high temperatures, whereas the synthesis of other proteins is turned on.

THERMOANAEROBACTER ETHANOLICUS

Earlier we reported (37) the isolation of two strains of a thermophilic bacterium, JW200 and JW201. The strains were obtained from hot springs in the Yellowstone National Park. They fermented glucose to ethanol and CO_2 with a stoichiometry similar to that of yeast. We have now proposed the name *Thermoanaerobacter ethanolicus* for this bacterium (38).

T. ethanolicus is a non-spore-forming, peritrichously flagellated rod. The cell size varies and coccoid-shaped or spheroplast-like forms appear. It grown between 37°C and 78°C with a temperature optimum at 69°C. The pH range is from 4.5 to 9.8, and the pH-optimum is broad: between 5.7-8.6. It ferments glucose, galactose, mannose, fructose, xylose, ribose, arabinose, cellobiose, sucrose, maltose, raffinose, starch and pectin.

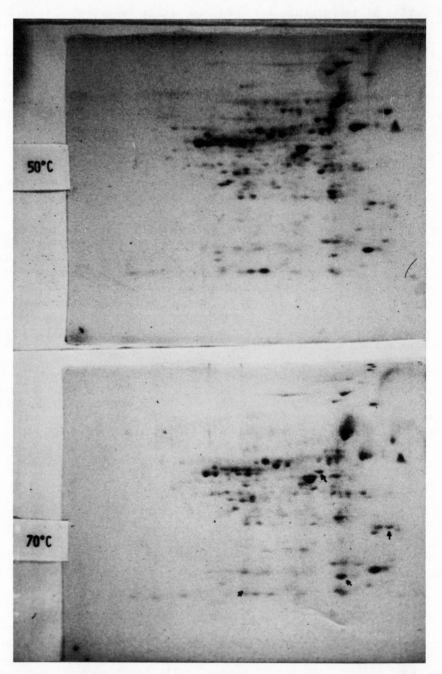

Figure 5. Two-dimensional protein maps of *C. thermohydrosulfuricum* grown at 50°C and 70°C. Proteins outstanding in the 70°C map are marked with arrows.

The fermentation balance obtained using 0.5% glucose as the substrate is represented by the following equation:

$$C_6H_{12}O_6 + 0.2 \ H_2O \longrightarrow$$

$$\underline{} 1.8C_2H_5OH + 0.1 \ CH_3COOH + 0.1 \ CH_3CHOHCOOH + 1.9 \ CO_2 + 0.2H_2$$

Thus, in addition to ethanol and CO_2, small amounts of acetate, lactate and hydrogen are produced. The same fermentation balance is obtained in fermentations of 0.5% starch or cellobiose.

T. ethanolicus grows well at substrate concentrations much higher than 0.5%; we have used media containing 20% starch. However, with strain JW200, the ethanol concentration, which is obtained, rarely exceeds 80 mM, although according to the amount of substrate fermented, much higher yields of ethanol were expected. We have now found that at substrate concentrations above 1% a shift in the fermentation occurs with the formation of more acetate and lactate and less ethanol.

In attemps to overcome the regulatory mechanism apparently operating at high substrate concentrations and to shift the fermentation toward ethanol formation with high substrate concentrations, we have exposed the wild type JW200 to UV-light and to media deficient in iron. Both these treatments have successfully produced apparent mutant strains which ferment starch at high concentration to ethanol and with reduced formation of acetate. Ethanol concentrations as high as 400 mM have been obtained. This is shown in Figure 6, using the mutant strain JW200 Fe, which was obtained after growth in iron-deficient medium.

The formation of ethanol in strain JW200, in addition to being controlled by the substrate concentration, is also affected by the alcohol dehydrogenase. This enzyme from the wild type has been studied to some extent (39). It catalyzes the following reaction:

$$CH_3CH_2OH + NADP^+ \xrightleftharpoons{} CH_3CHO + NADPH + H^+$$

The enzyme is specific for NADP; NAD is reduced at less than 0.5% of the rate of reduction of NADP. At high concentrations, NAD acts as an inhibitor. The enzyme has been purified to homogeneity. It has a Mr of 176,000 and it consists of four apparently identical subunits. The Mr of the subunits is 43,000. Like many other alcohol dehydrogenases (40), the enzyme from *T. ethanolicus* contains zinc. Analyses using atomic absorption indicate each subunit contains four Zn atoms. The enzyme is very heat stable and can be stored at 70°C for more than 2 days. At 80°C the enzyme is slowly denaturated. The optimum temperature for the enzyme reaction is at about 95°C.

The specificity for the alcohol-substrate is broad. This is

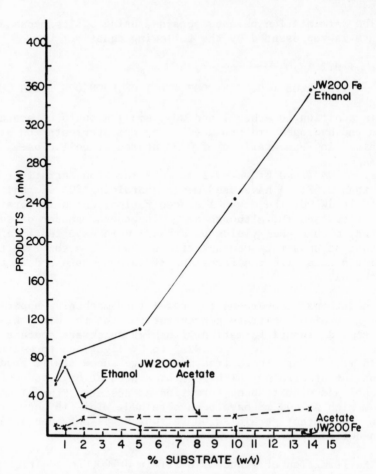

Figure 6.   Ethanol and acetate formation as dependent of the substrate concentration (starch) with *T. ethanolicus* wild type strain
JW200 and "mutant" strain JW200 Fe.   The incubations were for 77 h
at 68° and pH 6.8.

shown in Table I.   Interestingly, 2-propanol, allylalcohol and 2-
butanol appear to be better substrates than ethanol.   Kinetic
studies indicate that the enzyme may have allosteric control with
ethanol as the effector.   This is shown in Figure 7.   Clearly the
rate of the enzyme reaction is greatly influenced by the concentration of ethanol.   This fact may partly explain why a shift from
ethanol toward acetate and lactate occurs with the wild type substrate concentrations over 1%.   We have now started work with the
alcohol dehydrogenase from the mutant strains to elucidate this
point.

TABLE I

Substrates for Alcohol Dehydrogenase from
Thermoanaerobacter Ethanolicus

Substrate	Relative Activity
Ethanol	100
Methanol	75
1-Propanol	74
2-Propanol	1600
1-Butanol	4
2-Butanol	124
Allylalcohol	210
Ethylenglycol	2.6
Methoxy ethanol	4.0
2-Aminoethanol	0

ANAEROBIC, EXTREME THERMOPHILES FROM ICELAND

Encouraged by our successful isolation of strains of *C. ther-mohydrosulfuricum* and *T. ethanolicus* we have embarked on a screening program of anaerobic microorganisms indigenous to hot springs in Iceland. This work is being done in cooperation with the Agricultural Research Institute of Iceland and the help of Drs. Gretar Gudbergsson and Björn Sigurbjörnsson is greatfully acknowledged.

The hot springs in Iceland vary greatly in temperature and pH. This is shown in Table 2, which lists designation of samples that we are studying presently. The chemical contents of several of the springs have been determined and we will be able to correlate types of microorganisms with the chemical contents of the springs. At this meeting our intent is only to demonstrate the existence of the great variety of anaerobic microorganisms that live at extreme temperature and pH and to point out that to look for new microorganisms in nature is a fruitful endeavor. We have chosen the samples GG-1 and GG-13 for illustration. The samples were collected at 97°C, pH 5.0 and 90°C, pH 5.5., respectively.

GG-1 is from the Krysivik thermal area and originates from a mud pool. Most bacteria appear to be cocci of different sizes and possibly also similar to plasma. Very few rods were found in this sample. Ten ml of media containing lactate (60 mM), glucose (0.5%) or with a gas phase of CO_2/H_2 (20/80%) mixture, were inoculated with 0.1 ml sample and incubated for 90 h or 9 days at 90°C and pH 5. Gas chromatography analyses reveal the formation of methane and methanol and very little other volatile products. This is shown in Figure 8. Methane is dominant after 90 h of incubation in the glucose and CO_2/H_2 media, whereas methanol is high in the culture grown on lactate. After 9 days incubation at 90°C, the lactate culture shows a considerable increase in both methane and methanol over that of the 90 h culture.

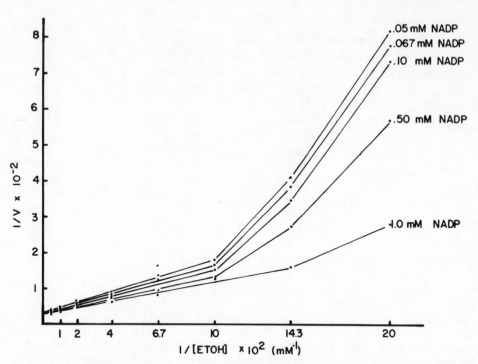

Figure 7. Double reciprocal plot of the initial rate of the alcohol dehydrogenase reaction, using ethanol as the varied substrate. The reactions were performed at 70°C at pH 9 in 50 mM Tris-buffer.

The GG-13 sample was collected in the Hveragardi thermal area from an open water spring. It contains small rods and small cocci. The latter clearly tend to lump together into packages. Samples of GG-13 were grown in exactly the same way as was described for the GG-1 sample. Gas chromatography tracings are shown in Figure 9. They were obtained after 90 h of incubation at 90°C and pH 5.5. Similarly to the GG-1 sample, methane and methanol were formed as products but, in addition, a relatively large amount of ethanol was produced. This especially was evident with glucose as the substrate. We believe that our result demonstrates that mixed populations of anaerobic, extreme thermophilic bacteria exist in thermal springs with temperatures of 90°C and higher. Furthermore, we believe that bacteria from such springs may be used industrially. We are now in the process of isolating pure cultures.

Recently, we have established enrichment cultures from samples obtained from Iceland that ferment cellulose. These cultures have been obtained from very different environments. This is shown in

TABLE II

Iceland: Sampling Conditions

Temperature	pH		
	3 → 4	4 → 7	8 → 9
40 → 50		GG - 23D; GG - 8C	
50 → 60	GG - 6A GG - 8 (A,B)	GG - 3 (A,B,C); GG - 23C	GG - 25D
60 → 70		GG - 4; GG - 12 (A,B)	GG - 22 (A,B,C) GG - 25C
70 → 80	GG - 2; GG - 6B	GG - 7 GG - 24; GG - 23 (A,B)	GG - 14 (A,B,C); GG - 25A; GG - 10; GG - 25B
80 → 97	GG - 5	GG - 1; GG - 13	

GG-1, GG-2, etc. represent established cultures of samples obtained.

Figure 10 which shows liquid chromatography tracings of carbohydrates obtained using a Hewlett-Packard 1084B HPLC instrument equipped with refractive index detector. The growth medium contained 0.1 g of filter paper per 10 ml as the only organic material. Yeast extract or vitamins were not added. The buffer solution contained 0.1 M sulfate ions which appear to promote growth of the cellulolytic cultures. The first tracing is of a culture incubated for 4 days at 84°C, pH 8.6, the second tracing from a 9-day culture at 56°C and pH 4, whereas the third culture is from a 9-day incubation at 37°C and pH 2. The first peak represents non-gaseous products such as acetate, ethanol, lactate, etc.; the second peak (clearly observed only with the pH 2 culture) is glucose; the third and larger peak obtained with all cultures is cellobiose. Trioses and larger oligomers are represented in the subsequent peaks. These results, although preliminary, demonstrate the existence of cellulolytic bacteria, which are capable of fermenting cellulose in environments as extreme as pH 2 and at temperatures as high as 84°C. Cellobiose accumulates in all three cultures. This is in agreement with the suggestion by Eriksson (41) and Peck (42) that cellobiose plays an important role in the degradation of cellulose.

SUMMARY

In this presentation, we have discussed that the acetogenic thermophilic bacterium, *Clostridium thermoaceticum*, ferments glucose almost quantitatively to acetate. That part of the acetate is formed from CO_2, which functions as the electron sink. We have demonstrated that enzymes in the acetate formation contain trace elements such as iron, cobalt, nickel, selenium and tungsten.

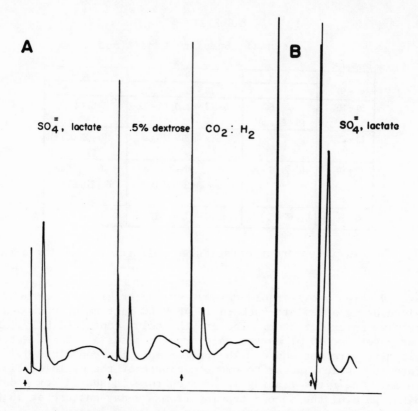

Figure 8. Gas chromatograph-tracings of volatile products found on media as indicated with culture GG-1 (Table II). Samples A were taken 90 h after inoculation and sample B after 9 days. The incubation temperature was 90°C and the initial pH was 5.0. Arrows indicate injection time. The peaks represent in order of appearance methane, methanol and ethanol. The column (Poropak GC) was run at 80°C with N_2.

Furthermore, we have indicated that this bacterium must have an electron transport system, which is not yet completely understood. With *Clostridium thermohydrosulfuricum* we have obtained results which indicate that this thermophile may selectively produce proteins dependent on the environmental temperature. We have presented a new bacterium, *Thermoanaerobacter ethanolicus*, which ferments several sugars including starch, cellobiose, and xylose to ethanol. We have demonstrated the existence in a thermal environment of anaerobic bacteria that grow at temperatures of around 90°C and which are capable of fermenting diverse substrates such as lactate, glucose, and cellulose.

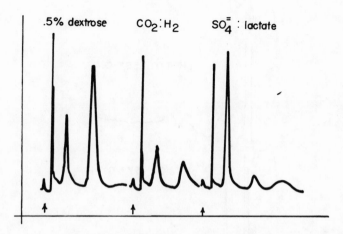

Figure 9. Gas chromatograph-tracings of volatile products found
on media as indicated with culture GG 13 (Table II). The initial
pH was 5.5. All other conditions were those described in the
legend of Figure 8.

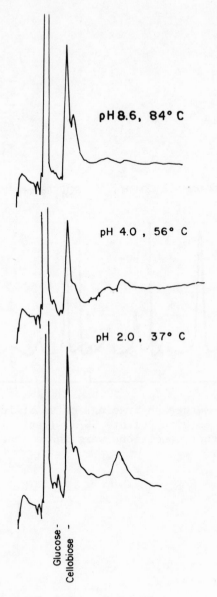

Figure 10.   Liquid chromatograph-tracings of carbohydrates formed by three Incelandic cultures grown on cellulose.   Details are given in the text.

ACKNOWLEDGEMENT

The work was supported by the U.S. Department of Energy under Contract No. DEAS-09-97 ER-10499, Public Health Service Grant AM27323 from the National Institute of Arthritis, Metabolic and Digestive Diseases; National Science Foundation Grant PCM-7726054 and by contributions from the University of Georgia, Research Foundation, Inc.

REFERENCES

1. Zeikus, J.G. (1980) Chemical and fuel production by anaerobic bacteria. Annu. Rev. Microbiol. 34, 423-464.
2. Ljungdahl, L.G. (1979) Physiology of thermophilic bacteria. Adv. Microbial Physiol. 19, 149-243.
3. Lymn, A.H., and Langwell, H. (1923) Discussion on the action of bacteria on cellulosic materials. J. Soc. Chem. Ind. pp280 T-283T.
4. Sandegren, E., Enebo, L. and Ljungdahl, L.G. (1953) Investigations on cellulase of barley and of bacteria connected with thermophilic cellulose fermentation. Proceedings from II Congress International des Industries de Fermentations. pp 139-146, Bruxelles, Belgium.
5. Ljungdahl, L.G. and Wood, H.G. (1969) Total synthesis of acetate from CO_2 by heterotrophic bacteria. Annu. Rev. Microbiol. 23, 515-538.
6. Ljungdahl, L.G., and Wood, H.G. (1980) Acetate Biosynthesis. in "Vitamin B_{12}" (Dolphin, D. ed.) John Wiley and Sons, Inc. N.Y. In press.
7. Wiegel, J., Ljungdahl, L.G. and Rawson, J.R. (1979) Isolation from soil and properties of the extreme thermophile *Clostridium thermohydrosulfuricum* J. Bacteriol. 139, 800-810.
8. Wiegel, J., and Ljungdahl, L.G. (1981) *Thermoanaerobacter ethanolicus* gen. nov., spec. nov. A new extreme thermophilic anaerobic bacterium. Arch. Microbiol. In press.
9. Fontaine, F.E., Peterson, W.H., McCoy, E., Johnson, M.J., and Ritter, G.J. (1942) A new type of glucose fermentation by *Clostridium thermoaceticum* n. sp. J. Bacteriol. 43, 701-715.
10. Andreesen, J.R., Schaupp, A., Neurauter, C., Brown, A., and Ljungdahl, L.G. (1973) Fermentation of glucose, fructose, and xylose by *Clostridium thermoaceticum*: Effect of metals on growth yield, enzymes, and the synthesis of acetate from CO_2.
11. Barker, H.A. (1944) On the role of carbon dioxide in the metabolism of *Clostridium thermoaceticum*. Proc. Nat. Acad. Sci. U.S. 30, 88-90.
12. Wood, H.G. (1952) A study of carbon dioxide fixation by mass determination of the types of C^{13}-acetate. J. Biol. Chem. 194, 905-931.
13. Schaupp, A., and Ljungdahl, L.G. (1974) Purification and

properties of acetate kinase from *Clostridium thermoaceticum*. Arch. Microbiol. 100, 121-129.

14. Schulman, M., Ghambeer, R.K., Ljungdahl, L.G. and Wood, H.G. (1973). Total synthesis of acetate from CO_2. VII. Evidence with *Clostridium thermoaceticum* that the carboxyl of acetate is derived from the carboxyl of pyruvate by transcarboxylation and not by fixation of CO_2. J. Biol. Chem. 248, 6255-6261.

15. Diekert, G.B., and Thauer, R.K. (1978) Carbon monoxide oxidation by *Clostridium thermoaceticum* and *Clostridium formicoaceticum*. J. Bacteriol. 136, 597-606.

16. Andreesen, J.R., Gottschalk, G., and Schlegel, H.G. (1970) *Clostridium formicoaceticum* nov. spec. Isolation, description and distinction from *C. aceticum* and *C. thermoaceticum*. Arch. Mikrobiol. 72, 154-174.

17. O'Brien, W.E., and Ljungdahl, L.G. (1972) Fermentation of fructose and synthesis of acetate from carbon dioxide by *Clostridium formicoaceticum*. J. Bacteriol. 109, 626-632 .

18. Diekert, G., and Thauer, R.K. (1980) The effect of nickel on carbon monoxide dehydrogenase formation in *Clostridium thermoaceticum* and *Clostridium formicoaceticum*. FEMS Microbiol. Lett. 7, 187-189.

19. Drake, H.L., Hu, S.-I., and Wood, H.G. (1980) Purification of carbon monoxide dehydrogenase, a nickel enzyme from *Clostridium thermoaceticum*. J. Biol. Chem. 255, 7174-7180.

20. Drake, H.L., Hu, S.-I. and Wood, H.G. (1979) Acetate synthesi by *Clostridium thermoaceticum*. Abstr. 04-3-599, p. 279. XIth Inter. Cong. Biochemistry, Toronto, Canada and Personal Communication.

21. Andreesen, J.R. and Ljungdahl, L.G. (1973) Formate dehydrogenase of *Clostridium thermoaceticum*: Incorporation of selenite, molybdate and tungstate on the enzyme. J. Bacteriol. 116, 867-873.

22. Ljungdahl, L.G. and Andreesen, J.R. (1976) Reduction of CO_2 to acetate in homoacetate fermenting clostridia and the involvement of tungsten in formate dehydrogenase. In "Microbial Production and Utilization of Gases" (Schlegel, H., Gottschal, G. and Pfennig, N., eds.) pp. 163-172. E. Goltze K. G. Gottinger.

23. Saiki, T., Shackleford, G., and Ljungdahl, L.G. (1981) Composition of tungsten-selenium containing formate dehydrogenase from *Clostridium thermoaceticum*. In "Proc. Symp. on Selenium in Biology and Medicine" (Martin, J.L. ed.) Chapter 20. AVI Publ. Comp. Westport, Conn. In press.

24. Yang, S.-S., Ljungdahl, L.G. and LeGall, J. (1977) A four-iron, four-sulfide ferredoxin with high thermostability from *Clostridium thermoaceticum*. J. Bacteriol. 130, 1084-1090.

25. Yang, S.-S., Lyngdahl, L.G., DerVartanian, D.V. and Watt, G.D. (1980) Isolation and characterization of two rubredoxins from *Clostridium thermoaceticum*. Biochim. Biophys. Acta. 590, 24-33.

26. Yang, S.-S., and Ljungdahl, L.G. (1977) Properties of two rubrodoxins and a NAD(P)H-rubredoxin reductase isolated from *Clostridium thermoaceticum*. Abstr. K. 135 Annu. Meet. Am. Soc. Microbiol. New Orleans.

27. Gottwald, M., Andreesen, J.R., LeGall, J., and Ljungdahl, L.G. (1975) Presence of cytochrome and menaquinone in *Clostridium formicoaceticum* and *Clostridium thermoaceticum*. J. Bacteriol. 122, 325-328.

28. Poston, J.M. and Stadtman, E.R. (1967) The conversion of carbon dioxide to acetate. III. Demonstration of ferredoxin in the system converting Co-^{14}CH$_3$-cobalamin to acetate. Biochem. Biophys. Res. Commun. 26, 550-555.

29. Thauer, R.K. (1972) CO$_2$-reduction to formate by NADPH. The initial step in the total synthesis of acetate from CO$_2$ in *Clostridium thermoaceticum*. FEBS Lett. 27, 111-115.

30. Tansey, M.R., and Brock, T.D. (1978) Microbial life at high temperatures: Ecological aspects. In "Microbial Life in Extreme Environments" (D.J. Kushner, ed) pp. 159-216, Academic Press, London.

31. Wiegel, J. and Ljungdahl, L.G. (1979) Ethanol as fermentation product of extreme thermophilic, anaerobic bacteria. In "4th Symp. Technische Mikrobiologie (Dellweg, H. ed) pp. 117-127, Verlag Versuchs-und Lehranstalt fur Spiritusfabrikation und Fermentationstechnologie, Berlin.

32. Klaushofer, H. and Parkkinen, E. (1965) Zur Frage der Bedeutung aerober und anaerober thermophiler Sporenbildner als Infectionsursache in Rubenzucker-fabriken. I. *Clostridium thermohydrosulfuricum* eine neue Art eines saccharoseabbauenden thermophilen schwefelwasser stoffbildenden Clostridiums. Z. Zuckerind. Boehm. 15, 445-449.

33. Hollaus, F. and Sleutr, U. (1972) On the taxonomy and fine structure of some hyper thermophilic saccharolytic clostridia. Arch. Microbiol. 88, 129-146.

34. Zeikus, J.G. (1981) This symposium.

35. Haberstich, H.U. and Zuber, H. (1974) Thermoadation of enzymes in thermophilic and mesophilic cultures of Bacillus *stearothermophilus* and *Bacillus caldotenax*. Arch. Microbiol. 98, 275-287.

36. O'Farrell, P.H. (1975) High resolution two-dimensional electrophoresis of proteins. J. Biol. Chem. 250, 4007-4021.

37. Wiegel, J. and Ljungdahl, L.G. (1979) Isolation and characterization of a new extreme thermophilic anaerobic bacterium. Abstr. I 63 Annu. Meet. Am. Soc. Microbiol. Los Angeles.

38. Wiegel, J. and Ljungdahl, L.G. (1981) *Thermoanaerobacter ethanolicus* gen. nov., spec. nov., a new extreme thermophilic anaerobic bacterium. Arch. Microbiol. In press.

39. Bryant, F.O., and Ljungdahl, L.G. (1981) NADP-dependent alcohol dehydrogenase from *Thermoanaerobacter ethanolicus*. Abstr. K44 Annu. Meet. Am. Soc. Microbiol. Dallas.

40. Brandeń, C.-I., Jornvall, H., Eklund, H., and Furngren, B. (1975) Alcohol dehydrogenases. In "The Enzyme" Vol. 11, Part A (Boyer, P.D. ed)pp. 103-190, Academic Press, New York.

41.   Eriksson, K.E. (1981) This symposium.
42.   Peck, H.D., Jr. (1981) This symposium.

DISCUSSION

Q.   LEADBETTER: In *Clostridium thermohydrosulfuricum*, for which
      you showed a biphasic temperature plot, are the fermentation
      products identical at 60°C and 70°C if you grow the organism
      at the two different temperature?

A.   LJUNGDAHL: Yes, they are. I would also like to mention that
      Thermoanaerobacter ethanolicus has a biphasic temperature
      plot. I believe we will find such plots in bacteria, which
      have large temperature spans like the two I have mentioned.
      They grow between 37°C and 78°C. Normally bacteria have only
      temperature ranges of 30° or less. I think it is possible
      that bacteria with a large temperature span need a mechanism
      to switch from low temperature growth to high temperature
      growth. The biphasic plot may reflect such a switch.

Q.   ERIKSSON: Lars, after having listened to your interesting pre
      sentation maybe many of us are thinking in the wrong direction
      We are trying to adapt bacteria to higher external concentra-
      tions of ethanol. Perhaps ethanol tolerance is regulated by
      the alcohol dehydrogenase.

A.   The evidence we have indicates that in *Thermoanaerobacter*
      ethanolicus this is the case. However, our results are pre-
      liminary. The enzyme has very strong "allosteric" properties
      and clearly it is "turned off" when the ethanol concentration
      increases.

Q.   WOLFE: Is there any evidence for a nickel co-factor in
      Clostridium thermoaceticum? Is the nickel on the protein or
      on some unique co-factor?

A.   LJUNGDAHL: I do not think that there is any evidence for a
      co-factor. Results from Harland G. Wood's laboratory indicate
      that the nickel is bound or closely associated with the pro-
      tein as has been demonstrated using labelled nickel. As far
      as I know a nickel co-factor like the one observed with methane
      bacteria has not been demonstrated in acetogenic bacteria.

Q.   GOTTSCHALK: I have a question in connection with the question
      by Dr. Eriksson. Is there anything known about the mechanism
      of the export of ethanol from the bacteria you discussed and
      about the concentration of ethanol inside the cells?

A.   LJUNGDAHL: We do not know much about this at all; actually, we know nothing. However, I can say that the bacteria tolerate 10% ethanol, and that bacteria stored for a period in 10% ethanol start to grow immediately when they are transferred to a regular medium. To me, that indicates that the ethanol is not destroying the bacterium, e.g., by effecting the membrane.

Q.   REDDY: In *Clostridium thermoaceticum* have you looked for hydrogen evolution? And a second question, is there any evidence for electron transfer phosphorylation?

A.   LJUNGDAHL: We have not observed hydrogen evolution in that bacterium. It does not have a hydrogenase, at least, nobody has found it. Although, the enzyme has been looked for by several investigators. As to the second question, the only evidence for electron transfer phosphorylation are high growth yields.

FORMATION OF HYDROCARBONS BY BACTERIA AND ALGAE

Thomas G. Tornabene

Solar Energy Research Institute

Golden, Colorado 80401

The chemical investigation of biologically synthesized hydro-carbons did not begin early in the history of the systematic study of fats. All the neutral or highly non-polar lipids were included in a category of compounds designated as waxes. The waxes were monoesters of fatty acids and long chain alcohols, hydrocarbons, long chain alcohols, and high molecular weight compounds. Systematic investigations into the derivation and chemical nature of the consti-tuents of waxes was started in 1942 by the American Petroleum Institute Project 43 which was designed to determine a) the part played by microorganisms in the formation of petroleum, b) the type hydrocarbons synthesized as animal and plant products to the extent and variety necessary to be able to form crude oil and c) whether radioactive and thermal sources of energy can transform organic matter into petroleum. The rationale for this project was apparently based on a number of factors. In 1899 it was proposed that complex organisms, such as trees, fish and animal fats could be a direct source of the hydrocarbons in petroleum (1). In 1906, the isoprenoid hydrocarbon squalene was isolated as the major constituent of shark liver oil (2-4). Diatom nobs in tertiary opal shales were reported in 1926 (5). These nobs were apparently secreted primarily by diatoms including the hydrocarbons and other organic matter found in them. Based on the field and microscopic studies of sediments and diatom blooms, Becking et al.(6) concluded in 1927 that diatoms directly produce hydrocarbon oils. Trask suggested in 1932 (7) on the basis of a laboratory experiment that bacteria are capable of creating reducing conditions for conversion of organic material into oil. Since these reports, simple organisms such as algae, foraminifera and bacteria were proposed as the sources of the hydrocarbons on the consideration of the age of petroleum (8) and the ability of the microorganism to survive under anaerobic and other adverse conditions (9).

Project 43A under the direction of Zobell investigated the
action of bacteria on organic substances and the possible hydrocarbons produced by bacteria as component parts of their cell substance (10-12). In a series of papers it was reported that a)
practically all hydrocarbons can be attacked under suitable conditions by some bacterial form (10), b) bacteria can convert caproic
acid to hydrocarbons of the C-20 to C-25 range (11), and c) marine
bacteria such as *Serratia marinorubra* contain appreciable amounts
of liquid and solid hydrocarbon substances (12). It was also
speculated that bacteria might contribute to the liberation and mi-
gration of oil by destroying organic and inorganic structures in
which the oil may be entrapped and by producing emulsion agents,
as fatty acids, that enabled oil to migrate. The finding that
caproic acid could be converted to hydrocarbons by bacteria was
considered a major breakthrough, offering a possible explanation
to earlier work in 1931 which had shown fatty acids to be transformed into methane and carbon dioxide (13). In a progress report
for A.P.I., Knebel (14) reported that a freshwater sediment contained
hydrocarbons, confirming that not all hydrocarbons in recent sediments are destroyed by bacterial action. The most significant part
of the report was that hydrocarbons extracted from bacteria and algae
exhibited optical properties comparable to the optical activity of
the active fractions of petroleum. Nevertheless, no information was
obtained concerning the nature and composition of microbial intracellular hydrocarbons. The A.P.I. project was terminated in 1952.
Some significant results emerged from this project but no clear,
definitive data were generated to support the concept of biotic
origin of petroleum hydrocarbons. Scattered reports on microbial
production of hydrocarbons continued to appear until 1967 but with
emphasis on the hydrocarbons as possible biological markers for
studying geologic time and geologic conditions (15).

A resurgence in the biotic theory of origin of petroleum resulted in the mid-1960's from the finding of large amounts of
alveolar "yellow bodies" in carboniferous limestone series of the
Scottish Lothian (Torbanite). These yellow bodies were identified
as the remains of an alga that appeared identical to those from the
contemporary alga *Botryococcus braunii*. It was subsequently shown
that 80% of the organic material of the brown resting stage of the
alga was acyclic hydrocarbon (16,17). "Each cell is embedded in a
cup of oil and when a cell divides into two daughter cells the
latter secrete oil, while remaining inside the cup of the mother
cell. Thus the matrix of the colony is built up of the cups of the
daughter cells" (16,18). It was believed that the Torbanite
orginated from *B. braunii*.

It is known today that isoprenoid and non-isoprenoid acyclic
hydrocarbons are components of most microorganisms. The concentrations of the hydrocarbons, however, vary from only trace constituents to major components of the cellular organic materials.

The hydrocarbon synthesizing capability of microorganisms that produce them as a major constituent are restricted to only few algal, bacterial and fungal species. Individual species that produce hydrocarbons as major components have been isolated from mesophilic, thermophilic, psychrophilic, acidophilic, alkalinophilic and halophilic environments under aerobic or anaerobic, autotrophic or hetertrophic conditions. The environmental distribution of hydrocarbon producers follows no discernible pattern that can be used as a guide for finding prolific hydrocarbon producers.

Hydrocarbons other than squalene generally occur as only trace constituents of marine animals, but may be major components of algae. In a variety of marine and freshwater algae, including a red, greens, browns, diatoms and phytoplankton, the hydrocarbon heneicosahexaene (C-21:6) exists in amounts inversely correlated with the abundance of the long-chain highly unsaturated fatty acid (C-22:6) (19-23). The all cis-3,6,9,12,15,18-heneicosahexaene was first isolated from the diatom *Skeletonema costatum* (24). Since then, the isomer all cis-1, 6,9,12,15,18-heneicosahexaene was reported in a variety of other algae (19-23), diatoms (19-23), and phytoplankton (19-23). It now appears that the Δ^1 isomer is produced by only the brown algae, that the Δ^3 isomer occurs in green algae and diatoms and with one exception, the red algae do not produce significant amounts of these polyunsaturated hydrocarbons (25). The exact structure of the positional isomer of the polyunsaturated hydrocarbon in phytoplankton is unresolved. This polyunsaturated hydrocarbon is produced in quantities exceeding 1% of the total dry weight of some species of brown and green algae. In contrast, nonphotosynthetic diatoms, dinoflagellates, cyanobacteria and photosynthetic bacteria contain traces of aliphatic hydrocarbons, but no C-21:6.

Blumer et al.(26) surveyed microalgae for hydrocarbon content. Their analyses of 23 species of algae belonging to 9 algal classes yielded results similar to those of Lee and Loeblich (19) and Youngblood et al.(27). Lee and Loeblich reported the distribution and quantitation of 21:6 hydrocarbons and 22:6 fatty acid within the major groups of algae in both marine and freshwater environments while Youngblood et al.(27) identified both the saturated and olefinic hydrocarbons of 4 green, 14 brown and 6 red benthic marine algae from the Cape Cod area of Massachusetts, USA (Table I). Their data indicated that n-pentadecane (C-15) predominates in brown algae, n-heptadecane (C-17) in red algae, olefins predominate in green and brown algae, and that polyunsaturated C-19 and C-21 hydrocarbons occur in brown and green algae and in only a few of the red algal species (20,25,27). A C-17 alkyl-cyclopropane was tentatively identified in two species of green algae. Among the unsaturated hydrocarbons, mono- and di-olefinic C-15 and C-17 hydrocarbons were common. Similar data were reported by Shaw and Wiggs (28) for Alaskan marine intertidal algae.

TABLE I

Principal Normal Hydrocarbons In Marine Algae

SPECIES	15:0*	15:1	17:0	17:1	17:2	17:3	19:5	19:6	21:5	21:6	23:0	24:0	25:0	26:0
Green Algae														
Enteromorpha compressa														
Ulva Lactuca				96										
Spongomorpha arcta				88					2.2	4.0				
Codium fragile			89.0	5.9			9.4	6.7	22.0	60.0				
Brown Algae														
Ectocarpus fasciculatus	7.0									91.0				
Pilayella littorales	59.0		3.6							98.0				
Leathesia difformis	85.0										5.7	13.0	6.0	5.4
Punctaria latifolia	38.0									5.9				
Scytosiphon lomentaria	38.0		11.0	15.0		4.2	19.0							
Chorda filum	31.0		2.3						37.0	10.0				
Chorda tomentosa	73.0						2.5	2.7	17.0	47.0				
Laminaria agardhii	64.0							9.7	2.8	3.8	2.4		4.2	5.0
Laminaria digitata	56.0				23.0	4.6	17.0							
Ascophyllum nodosum	98.0							5.8						
Fucus distichus														
Red Algae														
Porphyra leucosticta		15.0	17.0				62.0							
Dumontia incrassata			98.0											
Chondrus crispus			99.0											
Rhodymenia palmata			99.0											
Ceramium rubrum			96.0											
Polysiphonia urceolata			96.0											

Data taken from Ref. 27; *First number indicates chain length while the second number indicates number of double bonds.

The extremely halophilic green algae are considered important
organisms because of their capacity to synthesize glycerol and
provitamin A (29-31). The lipids of *Dunaliella salina*, excluding
glycerol, comprised some 50% of the cellular organic material; more
than 30% of the total lipids consisted of acyclic and cyclic hydrocarbons (32). Carotenes accounted for 21% of the cell mass. Another
3.5% was saturated and unsaturated C-17 straight chain hydrocarbons
and internally branched 6-methyl hexadecane and 4-methyl octadecane
(32). Methyl branched alkanes, other than the more common iso- and
anteiso-structures, are particularly significant because of their
restricted occurrence in microorganisms. The internally methyl
branched linear alkanes like those identified in *Dunaliella* had previously been reported a unique feature of only the cyanobacteria
(33-36).

The chlorophytes, such as *Coelastrum*, *Chlorella*, *Scenedesmus*
and *Tetraedron* that are contemporary algae found in sediments contain
saturated and unsaturated C-17 components typical of green algae
(33). Certain alga, however, contain in addition to C-17, the unsaturated C-27 (*Scenedesmus*) or saturated C-23, C-25 and C-27
(*Tetraedron*) chains (33). These findings are contrary to Han and
Calvin's prediction (37) that longer chain hydrocarbons, especially
ones that are also major constituents, are absent in algae. The
green alga *Botryococcus braunii*, implicated in the formation of
tertiary sediments (16), produces unusual hydrocarbons when in
particular physiological growth states. *B. braunii* is a freshwater
green colonial algae of widespread occurrence which has at least two,
and possibly three, physiologically distinct forms. The large green
resting cells synthesize negligible amounts of hydrocarbons while
the green fast growing cells (exponential growth) produce the un-
branched, diunsaturated hydrocarbons heptacosa-1,18-diene, nonacosa-1,
20-diene and hentriaconta-1,22-diene as the major components and
unsaturated heptadecane, trieicosene and pentaeicosene as the minor
constituents. These constituents in total account for approximately
17% of the cellular composition (27,38). Cells that are in a brown
resting stage, which often arise as massive rust-colored algal blooms
on the surface of lakes, contain two unsaturated isomeric hydrocarbons of the formula $C_{34}H_{58}$. The two components termed botryococcene and isobotryococcene (16) comprise between 70-90% of the
cellular composition. Hydrogenation of both hydrocarbons results
in the same hydrocarbon botryococcane structure 1 or 2 (16).

Structure 3 was proposed by Cox et al. (39) for botryococcene.
Although this alga can produce copious amounts of hydrocarbon oils
on a mass basis, an improved culturing system and prescribed growth
parameters will have to be developed before any realistic consideration can be given to the employment of this alga as a direct source
of hydrocarbon. The enormous difference in hydrocarbon content
among the different growth stages of *B. braunii* may have been the
origin of discrepancies among earlier reports and suggest the

(1) (C_4H_8) (C_3H_6) (C_7H_{14}) (C_3H_6)

(2) (C_4H_8) (C_7H_{14}) (C_3H_6) (C_3H_6)

(3)

possibility of inaccuracies that may exist in all previous reports on the evaluation of hydrocarbon biosynthesis in microorganisms when culture age and environmental parameters were not considered.

Cyanobacteria are similar to the green algae in that the concentration of cellular hydrocarbons ranges between 0.02 and 0.15% of the dry weight with the predominant hydrocarbons commonly being C-17 species. They are unlike all other algae, however, except for *Dunaliella*, with respect to the occurrence of linear hydrocarbon chains with an internal methyl branch (33-36,40). The hydrocarbon distribution in cyanobacteria is typically in the carbon range of C-15 to C-19 with the exception of *Anacystis montana* where the hydrocarbon range is from C-17 to C-29 with the major constituents being unsaturated C-25 and C-27 (33). Two blue green bacteria, *Coccochloris elabiens* and *Agmenellum quadruplicatum*, were reported to have neither C-17 nor branched hydrocarbon components but only mono- and diunsaturate C-19 components comprising the hydrocarbon fraction (40). The internally methyl branched linear hydrocarbons are particularly significant because of their limited occurrence. *Chlorogloea fritschii* contains 4-methyl heptadecane (34) similar to that described in *Dunaliella* (32), and 7- and 8-methylheptadecanes like those identified in *Nostoc* spp., *Anacystis* spp., *Phormidium luridum*, *Lyngbya aestuarii*, and *Chroococcus turgidus*, (33,34). In addition, 6- and 7-methyl hexadecane were identified in extracts of *C. turgidus* (33).

The n-C-7 hydrocarbon is common to most of the cyanobacteria studied. Since the cyanobacteria are supposedly significant to geochemical evolution, it would seem that geological samples should have an abundant C-17 hydrocarbon content; however, this is not the case. Perhaps, with time, the lighter molecular weight hydrocarbons were preferentially lost leaving the relatively heavier hydrocarbons in place.

Acyclic isoprenoid hydrocarbons are universal but generally exist as minor or trace constituents in cells. However, it is

important to point out that, except for the isoprenoids pristane
(C-19), phytane (C-20), and squalene (C-30), acyclic isoprenoid
hydrocarbons have been largely ignored in the systematic analysis of
fats and oils apparently because of their low quantities in most
organisms. Pristane and phytane have been most often sought because
of their geochemical significance; but, their distribution is limited
in bacteria (41) and they are not found in algae. On the other hand,
squalene ($C_{30}H_{50}$), the precursor to sterols, is a triterpene that
can be found as a major constituent in some algae (32,33) and it is
also widely distributed among bacteria (41-53) as well as in all
higher plants and animals. (See Faulkner and Anderson (47) for a
representative review on the occurrence of terpenoid hydrocarbons
and hydrocarbon pigments in the marine biota).

     Although the quantitative data on squalene are few, earlier
reports concerning levels in prokaryotes (0.001 to 0.1 mg/g cells)
are incorrect. Recent reports of squalene contents indicate *Halobacterium* (42,54) with 1 mg/g of cells, *Methylococcus capsulatus*
(48,49) 5.5 mg/g of cells, *Cellulomonas dehydrogenans* (52) 0.5 mg/g
of cells, and in the methanogens, *Sulfolobus* and *Thermoplasma*
10 mg/g of cells (44,45). These quantities exceed the squalene
concentrations in eukaryotic microorganisms (for example, *Aspergillus nidulans* which contains 0.3 mg/g of cells) (48,49).

     In addition to squalene, the neutral lipids of nine species
of methanogenic bacteria (including five methanobacilli, two methano-
cocci, a methanospirillum, one methanosarcina as well as two thermo-
acidophilic bacteria, *Thermoplasma* and *Sulfolobus*,) contained as
major components C-25 and/or C-20 acyclic iosprenoid hydrocarbons
with a continous range of hydroisoprenoid homologues (44,45). The
range of acyclic isoprenoids detected were from C-14 to C-30. Apart
from *Methanosarcina barkeri*, squalene and/or hydrosqualene derivatives were the predominant components in all species studied. The
components of *M. barkeri* were a family of C-25 homologues (44,45).
The structural differences among many of the isoprenoids found in
these bacteia, collectively referred to as archaebacteria, is seen
in the carbon skeletons of the individual isoprenoids. The carbon
skeleton of the C-30 isoprenoid is that expected from a tail to
tail (pyrophosphate end to pyrophosphate end) condensation product
of two farnesyl derivatives; however a positional isomer of a C-30
isoprenoid that is consistent with a head to tail condensation route
was also identified (44,45). The C-25 isoprenoid fraction comprises
constituents that result from tail to tail condensations of farnesyl
and geranyl derivatives as well as constituents from the condensation
of geranyl-geranyl pyrophosphate and one iso-pentenyl pyrophosphate.
With the exception of phytane (C-20), the remaining isoprenoids also
appear to be synthesized through condensations that involve more
than one biosynthetic pathway (44,45). The distribution of the
neutral lipid components and their specific variations in relative

concentrations emphasized the differences between the test organisms while the generic nature of the isoprenoid hydrocarbons demonstrated similarities between this diverse collection of bacteria (44,45). The neutral lipid compositions from these bacteria, many of which exist in environmental conditions like those described for the various evolutionary stages of the archean ecology, resemble the isoprenoid distribution isolated from ancient sediments and petroleum (55-60).

Halobacterium cutirubrum, cultivated under aerobic and micro-aerophillic conditions, contained cellular ratios of squalene to dihydro- and tetra-hydrosqualene that decreased proportionately with decreased aeration rates and lowered growth rates (54). The ratio of squalene to hydrosqualene conversely increased with increased aeration rates (54). Since electron carriers are lipophilic in nature and the squalenes were localized in the cellular subfraction containing the cytochromes, it was assumed that the electron transport carriers and the squalenes were held in close proximity (54).

Small amounts of nonisoprenoid hydrocarbons can be found in extracts from most bacterial cells. However, with appropriate precautions to eliminate extrinsic sources of hydrocarbons from the cultivation, extraction and analytical procedures, it is generally found that hydrocarbon biosynthesis is restricted to a relatively small number of bacteria. Numerous inconsistancies exist among the reports on the hydrocarbon synthesizing capabilities of bacteria. This is due, in part, to several reasons: a) the reporting of un-characterized or partially characterized mixtures consisting of primarily hydrocarbons; b) the use of organisms that were not ade-quately identified; c) the employment of cells from vastly different cultivation systems and at different physiological growth stages; and d) the absence of adequate controls and analytical procedures. The most thoroughly studied of the bacterial hydrocarbons have been those from the family *Micrococcaceae*. Kloos et al.(61) have demon-strated, however, that a large percentage of the members in the *Micrococcaceae* were misidentified. Thus, inconsistencies are obvious in the reported determinations of the hydrocarbon contents of micro-coccal strains many of which were assumed to be *Micrococcus luteus* (also known as *M. lysodeikticus* or *Sarcina lutea*) (41,61-70). The identities of the hydrocarbons of the micrococci (Table II) in the range from C-16 to C-30 has now been established as families of monounsaturated isomers containing methyl branches in the iso or anteiso or both configurations, symmetrically and asymmetrically disposed on the ends of the isomers (63,67,69). The double bond position is at or near the center of each hydrocarbon chain and some of the gas chromatographically resolved isomers were yet a mixture of positional isomers (67). The identification of the hydrocarbon composition of more than 50 micrococcal species and strains demon-strated that while the generic nature of the hydrocarbons were the same, the carbon distribution ranges were different (61,68).

For example, the major hydrocarbon constituents are C-24, C-25 for *Micrococcus roseus,* C-25, C-26, C-27 for *Micrococcus varians,* C-27, C-28, C-29 for *M. luteus* and C-30, C-31, and C-32 for *Micrococcus sedentarius* (61). The micrococcal species were subsequently differentiated on the basis of the carbon distribution ranges of the cellular hydrocarbons (61). The hydrocarbons of micrococci amount to 20 to 34% of the total lipids (61,66). Aliphatic hydrocarbons are apparently absent in the other members of the taxonomic family *Micrococcaceae* (61,68), which include the staphylococci, planococci and streptococci.

Uncharacterized or partially characterized non-isoprenoid hydrocarbons have been reported in *Pseudomonas spp.* (41,71); *Escherichia coli* (41,72); *Clostridium spp.* (41); *Desulfovibrio spp.* (41,73,74); *Rhodospirillum, Rhodopseudomonas, Chlorobium* and *Rhodomicrobium* (41); *Chromatium* (75); *Arthrobacter* and *Coryne-bacterium spp.* (61,70,76); *Mycobacterium* (70); *Vibrio marinus* (77) *Micrococcus spp.* (41,70); *Bacillus spp.* (70); and *Cellulomonas dehydrogenans* (52). The hydrocarbon chain length is generally from C-16 to C-30 and consists of normal alkanes with no predominance of even- or odd-numbered carbon chains, with the exception of *Pseudomonas maltophillia* (71), *Arthrobacter* strain CCM 1647 (61) and *Corynebacterium spp.* ATCC 21183 (61). These bacteria contain methyl branched unsaturated constituents that are similar in the distribution range and chemical configurations to those found in micrococci. For most of the bacteria listed in this group, however, the identities and quantities of hydrocarbons produced (which ranged from a trace to as much as 3% of cell dry weight of some bacteria (see Ref. 70) will have to be confirmed.

The first definitive investigation into the biosynthesis of hydrocarbons was reported by Sanderman and Schweers (78) who demonstrated acetate-^{14}C incorporation into n-heptane by *Pinus jeffreyi*. The n-heptane was the result of a condensation of four acetate units with an apparent decarboxylation. Since this report there have been numerous attempts to understand the biosynthesis of aliphatic hydrocarbons in microorganisms. There is virtually complete agreement that microbial hydrocarbons are derived from fatty acids. Biogenesis and chain elongation mechanism of normal, branched, saturated and unsaturated fatty acids have received intensive study and have been reviewed at frequent intervals (79, 80). The fatty acids converted to hydrocarbons may be either those comprising the cellular lipid pool or those that exist as a separate selective pool. With regard to the respective microbial systems, the hydrocarbons are derived from fatty acids by decarboxylation, elongation-decarboxylation, or decarboxylation-condensation reactions. The fatty acid decarboxylation mechanism in hydrocarbon biosynthesis exists in specific species of cyanobacteria (36), yeast (81), brown algae (19), and zooplankton (82). The decarboxylation and elongation-decarboxylation pathways are supported by

TABLE II

Relative Percentages of the Compositions of
C27, C28 and C29 Hydrocarbons of *M. luteus*.

Configuration	Per cent Hydrocarbons		
	C27	C28	C29
Iso-iso´	12.4	15.1	20.6
Anteiso-iso	32.8	22.5	39.6
Anteiso-anteiso´	44.3	--	37.4
Iso-normal	6.9	38.0	2.4
Anteiso-normal	--	24.3	--
Normal	3.6	--	--

labelling experiments (36,81). However, supporting evidence deriving from specific enzyme studies on decarboxylases, oxidases and
carboxyl reductases, necessary to reveal the exact mechanism have
not yet been described. Hydrocarbon biosynthesis by a carboxyl-
end to a carboxyl-end condensation of two fatty acids with one fatty
acid under going decarboxylation is well supported in *M. luteus*
(83,87). The hydrocarbon biosynthesis in *M. luteus* has been reviewed recently by Albro (88). The selectivity of the fatty acids
condensed into hydrocarbons of micrococci are to a degree dispro-
portional to their concentrations in the glyceride lipids (Table
III). This indicates the possibility of the existence of a specific pool of fatty acids (63,67,83) and lipid intermediates (83,87).
The specific pattern of normal and iso branched even-numbered carbon fatty acids (equations 1 and 2) and iso and anteiso branched
odd-numbered carbon fatty acids (equation 2) in micrococci predicts
the chemical nature of the ketones (equation 3) or the hydrocarbons
resulting from the combination of condensations of the different
fatty acids (equation 4). The inhibition of the pathway illustrated
by equation 4 by Pb^{2+} results in the synthesis of long chain ketones
(equation 3) with branching configurations and carbon numbers

1) $\begin{array}{c} \text{Propionic Acid} \\ \text{Acetic Acids} \end{array} \xrightarrow{\text{Acetate}} \text{n-Fatty Acids}$

2) Leucine, isoleucine or valine $\xrightarrow[NH_2]{} \xrightarrow[CO_2]{} \xrightarrow{\text{Acetate}} \begin{array}{l}\text{Branched-}\\\text{fatty acid}\end{array}$

3) $R-CH_2-*C\overset{\nearrow O}{\searrow_{OH}} + R'-{}^+CH_2-\bullet C\overset{\nearrow O}{\searrow_{OH}} \xrightarrow{\bullet CO_2} R-CH *\overset{O}{\overset{\|}{C}}-{}^+CH_2-R'$

4) $R-CH_2-*C\overset{\nearrow O}{\underset{OH}{}}$ + $R'-{}^+CH_2-{}^\bullet C\overset{\nearrow O}{\underset{OH}{}}$ $\xrightarrow{\quad\overset{\bullet CO_2}{\diagup}\quad}$ $C-CH=*C-{}^+CH_2-R'$

that were identical to the corresponding hydrocarbons (89). Normally,
the ketones exist as trace constituents of the cellular material.
The purified native, specifically radioactively labeled, ketones of
M. *luteus* were introduced into a cell free lysate of M. *luteus*. No
ketones were converted into hydrocarbons while a fraction of the
ketone pool was converted to free fatty acids, some of which were
further degraded (89). All lines of evidence support the idea that
the ketones are not precursors of hydrocarbons but constituents from
the metabolic regulation of the concentration of the cellular fatty
acid pool (equation 5).

5) Acetates $\overset{\leftarrow}{\rightarrow}$ fatty acids $\underset{\longrightarrow}{\overset{\longleftarrow}{\longrightarrow}}$ lipids
$\qquad\qquad\qquad\qquad\qquad\qquad\qquad$ ketones
$\qquad\qquad\qquad\qquad\qquad\qquad\qquad$ hydrocarbons

The hydrocarbons are an apparent end-product of the regulation of
the cellular fatty acid pool. This is supported by the result
obtained from the assay for enzymatic activity for hydrocarbon biosynthesis in cell free lysates of M. *luteus* (Figure 1). The fluctua-
tion in the biosynthesis of hydrocarbons in the course of cell
growth was a reproducible feature that was not altered by salt precipitation cuts of the lysates to remove possible endogenous inhibitors or by modifications in lysate preparations (89). These data
(Figure 1) indicate that the enzymes of the pathways of hydrocarbon
biosynthesis is a specifically regulated one. No evidence has been
obtained that demonstrates the oxidation and reutilization of the
hydrocarbons by M. *luteus*.

In studies on the modes of entry of a palmitic acid chain into
an alkane consisting of more than 16 carbon atoms, a suspected intermediate form of the acceptor moiety was identified as a neutral
plasmalogen (87,88,90). Studies in this laboratory with exogenous
labeled plasmalogens, however, did not support this concept (89).
Nonetheless, the direct participation of a neutral plasmalogen or
some similar intermediate as that illustrated in equation 6

6) $R-{}^+CH_2-*C\overset{\nearrow O}{\underset{OH}{}}$ + X $\rightarrow$ $R-{}^+CH=*CH-X$ + 0^{2-} + OH${}^-$

appears essential to form the type of monoene present in M. *luteus*
and described in equation 4.

Although it is established that specific microorganisms
synthesize hydrocarbons as natural cellular constituents, most
microorganisms do not and should not be expected to produce copious
amounts of hydrocarbon under natural conditions. Hydrocarbons

TABLE III

Fatty acids of *M. luteus*

Peak No.	Identification
1	i 12:0
2	12:0
3	i 13:0
4	ai 13:0
5	i 14:0
6	14:0
7	i 15:0
8	ai 15:0
9	i 16:0
10	16:0
11	i 17:0
12	ai 17:0
13	18:0
14	18:1

Symbols: i = iso; ai = anteiso. The first number represents the chain length; the second number represents the number of unsaturations.

reside in the hydrophobic regions of cells, namely cellular membranes. It is expected that the enzymes for hydrocarbon biosynthesis are membrane associated and that the biosynthesis occurs at the lipid-water interface. Since there are no apparent cellular transport mechanisms for the secretion of hydrocarbons from cells, the hydrocarbons remain immobilized in the hydrophobic structures of the cells. The cellular burden of hydrocarbons, therefore, must be limited to a relatively small quantity of the total membrane lipids. In addition to the physical-chemical limitations, there are the metabolic energy requirements for hydrocarbon biosynthesis. The biological energy demand to make a fatty acid is given in the stoichiometry of a representative fatty acid synthesis. The hydrocarbons made from the decarboxylation of a fatty acid or condensation of 2 fatty acids with a decarboxylation utilize a large quantity of biological energy. Since the hydrocarbons can not be metabolized by these cells, most organisms apparently do not store their energy reserves as hydrocarbons.

9) 8 Acetyl-CoA $+ 7$ $CO_2 + 14NADPH + 14H^+ + 7ATP \rightarrow$ palmitic acid

$+ 7CO_2 + 8CoASH + 14$ $NADP^+ + 7ADP + 7Pi + 6H_2O$

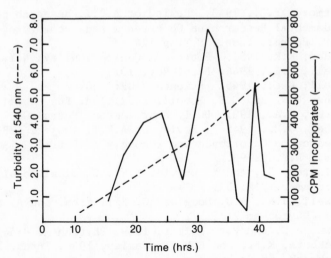

Figure 1. Changes in incorporation of $[(^{14}C)\ U]$ Palmitic acid into long chain, non-isoprenoid hydrocarbons (————) as a function of growth (--------). At the indicated times 1×10^6 cpm of palmitic acid was added to a cell-free extract prepared from an aliquot of cells corresponding to 1 gram dry weight. The cells were grown in 8 liters of Trypticase Soy broth at 25°C with aeration.

Although it is evident that most microorganisms do not synthesize significant quantities of hydrocarbons, there is the obvious exception. *Botryococcus braunii* accumulates hydrocarbons when in the stationary phase of growth in quantities that amount to 80% of its cellular dry weight. These cells embedded in a cup of "oil" release the oil from the cellular matrix when the cells divide. The question that remains is how many other organisms exist that have the equal potential to synthesize hydrocarbon? The current challenge in the field of hydrocarbon bioproduction is to identify the hydrocarbon producing organisms that exist among the immense number of yet "undiscovered" microbes and to determine the genetics and metabolic parameters that control hydrocarbon biosynthesis.

REFERENCES

1. Kramer, G., and A. Spilker. 1899. Ber 32: 2940.
2. Tsujimoto, M., 1906. Kogyo Kagaku Zasshi. 9:953.
3. Heilbron, I.M., W.M. Owens and I.A. Simpson. 1929. J.Chem.Soc.873.
4. Karrer, P. and A. Helfenstein. 1931. Helv.Chim.Acta. 14:78.
5. Tolman, C.F., 1926. Summary of results of symposium on the siliceous shales and the origin of oil in Calif. Geol.Soc. of Amer. Cordelleian Section.
6. Becking, L.B. and C.F. Tolman, H.C. McMillin, J. Field and T. Hashimoto. 1927. Econ. Geol., 22:356.
7. Trask, P.D., 1923. Origin and env. of source sediments of petroleum, Gulf Publ. Co., Houston, p. 233.

8. Whitmore, F.C., 1943. Review of A.P.I. Research project 43B:
    Fundamental Research on Occurrence and recovery of petroleum,
    Amer. Petrol. Inst., N.Y. p 124.

9. Landes, K.K. 1951. Petroleum Geology. Wiley, N.Y., p 135.

10. Zobell, C.E., 1946. Bact. Rev. 10:1.

11. Zobell, C.E., 1945. Science, 102: 346.

12. Stone, R.W. and C.E. Zobell, 1952. Ind. Eng. Chem; 44:2564.

13. Thayer, L.A., 1931. Bull. Amer. Assoc. Petro. Geol., 15: 441.

14. Knebel, G.M., 1946-7. Review of A.P.I. project 43B. Fundamental
    Research on Occurrence and recovery of Petrol.   Amer. Petrol.
    Inst., N.Y. p. 93.

15. Eglington, G., and M. Calvin. 1967. Chemical fossils. Scien-
    tific Amer. 216: 32.

16. Maxwell, J.R., A.G. Douglas, G. Eglington, and A. McCormick.
    1968. Phytochem 7: 2157.

17. Brown, A.C. and B.A. Knight. 1969. Phytochem. 8:543.

18. Blackburn, K.B., and B.N. Temperley, 1936. Trans. Roy Soc.
    Edinburgh, 58: 841.

19. Lee, R.F., and A.R. Loeblich. 1971. Phytochem. 10: 593.

20. Caccamese, S. and K. L. Rinehart, Jr., 1978. Experientia
    34: 1129.

21. Youngblood, W.W., and M. Blumer. 1973. Marine Biol. 21: 163.

22. Gregson, R.P., R. Kazlauskas, P.T. Murphy and R. J. Wells.
    1977. Aust. J. Chem. 30: 2527.

23. Blumer, M., M. M. Mullin and R.R.L. Guillard. 1970. Marine
    Biol. 6: 226.

24. Lee, R.F., J.C. Nevenzel, G.A. Paffenhofer, A.A. Benson, S.
    Patton and T.E. Kavanagh. 1970. Biochim. Biophys. Acta.
    202: 386.

25. Wright, J.L.C., 1980. Phytochem. 19: 143.

26. Blumer, M., R.R.L. Guillard and T. Chase. 1971. Marine Biol.
    8:183.

27. Youngblood, W.W., M. Blumer, R.L. Guillard and F. Fiore. 1971.
    Marine Biol. 8:190.

28. Shaw, D.G. and J.N. Wiggs. 1979. Phytochem. 18: 2025.

29. Ben-Amotz, A., and M. Avron. 1973. Plant Physiol. 51: 875.

30. Ben-Amotz, A. 1978. In Energetics and structure of Halophilic
    Microorganism. S.R. Caplan and M. Ginzburg, eds. Elsevier/
    North-Holland Biomedical press, p. 529.

31. Ben-Amotz, A. and M. Avron. 1980. In Genetic Engineering of
    Osmoregulation. D.W. Rains, R.C. Valentine and A. Hollaender,
    Plenum Publ. Corp., N.Y.,N.Y. p. 91.

32. Tornabene, T.G., G. Holzer and S.L. Petersen. 1980. Biochem.
    Biophy. Res. Comm. 96: 1349.

33. Gelpi, E., H. Schneider, J. Mann and J. Oro. 1970. Phytochem.
    9: 603.

34. Han, J., E.D. McCarthy, M. Calvin and M.H. Benn. 1968. J. Chem.
    Soc. (c), 2785.

35. Fehler, S.W.G., and R.J. Light. 1970. Biochemistry, 9: 418.

36.   Han, J., H.W.-S. Chan and M. Calvin. 1969. J. Amer. Chem. Soc.
       91: 5156.
37.   Han, J., and M. Calvin. 1969. Proc. Nat. Acad. Sci. 64: 436.
38.   Knight, B.A., A.C. Brown, E. Conway, and B.S. Middleditch.
       1970. Phytochem 9:1317.
39.   Cox, R.E., A.L. Burlingame and D.W. Wilson. 1973. J. Chem.
       Soc. Chem. Comm. 284.
40.   Winters, K., P.L. Parker and C. Van Baalen. 1969. Science 163:
       467.
41.   Han, J. and M. Calvin. 1969. Proc. Nat. Acad. Sci. 64: 436.
42.   Tornabene, T.G., M. Kates, E. Gelpi and J. Oro. 1969. J. Lipid
       Res. 10: 294.
43.   Tornabene, T.G. 1976. In Microbial Energy Conversion, H.G.
       Schlegel and J. Barnea eds. Oxford Engl: Pergamon Press p. 281.
44.   Tornabene, T.G., T.A. Langworthy, G. Holzer and J. Oro. 1979.
       J. Mol. Evol. 13: 73.
45.   Holzer, G., J. Oro and T.G. Tornabene. 1979. J. Chromatog.
       196: 795.
46.   Goldberg, I., and I. Shechter. 1978. J Bacteriol, 135: 717.
47.   Faulkner, D.J. and R.J. Andersen. 1974. In The Sea, Vol. 5,
       E.D. Goldberg ed., John Wiley and Sons. N.Y. p. 679.
48.   Bird, C.W., J.M. Lynch, F.G. Pirt, W.W. Ried, C.J.W. Brooks
       and B.S. Middleditch. 1971. Nature 230: 473.
49.   Bouvier, P., M. Rohmer, P. Benveniste and G. Ourisson, 1976.
       Biochem. J. 159: 267.
50.   Amdur, G.H., E.I. Szabo and S.S. Socransky. 1978. J. Bacteriol.
       135:161.
51.   Suzue, G., K. Tsukada and S. Tanaka. 1968. Biochim. Biophys.
       Acta 164: 88.
52.   Weeks, O.B., and M.D. Francesconi. 1978. J. Bacteriol. 136:
       614.
53.   Maudinas, B. and J. Villoutriex. 1976. C. R. Acad. Sci. Ser.
       D. 278: 2995.
54.   Tornabene, T.G., 1978. J. Mol. Evol. 11: 253.
55.   McCarthy, E.D. and M. Calvin. 1967. Tetrahedron. 23: 2609.
56.   Han, J. and M. Calvin. 1969. Geochim. Cosmochim. Acta. 33: 733.
57.   Spyckerelle, C., P. Arpino and G. Ourisson.1972. Tetrahedron.
       28: 5703.
58.   Spyckerelle, C., P. Arpino and G. Ourisson. 1978. Tetrahedron
       Letters, 595.
59.   Spyckerelle, C. P. Arpino and G. Ourisson. 1978. Nature 271:
       436.
60.   Moldowan, M., W.K. Seifert. 1979. Science 204: 169.
61.   Kloos, W.E., T.G. Tornabene and K.H. Schleifer. 1974. Intl.
       J. Syst   Bacteriol. 24:79.
62.   Albro, P.W. and C.K. Huston. 1964. J. Bacteriol. 88: 981.
63.   Tornabene, T.G., E. Gelpi, and J. Oro. 1967. J. Bacteriol. 94:333.
64.   Tornabene, T.G., E.O. Bennett and J. Oro. 1967. J. Bacteriol.
       94: 344.

65.   Tornabene, T.G., and J. Oro. 1967. J. Bacteriol. 94 :349.
66.   Tornabene, T.G., S. J. Morrison and W. E. Kloos. 1970. Lipids
       5: 929.
67.   Tornabene, T.G. and S.P. Markey. 1971. Lipid 6: 190.
68.   Morrison, S.J., T.G. Tornabene and W.E. Kloos. 1971. J.
       Bacteriol. 108: 353.
69.   Albro, P.W., 1971. J. Bacteriol. 108: 213.
70.   Jones, J.G., 1969. J. Gen. Microbiol. 59: 145.
71.   Tornabene, T.G. and S.L. Peterson. 1978. Can. J. Microbiol.
       24: 525.
72.   Naccarato, W.F., J.R. Gilbertson and R. A. Gelman. 1974.
       Lipids 9: 322.
73.   Davis, J.B. 1968. Chem. Geol. 3: 155.
74.   Jankowski, G.J. and C.E. Zobell. 1948. J. Bacteriol. 47: 447.
75.   Jones, J.G., and B.V. Young. 1970. Arch. Mikrobiol. 70: 82.
76.   LaCave, C., J. Asselineau and R. Toubiana. 1967. Eur. J.
       Biochem. 2: 37.
77.   Oro, J., T.G. Tornabene, P.W. Nooner, and E. Gelpi. 1967.
       J. Bacteriol. 93: 1811.
78.   Sanderman, W., and W. Schweers. 1960. Chem. Ber. 93: 2266.
79.   Volpe, J.J., and P.R. Vagelos. 1973. Ann. Rev. Biochem. 42: 21.
80.   Bloch, K. 1977. Ann. Rev. Biochem. 46: 263.
81.   Blanchardie, D. and C. Cassagne. 1976. C. R. Acad. Sc. Paris
       Ser D. 282: 227.
82.   Blumer, M. and D.W. Thomas. 1965. Science 148: 370.
83.   Albro, P.W. and J.C. Dittmer. 1969. Biochem. 8: 394.
84.   Ibid, p. 953.
85.   Ibid, p. 1913.
86.   Ibid, p. 3317.
87.   Albro, P.W., T.D. Meehan, and J.C. Dittmer. 1970. Biochem.
       9: 1893.
88.   Albro, P.W., 1976. In Chemistry of Natural Waxes, P. E.
       Kolatukuddy, ed. pp 419. Elsevier Publ. Co., Amsterdam.
89.   Tornabene, T.G., unpubl. results.
90.   Albro, P.W. and J.G. Dittmer. 1970. Lipids 5: 320.

DISCUSSION

Q.   TEMPEST: You seem to express a certain surprise that an
      organism can indulge in this sort of overflow metabolism
      which is energetically extremely expensive when growing in
      its natural environment. I'm not at all surprised; I think
      this is exactly what it should do because I think perhaps
      what you are overlooking, is the fact that in natural eco-
      systems there is frequently a limitation on cell synthesis
      imposed through the nonavailability of something other than
      carbon and energy in marine environments, for example, the
      nitrogen content generally is extremely low and under these

circumstances, where organisms are scavenging for nitrogen, there may well be an excess of energy either in a photo-synthetic form or in some heterotrophic form that could pose a problem. Anaerobically one finds a problem of redox balance over the oxidation of the reduced pyridine nucelo-tides, under excess energy conditions organisms have a prob-lem of recycling their adenine nucleotides. So what they need to have are energy spilling reactions, and we know that very many organisms (aerobes as well as anaerobes) have sys-tems for dissipating energy and turning over the adenine nucleotide pool. We're reluctant to believe that there can be some slip mechanism in the membrane ATP, but what you have demonstrated today, I think, is a superb example of an energy spilling reaction which would have real ecological significance not as a storage compounds, but as a means to dissipate its excess ATP.

A.   TORNABENE: I absolutely agree. However, we should not expect all microbial cells to have the same metabolic regulatory system. My intent was to demonstrate this point and to show cause for the many reports of microorganisms that do not synthesize hydrocarbons in appeciable quantities. Specific data presented, however, was consistent with what you are saying, namely that certain organisms synthesize hydrocarbons as a result of a metabolic regulatory mechanism.

TEMPEST: Well, it's probably more widely distributed than you imagine because you haven't exposed organisms to low nutrient environments.

TORNABENE: No, we have done that resulting in substantial increases in lipid yields. Unfortunately, the hydrocarbon formation was not one of the principle lipids made.

WOLFE: Dr. Tempest's point is that you should be using a chemostat, he didn't say it, but that's what he means.

ZABORSKY: I certainly concur with your view that there is a lot of confusion in the literature and especially when you go back, nomenclature and otherwise however, I would like to point out and I'm sure you'll have to agree that a lot of the studies that are reported in the literature especially in the 50's and even 60's and even now really are not concerned with optimization of these microbes for producing hydrocarbons so you see a low concentration but that concentration has really never been optimized to the point of really getting an assessment of the capability of these organisms to produce hydrocarbons.

TORNABENE: I agree. Many algae have been examined but not adequately. *Botryoccus* is a good example. Depending on which

growth phase one examines, you may find no hydrocarbons or a
hydrocarbon quantity that comprises 80% of the cell mass.

Q.   WOLFE: Do you really think these hydrocarbons act as a hydrogen sink?

A.   TORNABENE: No, not as a hydrogen sink.

WOLFE: I'm glad.

TORNABENE: I would like to point out, however, that no cellular
system has the luxury of making a compound for only one purpose.
I think hydrocarbons have a role in both the structure and function of a cell.   The only functional role demonstrated for
hydrocarbons has been *Halobacterium* where hydrogens are added
to hydrocarbons in anaerobic conditions and removed from the
hydrocarbons in the aerobic conditions.

WOLFE: Yes, I can see that for an aerobe.

TORNABENE: You know the other thing about *Halobacterium* ,
an organism that everyone has published as a strict aerobe,
is that it can in fact grow anaerobically as long as you
supply light to drive the ATP pump.

LIQUID PRODUCTS - CHAIRMAN'S REPORT

Anthony San Pietro

Indiana University

Bloomington, Indiana 47405

During the first two days of this symposium, we learned much
about the enzymatic degradation of biopolymers, such as cellulose,
lignin, etc.; the biochemical genetics of fermentations; and the
modification of fermentation pathways.

Today, the focus is on specific fermentations to provide
useful products. In this session, we will hear about the formation of useful liquid products; namely, ethanol production by
thermophilic organisms (Dr. Gregory Zeikus), butanol production
by *C. acetobutylicum* (Dr. Gerhard Gottschalk) and acrylate fermentations (Dr. Massey Akedo).

THERMOPHILIC ETHANOL FERMENTATIONS

J.G. Zeikus, Arie Ben-Bassat[1], Thomas K. Ng[2], and
Raphael J. Lamed[3]

Department of Bacteriology, University of Wisconsin
Madison, Wisconsin 53706

INTRODUCTION

The cost and availability of petroleum and natural gas has
generated interest in bioconversion processes that utilize renewable
biomass resources for the production of fuels and chemical feedstocks.
The bioconversion of biomass to ethanol via anaerobic fermentations
offers the promise of renewable liquid fuel and renewable chemical
feedstocks. The purpose of this presentation is to review some of
the recent studies in my laboratory on thermophilic ethanol fermentations. The emphasis of this review will be on understanding
fundamental aspects of the physiology and biochemistry of thermophilic anaerobes that may be of applied interest in developing
bioconversion technology for alcohol production. Most of the findings summarized here represent material published elsewhere (1-22).

Several factors account for technological interest in thermophilic bacterial fermentations as opposed to the use of yeast or
mesophilic bacteria in ethanol production. Bacterial fermentations
enable the direct fermentation of both cellulosic and hemi-cellulosic
components of delignified biomass into ethanol without pre-treatment
to depolymerize these substrates (1,2). As a consequence of growth
at high temperatures and unique macromolecular properties, obligately
thermophilic bacteria can possess: high metabolic rates, lower cell
growth yield and higher physical and chemical stability of enzymes
than in metabolically similar mesophilic species (see Table I).

1. Cetus Corporation, Berkeley, California
2. Biotechnology Branch, SERI, Golden, Colorado
3. Biotechnology and Biophysics Department, University of Tel Aviv,
   Israel

TABLE I

Advantages of Thermophilic Fermentation ($\geq 60^{\circ}C$)

A. MICROBIAL

1. HIGHER GROWTH AND METABOLIC RATES
2. LOWER CELLULAR GROWTH YIELD
3. HIGHER PHYSICAL AND CHEMICAL STABILITY OF ENZYMES AND ORGANISMS

B. PROCESS

1. INCREASED STABILITY
2. INCREASED PRODUCTION RATES
3. FACILITATED REACTANT ACTIVITY AND PRODUCT RECOVERY

GROWTH PROPERTIES OF THERMOPHILIC ETHANOLOGENS

Relatively little is known about the entire spectrum of thermophilic bacteria that may be of interest in bioethanol production. Thermophilic ethanologens are easily obtained (1,6-9) from a variety of self-heating environments (e.g., manure composts or soils) or volcanic features (e.g., thermal springs or decomposing bacterial-algal mats). Table II compares the general growth characteristics of several taxonomically described thermophilic anaerobic bacteria that produce ethanol during growth on a variety of saccharides including cellulose, starch, pentoses and hexoses. These species differ considerably in regard to their specific growth characteristics. Most notable is their substrate range for fermentation. *Clostridium thermocellum* actively ferments cellulose and cellulose hydrolysis products but not pentoses or starch (13). Growth of this species is noticably lower on cellulose (<7 h) than on cellobiose (∿2 h) which suggests that solubilization of the polymer is a rate limiting metabolic step (6). *C. thermohydrosulfuricum* utilizes a broad range of substrates as energy sources including pentoses and starch but does not ferment cellulose (8,19). *Thermoanaerobium brockii* and *Thermobacterioides acetoethylicus* display essentially the same substrate range; but, *T. acetoethylicus* is the most prolific thermophilic ethanologen described and has a doubling time around 20 min (7,8,9).

Figure 1 illustrates the relationship between end product formation and saccharide consumption during growth of *C. thermocellum* LQRI on cellobiose. All fermentation products (i.e., ethanol, acetate, lactate and H_2/CO_2) are formed as a direct consequence of growth but these products also continue to increase in concentration after growth ceases. *C. thermocellum* LQRI forms cellulase during growth on cellobiose; whereas, some strains do

TABLE II

Growth Characteristics of Thermophilic Saccharolytic Bacteria

CHARACTERISTIC	ORGANISM			
	CLOSTRIDIUM THERMOCELLUM LQRI	CLOSTRIDIUM THERMOHYDROSULFURICUM 39E	THERMOANAEROBIUM BROCKII HTD4	THERMOBACTEROIDES ACETOETHYLICUS HTB2
TEMP. RANGE FOR GROWTH:				
MIN.	40°C	40°C	40°C	40°C
OPT.	62°C	65°C	70°C	65°C
MAX.	70°C	75°C	80°C	80°C
SUBSTRATES SUPPORTING GROWTH	CELLULOSE CELLODEXTRINS CELLOBIOSE GLUCOSE	PYRUVATE XYLOSE GLUCOSE MANNOSE CELLOBIOSE SUCROSE STARCH	PYRUVATE GLUCOSE SUCROSE CELLOBIOSE STARCH	GLUCOSE MANNOSE SUCROSE CELLOBIOSE
SUBSTRATES NOT SUPPORTING GROWTH	PYRUVATE XYLOSE MANNOSE SUCROSE STARCH	CELLODEXTRINS CELLULOSE XYLAN MANNAN	CELLODEXTRINS CELLULOSE XYLOSE MANNAN	CELLODEXTRINS CELLULOSE XYLAN MANNAN
GROWTH RATE ON:				
GLUCOSE	0.44 HR^{-1}	0.55 HR^{-1}	0.69 HR^{-1}	1.38 HR^{-1}
CELLOBIOSE	0.5 HR^{-1}	0.5 HR^{-1}	-	-
CELLULOSE	0.15 HR^{-1}	-	-	-

not (6). All the thermophilic saccharolytic species described here produce ethanol during primary metabolism; whereas *C. thermosaccharlyticum* strains form butyrate during growth and produce ethanol in response to sporulation (1,2).

ENZYMES ASSOCIATED WITH SACCHARIDE CONVERSION TO ETHANOL

Growth of *Clostridium thermocellum* on crystalline cellulose or cellobiose is faster than that reported for *Trichoderma viride* (1,2). The cellulolytic enzyme outfit of *C. thermocellum* differ significantly from fungal cellulases (3,6,10). Table III compares the crude exocellular cellulase activies of *C. thermocellum* strain

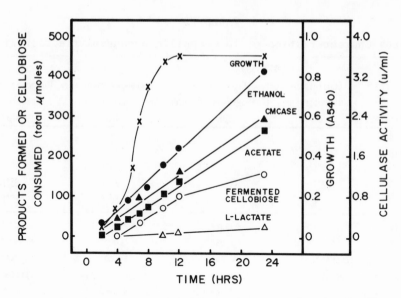

Figure 1.   Time course of cellobiose fermentation by *C. thermocellum*
AS39.   Anaerobic culture tubes contained 10 ml of CC medium and
were incubated at 60°C.

LQRI (virgin strain) and *T. reesei* QM 9414 (hypercellulase mutant
strain).   The fungal cellulase was considerably more active than
the thermophile under reaction conditions optimized for each enzyme.
The following comparative enzymatic features are worth noting: the
ratio of endo-glucanase to exo-glucanase activity is higher for
C. thermocellum; *T. reesei* contained detectable cellobiase and
xylobiase activity; and the cellulose solubilizing activity [i.e.,
as measured by the continuous spectrophotometric assay method (11)]
of the *T. reesei* mutant was only two-fold greater than this virgin
strain of *C. thermocellum*.   Detailed kinetic comparison of the
hydrolysis of defined degree of polymerization cellooligosaccharides; however, demonstrated that the rates of cellohexaose
conversion to cellotriose were equivalent for both the thermophile
and the fungal cellulase (10).   From analysis of the crude cellulase data at hand it appears that the faster rate of cellulose
hydrolysis during growth of *C. thermocellum* is more related to the
mechanism of saccharide uptake because the fungal exocellular
cellulase is clearly more active.   Also, note that crude cellulase
of *C. thermocellum* contained significant activity of xylanase but
xylobiase was not detectable.   Figure 2 compares the thermal stability of cellulose solubilizing activity of *C. thermocellum* and *T.
reesei*.   As expected the crude thermophilic enzyme was active and
stable at temperature <70°C; whereas, the fungal enzyme was readily
denatured at 60°C.

TABLE III

Exocelluar Cellulase Activities of *C. Thermocellum* LQRI and *T. Reesei* QM9414

	ACTIVITY (μMOL/MIN/MG)	
ENZYME-SUBSTRATE	LQRI	QM9414
EXOGLUCANASE		
AVICEL	0.09	0.37
ENDOGLUCANASE		
CMC-NA	4.63	7.86
CELLULOSE SOLUBILIZING ACTIVITY		
DYED-AVICEL	0.19	0.36
XYLANASE		
XYLAN	0.53	1.00
CELLOBIASE		
PNPG	0.03	0.09
CELLOBIOSE	N.D.	0.08
β-XYLOSIDASE		
PNPX	N.D.	0.20

N.D. MEANS NOT DETECTED.

The major activity component in crude exocellular cellulase of *C. thermocellum* was purified to ultracentrifugation homogenity by differential chromatographic and electrophoretic techniques (12). The purification procedures used were tedious and yielded low amounts of enzyme because a specific affinity purification step was not discovered. The substrate-activity relationships of the purified endo-glucanase are shown in Table IV. The purified enzyme produced reducing sugars from Avicel or carboxymethyl cellulose. Most notably the endo-glucanase was not active on cellobiose or cellotriose and the apparent $[S]_{0.5V}$ decreased while the V_{max} increased as the substrate cellooligosaccharide degree of polymerization increased from C_4 to C_7.

Table V compares the effect of temperature on the enzymes involved in pyruvate conversion to alcohol by *T. brockii* and *C. thermocellum* strains. Note that all enzymes examined were active at 40°C or 60°C and displayed calculated Q_{10} values that from 1.5 for pyruvate dehydrogenase to 2.7 for hydrogenase in *T. brockii* (18).

The examined enzyme activities of thermophilic saccharolytic bacteria (15,18), as well as tricarboxylic acid cycle related enzymes and hydrogenase of *Methanobacterium thermoautotrophicum* (14)

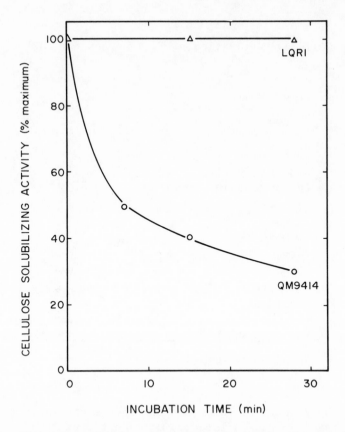

Figure 2. Thermal stability of *T. reesei* and *C. thermocellum* cellulase at 60°C. Cellulase (2 mg/ml buffer) was heated for the time
indicated, chilled on ice and then assayed for cellulose solubilizing activity. 100% activity (0% denaturation) corresponding to 0.15
μmol/min/mg protein for *C. thermocellum* and *T. reesei* cellulase
respectively.

are easily quantified at 40°C. Thus, understanding the metabolic
machinery of thermophiles does not obligately require the use of
extremely high temperatures that often destroy reaction mixture cofactors or components. The differences in alcohol dehydrogenase
activity of *T. brockii* and *C. thermocellum* strains are of special
importance. Ethanol dehydrogenase in *C. thermocellum* was uni-
directional, specific for NADH, and noticably inhibited by ethanol
and NAD. *T. brockii* alcohol dehydrogenase was reversible and
displayed activity towards both NAD(P) and NAD(P)H.

    The NADP-linked alcohol dehydrogenase of *T. brockii* appeared
interesting and was readily purified in high yield by differential
chromatographic procedures that included an affinity step with Blue

TABLE IV

Substrate-Activity Relationships of Purified *C. Thermocellum*
Endo-Glucanase

SUBSTRATE	SPECIFIC ACTIVITY (μMOL/MIN/MG)	$S_{0.5V}$ (μM)	V_{MAX} (U AT 60°C)
CMC	65.05	-	-
DYED AVICEL	5.33	-	-
AVICEL	0.17	-	-
CELLOBIOSE	0.01	-	-
CELLOTRIOSE	0.01	-	-
CELLOTETRAOSE	0.63	-	-
CELLOPENTAOSE	11.21	2.30	39.25
CELLOHEXAOSE	19.06	0.56	58.7
CELLOHEPTAOSE	25.13	N.D.	N.D.

N.D. MEANS NOT DETECTED.

Dextran Sepharose (15). The purified alcohol dehydrogenase displayed one protein band (38,000 M.W.) after SDS-polyacrylamide gel
electrophoresis and was specific for NADP(H). Figure 3 shows the
relation of activity to substrate concentration of purified *T.
brockii* alcohol dehydrogenase. *T. brockii* enzyme is more appropriately called an NADP linked, alcohol-aldehyde/ketone oxidoreductase that displays wide substrate range for 1° or 2° alcohols

TABLE V

Effect of temperature on enzymes involved in pyruvate
catabolism of *T. brockii* and *C. thermocellum*

Enzyme	Sp act (μmol/min per mg of protein)								
	T. brockii			*C. thermocellum* LQRI			*C. thermocellum* AS39		
	40°C	60°C	Q_{10}	40°C	60°C	Q_{10}	40°C	60°C	Q_{10}
L-Lactate dehydrogenase	0.55	1.59	1.7	0.44	2.33	2.3	0.31	1.50	2.2
Pyruvate dehydrogenase (CoA acetylating)	0.53	1.19	1.5	0.48	2.12	2.1	0.60	1.94	1.8
Hydrogenase (methyl viologen reducing)	3.3	24.0	2.7	13.0	—	—	11.0	74.0	2.6
Acetate kinase	1.50	—	—	0.78	—	—	0.30	—	—
Acetaldehyde dehydrogenase (CoA acetylating)	0.15	—	—	0.35	—	—	0.39	—	—
Ethanol dehydrogenase									
NADH oxidizing	0.48	—	—	0.45	2.02	2.1	0.24	1.06	2.1
NAD reducing	0.4	—	—	<0.005	<0.005	—	<0.005	<0.005	—
NADP reducing	1.57	6.92	2.1	<0.005	<0.005	—	<0.005	<0.005	—
NADPH oxidizing	1.50	6.9	2.1	<0.005	<0.005	—	<0.005	<0.005	—

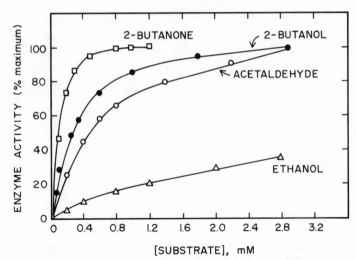

Figure 3. Dependence of *T. brockii* NADP linked alcohol-aldehyde/ketone oxidoreductase on substrate concentration. Reaction conditions: 40°C, 1 ml reaction mixture that contained 0.1 M Tris-HCl buffer (pH 7.8), 0.5 mM NADP or 0.2 mM NADPH, the substrate; and, 2.5 μg purified enzyme. Maximal activity represents (in μmole/min/mg protein): sec-butanol, 78; 2-butanone, 7.6; ethanol, 3.2; acetaldehyde, 7.8.

and ketones. The enzyme is more active towards ketones (e.g. 2° alcohols butanol) than 1° alcohols (e.g., ethanol). This same enzyme activity is found in *C. thermohydrosulfuricum* but not in *C. thermocellum* or *T. acetoethylicus* (15).

The extreme temperature stability of *T. brockii* alcohol dehydrogenase is illustrated in Figure 4. Enzyme activity was only significantly decreased at temperature >86°C. High solvent stability of the enzyme was found in association with lower temperature (see Figure 5). Note that at 40°C the NADP linked alcohol-aldehyde/ketone oxidoreductase was active with 2-propanol concentration as high as 50%. However, preincubation of the enzyme with 30% 2-propanol and temperature >52°C rapidly denatured the enzyme. The extreme solvent stability of the enzyme at moderate temperature was used to demonstrate practical applications that included immobilized enzyme NADPH synthesis, enzymatic NADP/NADPH coenzyme regeneration and enzymatic chiral alcohol production. It is of interest to note that the thermophile enzyme is unlike yeast alcohol dehydrogenase and has the rare carbonyl si-face stereospecificity in hydrogen transfer reactions (17).

All saccharolytic thermophiles examined to date employ the Embden-Meyerhof-Parnas Pathway (2,9,13,18,19). Figure 6 compares

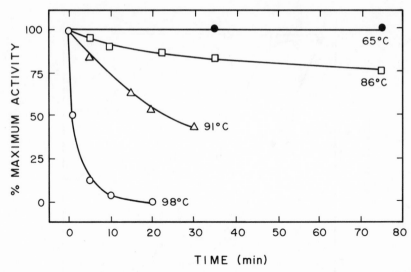

Figure 4. Thermal stability of *T. brockii* secondary alcohol dehydrogenase. Purified alcohol dehydrogenase (16 µg protein/ml 25 mM potassium phosphate, pH 7.1) was heated for the time and temperature indicated, and assayed for sec-butanol dehydrogenase activity.

the biochemical routes of hexose and pentose metabolism of *C. thermohydrosulfuricum*. This pathway is based on finding significant $^{14}CO_2$ production during growth on differentially labelled glucose from position C_3 and C_4 alone and detection of catabolic levels (i.e., > 200 nmol/min/mg protein at 40°C) of hexokinase, fructose 1-6 diphosphate aldolase; glyceraldehyde 3-phosphate dehydrogenase, pyruvate dehydrogenase, lactate dehydrogenase and hydrogenase in glucose grown cells and in addition, xylose isomerase and xylulose kinase in xylose grown cells (19). Note that conversion of 1.0 mol hexose leads to 2 mol glyceraldehyde-3 phosphate via aldolase; whereas, 1.2 mol of pentose yields the same amount of product via transaldolase and transketolase.

METABOLIC CONTROL OF SACCHARIDE FERMENTATION

Table VI compares the balanced cellobiose fermentation product ratios of *T. brockii*, *C. thermohydrosulfuricum*, *C. thermocellum* and *T. acetoethylicus* grown on the same yeast extract containing complex medium (7,8,9,13). Note that each species, except for *T. acetoethylicus*, which does not form lactate, produces the same end products but in totally different proportions. Under the batch fermentation conditions employed, the major reduced end products (i.e., total µmol formed) of these thermophilic ethanologens were: lactate for *T. brockii*; ethanol for *C. thermohydrosulfuricum* and

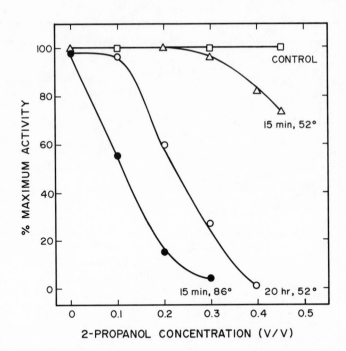

Figure 5. Temperature and 2-propanol stability of *T. brockii* alcohol dehydrogenase. Experimental conditions: purified enzyme was dissolved (16 μg/ml) in 50 mM potassium phosphate buffer (pH 7.1), 2mM DTT, 0.05 mM NADP and the 2-propanol concentrations indicated; the solution was heated aerobically in sealed tubes at the indicated times the solution was cooled and assayed for activity at 40°C: Δ, 15 min, 52°C; o, 20 h, 52°C; •, 15 min, 86°C; □, control. 100% activity (unheated control) represents μmoles min^{-1} mg^{-1} protein of secondary alcohol dehydrogenase at 40°C.

T. acetoethylicus; and hydrogen for *C. thermocellum*. *C. thermohydrosulfuricum* strain 39E notably produced the highest ethanol yield reported (8) for thermophiles (~1.9 mol ethanol/mol glucose).

The biochemical basis for different reduced end product ratios in thermophilic bacterial species that possess the same glycolytic pathways is related to subtle differences in the specific activities and regulatory properties of the enzymes which control carbon and electron flow during fermentation. Figure 7 demonstrates the relation of catabolic enzyme activities to reduced end product ratios of cellobiose fermentations of *T. brockii* strain HTD4 and *C. thermocellum* strain LQRI. The numbers above the arrows represents the specific activity of the enzyme reaction indicated in μmol/min/mg protein at 40°C. The numbers above the reduced end product represent the total μmol product formed in batch cultures (see Table VI).

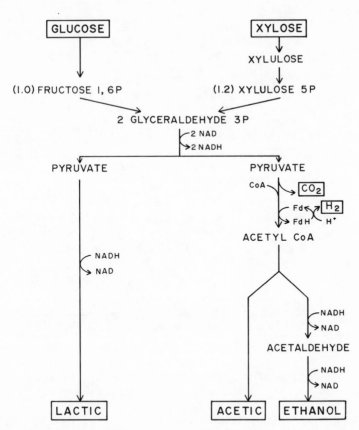

Figure 6. Hexose and pentose metabolism pathways of thermophilic ethanologens.

TABLE VI

Cellobiose Fermentation Products of Saccharolytic Thermophiles

| | ORGANISM | | |
| | (TOTAL μMOLE FORMED) | | |
PRODUCT	_T. BROCKII_ HTD4	_C. THERMOHYDROSULFURICUM_ 39E	_C. THERMOCELLUM_ LQRI	_T. ACETOETHYLICUS_[B] HTB2
ETHANOL	224	543	157	139
ACETATE	48	31	165	134
L-LACTATE	352	50	24	0
CO$_2$	230	580	346	190
H$_2$	20	31	286	29

[A]CULTURES WERE INCUBATED IN COMPLEX MEDIUM AT 60-65°C.

[B]BUTYRATE AND ISOBUTYRATE WERE TRACE PRODUCTS.

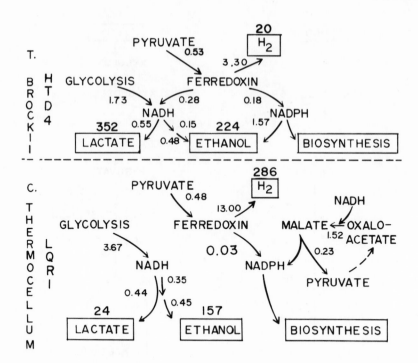

Figure 7.   Relation of the catabolic enzyme activities and proposed electron flow scheme to the reduced fermentation product yields of *T. brockii* HTD4 and *C. thermocellum* LQRI.   Numbers represent final end-product yields (total micromoles formed) of cellobiose fermentations and the specific activities of the enzymes indicated by the arrows in micromoles per minute per milligram of protein at 40°C.

We related the high hydrogen yield of *C. thermocellum* to the absence of electron flow from pyruvate to lactate or ethanol because of: the absence of detectable ferredoxin-NAD reductase and NADPH linked acetaldehyde reductase activities; and high relative hydrogenase activity.   In *T. brockii* fermentations low H_2 yield corresponded to low relative hydrogenase activity and the interconnected flow of electrons from pyruvate to: reduced ferredoxin via pyruvate dehydrogenase, reduced pyridine nucleotides via ferredoxin NAD(P) reductases; lactate via pyruvate reductase; and to ethanol via acetyl CoA reductase and both NADPH and NADH linked acetaldehyde reductases.   The difference in lactate yields was in part related to the flow of electrons from pyruvate to lactate as described above and, more importantly, to the regulatory properties of lactate dehydrogenase.   Lactate dehyerogenase in these thermophiles is an allosteric enzyme and fructose 1,6-diphosphate is a specific enzyme activator (13).   During cellobiose fermentation the intracellular fructose 1,6-Diphosphate concentration is about 9 fold higher in

TABLE VII

Relation of Energy Sources to Growth, [FDP] and
Fermentation Product Yields of *T. Brockii*

ADDITIONS	GROWTH (A$_{540}$)	[FDP] (NMOL/MG CELLS)	H$_2$	ETHANOL	ACETATE	LACTATE	ETHANOL/LACTATE
				END PRODUCTS FORMED (TOTAL µMOL/TUBE)			
NONE	0.15	--	8	33	11	16	2.0
GLUCOSE	1.3	52	11	110	15	162	0.70
STARCH	1.0	2	20	215	29	81	2.65
ACETONE	0.40	--	3	3	90	15	0.2
GLUCOSE + ACETONE	2.3	21	4	15	262	20	0.75

CONDITIONS: ANAEROBIC CULTURE TUBES CONTAINED COMPLEX MEDIUM WITH 0.3% YEAST EXTRACT.

T. brockii than *C. thermocellum*. These findings correlated with 2
fold higher activities of glyceraldehyde-3-phosphate dehydrogenase
and thus helps to explain the different lactate yields of these
species.

Table VII compares the relation of energy source to growth,
[FDP] and fermentation product yields of *T. brockii* in batch culture
(20). The ethanol/lactate ratio was 0.7 on glucose as compared to
2.7 on starch, the more slowly metabolized energy source . Note
that this finding corresponded with dramatically lower intracellular
fructose 1,6-diphosphate concentrations (>10 fold decrease) on
starch as the energy source. Most importantly, the addition of
acetone (100 mM), and exogenous electron acceptor recognized with
high specificity by the NADP linked alcohol dehydrogenase, nearly
doubles the growth yield and rate (data not shown), while it only
lowers the [FDP] by about one-half. The drastic decrease in
ethanol, H$_2$ and lactate yield during glucose fermentation corresponded with the production of isopropanol as the major reduced end
product (data not shown). Thus this lactic acid bacterium can be
regulated so as to make isopropyl alcohol as the only significant
reduced end product (20).

Figure 8 illustrates the relation between metabolic control
of electron flow in *T. brockii* fermentations and key reversible
oxidoreductases. This information is used to explain how the
direction of electron flow relates to differences in specific
fermentation conditions. Growth of *T. brockii* but not *C. thermocellum* is totally inhibited by 1 atm of exogenous H$_2$. The biochemical explanation for this phenomena is as follows: because of
interconnected oxidoreductases electrons flow from H$_2$ and reduce

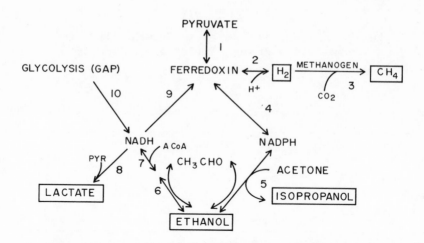

Figure 8. Metabolic control of catabolic electron flow by reversible oxidoreductases in *T. brockii*. The numbers refer to the following enzyme activities: 1, pyruvate ferredoxin oxidoreductase; 2, hydrogenase; 3, "methanogenases"; 4, ferredoxin-NADP oxidoreductase; 5, ethanol-NADP oxidoreductase; 6, ethanol-NAD oxidoreductase; 7, NADH-acetyl CoA oxidoreductase; 8, NADH-pyruvate reductase; 9, ferredoxin-NAD oxidoreductase; and 10, glyceraldehyde 3 P dehydrogenase, ACoA means acetyl CoA; GAP means glyceraldehyde 3 phosphate. Note the specific product of enzyme 5 depends on the substrate (i.e., acetaldehyde, ethanol or acetone).

NAD which is needed to perform the key oxidation of glycolysis (i.e. glyceraldehyde 3-phosphate dehydrogenase). Hydrogen is not a metabolic inhibitor in the presence of acetone because this exogenous electron acceptor is reduced via acetaldehyde-NADP reductase to isopropanol, and thus allows for re-generation of oxidized pyridine nucleotides. *T. brockii* but not *C. thermocellum*, grows on ethanol as an energy source in the presence of *Methanobacterium thermoautotrophicum*, a hydrogen consuming species, because of reversible NAD and NADP linked alcohol dehydrogenases, interconnected ferredoxin-NAD(P) linked oxidoreductases and hydrogenase. The methanogen, an exogenous electron acceptor, enables growth to occur as a consequence of hydrogen consumption because H_2 is a potent metabolic inhibitor of *T. brockii* fermentations.

The foregoing fermentation data were all representatives of metabolism in batch cultures. Saccharide fermentations of *C. thermohydrosulfuricum* were also examined in continuous culture under carbon or nitrogen limitation. Figure 9 illustrates the effect of dilution rate on the fermentation product ratio during xylose fermentation. The ethanol product ratio was not significantly altered by the specific xylose concentration of the chemostat, but it was significantly lowered under nitrogen limited conditions and lactate

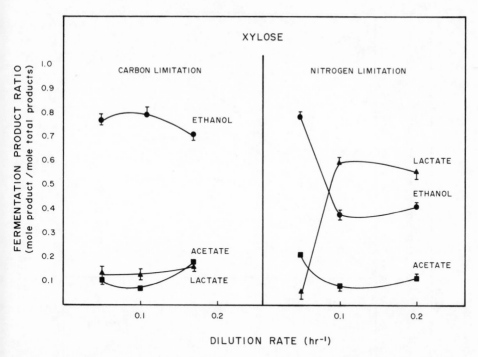

Figure 9. Continuous culture fermentation of xylose by *Clostriduim thermohydrosulfuricum*.

became the major end product, when the nitrogen level increased in the chemostat. The results of glucose fermentation in chemostat culture demonstrated that increasing the dilution rate significantly increased the lactate product ratio under carbon or nitrogen limited conditions. These data are consistent with a mechanism for control of reduced end product yield such that less rapidly metabolized substrates (i.e., xylose or starch in lieu of glucose) and limiting nitrogen decrease the intracellular frucose 1,6-diphosphate concentration and increase ethanol yield in lieu of lactate (19).

Another approach to achieve metabolic control of saccharide conversion to ethanol in lieu of varying chemical and physical fermentation parameters is to alter the microbial population.

Figure 10 shows the kinetics of product formation during Solka Floc cellulose fermentation in *C. thermocellum* mono-culture and in co-cultures with *C. thermohydrosulfuricum* (22). Solka Floc is a wood cellulose that contains both cellulose and hemicellulose. Ethanol, acetate, cellulase and reducing sugars were formed by the co-culture but at drastically different rates than those observed in mono-culture. Reducing sugar accumulation in the co-culture was 10-fold lower than in the mono-culture. At 1% Solka Floc the

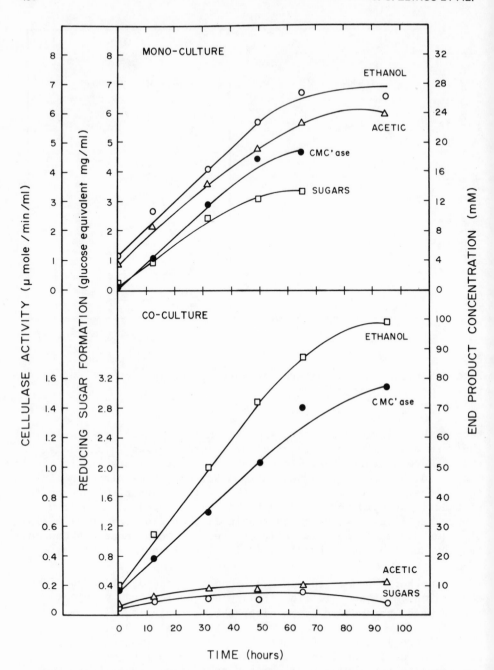

Figure 10.   Time course of cellulose fermentation in mono-culture of
C. thermocellum LQRI and in co-culture with *C. thermohydrosulfuricum*
strain 39E.   Experiments were performed in anaerobic serum vials that
contained 80 ml of GS medium with 1% Solka Floc.   Experiments were
incubated at 60°C without shaking and pH control.

TABLE VIII

Comparison of the mono- and co-culture fermentations of cellulosics
by *C. thermocellum* and *C. thermohydrosulfuricum*[a]

SUBSTRATES	CULTURE	PRODUCTS FORMED (MM) ETHANOL	ACETATE	CMCASE (U/ML)	REDUCING SUGAR (MG/ML)	SUBSTRATE CONSUMED (%)	ETHANOL/ACETATE RATIO (MOLE/MOLE)
CELLULOSE (7%)	MONO-	31.2	22.5	2.66	1.28	60	1.39
	CO-	88.9	4.2	0.79	0.08	100	21.1
FLOC (1.0%)	MONO-	30.8	27.3	4.61	2.89	50	1.13
	CO-	98.7	11.3	1.54	.15	80	8.73
TREATED PEN WOOD	MONO-	16.9	13.6	2.14	1.55	-	1.24
	CO-	54.3	11.2	1.0	.64	-	4.85
EXPLODED D (1.0%)	MONO-	14.9	15.2	2.97	1.58	-	0.98
	CO-	63.9	6.6	0.72	0.12	-	9.68
WOOD TREATED)	MONO-	2.2	6.4	-	-	-	0.34
	CO-	8.4	9.3	-	-	-	0.90

ERIMENTS WERE PERFORMED IN ANAEROBIC CULTURE TUBES THAT CONTAINED 10 ML OF GS MEDIUM AND 1.0%
TRATE EXCEPT FOR MN300 CELLULOSE (0.7%). TUBES WERE INCUBATED WITHOUT SHAKING AT 62°C FOR 120 H.

accumulated sugars consisted mainly of xylobiose, lower amounts of
glucose and xylose, and only traces of cellobiose. Carboxymethyl-
cellulase (CMCase) was produced during the fermentation but the
rate of production was three times lower in the co-culture than the
mono-culture. Despite the lower production of CMCase, the co-culture fermented cellulose (as measured by residual cellulose) at
similar rates ot that of *C. thermocellum* alone (data not shown).
Most importantly, the rate of ethanol production in co-culture
increased three fold; whereas, acetate production ceased early in
the fermentation (~30 h) and the final acetate concentration was
less than one half than that of the mono-culture. The co-culture
was very stable at 62°C, repeatably transferable and contained
approximately equal numbers of each species. Essentially the same
high ethanol production rates and yields were obtained in *C. thermohydrosulfuricum* mono-culture fermentations of Solka Floc cellulose
that contained cellulase from *C. thermocellum*. Several physiological and biochemical properties of *C. thermocellum* and *C. thermohydrosulfuricum* help explain the basis for enhanced fermentation of
Solka floc cellulose to ethanol in co-culture. These features
include: the ability of *C. thermocellum* cellulase to degrade β-1-
4-xylans or glycans; the ability of *C. thermohydrosulfuricum* to
ferment xylose and xylobiose and to incorporate cellobiose and

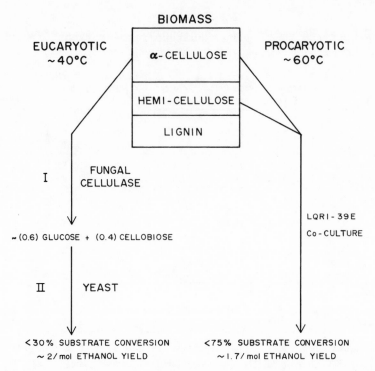

Figure 11.   Comparison of hypothetical schemes for production of
ethanol by eukaryotic or thermophic bacterial fermentations.

glucose faster than *C. thermocellum*; and a lower proton concentration associated with fermentation of equivalent amounts of cellulose
by the co-culture.

In batch culture fermentations the co-culture significantly
increased the amount of cellulosic substrate degraded and the
ethanol yield when compared to *C. thermocellum* fermentations in mono
culture.   Table VIII compares the fermentation of various cellulosic substrates in mono- and co-culture.   In addition to MN300 and
Solka Floc cellulose, the cellulosic components of Aspen wood with o
without SO_2 treatment and steam explosion were used as test substrates.   As expected, untreated wood was not significantly fermented by the co-culture or mono-culture.   However, alteration of
the chemical-structural conformation of lignin in wood by the steam
explosion or SO_2-treatments significantly rendered the wood fermentable. The ethanol/acetate ratio was considerably higher for all
fermentable cellulosics in co-culture than mono-culture.   As a
consequence of lower acetate formation in co-culture , the final pH
was 0.5 units higher than in mono-culture and this in part accounts
for the greater amount of substrates consumed and the higher total
end products concentration.   Cellulase activity and reducing sugar

TABLE IX

Key Control Parameters of Thermophilic Ethanol Production

RATE LIMITATION (MOL/H/G CELL)

BIOPOLYMER SOLUBILIZATION
SUBSTRATE UPTAKE
ELECTRON ACCEPTOR OXIDATION
PRODUCT EXCRETION

YIELD LIMITATION (MOL/G SUBSTRATE)

ELECTRON FLOW CONTROL
ENERGY METABOLISM EFFICIENCY
SUBSTRATE CONSUMPTION RANGE

CONCENTRATION LIMITATION (MOL/L)

PRODUCT FORMATION RATE
GROWTH RATE
VIABILITY

accumulation were considerably higher in all mono-culture fermentations. The final ethanol concentration observed in co-culture
cellulose fermentations with non-ethanol adapted strains (i.e., LQRI
and 39E) of *C. thermocellum* and *C. thermohydrosulfuricum* did not
exceed 1%.

SUMMARY

Thermophilic ethanol fermentations are of interest to industrial alcohol production because both the pentose and hexose fraction of biomass can be directly fermented in high yield (i.e., mol
ethanol/mol substrate consumed), and because of potential novel
process features associated with high temperature operation. As a
net result, the co-culture cellulose fermentations described here
may have the potential to convert more substrate to alcohol than
some other bioconversion systems described [see Figure 11, (2)].
However, considerably more fundamental and applied research is
required before realistic economic assessments can be made.

Detailed analysis of the data presented above suggests key
control parameters for thermophilic ethanol production (see Table
IX). Understanding in detail the physiological and biochemical
features that control rate limitation, yield limitation and concentration limitation appears to me as trends for future applied
and fundamental studies on thermophilic ethanologenic bacteria. It
is worth noting from the data reviewed here that understanding
control of any one of these 3 major limitations is complex and
multi-faceted. Indeed, improvement of ethanol tolerance (i.e. the

ability to produce greater than 1% ethanol at high rates) in these
bacteria appears to involve challenges by all three limitations.
Furthermore, the biochemical basis for alcohol tolerance in thermophilic ethanologens appears to vary in different species. For
example, the ethanol dehydrogenase of *C. thermocellum* is inhibited
by physiological concentrations of alcohol (i.e. 1%) whereas, the
reversible activity of *T. brockii* or *C. thermohydrosulfuricum* enzyme
is increased by higher solvent concentration (>5%).

REFERENCES

1.   Zeikus, J.G. 1979. Thermophilic bacteria: Ecology physiology
     and technology. Enzyme Microb. Technol. 1: 243-252.
2.   Zeikus, J.G. 1980. Chemical and fuel production by anaerobic
     bacteria. Ann. Rev. Microbiol. 34: 423-64.
3.   Ng, T.K., A. Ben-Bassat, R. Lamed and J.G. Zeikus. 1979.
     Cellulose Fermentation by Thermophilic Anaerobic Bacteria.
     Proc. U.S. Conference. Fundam. Microb. Processes, Oct. 29,
     Boston, MA.
4.   Ben-Bassat, A., R. Lamed, T.K. Ng and J.G. Zeikus. 1980.
     Metabolic Control for Microbial Fuel Production during
     Thermophilic Fermentations of Biomass. Inst. Gas. Technol.
     2nd Ann. Symp. Energy from Biomass and Wastes IV. p. 275-301.
5.   Zeikus, J.G., T.K. Ng, R.J. Lamed and A. Ben-Bassat. 1980.
     Microbial Fuel and Enzyme Production from Thermophilic Biomass
     Fermentations. In: II International Symposium on Bioconversion
     and Biochemical Engineering Delhi, India. March.
6.   Ng, T.K., P.J. Weimer and J.G. Zeikus. 1977. Cellulolytic and
     Physiological Properties of *Clostridium thermocellum*. Arch.
     Microbiol. 114: 1-7.
7.   Zeikus, J.G., P.W. Hegge and M.A. Anderson. 1979. *Thermoa-
     naerobium brockii* gen. nov. and sp. nov., a new chemoorgano-
     trophic caldoactive anaerobic bacterium. Arch. Microbiol.
     121: 41-58.
8.   Zeikus, J.G., A. Ben-Bassat and P. Hegge. 1980. Microbiology
     of Methanogenesis in thermal volcanic environments. J.
     Bacteriol. 143: 432-440.
9.   Ben-Bassat, A. and J.G. Zeikus. 1981. *Thermobacteroides aceto-
     ethylicus* gen. nov. and spec. nov., a new chemoorganotrophic,
     anaerobic, thermophilic bacterium. Arch. Microbiol. (in press)
10. Ng, T.K. and J.G. Zeikus. 1981. Comparison of Exocellular
     Cellulase Activities of *Clostridium thermocellum* LQRI and
     Trichoderma reesei QM9414. (Manuscript submitted to Appl.
     Environ. Microbiol.)
11. Ng., T.K. and J.G. Zeikus. 1980. A continuous spectrophoto-
     metric assay for the determination of cellulose solubilizing
     activity. Analy. Biochem. 103: 42-50.
12. Ng, T.K. and J.G. Zeikus. 1981. Purification and partial
     characterization of B1-4 endo-glucanase from *Clostridium*

thermocellum (manuscript prepared for submission to Biochemical Journal).

13. Lamed, R. and J.G. Zeikus, 1980. Ethanol Production by
Thermophilic Bacteria: Relationship between Fermentation
Product Yields and Catabolic Enzyme Activities in *Clostridium
thermocellum* and *Thermoanaerobium brockii*. J. Bacteriol. 144-
569-578.

14. Zeikus, J.G., G. Fuchs, W. Kenealy and R.K. Thauer. 1977.
Oxidoreductases Involved in Cell Carbon Synthesis of
Methanobacterium thermoautotrophicum. J. Bacteriol. 132: 604-
613.

15. Lamed, R. and J.G. Zeikus. 1981. Novel NADP-linked alcohol-
aldehyde/ketone oxidoreductase in Thermophilic, Ethanologenic
Bacteria. Biochemical Journal (in press).

16. Lamed, R. and J.G. Zeikus. 1981. Thermostable Ammonium
Activated Malic Enzyme of *Clostridium thermocellum*. (Manuscript submitted to Biochem. Biophys. Acta).

17. Lamed, R.J., E. Keinan and J.G. Zeikus. 1981. Potential
Applications of an Alcohol aldehyde/ketone oxidoreductase
from Thermophilic Bacteria. (In Press, Enzyme Microbiol.
Technol.).

18. Lamed, R.J. and J.G. Zeikus. 1980. Glucose Fermentation Pathway of *Thermoanaerobium brockii*. J. Bacteriol. 141: 1251-1257.

19. Ben-Bassat, A. and J.G. Zeikus. 1981. Saccharide Metabolism
of *Clostridium thermohydrosulfuricum*: Relation of substrate
utilization to enzmatic activities, and comparison of batch
and continuous culture fermentations. (Manuscript prepared
for submission to Appl. Environ. Microbiol.)

20. Ben-Bassat, A., R. Lamed and J.G. Zeikus. 1981. Ethanol
Production by Thermophilic Bacteria: Metabolic Control of
End Product Formation in *Thermoanaerobium brockii*. (In press.
J. Bacteriol.)

21. Weimer, P.J. and J.G. Zeikus. 1977. Fermentation of Cellulose
and Cellobiose by *Clostridium thermocellum* in the absence and
presence of *Methanobacterium thermoautotrophicum*. Appl.
Environ. Microbiol. 33: 289-297.

22. Ng, T.K., A. Ben-Bassat and J.G. Zeikus. 1981. Ethanol Pro-
duction by Thermophilic Bacteria Fermentation of Cellulosic
Substrates by Co-cultures of *Clostridium thermocellum* and
C. thermohydrosulfuricum. (Manuscript submitted to Appl.
Environ. Microbiol.)

FEASIBLE IMPROVEMENTS OF THE BUTANOL PRODUCTION

BY *CLOSTRIDIUM ACETOBUTYLICUM*

Gerhard Gottschalk and H. Bahl

Institut für Mikrobiologie der Universität Göttingen
Grisebachstrasse 8, D-3400 Göttingen
West Germany

Butanol as a fermentation product was discovered by Pasteur (7) in 1862 and the formation of acetone by a "Rottebacillus" was described by Schardinger (9) in 1905. Later a fermentation process for the production of acetone and butanol from carbohydrates was patented (4). Thereafter, Weizmann (13) isolated *Clostridium acetobutylicum* which was especially suitable for the production of these solvents from corn starch. A number of factories were operated on the basis of this fermentation in various countries. With the increasing availability of low-cost petrochemical raw materials and the growth of the chemical industries the fermentation process became uneconomical in industrialized countries and was discontinued. At present only a few plants are in operation, mostly in agricultural countries. Excellent reviews on the development of this process and on its operation have been published (2, 8, 10).

Because of the enormous increase of the price of oil during the last years the situation has changed. It now seems reasonable to consider the fermentation process for butanol production again and think about possible improvements. In this context one realizes immediately that very little research has been devoted to this process in recent years.

The acetone-butanol fermentation as carried out by *C. acetobutylicum* is not directly comparable with the ethanol fermentation. When yeast is confronted with a glucose-containing medium under anaerobic conditions it will inevitably produce ethanol and carbon dioxide. *C. acetobutylicum* cultures transferred several times in the laboratory or grown from lyophylized stock cultures will usually produce only butyrate, acetate, carbon dioxide and molecular hydrogen from glucose or other sugars. O'Brien and Morris (6) studied

463

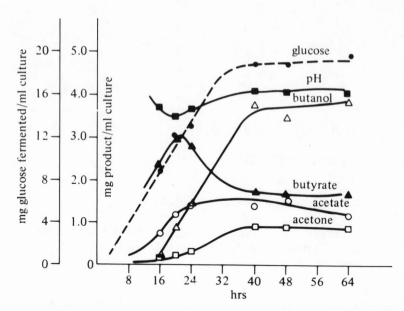

Figure 1.   Course of acid and solvent production by *C. acetobutylicum*
(from Davies, R. and Stephenson, M. (1941), Biochem. J. 35, 1320).

the effect of oxygen on growth and survival of *C. acetobutylicum*.
As is apparent from the fermentation balances given only trace
amounts of solvents were produced by their cultures which, of course,
was not the purpose of this investigation. Even solvent-producing
strains produce acetate and butyrate before forming acetone and
butanol. As was shown by Davies and Stephenson (3) in the classical
experiment depicted in Figure 1, acids are produced first followed
by a shift in the fermentation to acetone and butanol as final
products. The timing and magnitude of this shift tends to be somewhat variable. It certainly depends on the composition of the
growth medium, the pH in the culture and most importantly on the
"history" of the inoculum. Sivey (10) describes the preparation of
the inoculum cultures as follows: "Sporulation is used as a convenient method of preserving or maintaining stock cultures on a routine
basis. The organisms are inoculated into potato/glucose medium
either directly from a spore culture or from vegetative cells and
allowed to grow at 34°C for 48 hours. A small portion of this
culture is transferred to a similar medium after a heat shock treatment at 70°C for 90 seconds. The subsequent culture is then allowed
to stand at 34°C for 3-4 days to induce sporulation whereupon a
portion is transferred to sterile sand/soil and allowed to dry.
Several cycles of heat shocking may be needed to produce an acceptable culture." Ross (8) mentions: "When spores are used to start

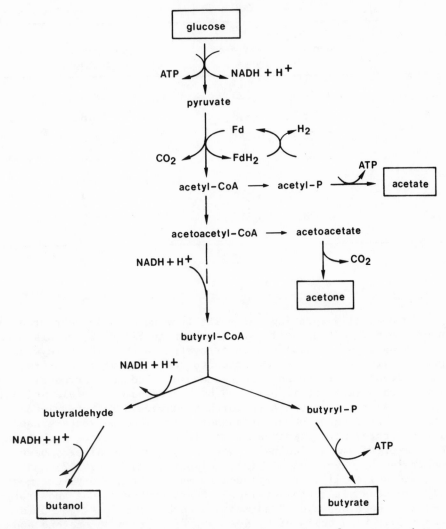

Figure 2.   Reactions involved in the formation of acetate, butyrate, butanol and acetone from glucose.

a fermentation, it is common practice to subject them to a heat shock, the duration of which may be from 1 to 3 minutes at a temperature of 65.5 - 100°.   This kills the weaker spores and is believed to produce a better fermentation."

This procedure is very unsatisfactory to a microbiologist because it is difficult to imagine how cycles of heat shocking could have an effect on the patternof fermentation products and the yields of acetone and butanol.

TABLE I

Growth rate μ	Products acetate butyrate (mol/mol glucose)		$Y_{glucose\ diss.}$ (g dry weight/mol glucose)
0.140	0.410	0.620	48.5
0.236	0.368	0.578	55.8
0.332	0.350	0.541	61.3
0.426	0.343	0.529	64.0
0.475	0.339	0.526	64.7
0.600	0.331	0.518	67.3
0.720	0.326	0.515	68.5

Biochemically speaking the shift from acid to solvent production presents itself as follows: As shown in Figure 2, sugars are fermented by C. acetobutylicum to pyruvate via the Embden–Meyerhof pathway. Pyruvate is then converted to acetyl-coenzyme A by the enzyme pyruvate: ferredoxin oxidoreductase. Reduced ferredoxin formed in this reaction is oxidized by hydrogenase to yield molecular hydrogen. Acetyl-coenzyme A is further converted to butyryl-CoA which by the action of phosphotransbutyrylase and butyrate kinase yields butyrate. The presence of the latter two enzymes in butyrate producing organisms including C. acetobutylicum has already been demonstrated by Gavard et al. (5); Valentine and Wolfe (12) and Twarog and Wolfe (11). Butyryl-CoA formation from acetyl-CoA most likely proceeds via acetoacetyl-CoA, β-hydroxybutyrl-CoA and crotyonyl-CoA as been shown by Stadtman and Barker for C. kluyveri (see Barker (1)). When cells of C. acetobutylicum turn on acetone and butanol formation the metabolic flux is diverted at two points:

First, part of the acetoacetyl-CoA is used to produce acetone via acetoacetate. Whereas the enzyme acetoacetate decarboxylase has been studied extensively (14), it is not known how acetoacetate is formed from aceto-acetyl-CoA. This could be either by hydrolysis or by transfer of coenzyme A to another acid such as acetate or butyrate. In some preliminary experiments we obtained evidence for the presence of a coenzyme A transferase in C. acetobutylicum under certain growth conditions.

Second, butyryl-CoA is no longer converted to butyrate via butyryl phosphate but is reduced to butyraldehyde and further to

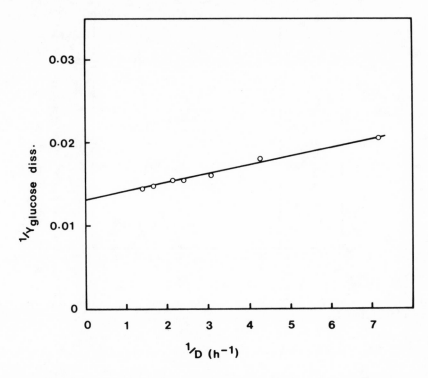

Figure 3. Double reciprocal plot of the growth yield (^{Y}glucose diss.) against the dilution rate.

butanol. Nothing is known about the regulation at this branch point. Two enzymes compete for butyryl-CoA: phosphotransbutyrylase and butyraldehyde dehydrogenase, the former being extremely active in cell extracts. The specific activity of this enzyme in extracts of acid-producing cells is in the order of 8 U per mg of protein; it is much lower in extracts of solvent-producing cells (0.1 to 1.2 U/mg protein). Thus it seems that the activity of this enzyme is somehow adjusted to the fluxes of metabolites to either butyrate or butanol. These investigations on the level of certain key enzymes in *C. acetobutylicum* have to be extended so that the biochemistry of the shift can be understood.

Another question is how acetone and butanyol formation is initiated. To study this we have grown *C. acetobutylicum* in continuous culture with glucose as the growth-limiting substrate. Its concentration in the reservoir was 19 mM. Table I summarizes data obtained at various dilution rates. It is apparent that *C. aceto-butylicum* is a fast growing organism; a growth rate of 0.72 could be achieved. ^{Y}glucose diss. was in the order of 48 to 68 g dry weight/mol glucose depending on the growth rate. The fermentation

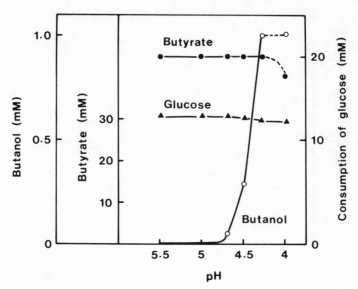

Figure 4.   Effect of a decrease in pH on butanol formation in continuous culture.

products were acetate, butyrate, CO_2 and molecular hydrogen. On the
basis of the concentrations in which acetate and butyrate were present in the effluent it could be calculated that the organisms
coupled the breakdown of 1 mol of glucose with the phosphorylation
of 3.5 mol ADP.   The maximum growth yield ($Y^{max}_{glucose\ diss.}$) as
calculated from a Pirt plot (Figure 3) amounted to 74 g dry weight
per mol glucose.

     Why should these organisms form butanol?   The production of
butanol instead of butyrate yields less ATP and results in lower
growth yields.   The shift toward solvent formation, therefore, must
be the response to an unfavorable environment or it must be connected to a growth stage of these organisms in which maximum growth
of the cells is no longer necessary, as, for instance, in the
sporulation stage.   To create unfavorable growth conditions, the
pH of the continuous culture was gradually decreased.   It is
apparent from Figure 4 that at pH 4.7 butanol appeared as a product
in the effluent, it reached its maximum steady state concentration
at pH 4.3.   Figure 5 shows that a shift back to pH 5.0 decreased
the butanol concentration but butanol went up again when a pH of
4.3 was reestablished.   Acetone was not formed in detectable amounts
under these conditions.   The final butanol concentration was still
low.   However, it must be considered that the culture was run with
carbon limitation.

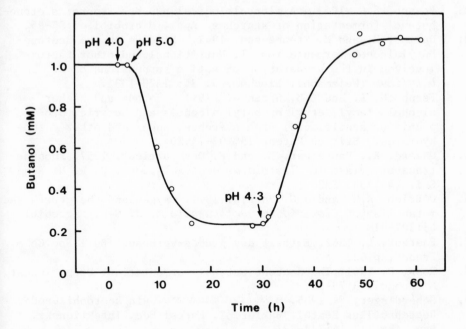

Figure 5. Effect of pH changes on the steady state concentration of butanol.

This is an interesting result. The technique allows us to determine the pH optimum of butanol formation for various strains of *C. acetobutylicum* and under various conditions. Moreover, it permits the study of the effect of medium components as well as the optimum sugar concentration. It may even lead to conditions under which solvent production is not preceded by acid production. In batch culture, as it is usually carried out, the conditions for solvent production are established through acid production. The latter is accompanied by H_2-evolution. This molecular hydrogen is lost as reducing agent for butanol production. In a process in which butanol is formed from the beginning the molecular hydrogen might be recycled for the reductive processes leading to butanol.

ACKNOWLEDGEMENT

This work was supported by a grant of the "Bundesministerium für Forschung und Technologie".

REFERENCES

1.   Barker, H.A. 1956. Bacterial Fermentations, John Wiley and Sons Inc., New York, p. 28.

2.   Beesch, S.C. 1953. A microbiological process report: acetone-
      butanol fermentation of starches. Appl. Microbiol. 1:85-95.
3.   Davies, R. and M. Stephenson. 1941. Studies on the acetone-
      butylalcohol-fermentation: 1. Nutritional and other factors
      involved in the preparation of active suspensions of *C. aceto-
      butylicum* (Weizmann). Biochem. J. 35: 1320-1331.
4.   Fernbach, A. and E.H. Strange. 1911. Acetone and higher
      alcohols (amyl, ethyl or butyl alcohols and butyric, pro-
      pionic or acetic acid) from starches, sugar and other carbo-
      hydrates. British Patent 15.203-15.204.
5.   Gavard, R., Hautecoer, B. and H. Descourtieux. 1957. Phospho-
      transbutyrylase in *Clostridium acetobutylicum*. C. R. H. Acad.
      Sci. 244:2323-2326.
6.   O'Brien, R.W. and J.G. Morris. 1971. Oxygen and the growth and
      metabolism of *Clostridium acetobutylicum*. J. Gen. Microbiol.
      68:307-318.
7.   Pasteur, L. 1862. Extrait des proces-verbeaux. Bull.Soc.Chim.
      France, p.52.
8.   Ross, D. 1961. The acetone-butanol fermentation. Prog. Indust.
      Microbiol. 3:73-90.
9.   Schardinger, F. 1905. *Bacillus macerans,* ein acetonbildender
      Rottebacillus Zentbl. Bakteriol. Parasitkde. Infektionskr.
      Hyg. Abt. II 14:772-781.
10.   Spivey, M.J. 1978. The acetone/butanol/ethanol fermentation.
      Process Biochem. 13: 2-15.
11.   Twarog, R. and R.S. Wolfe. 1962. Enzymatic phosphorylation of
      phosphotransbutyrylase. J. Biol. Chem. 237:2474.
12.   Valentine, R.C. and R.S. Wolfe. 1960. Purification and role
      of phosphotransbutyrylase. J. Biol. Chem. 235: 1948-1952.
13.   Weizmann, C. 1945. British Patent 4845.
14.   Zerner, B., Coutts, S.M., Lederer, F., Waters, H.H. and F.H.
      Westheimer. 1966. Acetoacetate decarboxylase. Preparation of
      the enzyme. Biochemistry 5:813-816.

DISCUSSION

Q.   REDDY: When your butanol production is maximum, are you also
      allowing for a certain level of butyrate or acetate so the
      organisms get some energy for growth?

A.   GOTTSCHALK: Under chemostat conditions they keep on producing
      acetate and butyrate under these conditions but this is done,
      as I said, under glucose limitation. The next thing we plan
      is to set up a system where substrate is in excess.

B.   TEMPEST: I would have been very dissappointed had you not
      used continuous culture, but my question really relates to the
      question of fatty acids and pH. With acidic pH you can have
      quite devastating consequences because the acids become

unionized and as such cross the plasma membrane and dissipate
the trans membrane pH gradient. So do you see this in that
context as a mechanism for a neutralization kind of reaction?
Do you think that the control mechanism possibly could be or
result in a dissipation of the trans membrane pH gradient?

A.   GOTTSCHALK: I think the problem is, as I mentioned at the
      beginning: If you take a culture of *Clostridium acetobutylicum*
      it simply won't produce butanol in high yields. I didn't talk
      about how we have to prepare our inoculum in order to get the
      cells to produce butanol in batch culture. If you set up a
      culture the organisms often lower the pH to 3.5, they don't
      sporulate under these conditions and they don't produce buta-
      nol. Therefore, the switch is more complicated. It is not
      just the pH.

Q.   WOOD: In all that old work that was done on this fermentation
      and all the industrial concerns that made butanol acetone
      this way, did anybody ever find or report cellulytic or
      thermophilic variants or membrs of this fermentation family?

A.   GOTTSCHALK: Yes, I think they were patented in the 19's I
      can't remember the name but there are at least 30 or 40 sub-
      species that are mentioned in patents and some of them are
      thermophiles. Also, they vary with respect to the substrates
      which they can use. You have organisms which use starch,
      others which are not able to use starch but go with molasses,
      and so on. There's quite a variation with respect to the
      nutrients and temperatures.

ACRYLATE FERMENTATIONS

A. J. Sinskey, M. Akedo, and C. L. Cooney

Department of Nutrition and Food Science
Massachusetts Institute of Technology
Cambridge, Massachusetts 02139

INTRODUCTION

It is well recognized that non-renewable resources such as natural gas and oil are limited in availability. As a consequence, considerable effort is being expended to develop alternative technologies for the manufacture of industrial chemicals (ethanol, acetic acid, 2,3-butanediol, and acetone/butanol) which utilize renewable raw materials. It is in this context that we have sought to investigate the potential of microbially catalyzed reactions for the production of acrylic acid from a biomass which is one of renewable solar energy resources.

Acrylic acid and its esters are industrial chemical feedstock of considerable value and are primarily used in the form of polymers. Starting materials for commercial synthesis of the acrylates include acetylene, propylene and ethylene.

Acrylate, in the form of the activated coenzyme A thiolester, is known to occur as an intermediate in several microbial pathways (Table I). For example, the catabolic metabolism of propionate by *Escherichia coli* includes acrylyl-CoA (29). For propionate formation as a major end product of fermentations, acryly-CoA exists as an intermediate in the so-called "direct reductive pathway" or the "acrylate pathway", in which lactate is reduced to propionate without succinate being an intermediate. This pathway is exhibited by at least two anaerobic bacteria, *Clostridium propionicum* (4,11) and *Megasphaera (Peptostreptococcus) elsdenii* (8,13). The occurence of the direct reductive pathway was also observed in *Bacteroides ruminicola* (27,28). Because of the relative simplicity of the fermentation metabolism and by pursuing preliminary results obtained in our laboratory, we have chosen to work with *C. propionicum*.

473

TABLE I

Acrylyl-CoA as an Intermediate
(excluded plant and animal tissues)

Propionate Oxidation

Escherichia coli (Wegener and coworkers, 1967)
Pseudomonas aeruginosa (Sokatch and coworkers, 1968)
Clostridium kluyveri (Stadtman and Barker, 1950)
Moraxella lwoffi (Hodgson and McGarry, 1968)

Propionate Formation (direct reductive pathway)

Clostridium propionicum (Cardon and Barker, 1947)
Megasphaera eladenii (Elsden and coworkers, 1956)
Bacteroides ruminicola (Wallnöfer and coworkers, 1966)

The objective of this paper is to demonstrate accumulation
of a catabolic intermediate that is not normally a metabolic end
product, acrylic acid, from the breakdown products of biomass as
well as to discuss the significance of acrylate accumulation in
propionate fermentation pathway in *C. propionicum*.

CLOSTRIDIUM PROPIONICUM AND ACRYLATE AS A BIOCHEMICAL INTERMEDIATE

C. propionicum is a strict anaerobe which can grow in a
medium containing α-alanine or β-alanine as sources of carbon and
nitrogen (3). Resting cells can readily ferment lactate, acrylate,
pyruvate and some other amino acids including serine, threonine,
cysteine, and methionine to acetate and propionate as fermentation
end products (propionate and butyrate for threonine and methionine)
in ratios governed by intermolecular electron balances (Table II)
These fermentations constitute the first indication of the occurrence of the direct reductive pathway for propionate formation.

One hypothesis of long standing as to the mechanisms of
propionate formation involves dehydration of lactate to acrylate
and reduction of acrylate to propionate. Rapid conversion of
acrylate to propionate gives some support to acrylate as an intermediate. *C. propionicum* lacks the ability to decarboxylate
succinate and does not fix $^{14}CO_2$ into the carboxyl carbon of propionate (11). Cell suspensions do not ferment fumarate, malate or
succinate (4). No succinate is formed. Thus it has been established that *C. propionicum* produces propionate by a type of fermentation different from that observed with *Propionibacteria*. Evidence
for the reduction of lactate to propionate via acrylate has derived
principally from isotopic studies. In contrast to *Propionibacterium
arabinosum*, lactate $3-^{14}C$ is fermented to acetate and propionate
labelled almost exclusively in the methyl or methylene carbons, and
randomization between α- and β-carbon atoms of propionate was not
observed (15). Such a distribution of labelling suggests the direct

TABLE II

Anaerobic Fermentation of Various Substrates by Cell Suspensions of *C. propionicum* (molar ratios)

	α-alanine β-alanine	pyruvate	lactate	serine	acrylate	threonine	cysteine	methionine
Ammonia	3	—	—	3	—	3	3	3
Carbon dioxide	1	2	1	2	1	2	2	2
Acetic acid	1	2	1	2	1	—	2	—
Propionic acid	2	1	2	1	2	2	1	2
Butyric acid	—	—	—	—	—	1	—	1
Hydrogen sulfide	—	—	—	—	—	—	3	3

(Cardon and Barker, 1947)

reduction of lactate to propionate in *C. propionicum*. However, these experiments only tell us that the carbon skeleton of lactate is intact in propionate.

In view of the fact that the butyrate formation has been shown to occur via the acyl-CoA esters of the respective inter- mediates rather than free acids (20), it was postulated that the intermediates in propionate formation via the direct reductive pathway involved the CoA derivatives of lactate, acrylate and pro- pionate in *C. propionicum* (21) and in *M. elsdenii* (8). Since then, evidences for CoA intermediates and acrylate intermediate have been accumulated. The overall proposed metabolic pathway is summarized in Figure 1. A part of each substrate is oxidized to acetate and carbon dioxide, while another part is reduced to propionate. Energy for growth is presumably obtained solely through the phosphoro- clastic reaction involving phosphotransacetylase and acetate kinase. No hydrogen is formed. The oxidation of pyruvate to carbon dioxide and acetyl-CoA is tightly coupled to the reduction of acrylyl-CoA to propionyl-CoA. To maintain this oxidation-reduction balance, three moles of α-alanine, for example, are fermented to two moles of propionate and one mole of acetate yielding one mole of ATP. β-alanine is readily metabolized by β-alanine grown cells via β- hydroxy-propionate (9). The reactions including-acrylyl-CoA as an intermediate which are believed to occur in *C. propionicum* are summarized in Figure 2. To date, all the available evidence for acrylate as an intermediate so far obtained by various workers has been indirect, or in other words, acrylate itself has never been directly demonstrated. In the following sections, we will demon- strate and discuss experimental evidences for an acrylate inter- mediate with three primary substrates, i.e. propionate, β-alanine and lactate, and at the same time, suggest possible routes to acrylate production.

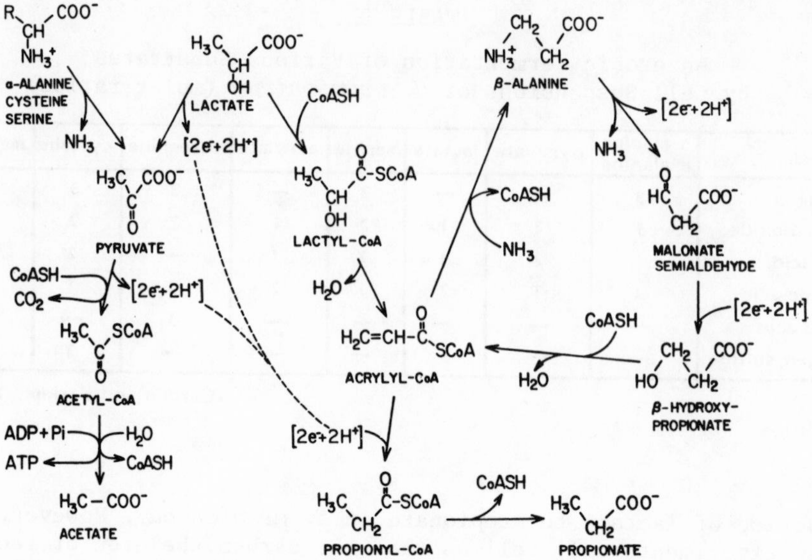

Figure 1. Metabolic pathways in *Clostridium propionicum*

β-ALANINE TO ACRYLATE

C. propionicum can grow on β-alanine as a carbon and nitrogen
source as well as α-alanine. Growing or resting cells are capable
of fermenting β-alanine to propionate and acetate. The conversion
of acrylate to β-alanine was observed in the presence of acetyl-CoA
and ammonia salt with the use of an enzyme, acrylyl-CoA aminase
(22,26), that catalyzes amination of acrylyl-CoA to form β-alanyl-
CoA. The purified enzyme also catalyzes the reaction, acrylyl-
pantetheine (Pa) and ammonia to form β-alanyl-pantetheine (Pa)
(25). Evidence that β-alanine is actually formed has been obtained
by showing that in the presence of added ammonia salt, acrylyl-Pa
disappeared as measured by a decrease in optical density at 263nm
and the oxidation of carboxyl-labelled propionate leads to the
accumulation of a ^{14}C-labelled non-volatile compound which was then
identified as β-alanine by paper chromatography and ninhydrin reaction (23,24).

For the reverse reaction, β-alanine to acrylate, β-alanyl-Pa
was added to the purified enzyme from β-alanine grown cells. An
increase in optical density at 263nm was observed, indicating the
formation of acrylyl-Pa, and hydroxamic acid derivative of acrylyl-
Pa was identified by chromatography. However all the above evidence
did not directly show acrylyl-Pa or acrylate itself from β-alanine,
although strongly suggesting that acrylyl-CoA is involved as an
intermediate.

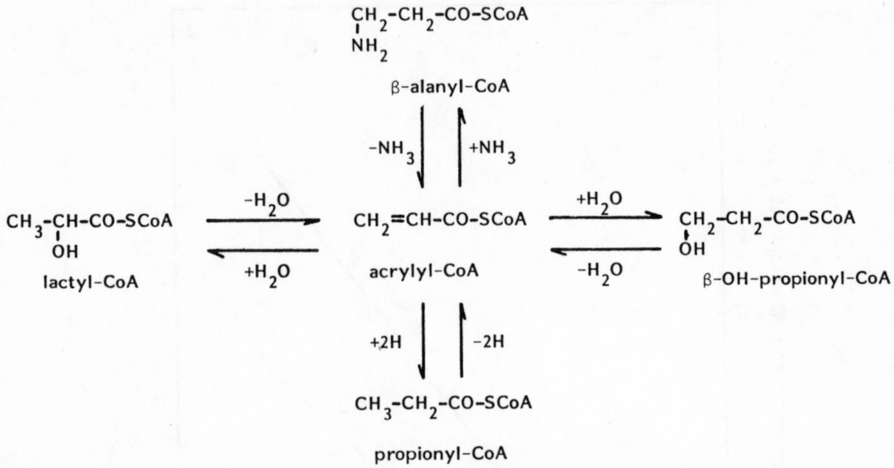

$$CH_2-CH_2-CO-SCoA$$
$$|$$
$$NH_2$$

β-alanyl-CoA

$$-NH_3 \Big\uparrow \quad \Big\uparrow +NH_3$$

$$CH_3-CH-CO-SCoA \xrightarrow{-H_2O} CH_2=CH-CO-SCoA \xrightarrow{+H_2O} CH_2-CH_2-CO-SCoA$$
$$| \qquad\qquad\quad \xleftarrow{+H_2O} \qquad\qquad\qquad\quad \xleftarrow{-H_2O} \qquad |$$
$$OH \qquad\qquad\qquad\qquad\qquad\qquad\qquad\qquad\qquad\qquad\qquad OH$$

lactyl-CoA   +H_2O   acrylyl-CoA   -H_2O   β-OH-propionyl-CoA

$$+2H \Big\downarrow \quad \Big\uparrow -2H$$

$$CH_3-CH_2-CO-SCoA$$

propionyl-CoA

Figure 2.   Acrylyl-CoA as a Biochemical Intermediate

When fermentation of β-alanine by β-alanine grown cells under
anaerobic conditions was conducted (Figure 3), in addition to the
accumulation of acetate and propionate, there was a transient
accumulation of acrylate. This result represents the first demonstration of acrylate being detected in *C. propionicum* and demonstrates that acrylate is indeed a fermentation intermediate. From
knowledge of the metabolic pathway in *C. propionicum* (Figure 1),
acrylyl-CoA serves as a terminal electron acceptor in order to
maintain reduction-oxidation balance. Since *C. propionicum* is an
obligate anaerobe which is primarily distinguished by its sensitivity to molecular oxygen, it is interesting to know that many of the
obligate anaerobes contain electron-transport soluble flavoproteins
capable of functioning as NADH oxidases which can utilize molecular
oxygen as a terminal electron acceptor (6,7). Thus, experiments
were conducted to evaluate the effect of a variety of electron
acceptors on the fermentation by resting cells of *C. propionicum*.
When β-alanine grown cells were incubated with β-alanine in the
presence of air, acrylate accumulation was stimulated and stablized,
suggesting that oxygen can serve as an alternate electron acceptor
(Figure 4). This is consistent with the fact that *C. propionicum*
has an active terminal oxidase system (24). Propionate production
was greatly decreased and little or no acetate was produced. A
similar pattern of acrylate accumulation was obtained when β-alanine
was fermented under anaerobic conditions in the presence of artificial electron acceptors such as methylene blue and triphenyl-tetrazolium chloride (Figure 5). These results further support the
hypothesis that oxygen is acting as an electron acceptor and "short-
circuit" electron flow (17). Therefore, it appears that exogenous
electron acceptors including oxygen may be used to alter the metabolic activity of the organism so as to prevent the reduction of

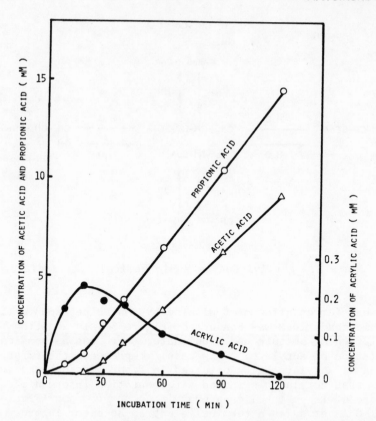

Figure 3.   Anaerobic fermentation of β-alanine by resting cells of
C. propionicum grown on β-alanine.   Cells were grown at 37°C
anaerobically on β-alanine and harvested at late exponential phase.
Reaction mixture (total volume 1ml) contained: triethanolamine-HCl
buffer (pH 7.5), 50 mM; β-alanine, 50 mM; resting cells, 0.1g wet
wt./ml.   Incubation was carried out 37°C under nitrogen atmosphere
with magnetic stirring.   Samples (100 µl) were taken at each time
interval and transferred to a tube containing 20 µl of 50% H_2SO_4.

acrylate to propionate. Furthermore, these results demonstrate
acrylate as an intermediate and the role of acrylate in the metabolic pathway.

PROPIONATE TO ACRYLATE

        Conversion of acrylate to propionate implied that acrylate
is an intermediate in the direct reductive pathway in *C. proionicum*
(3). The reduction of acrylyl-Pa to propionyl-Pa was also observed
using reduced safranin dye as an electron donor with extracts of
C. propionicum.   The product of acrylyl-Pa reduction was identified

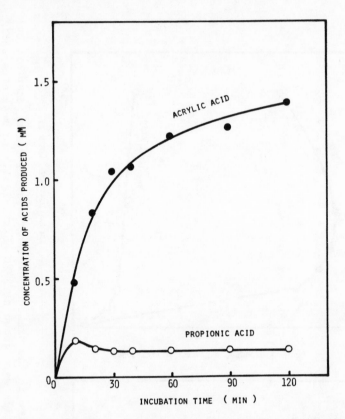

Figure 4. Aerobic fermentation of β-alanine by β-alanine grown cells of *C. propionicum*. Cells were grown at 37°C anaerobically on β-alanine and harvested at late exponential phase. Reaction mixture (1 ml) contained: triethanolamine-HCl buffer (pH 7.5), 50 mM; β-alanine, 50 mM; resting cells, 0.1g wet wt./ml. Incubated at 37°C under air atmosphere with magnetic stirring. Samples (100 µl) were taken at each time interval and transferred to a tube containing 20 µl of 50% H_2SO_4.

as propionyl-Pa by paper chromatography of the hydroxamic acid derivatives (19). Acetone powder of *M. elsdenii* reduced acrylyl-CoA to propionyl-CoA (16). For the reverse reaction, propionate to acrylate, extracts of *M. elsdenii* converted propionyl-Pa to acrylyl-Pa as identified by paper chromatography of hydroxamic acid derivatives (1). With cell-free extracts of *C. propionicum*, the reaction propionyl-Pa to acrylyl-Pa was demonstrated in the presence of a trapping agent, glutathione, and final product was identified as acrylate-glutathione complex (24). In the presence of ammonia and catalytic amounts of acetyl-phosphate (acetyl-P) and coenzyme A, *C. propionicum* cell-free extracts catalyzed the oxidation of

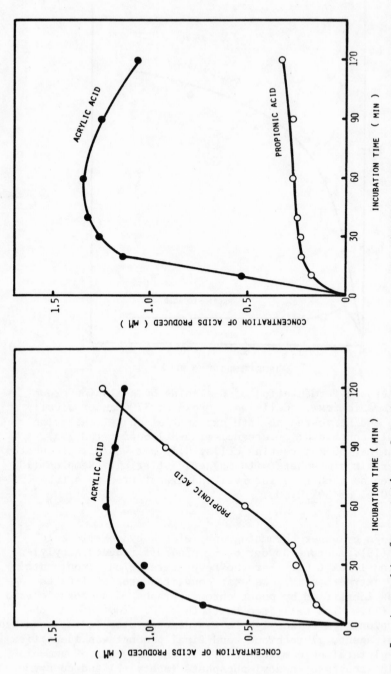

Figure 5. Anaerobic fermentation of β-alanine in the presence of artificial electron acceptors by β-alanine grown cells of *C. propionicum*. Cells were grown at 37°C anaerobically on β-alanine until early stationary phase. Reaction mixture (1 ml) contained: triethanolamine-HCl buffer (pH 7.5), 50 mM; β-alanine, 50 mM; methylene blue or triphenyl-tetrazolium chloride, 0.1%; resting cells, 0.1g wet wt./ml. Incubation was carried out at 37°C under nitrogen atmosphere with magnetic stirring. Samples (100μl) were withdrawn at each time interval and transferred to a tube containing 20 μl of 50% H_2SO_4.

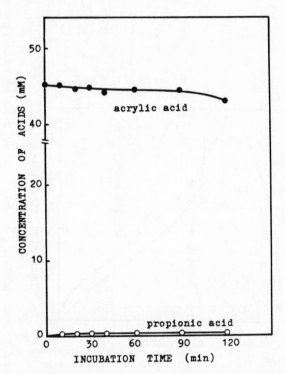

Figure 6. Aerobic fermentation of acrylate by resting cells of *C. propionicum*. Cells were grown at 37°C anaerobically on α-alanine and harvested at late exponential phase. Reaction mixture (total volume 1ml) contained: triethanolamine-HCl buffer (pH 7.5), 50 mM; acrylate, 50 mM; resting cells, 0.1g wet wt./ml. Incubation was carried out at 37°C with magnetic stirring under air atmosphere. Samples (100 μl) were taken at each time interval and acidified with 20 μl of 50% H_2SO_4.

[14]C-labelled propionate to ^{14}C-labelled β-alanine (23). Even though the formation of β-alanine from propionyl-Pa in the presence of ammonia is presumptive evidence that acryly-CoA is an intermediate in propionate oxidation, the immediate product of propionyl-CoA dehydrogenation in the absence of ammonia has not been directly identified.

Having demonstrated that oxygen is able to accept available electrons during β-alanine fermentation, studies on fermentation of other metabolites were conducted with resting cells of *C. propionicum* in the presence of oxygen. It is interesting to note that under an aerobic atmosphere, acrylate was not fermented by resting cells (Figure 6). This result is consistent with an observation of a stable acrylate accumulation from β-alanine in the presence of electron acceptors. Since propionate is one of the fermentation

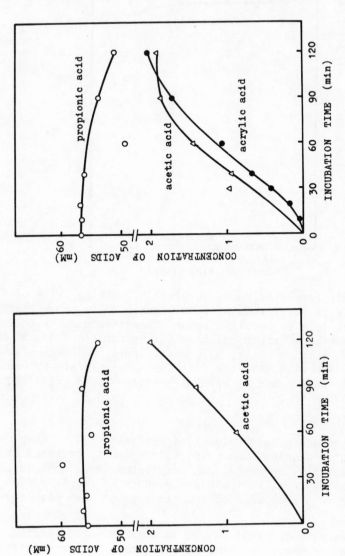

Figure 7. Effect of experimental atmosphere on the fermentation of propionate by resting cells of *C. propionicum*. Cells were grown at 37°C anaerobically on α-alanine until late exponential phase. Reaction mixture (total 1 ml) contained: triethanolamine–HCl buffer (pH 7.5), 50 mM; propionate, 50 mM; resting cells, 0.1g wet wt. cells/ml. Incubation was carried out at 37°C with magnetic stirring under either nitrogen or air atmosphere. Samples (100 µl) were taken at each time interval and reactions were stopped with 20 µl of 50% H_2SO_4.

end products, it is normal that propionate is not metabolized under
anaerobic conditions. However, when the fermentation was carried
out in the presence of air, acrylate accumulation was observed
(Figure 7). This result clearly showed that one can in fact reverse
the reaction of acrylate reduction to propionate. With the same
principle in aerobic fermentation of β-alanine, molecular oxygen
can serve as an electron acceptor for the propionate oxidation. This
concept was supported by an observation that *C. propionicum* cells
can oxidize propionate to acrylate anaerobically in the presence
of methylene blue as an alternative electron acceptor replacing
oxygen (Figure 8). Without methylene blue there was no acrylate
accumulation. Increasing concentrations of methylene blue resulted
in increased amounts of acrylate. Once the methylene blue was fully
reduced, as observed by a color change from blue to colorless, the
accumulated acrylate was rapidly metabolized and disappeared. This
observation can be explained by considering that the role of
acrylyl-CoA is as an electron acceptor in the metabolic pathway of
C. propionicum. In the presence of both methylene blue and air,
acrylate accumulation was stable and methylene blue remained in the
reduced state.

    In the course of lactate fermentation studies, it was found
that lactate addition to a resting cell preparation oxidizing
propionate to acrylate stimulated acrylate accumulation when both
methylene blue and air were present (Figure 9). When one of the
components was removed from the reaction mixture, stimulation of
acrylate accumulation was not observed. To test this finding with
other metabolites in the pathway, the experiment was carried out
with α-alanine, pyruvate, β-alanine, and β-hydroxy-propionate
(Table III). Like lactate, incubation with α-alanine or pyruvate
resulted in an increased amount of acrylate. β-alanine or β-hydroxy-
propionate showed no effect. Since β-alanine was poorly metabolized
by α-alanine grown cells, experiments were also conducted with β-
alanine grown cells. Similar to α-alanine grown cells, α-alanine
and pyruvate as well as lactate showed a stimulatory effect. To
explain this observation, there are two possibilities: 1. lactate
(α-alanine or pyruvate) serves as an additional substrate, or 2.
not as a substrate, but stimulates reactions by some other mechanism. In order to elucidate this point, radioactive ^{3}H-α-alanine
and ^{14}C-propionate were used (Figure 10). Even though acrylate
was not clearly separated from propionate on the paper chromatogram,
the acrylate-propionate peak was not associated with ^{3}H activity.
Thus, role of lactate was not as an additional substrate for acrylate
accumulation.

    With cell-free preparations of *C. propionicum*, propionate oxi-
dation to acrylate was examined with high energy compounds and coenzyme A together with these metabolites under conditions where both
air and methylene blue were present (Table IV). Little accumulation

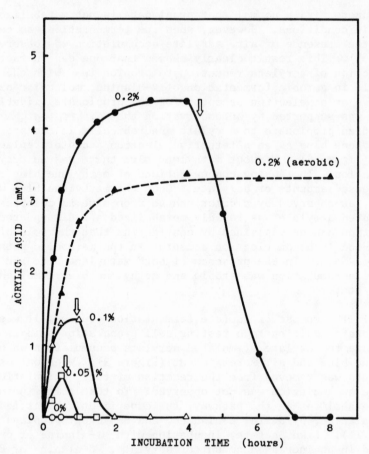

Figure 8. Effect of methylene blue on the conversion of propionate
to acrylate under anaerobic conditions. Reaction mixture (total
2 ml) contained: triethanolamine-HCl buffer (pH 8.5), 50 mM; propionate, 200 mM; methylene blue, 0 - 0.2%. Incubated at 37°C under
nitrogen atmosphere with mechanical agitation. Samples (200 µl)
were taken at each time interval and reaction was stopped with 40µl
of 50% H_2SO_4.

          —o— 0%   methylene blue (control)
          —□— 0.05%   methylene blue
          —△— 0.1%   methylene blue
          —●— 0.2%   methylene blue
          --▲-- 0.2%   methylene blue (under
                          aerobic condition)

arrow (⇓) indicates the color change of methylene blue from blue
to colorless.

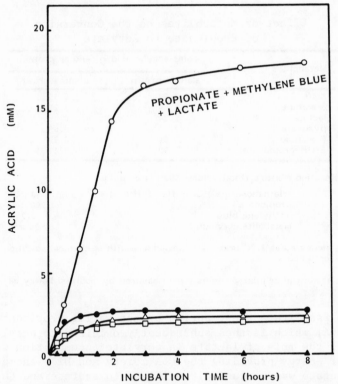

Figure 9.   Conversion of propionate to acrylate in the presence of methylene blue and lactate.   Reaction mixture (2 ml) contained triethanolamine-HCl buffer (pH 8.5), 50 mM; propionate, 200 mM; methylene blue, 0.2%; lactate, 25 mM. Incubated at 37°C under air atmosphere with mechanical agitation. Samples (200 μl) were taken at each time interval and acidified with HO μl of 50% H_2SO_4.

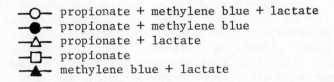

—○— propionate + methylene blue + lactate
—●— propionate + methylene blue
—△— propionate + lactate
—□— propionate
—▲— methylene blue + lactate

of acrylate was observed when propionate was incubated with CoASH or high energy phosphate compounds separately. However, when CoASH was used together with acetyl-P or ATP, acrylate production from propionate greatly increased. ADP was less effective than ATP. The same observation was true when acetyl-CoA was added to propionate or pyruvate and CoASH were added to propionate.   These results clearly indicated that cell-free extracts of *C. propionicum* were unable to catalyze the oxidation of propionate unless the CoA moiety and high energy compounds were present in the reaction mixture in

TABLE III

Effect of Metabolites on the Conversion
of Propionate to Acrylate

Metabolites	m moles acrylic acid/g cellular protein	
	α-alanine grown	β-alanine grown
none	0.91	0.15
α-alanine	4.34	3.25
lactate	2.24	0.49
pyruvate	2.47	0.65
β-alanine	0.84	0.23
β-OH-propionate	0.90	0.17

Reaction mixture (total volume 500 μl) contained:

triethanolamine-HCl buffer (pH 8.5)	50 mM
propionate	200 mM
methylene blue	0.2%
metabolite compound	20 mM

Incubated at 37°C under air atmosphere with mechanical agitation
for 4 hours.

Amount of cellular proteins were measured by modified Lowry method.

order to facilitate the reaction by activating propionate to propionyl-CoA, which is then subsequently oxidized to acrylyl-CoA.
Moreover, the role of lactate in acrylate accumulation was as a
source of energy providing the CoA moiety and high energy compound
while lactate was exclusively oxidized to acetate and CO_2 under
these experimental conditions. This conclusion was supported by
the observation (23) that propionate oxidation to β-alanine was
achieved only when acetyl-P, CoA moiety and ammonia were present.

The hypothesized lactate reduction pathway in *C. propionicum*
is in many respects similar to the metabolic sequence involving
butyrate formation via crotonyl-CoA occurring in *Clostridium buty-
ricum*. Threonine metabolism by *C. propionicum* resulted in the
formation of propionate and butyrate, much as serine metabolism
resulted in acetate and propionate formation. This prompted efforts
to obtain crotonate as a result of buyrate dehydrogenation. Using
a system similar to that observed for acrylate from propionate,
resting cells of *C. propionicum* produced crotonate from butyrate.
This resting cell bioconversion system was further employed to
produce methacrylate from isobutyrate (5).

LACTATE TO ACRYLATE

Efforts have been made by various workers to show evidences
for acrylate intermediate in lactate reduction to propionate. Lactate and acrylate were rapidly metabolized by cell-free extracts of
M. elsdenii at identical rates and to the same products in identical

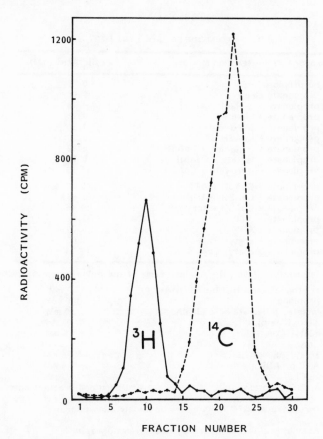

Figure 10. Substrate flux. Reaction mixture (1 ml) contained:
triethanolamine-HCl buffer (pH 8.0), 50 mM; propionate, 100 mM;
α-alanine, 25 mM; methylene blue, 0.2%; [3-^{3}H]-α-alanine, 10 µCi;
[3-^{14}C]-propionate, 1 µCi; cellular protein, 15 mg/ml. Incubated
at 32°C for 4 hours under air atmosphere. Acids were extraced with
ethyl ether and concentrated by flushing nitrogen. Ammonium salts
of acids were separated by paper chromatography and radioactivity
was measured after development.

proportions (12). For the reaction of lactate to acrylate, extracts
of *M. elsdenii* catalyzed the reaction of ^{14}C-lactyl-Pa to acrylyl-
Pa as identified on paper chromatography of hydroxamic acid derivatives (1). Evidence for lactyl-CoA dehydrase with *M. elsdenii* was
presented by showing that purified enzyme catalyzed the reaction
lactyl-CoA to acrylyl-CoA in the presence of acyl-CoA dehydrogenase,
reduced safranin and ^{14}C-lactyl-CoA by measuring an increase in
optical density at 540nm due to the formation of oxidazed safranin
and by paper chromatography of the hydroxamates (2). But a reaction
product in the absence of acyl-CoA dehydrogenase and reduced
safranin was not mentioned.

TABLE IV

Propionate Activation

Components in Reaction Mixture	Acrylic Acid (mM)
no propionate	0.00
propionate alone	0.05
propionate + α-alanine	0.16
propionate + lactate	0.11
propionate + pyruvate	1.20
propionate + CoASH	0.78
propionate + α-alanine + CoASH	0.12
propionate + lactate + CoASH	0.72
propionate + pyruvate + CoASH	16.46
propionate + CoASH + ATP	15.90
propionate + CoASH + ADP	8.95
propionate + CoASH + acetyl-P	14.76
propionate + ATP	2.24
propionate + ADP	0.79
propionate + acetyl-P	1.65
propionate + acetyl-CoA	14.71

Reaction mixture (200 µl) contained some of the following compounds:

triethanolamine-HCl buffer (pH 8.0)	50 mM
propionate	100 mM
lactate, pyruvate or α-alanine	20 mM
methylene blue	0.2%
acetyl-CoA	5 mM
CoASH	5.5 mM
acetyl-phosphate	5 mM
ATP or ADP	5 mM
MgCl$_2$	3 mM
cellular protein	4.42 mg/ml cell-free extracts

Incubated at 32°C for 4 hours under air atmosphere.

Acrylic acid was analyzed by gas chromatography.

In an attempt to demonstrate the conversion of acrylate to lactate, cell-free extracts of *C. propionicum* failed to show the conversion of acrylyl-Pa to lactyl-Pa (25). However, this α-addition of water molecule to the double bond in acrylyl-CoA was found to occur in extracts of a propionate oxidizing *Pseudomonas* and in pigeon heart muscle extracts. With extracts of *Clostridium kluyveri*, a β-addition of water to acrylyl-CoA to form β-hydroxy-propionyl-CoA was observed. Cell-free extracts of *M. elsdenii* showed that acrylate conversion to lactate occurred in the presence of NAD, extracts, lactate dehydrogenase, CoA transferase, and ^{14}C-acrylyl-CoA, and ^{14}C-pyruvate was identified as a final product. However, lactate formation in the absence of lactate dehydrogenase has never been mentioned. Instead, it says that D-lactate dehydrogenase was inactive indicating that the product formed by hydration was L-lactate. All the above studies have never shown the immediate

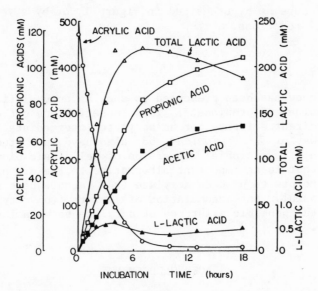

Figure 11. Anaerobic fermentation of acrylate by resting cells of
C. propionicum. Cells were grown at 37°C anaerobically on α-alanine
to late exponential phase. Reaction mixture (total volume 7.5 ml)
contained: triethanolamine-HCl buffer (pH 7.5), 50 mM; acrylate,
500 mM; resting cells, 0.15g wet wt./ml. Incubation was carried
out at 35°C under nitrogen atmosphere. At appropriate time intervals, samples were withdrawn and assayed for volatile acids and
lactate.

reaction product, acrylate from lactate or lactate from acrylate.

        The same strategy did not result in acrylate as an intermediate
in lactate reduction to propionate and thus no accumulation of acrylate from lactate in the presence of electron acceptors including
oxygen could be demonstrated. In spite of the fact that acrylate cannot be utilized as a carbon source by *C. propionicum* and even is
toxic to its growth, resting cells were capable of fermenting acrylate very rapidly to propionate and acetate (Figure 11). Besides
these two end products, a large amount of lactate was found to
accumulate, accounting for the material balance. When the concentration of lactate was assayed by the L-lactate dehydrogenase system,
only a small amount of lactate was detected. Thus, it was concluded
that the majority of the accumulated lactate from acrylate was D-
lactate. This demonstration strengthened a belief that lactate reduction to propionate occurred via acrylate, but yet no acrylate
formation has been shown from lactate. It is interesting to know
that α-addition of water molecule to the double bond in acrylate is
very unlikely from the thermodynamical point of view. There is still
considerable speculation as to whether the conversion of lactate to

acrylate occurs as hypothesized in Figure 1, or by a yet unconfirmed sequence of reactions.

CONCLUSIONS

Evidence has been presented to show an accumulation of acrylate from β-alanine and propionate. These observations not only serve as the first direct evidence for an acrylate intermediate in the metabolic pathway of *C. propionicum*, but also have indicated a possible application of a microbial conversion of cellulosic biomass to acrylate, that is an important alternative to the use of fossil fuels. Attempts to produce acrylate from lactate have so far not been successful. But accumulation of lactate from acrylate strongly suggested the possible existence of acrylate between lactate and propionate.

ACKNOWLEDGEMENTS

This study was supported by a grant from the United States Department of Energy, contract number EG-77-S-02-4198. M. Akedo is supported by a fellowship from the National Distillers and Chemical Corporation.

REFERENCES

1. Baldwin, R.L., W.A. Wood and R.S. Emery. Conversion of lactate-^{14}C to propionate by the rumen microflora. J. Bacteriol. 83:907-913(1962).
2. Baldwin, R.L., W.A. Wood and R.S. Emery. Lactate metabolism by *Peptostreptococcus elsdenii*: Evidence for lactyl coenzyme A dehydrase. Biochim. Biophys. Acta 97:202-213 (1965).
3. Cardon, B.P. and H.A. Barker. Two new amino-acid-fermenting bacteria, *Clostridium propionicum* and *Diplococcus glycinophilus*. J. Bacteriol. 52:629-634(1946).
4. Cardon, B.P. and H.A. Barker. Amino acid fermentations by *Clostridium propionicum* and *Diplococcus glycinophilus*. Arch. Biochem. 12:165-180 (1947).
5. Dalal, R.K., M. Akedo, C.L. Cooney, and A.J. Sinskey. A microbial route for acrylic acid production. Biosources Digest 2:89-97 (1980).
6. Dolin, M.I. Survey of microbial electron transport mechanisms. In: I.C. Gunsalus and R.Y. Stanier (ed.). The Bacteria. Academic Press, New York, Vol. II, pp. 319-363 (1961a).
7. Dolin, M.I. Cytochrome-independent electron transport enzymes of bacteria. In: I.C. Gunsalus and R.Y. Stanier (ed.). The Bacteria. Academic Press, New York. Vol. II, pp. 425-460 (1961b).

8. Elsden, S.R., B.E. Volcani, F.M.C. Gilchrist, and D. Lewis. Properties of a fatty acid forming organism isolated from the rumen of sheep. J. Bacteriol. 72:681-689 (1956).

9. Goldfine, H. and E.R. Stadtman. Propionic acid metabolism. V. The conversion of β-alanine to propionic acid by cell-free extracts of *Clostridium propionicum*. J. Biol. Chem. 235:2238-2245 (1960).

10. Hodgson, B. and J.D. McGarry. A direct pathway for the conversion of propionate into pyruvate in *Moraxella Iwoffi*. Biochem. J. 107:7-18 (1968).

11. Johns, A.T. The mechanism of propionic acid formation by *Clostridium propionicum*. J. Gen. Microbiol. 6:123-127 (1952).

12. Ladd, J.N. and D.J. Walker. The fermentation of lactate and acrylate by the rumen micro-organism LC. Biochem. J. 71:364-373 (1959).

13. Ladd, J.N. and D.J. Walker. Fermentation of lactic acid by the rumen microorganism, *Peptostreptococcus elsdenii*. Ann. N.Y. Acad. Sci. 119:1038-1045(1965).

14. Leaver, F.W. and H.G. Wood. Evidence from fermentation of labeled substrates which is inconsistent with present concepts of the propionic acid fermentation. J. Cell and Comp. Physiol. 41:suppl. 1. 225-240(1953).

15. Leaver, F.W., H.G. Wood and R. Stjernholm. The fermentation of three carbon substrates by *Clostridium propionicum* and *Propionibacterium*. J. Bacteriol. 70:521-530(1955).

16. Lewis, D. and S.R. Elsden. The fermentation of L-threonine, L-serine, L-cysteine, and acrylic acid by a Gram-negative coccus. Biochem. J. 60:683-692 (1955).

17. Morris, J.G. The physiology of obligate anaerobiosis. In: A.H. Rose and D.W. Tempest (ed.). Advances in Microbial Physiology. Academic Press, New York. Volume 12. pp. 169-246 (1975).

18. Sokatch, J.R., L.E. Sanders and V.P. Marshall. Oxidation of methylmalonate semialdehyde to propionyl-coenzyme A in *Pseudomonas aeruginosa* grown on valine. J. Biol. Chem. 243:2500-2506 (1968).

19. Stadtman, E.R. and H.A. Barker. Fatty acid synthesis by enzyme preparations of *Clostridium kluyveri*. VI. Reactions of acyl phosphates. J. Biol. Chem. 184:769-793 (1950).

20. Stadtman, E.R. Studies on the biochemical mechanism of fatty acid oxidation and synthesis. Record Chem. Progr. Kresge-Hooker Sci. Lib. 15:1-17 (1954).

21. Stadtman, E.R. Fermentations de l'acide propionique. Bull. Sté. Chim. Biol. 37:931-938 (1955a).

22. Stadtman, E.R. The enzymatic synthesis of β-alanyl coenzyme A. J. Am. Chem. Soc. 77:5765-5766 (1955b).

23. Stadtman, E.R. Propionate oxidation by cell-free extracts of *Clostridium propionicum*. Federation Proc. 15:360-361 (1956).

24.   Stadtman, E.R. and P.R. Vagelos. Propionic acid metabolism.
      Proceedings of the International Symposium on Enzyme Chemistry,
      Tokyo and Kyoto, 1957. Maruzen, Tokyo. pp. 86-92 (1958).

25.   Vagelos, P.R. and E.R. Stadtman. Enzymatic conversion of
      acrylyl-pantetheine to beta-alanyl-pantetheine and lactyl-
      pantetheine. Abstracts of papers of the 131st meeting of
      the American Chemical Society, American Chemical Society,
      Washington, pp. 24C-25C (1957).

26.   Vagelos, P.R., J.M. Earl and E.R. Stadtman. Propionic acid
      metabolism. I. The purification and properties of acrylyl
      coenzyme A aminase. J. Biol. Chem. 234:490-497 (1959).

27.   Wallnöfer, P., R.L. Baldwin and E. Stagno. Conversion of
      ^{14}C-labeled substrates to volatile fatty acids by the rumen
      microbiota. Appl. Microbiol. 14:1004-1010 (1966).

28.   Wallnöfer, P. and R.L. Baldwin. Pathway of propionate forma-
      tion in *Bacteroides ruminicola*. J. Bacteriol. 93:504-505
      (1967).

29.   Wegener, W.S., H.C. Reeves and S.J. Ajl. Propionate oxidation
      in *Escherichia coli*. Arch. Biochem. Biophys. 121:440-442
      (1967).

DISCUSSION

WOOD: I'd just like to make a few comments. First of all
it looks to me as though the *Clostridium* system must be very
similar, if not identical to, the system in *Megasphera* (or
as we used to call it *Peptostreptococcus*. With regard to the
oxidation process that you see where electrons go up to water,
there are two electron transport components in *Megasphera*,
and the arrangement might be the same in *Clostridium propionicum*. One is the acyl CoA dehydrogenase which you
mentioned, and the other is an electron transfer protein which
mediates between acyl CoA dehydrogenase and oxygen, as least
in *Megasphera*. Another point you mentioned several times is
the fact that the lactyl CoA-acrylyl CoA reaction catalyst
has been very difficult to isolate. Every test for lactyl
CoA dehydration or acryly CoA hydration has been frustrated
by the extremely high levels of crotonase that are present in
both of these organisms. Thus, if one could remove crotonase,
we might be able to make progress. As you have pointed out,
removal of the α-hydroxyl group or an anti-Markonikov's rule
hydration-dehydration reaction has everyone puzzled and it
may not go as a one-step process. Finally, we attempted to
establish phospholactyl CoA as being an intermediate, but I
don't really believe we have the evidence.

MICROBIAL ADAPTATIONS TO STRESS:

SOME LESSONS TO BE LEARNED FROM AEROBES

Terry Ann Krulwich and Richard J. Lewis

Department of Biochemistry, Mount Sinai School of
Medicine of the City University of New York
New York, New York 10029

There are microbial adaptations to "stress" or unusual conditions that would seem to be of obvious importance for optimizing
fermentative capacities for the production of fuels. Three of these
areas are the specific topics of talks in this session. There are
two other environmental constraints upon microbial viability and
metabolism that have been the subjects of investigations in our
laboratory. These are the problem of pH---both extremely acidic
and extremely alkaline---and the problem of the controls regulating
aerobic vs. a more fermentative mode of metabolism. While all these
studies have been conducted in aerobes, they touch upon concerns
with respect to the issues at hand.

The studies of regulation of aerobic vs. fermentative metabolism emerged from work on alternate sugar transport systems in the
coryneform bacterium *Arthrobacter pyridinolis*. Coryneforms are
generally aerobic, although some species are relatively facultative
and/or can withstand long periods of nutrient deprivation (reviewed
in 1). *A. pyridinolis* was among the first aerobic bacteria in which
a phosphoenolpyruvate:hexose phosphotransferase system (PTS) was
documented (2,3). Theretofore, the PTS was a transport system that
was associated with facultative or obligately anaerobic organisms
(4). More recently, *A. pyridinolis* as well as certain other
aerobes (5-8) have been found to possess PTS activity for D-fructose
and some other carbohydrate substrates. Could the PTS have some
special role in these aerobic species? In *A. pyridinolis,* inducible
PTS activity for D-fructose and L-rhamnose is present in addition
to respiration-coupled transport systems for each of these hexoses
(9-11). Several interesting regulatory effects are associated with
these alternate transport systems: first, free hexose must be transported into the cell in order for induction of the PTS to occur

(12,13); second, the respiration-coupled transport system for D-fructose is active until the mid-log phase of growth, whereas the PTS activity for D-fructose begins to appear at about that same time; and third, studies of a ʃ-aminolevulinic acid auxotroph indicate that PTS activity is highest under conditions in which the respiratory capacity is suboptimal for aerobic growth (14). These observations suggest that the two transport systems are controlled in such a way as to result in a temporal pattern, with the PTS expressed as cultural conditions become less highly aerobic. There are at least certain indications that indeed the period of PTS activity is also a period in which D-fructose metabolism is somewhat more fermentative (14). Current studies (15) are directed towards the elucidation of metabolic signals that are involved in the transition between a highly aerobic metabolic mode and a more fermentative metabolism.

Our other area of investigation involving adaptations to an environmental contraint is that of external pH. Since there are important bioconversions that occur at both extremes of pH, or result in acid or base production, the mechanisms for tolerance of extremes of pH are of general interest. In 1977, Garland (16) rather perceptively outlined the particular bioenergetic problems that would be expected to confront acidophiles and alkalophiles. Acidophiles (optimal pH 1.5-4.0) must be able to maintain a large transmembrane ΔpH, outside acid, i.e. they must be able to keep their cytoplasm at a considerably higher pH than the external milieu. Indeed, the intracellular pH of *Thermoplasma acidophilum* (17,18), *Thiobacillus ferro-oxidans* (19), and *Bacillus acidocaldarius* (20) is maintained between pH 5.5 and 6.9 over a range of highly acidic external pHs. The large ΔpH of the acidophiles is apparently a chemiosmotic energy form and can energize solute transport (20) and ATP synthesis (21). Abolition of the ΔpH results in rapid loss of viability (22). In all of these obligate acidophiles, a transmembrane electrical potential (Δψ), inside positive, exists (19,20,23). This Δψ is the reverse of the usual direction (inside negative) (Figure 1), and is probably a special and necessary bioenergetic feature of acidophiles. The ionic fluxes that are involved in the maintenance of the large ΔpH and "reversed" Δψ will be a fundamental aspect of this pattern of gradients. These ionic fluxes are not as yet known. Similarly, knowledge of the respiratory chains of the acidophiles is only fragmentary (e.g. 24,25), but will be important to the understanding of acid tolerance. Interestingly, recent studies of the facultative species *Streptococcus faecalis* suggest that mutational loss of a cation transporter results in unusual acid sensitivity (26).

In extreme obligate alkalophiles, the converse problem was anticipated, i.e. such organisms must maintain a cytoplasmic pH that is lower than that of the external *milieu* (16). Indeed, obligate alkalophiles grow optimally at pH 10.5 and can grow up to pH 11.5, but exhibit cytoplasmic pHs no higher than pH 9.5 (27,28). The

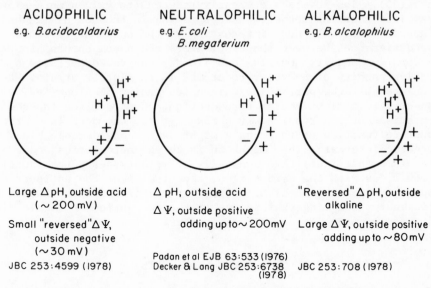

Figure 1.   Protonmotive force in whole cells.

latter pH is probably the upper limit that is compatible with viability.   Non-alkalophilic mutant strains can be isolated (28,29).
These strains have lost the ability to grow above pH 9.0, but can
grow in the neutral range of pH.   They are found to have lost the
activity of an electrogenic Na^+/H^+ antiporter (28-30), which is thus
associated with the generation of the "reversed" ΔpH in the wild
type strains.   That reversed ΔpH, however, poses a problem with
respect to the energetics of the alkalophiles.   Although a substantial electrical potential ($\Delta\psi$) exists in these organisms, the
sum of the $\Delta\psi$ and the reversed ΔpH is a rather low total protonmotive force (Figure 1) (27,28).   How, then, are processes such as
solute transport and ATP synthesis energized?   For many of the
solute systems, in several alkalophiles, the problem of a low protonmotive force is bypassed by use of a sodium-motive force i.e.
Na^+/solute symport systems (27,31,32).   For at least one fermentable
carbon source (and its analogue), *Bacillus alcalophilus* utilizes a
transport system that depends upon ATP per se rather than the
protonmotive force (33).   The resolution of the problems of the low
protonmotive force in connection with ATP synthesis is less clear.
The evidence so far indicates that the F_1 subunit of the ATPase of
alkalophiles is conventional (34) and that a proton-translocating
ATPase catalyzes the ATP production at low protonmotive forces (35).
The energetics of this synthesis requires further investigation.
It is notable that obligately alkalophilic bacteria have been found
to possess extraordinarily high levels of respiratory chain compo-

nents (36). The levels are greatly reduced (to values more closely resembling those of conventional bacteria) in the non-alkalophilic mutant derivatives. Most interestingly, there appear to be qualitative differences between the respiratory chain components of *B. alcalophilus* and its non-alkalophilic derivative, especially a relative paucity of *b*-type cytochromes in the latter strain. We would speculate that the particular exigencies facing alkalophiles, with respect to efficient energy transduction, have resulted in specific adaptations of the respiratory chain. If so, the details of the structure/function of that chain might be of considerable bioenergetic interest. They might indicate characteristics and mechanisms that facilitate unusually efficient energy transduction. Moreover, as with the acidophiles, the studies of the antiport and symport systems in the alkalophiles can clarify aspects of chemiosmotic energy coupling that relate to the energetics of facultative and anaerobic species as well as aerobes.

ACKNOWLEDGEMENTS

This work was supported by research grants PCM7725586 and PCM7810213 from the National Science Foundation. Richard Lewis is a trainee on Medical Scientist Training Grant GM07280 from the National Institutes of Health.

REFERENCES

1.   Krulwich, T.A., and Pelliccione, N.J. (1979) Ann. Rev. Microbiol. 33:95.
2.   Sobel, M.E., and Krulwich, T.A. (1973) J. Bacteriol. 113:907.
3.   Wolfson, E.B., Sobel, M.E., and Krulwich, T.A. (1973) Biochim. Biophys. Acts 321:181.
4.   Romano, A.H., Eberhard, S.J., Dingle, S.L., and McDowell, T.C. (1970) J. Bacteriol. 104:808.
5.   Dills, S.S., Apperson, A., Schmidt, M.R., and Saier, M.H.,Jr. (1980) Microbiol, Revs. 44:385.
6.   Marquet, M., Creignou, M.-C., and Dedonder, R. (1976) Biochimie 58:435.
7.   Sawyer, M.H., Baumann, P., Baumann, L., Berman, S.M., Canovas, J.L., and Berman, R.H. (1977) Arch. Microbiol. 112:49.
8.   Sawyer, M.H., Baumann, P., and Baumann, L. (1977) Arch. Microbiol. 112:169.
9.   Krulwich, T.A., Sobel, M.E., Wolfson, E.B. (1973) Biochem. Biophys. Res. Commun. 53:258.
10. Wolfson, E.B., Sobel, M.E., Blanco, R., and Krulwich, T.A. (1974) Arch. Biochem. Biophys. 160:440.
11. Levinson, S.L. and Krulwich, T.A. (1974) Arch. Biochem. Biophys. 160:445.

12.   Wolfson, E.B. and Krulwich, T.A. (1974) Proc. Natl. Acad. Sci.
      U.S.A. 71:1739.
13.   Levinson, S.L. and Krulwich, T.A. (1976) J. Gen. Microbiol.
      95:277.
14.   Pelliccione, N., Jaffin, B., Sobel, M.E., and Krulwich, T.A.
      (1979) Eur. J. Biochem. 95:69.
15.   Pelliccione, N.J. and Krulwich, T.A. (1981) Eur. J. Biochem.,
      in press.
16.   Garland, P.B. (1977) Symp. Soc. Gen. Microbiol. 27:1.
17.   Hsung, J.C. and Haug, A. (1975) Biochim. Biophys. Acta 389:
      477.
18.   Searcy, D.G. (1976) Biochim. Biophys. Acta 451:278.
19.   Cox, J.C., Nicholls, D.G., and Ingledew, W.J. (1979) Biochem.
      J. 178:195.
20.   Krulwich, T.A., Davidson, L.F., Filip, S.J., Jr., Zuckerman,
      R.J., and Guffanti, A.A. (1978) J. Biol. Chem. 253:4599.
21.   Apel, W.A., Dugan, P.R., and Tuttle, J.H. (1980) J. Bacteriol.
      142:295.
22.   Guffanti, A.A., Davidson, L.F., Mann, T. and Krulwich, T.A.
      (1979) J. Gen. Microbiol. 114:201.
23.   Hsung, J.C. and Haug, A. (1977) FEBS Lett. 73:47.
24.   Belly, R.T., Bohkul, B.B., and Brock, T.D. (1973) Ann. N.Y.
      Acad. Sci. 225:94.
25.   Hollander, R. (1978) J. Gen. Microbiol. 108:165.
26.   Kobayashi, H., and Unemoto, T. (1980) J. Bacteriol. 143:1187.
27.   Guffanti, A.A., Susman, P., Blanco, R., Krulwich, T.A. (1978)
      J. Biol. Chem. 253:708.
28.   Guffanti, A.A., Blanco, R., Benenson, R.A., and Krulwich,
      T.A. (1980) J. Gen. Microbiol. 119:79.
29.   Krulwich, T.A., Mandel, K.G., Bornstein, R.F., and Guffanti,
      A.A. (1979) Biochem. Biophys. Res. Commun. 91:58.
30.   Mandel, K.G., Guffanti, A.A., and Krulwich, T.A. (1980) J.
      Biol. Chem. 255:7391.
31.   Koyama, N., Kiyomuja, A., and Noshoh, Y. (1976) FEBS Lett.
      72:77.
32.   Kitada, M., and Horikoshi, K. (1977) J. Bacteriol. 131:784.
33.   Guffanti, A.A., Blanco, R., and Krulwich, T.A. (1979) J.
      Biol. Chem. 254:1033.
34.   Koyama, N., Koshiya, K. and Nosoh, Y. (1980) Arch. Biochem.
      Biophys. 199:103.
35.   Guffanti, A.A. and Krulwich, T.A. (1979) Abstr. XIth Intl.
      Cong. Biochem., p. 422.
36.   Lewis, R.J. Belkina, S., and Krulwich, T.A. (1980) Biochem.
      Biophys. Res. Commun. 95:857.

THERMOPHILY

H. Zuber

Institut für Molekularbiologie und Biophysik
Eidg. Technische Hochschule
Zürich, Switzerland

Life at high temperature has been a subject of interest and
of studies for many years, the first work in this area having been
done in the last century - e.g. by F. Cohn and F. Hoppe-Seyler.
However, the presence of life in hot springs has been described
already by the Romans, e.g. by Pliny, the Elder. It has also been
known for a long time that temperature is one of the most important
environmental factors controlling the activities and the evolution
of organisms. In the living cell, temperature determines not only
the rates of enzyme-catalyzed chemical reactions, but also the state
of active structures of the important biopolymers (proteins, nucleic
acids, lipid-membranes) and of water. In order to live within a
particular temperature range, organisms have to adapt structurally
and functionally to the environmental temperature. This means they
must "love" these temperatures: to be alive at high temperatures,
they must be thermophiles. Temperature adaptation is especially
important for heterothermal organisms (the poikilotherms). for
example the microorganisms, in which the cell temperature follows
the varying environmental temperature. In contrast, at a higher
phase of evolution, mammals and birds as homoiothermal organisms
have developed a metabolic system to insure a constant cell temperature, and thus to avoid this problem of adaptation to varying
temperatures.

EXTREME THERMAL ENVIRONMENTS, NUMBER AND TYPES OF ORGANISMS IN THERMAL ENVIRONMENTS, EVOLUTION OF THESE ORGANISMS

Where in the biosphere do we find extremely high temperatures?
The average temperature on the surface of the earth is about 12°C.
The majority of organisms have adapted to a moderate temperature

TABLE I

Upper Temperature Limits for Life of Various Organisms

Organisms	Approximate upper temperature ($^{\circ}$C)
Animals	
Fish	35-40
Insects	45-50
Ostracods (Crustaceans)	50
Plants	45
Mosses	50
Microorganisms (Eucaryotes)	
Protozoa	50-55
Algae	55-60
Fungi	55-60
Microorganisms (Procaryotes)	
Cyanobacteria	70-75
Photosynthetic bacteria	70-75
Chemolithotrophic bacteria	> 90
Heterotrophic bacteria	> 90

around this average. Although frequent on earth, high temperature environments are restricted to relatively few limited regions.

Extreme thermal environments are found in regions with geo-thermal energy - in hot springs (USA, Japan, Iceland, New Zealand, etc.), in small bays warmed by the sun, in solar heated soil and in heating systems and power stations (1).

Biological combustion processes represent a particularly high temperature ecosystem, for here heat from cell metabolism is released by mostly thermophilic soil bacteria and fungi, and heats the organic material (leaves, grass, hey) (2). By this process of thermogenesis, these thermophilic microorganisms create their own ecosystem. It is interesting that these thermophilic soil bacteria which are moderate thermophiles are found all over the earth, even in zones with relatively low average temperatures (2).

Regions with a high environmental temperature are of particular interest from the viewpoint of the evolution of microorganisms since such regions give insight both into a specific ecosystem with a restricted number of species (a situation that corresponds to the definition of an extreme environment), and to new types of micro-organisms especially adapted to high temperatures.

It has been found that in a high temperature habitat only a few types of organisms are able to live, and as seen in Table I, only procaryotic microorganisms with an upper temperature limit above 60-70°, can grow. Higher organisms can exist only up to 50°C. A group of eucaryotic microorganisms e.g. some moderate thermophilic fungi are found in between these temperatures. Considering the upper temperature limit of organisms the question arises: Is there an upper temperature for life? This question is not answered easily. Not only temperature, but also other factors, such as pH, nutrient concentration, salinity will strongly influence this limit. Thus, we can only circumscribe the upper temperature at which all conditions for life on earth are possible (1).

Accordingly only bacteria can adapt optimally to extreme temperatures. Since they are found from 0° - 100°C, their viability appears only to be limited to the liquid state of the water. This, of course, does not mean that all bacteria can grow in the entire temperature range. In any given case cell metabolism and cell components are optimally adapted to one particular temperature range between the freezing and boiling point of water. As in the case of the other organisms, every species of bacteria has a relatively limited temperature optimum for growth, rarely exceeding 30°C. On this basis, with a somewhat arbitrary classification system one can differentiate between:

    1.) thermophiles living between 45° and 100°C
    2.) mesophiles living between 20° and 45°C
    3.) psychrophiles living between -5° and 25°C

(minimal and maximal temperature, the optimal temperature lies in between). All three groups overlap.

In bacteria, the number of species decreases grossly as the environmental temperature increases. However, a considerable number of thermophilic bacteria species has been found, especially, in recent years (Table II). One can distinguish between extreme and more moderate thermophilic bacteria (1). Extreme types are among the heterotrophic bacteria, some spore-forming bacilli and the gram-negative aerobes in the Thermus series (temperature optimum: 70-80°C). Studies on heterotrophic, moderate thermophilic bacteria concentrated on bacilli, and here mainly on *B. stearothermophilus*. This group also includes the clostridia and lactic bacteria (temperature optimum 40-60°C) and Thermoplasma (acidophilic). Chemolithotropic thermophiles are *Thiobacillus thioxydans*, *Sulfolobus acidocaldarius* and the *methanogenic bacteria*. Photo-

TABLE II
Growth Temperatures of Thermophilic Bacteria
(selection of typical species).

Group, Genus, Species	(Temperature ^{o}C)	
	optimum	maximum
Bacilli (spore former)		
B. stearothermophilus	50-65	70-75
B. caldotenax (YT-G)	65-80	85
B. caldolyticus (YT-P)	72	82
B. subtilis var.	45-50	55-65
B. acidocaldarius	60-65	70 (acidophilic)
Clostridia		
C. thermosaccharolyticum	55	70
C. thermoaceticum	55-60	65
C. thermocellum	60	70
Lactic acid bacteria		
Lactobacillus thermophilus	50-60	65
Streptococcus thermophilus	40-45	50
Gram-negative aerobes		
Thermus aquaticus	70	80
Thermus thermophilus	70	85
Thermomicrobium roseum	70-75	85
Sulfur-oxidizing bacteria		
Sulfolobus acidocaldarius	70-75	85-90 (acidophilic)
Thiobacillus sp.	50	55-60
Sulfate-reducing bacteria		
Desulfcvibrio thermophilus	65	85
Myoplasma		
Thermoplasma acidophilus	60	65 (acidophilic)
Methane-producing bacteria		
Methanobacterium thermoautotrophicum	65-70	75

Group, Genus, Species	(Temperature $^{\circ}$C) optimum	maximum
Photosynthetic bacteria		
Chloroflexus auranticus	55	70-73
Cyanobacteria		
Synechococcus lividus	60-65	75
Mastigocladus laminosus	55-65	65
Phormidium laminosum		60

trophic forms of thermophilic bacteria have a relatively low temperature optimum, which implies that the photosynthetis apparatus is a
rather heat sensitive membrane system. Instances of photosynthetic
thermophilic cyanobacteria are *Synechococcus lividus*, *Mastigocladus
laminosus* and the facultative photoheterotrophic flexibacterium:
Chloroflexus auranticus, found in hot springs. In recent years, a
series of bacteria was discovered in hot springs above 90°C by T.
Brock (Yellowstone Park, New Zealand, Iceland) (1). These rod shaped
bacteria were characterized morphologically. Although their growth
was established in situ, it has proved impossible up to this day to
cultivate them in the laboratory. Some appear to be chemolitho-
trophs with a sulfide-stimulated CO_2-incorporation, others absorb
amino acids or organic compounds at 90°C (radioactively labeled) and
others may possibly be autotrophs capable of oxydizing hydrogen.
Under favorable pressure conditons these bacteria are also found
in boiling water above 100°C.

The taxomy of most thermophilic bacteria is far from complete
at the present time. In this case it seems to be especially difficult to differentiate between species and mutants. What is certain,
is that thermophilic bacteria do not belong to one particular genus
or group. They occur in different genera or groups, similar to
those of the mesophilic bacteria (3). This wide-spread distribution
of thermophiles, as well as the fact that the metabolic processes
and the structures (e.g., the amino acid sequences of the proteins)
are very similar, suggest that thermophilic and mesophilic bacteria
have a common origin. However, the origin of thermophlic bacteria
is still uncertain and it is still open which was first: the mesophiles or the thermophiles? It may be possible to obtain insight
into their origin by comparing their protein structures. It is
improbable that phylogenetic transitions between thermophilic and
mesophilic bacteria (and microorganisms) can result from the
spontaneous mutation of one single protein. To adapt to new environmental temperatures, the majority - if not all - of the enzymes and
proteins has to undergo acceptable mutations, with the corresponding variation in thermostability and biological activity. These are

slow processes in evolution. In recent years, spontaneous transitions were observed between thermophilic and mesophilic bacilli (variation in temperature optimum of growth) (4) (5). Because of these fast adaptations, a hypothesis was proposed according to which thermophily is controlled genetically. The thermophilic properties of thermophilic bacteria appear to be coded in a small number of adaptorgenes controlling the structure genes (4). The possible existence of thermophilic plasmids has been discussed in this context. However, no concrete conclusion has been achieved in this field, as the majority of experiments - transformation of the thermophilic properties by DNA-transformation or temperature adaptation experiments with bacilli could not be reproduced. The facultative thermophilic bacteria, described a number of times (1) (6), can live at a broader temperature range (broad temperature optimum). Under certain conditions, the metabolism of these bacteria adapts rapidly to different temperatures. It is conceivable to assume that changes in thermostability and biological activity of the cell components during temperature adaptation are a consequence of variations of the inner-cellular micro-environment, e.g. of pH, ion concentration and water content.

EFFECTS OF TEMPERATURE AND THE STRUCTURE AND FUNCTION OF THERMOPHILIC CELL COMPONENTS

Changes in temperature, that is changes in average kinetic energy, will result in an alternation of the rate of the enzyme catalyzed chemical reactions and consequently of the overall rate of metabolism. Moreover, once the structure and function of the biopolymers (proteins, nucleic acids, lipid membranes) is based on the number and distribution of non-covalent bonds, even slight changes in the input of kinetic energy into the living system can have large influence. This applies especially to proteins and to the metabolically important enzymes. Such weak bonds are essential not only for the stability and functional state of the proteins, but also for the specific interactions between these macromolecules or between macromolecules and ligands. In the case of the enzymes these interactions are fundamental for catalytic function (substrate binding, transition state). Since the low bond-energies for the noncovalent bonds (1-5 Kcal/mol) exceed the thermal energy (∿ 0.6 Kcal/mol at 25°C) by less than an order of magnitude, and the free energies of activation associated with the formation of breaking of non-covalent bonds are also small, these bonds are very sensitive to changes in temperature. Large temperature shifts are followed by drastic structural and functional changes (thermal denaturation). On the other hand, the small bond-energies or activation-energies of the non-covalent bonds allow the fast formation or breaking of bonds, which forms the basis for the biological activities of the proteins - e.g. the rate of enzyme catalysis. Indeed, the structural flexibility of proteins, enzymes and other

cell components at a certain temperature is essential for their biological activity (dynamics of protein structure). Therefore, the
biopolymers have to adapt their structures, that is, the network of
non-covalent bonds to a certain environmental temperature. This
adaptation must satisfy not only thermal stability which determines
the life time of these molecules, but also a certain degree of flexibility (mobility) which is necessary to gain optimal biological
activity. This specific equilibrium between thermostability (rigid-
ity) and flexibility (mobility = activity) in biological active
proteins is manifested by: 1.) the low free energy of polypeptide-
folding (5-10 Kcal/mol), demonstrating a delicately balanced protein
molecule; 2.) the rather narrow temperature optima, which have
actually been found in all organisms.

Temperature also effects a wide variety of properties of water,
important as solvent for all life processes and important also for
the structures of the biopolymers. Some of these temperature effects
on the structure of water very strongly influence the structure and
function of cell components (especially of the proteins, dissolved
in water), e.g. the density, surface tension, heat capacity, dielec-
tric constant and ionization.

After all, temperature adaptation, love for a certain temperature, means shifting the narrow temperature optimum to a certain
preferred temperature range. In the case of thermophilic bacteria
this adaptation means a shift of the temperature optimum for growth
of the metabolism and of the biological active cell components
(especially the proteins, enzymes) to higher temperatures, compared
to that of the mesophiles. These thermophilic cell components
should be more thermostable at high temperatures and less active
(effective) at low temperatures (7)(8).

This implies also that the thermophilic properties – thermostability and structural mobility, which differ in thermophiles and
mesophiles, could probably be explained at the molecular level by
the particular structure of the thermophilic or mesophilic cell
components (structural cause of thermophily). One hypothesis, often
contemplated in the past, that continual and fast *de novo* resynthesis
of thermolabile cell components takes place in thermophilic bacteria
– that is the dynamic origin of thermophily (1) – hardly appears
probable today.

A large number of proteins (more than 100, mainly enzymes)
but also nucleic acids and lipid membranes have been isolated from
thermophilic organisms and are thermostable or thermophilic per se:
their thermophilic properties are structurally inherent (3),(9),
(10). Furthermore, the hypothesis of resynthesis of thermolabile
cell components does not explain the minimal growth of thermophilic
bacteria at low temperature, as these should also be active at low

temperatures. It is conceivable that at extreme temperatures, e.g.
at the upper temperature limit of a thermophilic bacterium, an
increase in denaturation will cause an increase in resynthesis
(extreme conditions for functional uncoupling of metabolism).

What are the detailed functional and structural differences
between thermophilic and mesophilic cell components? Probably these
differences are most characteristic in the case of the biologically
active proteins, and especially in enzymes, the active molecules in
cell metabolism. It has been found that enzymes have temperature
optima which normally coincide with those of the whole organism.
For thermophilic enzymes these temperature optima are at higher
temperatures with an increase of thermostability (descending branch
of temperature optimum), but also with a decrease of catalytic efficiency at lower temperatures (ascending branch of temperature optimum). It follows that for investigations of the properties of thermo
philic enzymes, it is important to measure and to compare both the
thermostability and activity.

Thermostability can be determined by various methods of measuring the degree and rate of heat denaturation (7), (thermophilic
enzymes show a lower rate of heat denaturation):

1.) by heating to various temperatures and measurement
     of residual enzyme activity (irreversible denatur-
     ation);
2.) by following the unfolding of the entire enzyme
     (protein) molecule at a certain temperature, by
     circular dichroism and by fluorescence measurements
     which determine the extent of native or denatured
     conformation;
3.) by determining the pH-changes of unbuffered pro-
     tein (enzyme) solutions at different temperatures
     which reflect normalization of abnormal pK-values
     of buried ionizable groups during unfolding (exposed
     during unfolding).

The denaturation points - points of unfolding of thermophilic
enzymes - lie between 70°C and 90°C, compared to those of mesophilic
types, denaturing between 40°-50°C. On the basis of these denaturation point differences, or better on that of the differences between
the rates of denaturation, the differences in the free activation
energies (ΔG^*) of denaturation of thermophilic and mesophilic enzymes
can be calculated. Accordingly only values between 2-5 Kcal/mol were
found. This could mean only that small structural differences (only
amounting to a few non-covalent bonds) exist between thermophilic and
mesophilic enzymes. However, as we found in the case of thermophilic
LDH (lactic dehydrogenase) the activation enthalpies and activation
entropies of denaturation are much greater in the thermophilic enzyme
than in the mesophilic types (increasing with denaturation temperature

This seems to indicate rather large structural differences between
thermophilic and mesophilic LDH. On the other hand, the denaturation at the active site of the thermophilic enzymes (as also found
with LDH) starts at lower temperatures than that of the unfolding
of the whole enzyme molecule (7). The decrease in enzyme activity
for thermophilic LDH from *B. stearothermophilus* begins at 55°C
(pyruvate reduction) resp. 65°C (lactate oxidation, different
temperature optima for the forward and reverse reaction), whereas
unfolding starts above 80°C. The thermal stability of the active
site of the enzyme-substrate complex is the important stability in
respect to the temperature optimum. The active site lies in the
interface: polypeptide chain-water, it is more hydrated, it is more
thermolabile, but also more mobile or flexible. The same is true
for the surface of the whole enzyme molecule. The increased surface
denaturation at lower temperatures (above 55°C) can be shown by
light scattering (7) (laser beam). With this method the state of
aggregation of the enzyme (protein) molecule (e.g. of the LDH) is
measured depending on temperature. With a rise in temperature,
before the entire protein unfolds, the protein surface (surface
of the whole LDH molecule or of the LDH subunits) denatures initially and the molecules start to aggregate. The temperature at
which the aggregation begins is referred to as the surface denaturation temperature. This surface denaturation temperature,
55°C for thermophilic LDH, is practically identical to the active
site denaturation, it is, of course, higher for thermophilic
enzymes.

   As the ascending activity curve in the temperature optimum
shows thermophilic enzymes are less efficient biocatalysts at low
temperatures. However, the specific activities of thermophilic and
mesophilic enzymes are very similar at their respective temperature
optima (35° or 55°C). This means that there exists an adaptation of
catalytic function to the various temperatures. Correspondingly, as we
found, the kinetic parameters are varied, for instance of LDH-cataly-
sis (pyruvate reduction, the activation step is rate limiting). The
values for free activation energy (ΔG^*) of LDH catalyzed pyruvate reduction for the thermophilic enzyme are about 500-1000 cal/mol higher
than those of mesophilic LDH (7). This causes a substantial reduction of specific activity at low temperatures. Of interest also are
the values obtained for the activation enthalpy (ΔH^*) and activation
entrophy (ΔS^*)(7). These parameters are much smaller for thermophilic LDH at the temperature optimum (55°C) than for mesophilic
LDH: ΔH^*:1-2 Kcal/mol compared to 7-9 Kcal/mol and ΔS^*: -36 - 38 e.u.
compared to 11-20 e.u. These data seem to reflect the specific and
characteristic situation of thermophilic enzyme catalysis. Apparently,
to judge from the low ΔH^* and large negative ΔS^* values, during
catalysis thermophilic LDH primarily uses the water-protein interactions as entropy contribution (ΔS^*) to the free energy of activation, rather than the exchange of energy (ΔH^*) with the environment

(high temperature environment). The system is thus less temperature
dependent than the mesophilic catalytic system. It is interesting
that during transition to low temperatures, at 45°C, thermophilic
LDH undergoes a conformational change, which also changes the cataly
tic site and leads to a substantial increase of ΔH* and to a more
positive ΔS* (at e.g. 37°C). The system then is similar to the meso
philic LDH energetically and more temperature dependent. This change
at 45°C is related to a change in heat capacity of the LDH-molecule
(energy content, energy for energy transduction in catalysis). A
corresponding conformational change cannot be measured for mesophili
enzymes (LDH), since these denature at this temperature range.
Thermophilic enzymes (e.g. LDH) show increased apparent K_m-values
(Michaelis constants) for substrate and coenzyme: e.g. in the case
of LDH the K_m for pyruvate is 10-70 times larger, which might perhaps imply a smaller affinity for the substrate (11). As opposed
to the mesophilic LDH, the K_m-values remain constant at various
temperatures, up to the denaturation temperature of the active site
at 55-60°C. These catalytic properties seem to be caused mainly by
the higher thermostability of the whole protein molecule of the
thermophilic LDH which also affects the active site.

As mentioned before, the properties of thermophilic and also
of mesophilic proteins and of the other cell components should be
based on characteristic structures. This implies that thermophilic
and mesophilic proteins should differ in respect to the number and
distribution of their non-covalent bonds, that is to say in respect
to the number, distribution and position of their amino acid residues
in the three-dimensional structure. An important objective in the
thermophilic field is to explore these structural differences.

First structural investigations on thermolysin (thermophilic
neutral protease) (12), thermophilic glyceraldehyde-3-phosphate-
dehydrogenase (GPDH) (13) and lactate dehydrogenase (LDH) (7) have
shown that the amino acid sequences and the three-dimensional
structures are very similar to those of the mesophilic types.
Extensive and pronounced structural differences have not been
detected. In the case of thermolysin it could be demonstrated that
the strong binding of Ca^{2+} ions in the form of Ca^{2+}- chelates
stabilizes the enzyme. In thermophilic GPDH from *B. stearothermophilus* two stabilizing ionic bonds between the subunits have been
found. Further major differences in the amino acid composition
and in the amino acid sequences were not detected. The structural
differences between thermophilic and mesophilic enzymes and proteins seem to be subtle and probably difficult to detect. For
thermodynamic and kinetic reasons in respect to denaturation this
is not unexpected. The free energy of folding (ΔG) and of the
activation of denaturation (ΔG*) of the thermophilic proteins is
not much higher (~2-5 Kcal/mol) than in the mesophilic types. A
difference of only a few non-covalent bonds has the potential to alte
the free energy (ΔG) of folding. However, for phylogenetic reasons

to allow the adaptation of the enzyme (protein) structure in stability and functionality – a larger number of minor structural changes can be expected. The results obtained by the denaturation studies with the ΔH*, ΔS* values of LDH indicate more extensive structural differences. It is, however, probable that when thermophilic bacterial enzymes (proteins) and mesophilic enzymes (proteins) from higher organisms are compared, the species differences may conceal the structural differences caused by temperature. This should be especially the case when comparing the amino acid sequences: the thermophilic-mesophilic differences are part of the overall species differences in sequence.

To overcome this problem we compared, for example, thermophilic and mesophilic LDH from phylogenetically closely related bacilli (sequence homology > 60%). By comparing thermophilic and mesophilic LDH-pairs and analyzing the differences in an antisymmetric matrix system we typically found thermophilic and mesophilic amino acid residues. It appears that thermophilic amino acid residues are hydrophobic and include alanine (14) – and mesophilic residues consist of serine-threonine residues. Further, in the thermophilic LDH charged residues are more frequent but polar residues are more frequent in the mesophilic sequence. A substantial proportion of amino acid residues, an average 15% of total residues, is exchanged in the course of the structural change. Interesting are the positions of the typical residues or of the respective amino acid exchanges. Inside the LDH molecule the positions of hydrophobic residues in the enzymes from the thermophilic organs or of the corresponding serine-, threonine residues are found mostly in helical and intersubunit contact regions which interact with the active site. An exchange of serine-, threonine residues for hydrophobic residues during transsition from mesophilic to thermophilic LDH in this region would probably mean an increase in thermostability, a decrease in mobility of the helical and active site structures. In other words, in the thermophilic LDH we have more hydrophobic bonds which means an increase of stabilizing entropy contributions, to overcome the destabilizing chain entropy, which increases with temperature. On the other hand, in the mesophilic LDH this region with the serine-, threonine residues is probably more hydrated, has lower stability, but higher mobility and therefore higher activity at lower temperatures. This could provide the structural explanation for the functional changes, e.g. the shift of the temperature optimum, going from mesophilic to thermophilic LDH (and vice versa).

At the surface of the LDH molecule, a second type of thermostabilizing residue consists of the charged residues; these should form stabilizing ion pairs (salt bridges). Such stabilizing ion pairs have been discussed in the case of ferredoxins from clostridia and of some enzymes (7),(8),(15). We found a large increase of ion pairs, containing arginine, in the thermophilic LDH (12 arginine

compared to 1-3 in mesophilic LDH). These ionic pairs are especially
strong. Also with ion pairs we should have an increase of stabilizing entropy contributions, a point especially important for surface
stability.

Besides the smaller thermophilic enzymes (proteins), complicated multienzyme (multiprotein) complexes also show thermophilic
properties. This has been demonstrated for instance for membrane
bound ATPase from the thermophilic bacterium PS3 (16).

For life at high temperatures, the thermostability and the
adapted functionality of the membranes are also important. It has
been found that the "melting point" (T_m of the phase transition
gel crystalline/liquid) is at higher temperatures for the thermophilic membrane from thermophilic bacteria than that of mesophiles
(17). On the other hand, it has been established for both thermophilic and mesophilic membranes that the melting point of membranes
increases with the growth temperature (3)(10)(18). The melting
point of a membrane, and thus also the phase distribution below and
above this point, is determined by: 1.) the composition of the
phospholipids 2.) the length of the fatty acids, the degree of their
saturation and charge and size of the polar head, 3.) the species
of neutral lipids. In thermophilic membranes (lipids) practically
no unsaturated fatty acids (or hydroxy fatty acids) were found, but
larger quantities of saturated and branched fatty acids (C_{15},C_{16},
C_{17}, were found (1),(3),(10),(17). The optimal cell growth of
bacteria and thus also the temperature optimum of the membranes lies
above or close to the melting point. Inactivation apparently does
not occur until a particular state in the liquid membrane system is
disturbed at high temperatures. It is hypothetically assumed that
at high temperature, the lipid-protein interactions are eliminated.
Thus adaptation of membranes to high temperatures would, to a large
extent, depend on an improved lipid-protein interaction brought
about by a change in the lipid pattern (thermophilic properties of
the membranes). Here, an important role may be placed by the
branched fatty acids.

In addition to the proteins, thermostability of the nucleic
acids is important for the replication processes in the genome and
for protein biosynthesis. Nucleic acids have a characteristic sharp
melting point - especially DNA. The melting point rises in proportion to the C-G content. The DNA and t-RNA of thermophilic bacteria
have a higher melting point and a corresponding higher C + G content
than mesophiles (3,10,19). (DNA of Mesophilic bacteria $E.$ $coli$ T_m
87°-90°, C + G : 45-48%; DNA of thermophilic bacteria T_m up to 97^oC,
$B.$ $stearothermophilus$ C + G : 51-56%, $Thermus$ $aquaticus$ C + G : 66-
69%). As the melting points for the DNA from mesophilic bacteria
already lie far above the temperature optimum of most thermophilic
bacteria, the higher melting point (higher thermostability), should
not be really necessary. It may be that DNA already undergoes

structural changes below the actual melting point and that these
changes influence its functionality, that is the interaction with
proteins. Thermophilic proteins can also stabilize nucleic acids:
the ribosomal RNA is stabilized by the thermophilic ribosomal
proteins yielding thermophilic and thermostable ribosomes (20,21).

ACKNOWLEDGEMENT

The studies on the structure and function (properties) of
thermophilic and mesophilic LDH were supported by the SWISS National
Science Foundation, project no. 3.005-0.76 and 3.361-0.78 and by
the ETH Zürich, Kredit Unterricht und Forschung, project no. 0.330.
078.06/4.

REFERENCES

1. Brock, T.D. (1978), Thermophilic Microorganisms and life at
    high temperatures, Springer, New York, Heidelberg, Berlin.
2. Allen, M.B. (1953), Thermophilic aerobic sporeforming bacteria.
    Bacteriol. Revs. 17, 125.
3. Ljungdahl, L.G. (1979), Physiology of thermophilic bacteria,
    Adv. Microbiol. Physiol. in press.
4. Haberstich, H.U. and Zuber, H. (1974), Thermoadaptation of
    enzymes in thermophilic and mesophilic cultures, Arch. Micro-
    biol. 98, 275.
5. Lindsay, J.A. and Creaser, E.H. (1975), Studies on the geneti-
    cal and biochemical basis of thermophily, in Enzymes and
    proteins from thermophilic microorganisms (ed. H. Zuber),
    Birkhauser, Basel, p. 391.
6. Williams, R.A.D. (1975), Caldoactive and thermophilic bacteria
    and their thermostable proteins, Sci. Prog. Oxford 62, 373.
7. Zuber, H. (1979), Structure and function of enzymes from thermo-
    philic microorganisms, in Strategies of microbial life in
    extreme environments (ed. M. Shilo), Verlag Chemie, p. 393.
8. Zuber, H. (1978), Comparative studies of thermophilic and
    mesophilic enzymes objectives, problems, results, in Bio-
    chemistry of thermophily (ed. S.M. Friedman) Academic press,
    p. 267.
9. Singleton, R. and Amelunxen, R.E. (1973), Proteins from ther-
    mophilic microorganisms, Bacteriol. Revs. 37, 320.
10. Amelunxen, R.E. and Murdock, A.L. (1978), Mechanism of thermo-
    phily, CRC Critical reviews microbiol. p. 343.
11. Schar, H.-P. and Zuber, H. (1979), Structure and function of
    L-lactate dehydrogenases from thermophilic and mesophilic
    bacteria, I. Isolation and characterization of lactate dehy-
    drogenases from thermophilic and mesophilic bacilli, Hoppe
    Seyler's Z. Physiol. Chem. 360, 795.
12. Coleman, P.M., Jansonius, J.N., and Matthews, B.W. (1972), The
    structure of thermolysin: an electron density map at 2.3 Å
    resolution, J. Mol. Biol. 70, 701.

13. Biesecker, G., Harris, J.I., Thiery, J.C., Walker, J.E., and
     Wonacott, A.J. (1977), Sequence and Structure of D-glyceralde-
     hyde-3-phosphate dehydrogenase from Bacillus stearothermophilus
     Nature <u>266</u>, 328.

14. Argos, P., Rossmann, M.G., Grau, U.M., Zuber, H., Frank, G.,
     and Tratschin, J.D. (1979), Thermal stability and protein
     structure, Biochemistry <u>18</u>, 5698.

15. Perutz, M.F., and Raidt, H. (1975), Stereochemical basis of
     heat stability in bacterial ferredoxins and in haemoglobin A
     2, Nature <u>255</u>, 256.

16. Kagawa, Y., Sone, N., Hirata, H. and Yoshida, M. (1976), The
     membrane of thermophilic bacterium PS3, in Biochemistry of
     thermophily, (ed., S.M. Friedman), Academic press p. 61.

17. Esser, A.F.,(1979(Physical chemistry of thermostable mem-
     branes, in strategies of microbial life in extreme environ-
     ments, (ed. M. Shilo), Verlag Chemie p. 433.

18. M. Elhaney, R.N. and Soriza, K.A. (1976), The relationship
     between environmental temperature, cell growth and the fluidity
     and physical state of the membrane lipids in B. *stearothermo-
     philus*, Biochem. Biophys. Acta <u>443</u>, 348.

19. Oshima, T., (1979), Molecular basis of unusual thermostabili-
     ties of cell components from an extreme thermophile, Thermus
     thermophilus, in Strategies of microbial life in extreme en-
     vironments, (ed. M. Shilo), Verlag Chemie p. 455.

20. Friedman, S.M., (1978), Studies on heat-stable ribosome from
     thermophilic bacteria, in Biochemistry of thermophily (ed.
     S.M. Friedman, Academic press, p. 151.)

21. Yaguchi, M., Visentin, L.P., Nazar, R.N., and Matheson, A.T.
     (1978), Structure and thermal stability of ribosomal components
     from thermophilic bacteria, in Biochemistry of thermophily,
     (ed. SmM. Friedman), Academic press, p. 169.

END-PRODUCT TOLERANCE AND ETHANOL

Anthony H. Rose and Michael J. Beavan

Zymology Laboratory, School of Biological Sciences
Bath University
Bath, Avon, England

INTRODUCTION

Fossil fuels, and in particular oil and its derivatives, are the source of the vast proportion of fuels and chemicals used today in developed countries of the World. However, fossil fuels have two insurmountable drawbacks which restrict their production and utilization. The first of these, all too well known to inhabitants of both developed and underdeveloped countries of the World, is that the sources of most of the more desirable fossil fuels are approaching exhaustion, so that they are fast becoming a precious and expensive commodity. Secondly, their continued and increasing use has brought with it environmental pollution problems.

Scientists, economists and politicians in very many countries of the World are actively examining alternative sources of fuels and chemicals. An attractive long-term solution to the problem is to convert major continuously renewable non-fossil carbon sources - principally products of plant photosynthesis - into fuels and chemicals (1). In this connection, production of ethanol by microbiological processes using renewable plant products figures prominently in the majority of proposed programmes.

The use of ethanol as a fuel and as a source of industrial chemicals is not new. The text by Brachvogel, written in 1907 (2), gives a comprehensive account of early work on the manufacture of industrial alcohol by yeast fermentation, and of the many uses to which this product was put. He described several motors, heating and lighting appliances, and even a coffee roaster, that were fuelled with industrial alcohol. In the 1930s, use of ethanol in admixture with petroleum as a motor fuel became very extensive in

Europe (3). During World War II, tractors in Normandy in France were run on occasions using a fuel that bore an uncanny resemblance to calvados. The decline of fermentation ethanol dates principally from the late 1940s when ethylene began to be produced on a large scale from petrochemicals mainly for polymer manufacture.

There are many detailed accounts of programmes that have been planned, or are in operation, in various countries of the World, to produce industrial ethanol by fermentation, in almost all instances using strains of yeast (4,5). Foremost among these is the Brazilian National Alcohol Program, the most extensive of its kind in the World. The programme was initiated in November 1975, with the objective of attaining a total production of three million cubic metres of anhydrous ethanol per annum in early 1982 (6). In the United States, a fast-developing programme based on corn has also received much publicity (5), although in Europe, where the preferred substrate is beet molasses or cellulosic materials, there is somewhat less enthusiasm about industrial alcohol programmes (7). Many international agencies look to underdeveloped countries of the World, such as Thailand, where starchy roots such as cassava are relatively plentiful.

Ethanol is in many respects superior to gasoline as a liquid fuel particularly for vehicle propulsion. It is safer to handle, burns cleaner and does not cause the same level of atmospheric pollution. Moreover, ethanol has a high octane number, around 106, and is not likely to require tetraethyl lead for satisfactory engine performance. As a source of industrial chemicals, ethanol can easily be converted into ethylene, a starting material in the synthesis of many chemicals.

Any microbiological process for the manufacture of ethanol is made up of three basic unit processes, namely provision and preparation of the substrate, fermentation of sugars in the substrate to produce ethanol and carbon dioxide, and removal of ethanol from the fermented substrate usually by distillation. The first of these unit processes is reviewed in detail by Harrison and Graham (8) and Ng et al. (5), while distillation is comprehensively covered in the article by Hofslund (9). The present article deals with aspects of the second unit process, namely alcohol fermentation of sugars, by far the most complex and least understood of the three unit processes. If processes for microbiological production of industrial ethanol are to operated with maximum efficiency, a great deal more needs to be learned about the physiology of this process.

The process of alcoholic fermentation is almost inevitably associated with yeasts, and particularly with strains of *Saccharomyces cerevisiae*. The present article deals exclusively with

ethanol production and tolerance in strains of this yeast. Other
microorganisms have, however, been considered for large-scale production of ethanol. The bacterium *Zymomonas mobilis* is traditionally
used in tropical countries for making palm and cactus wines (10),
and some 50 years ago, Kluyver and Hoppenbrouwers (11) reported that
it could produce 10% (w/v) ethanol from 25% solutions of glucose.
Ethanol production by this bacterium, with a view to scale up to an
industrial process, has been studied by several workers, the most
extensive examination having been made in the University of New
South Wales in Australia (12,13,14). Interest has also been shown
in other bacteria as a source of industrial ethanol. Some of these
bacteria form the subject of Dr. Zeikus's contribution to the present
text.

ETHANOL AS A FERMENTATION PRODUCT

The Glycolysis Pathway

The classical studies of Louis Pasteur, over a century ago (15),
established that, when grown under anaerobic conditions, strains of
Sacch. cerevisiae convert a large proportion of the glucose supplied
in the medium to ethanol and carbon dioxide. In the last quarter of
the 19th Century and the first quarter of the present century, the
metabolic pathway by which glucose is converted into ethanol and
carbon dioxide was charted. This was the first biochemical pathway
to be fully described, and the work was carried out by some of the
founders of modern-day biochemistry, including Gustav Embden, Otto
Meyerhof, Sir Arthur Harden and Edouard Buchner. The pathway is
shown in Figure 1. A comprehensive account of the pathway - known
as the Embden-Meyerhof-Parnas pathway - as it operates in yeasts, and
of the enzymes which catalyse individual reactions on the pathway,
has come from Sols et al. (16).

Despite the fact that the glycolytic pathway in *Sacch. cerevisiae* was the first biochemical pathway to be charted, we are today
still woefully ignorant of many aspects of this pathway. These
aspects are discussed briefly in the following paragraphs.

Location of Glycolytic Enzymes in *Saccharomyces cerevisiae*

Biochemistry text books tell us that the enzymes of the Embden-
Meyerhof-Parnas pathway of glycolysis are soluble enzymes. They
certainly appear in the soluble fraction when cells, including those
of *Sacch. cerevisiae*, are mechanically disrupted and the cell homo-
genate submitted to differential centrifugation. However, there are
both theoretical and experimental reasons to believe that, in many
organisms, these enzymes are not necessarily molecularly dispersed
in intracellular water but may be aggregated into multienzyme

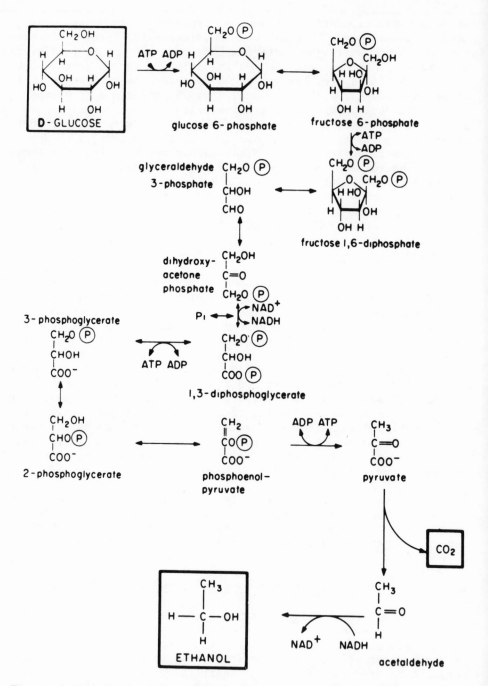

Figure 1. Embden–Meyerhof–Parnas pathway for catabolism of glucose to ethanol and carbon dioxide by *Saccharomyces cerevisiae*.

complexes. On theoretical grounds, Atkinson (17) suggested that the solvent capacity of a cell may be so limited that it would not be possible to reconcile the capacity to solvate all so-called soluble enzymes at a concentration that would allow each enzyme sufficient catalytic activity. Moreover, Sols and Marco (18) concluded, from a study of binding constants and available binding sites, that, in eukaryotic cells, many metabolic intermediates, including several glycolytic intermediates, probably remain bound to proteins. Experimental evidence has come from Rothstein et al. (19) and from Green and his colleagues (20) that, in *Sacch. cerevisiae*, several enzymes of the Embden-Meyerhof-Parnas pathway are membrane-bound. The most convincing evidence for the existence of multienzyme complexes of glycolytic enzymes has come, however, from Moses and his colleagues (21,22) working with *Escherichia coli*. A search for similar complexes in *Sacch. cerevisiae* is now urgently required if regulation of the activity of these enzymes and their tolerance of ethanol is to be fully understood.

Regulation of Glycolytic Enzymes in *Saccharomyces cerevisiae*

The principal metabolic functions of the glycolytic pathway in anaerobically growing *Sacch. cerevisiae* are to provide the cell with energy, in the form of ATP from substrate-level phosphorylation, and with a supply of low molecular-weight compounds for synthesis of cell components. On comparative biochemical grounds, it would be expected that the activity and possibly synthesis of many of the enzymes that catalyse reactions on the pathway would be subject to the various types of control that operate on other biochemical pathways. However, information on this control, for *Sacch. cerevisiae*, is limited. As might be expected, adenine nucleotides, including ATP, have effects on some of the enzymes, effects which have been reviewed by Sols and his colleagues (16).

Although ethanol is a major end-product of anaerobic glycolysis in *Sacch. cerevisiae*, the amount of available information on feedback effects of the alcohol on activity and synthesis of glycolytic enzymes is meagre. Some years ago, Augustin and his colleagues (23) provided circumstantial evidence that ethanol has a feedback effect on hexokinase activity, but firm evidence was not forthcoming until Nagodawithana and his associates (24) published kinetic data. They reported non-competitive inhibition of the activities of hexokinase and α-glycerophosphate dehydrogenase, but not of phosphofructokinase, in extracts of *Sacch. cerevisiae* (Table 1). With the first two enzymes, a reversible inhibitor-enzyme complex is formed, and assay procedures had to be devised to avoid dilution of the cell extract. As seen in Table 1, the inhibitory effect is on the V_{max} values for enzyme activity, the K_m values remaining unaltered. Navarro (25) has also shown an inhibitory effect of ethanol on hexokinase from *Sacch.*

TABLE I

EFFECT OF ETHANOL ON KINETIC VALUES FOR SELECTED GLYCOLYTIC ENZYME
ACTIVITIES IN EXTRACTS OF *SACCHAROMYCES CEREVISIAE*

Enzyme	K_m Value (M)		V_{max} Value (μmol 1^{-1} min^{-1})	
	No Ethanol	15% Ethanol	No ethanol	15% Ethanol
Hexokinase	$7.6 \cdot 10^{-5}$	$7.6 \cdot 10^{-5}$	1176	532
Phosphofructokinase	$1.3 \cdot 10^{-4}$	$1.3 \cdot 10^{-4}$	73.0	61.0
α-Glycerophosphate dehydrogenase	$5.7 \cdot 10^{-5}$	$5.7 \cdot 10^{-5}$	92.8	59.4

From Nagodawithana et al. (24)

cerevisiae. If a deeper understanding of the ability of strains of
Sacch. cerevisiae to tolerate ethanol is to be acquired, more information must be sought on the effect of the alcohol on activity and
synthesis of glycolytic enzymes in yeast.

Ethanol Tolerance of *Saccharomyces cerevisiae*

Ethanol differs from many other end products of catabolic and
anabolic pathways in cells in that it is a compound which is known
to denature proteins (26). Unlike some other compounds which are
excreted by micro-organisms, ethanol is, moreover, accumulated in
the yeast cell (see Section on "Kinetics of Ethanol Production by
Saccharomyces cerevisiae"). It follows that both intracellular proteins, as well as those in the plasma membrane, will in anaerobicall
growing *Sacch. cerevisiae* be exposed to fairly high concentrations
of ethanol. Moreover, since the concentration of ethanol inside
cells is probably greater than that in the surrounding medium, intra
cellular proteins will be bathed in a higher concentration of the
alcohol than those exposed in the outer envelope layers of the cell.

It has long been appreciated that strains of *Sacch. cerevisiae*
differ in their ability to remain viable in the presence of ethanol
(2). In general, strains used in beer brewing have only moderate
alcohol tolerance (27), while those employed in distilleries, predictably, have a greater tolerance (8). Unfortunately, there is no
recognized method for measuring the ethanol tolerance of yeast
strains, and not a little confusion pervades this area of investigation. Easiest, of course, is to assess the effect of ethanol, incorporated into the medium, on batch growth of strains of *Sacch.
cerevisiae*. The first data on ethanol tolerance of strains of *Sacch
cerevisiae* were obtained in this way and, as Innoue et al. (28) and

TABLE II

RANGE OF ETHANOL TOLERANCES IN SOME STRAINS OF
SACCHAROMYCES CEREVISIAE

Strain	Lowest concentration of ethanol which just prevents aerobic growth in 72 hours in a defined medium		
	w/v	v/v	molar
NCYC 366	7.0	5.4	1.2
NCYC 431	13.0	10.1	2.2
NCYC 478	12.0	9.3	2.0
NCYC 479	13.0	10.1	2.2
CBS 1198	12.0	9.3	2.0

Day and his colleagues (27) have shown, the method is still employed. Table II shows data on the ethanol tolerance of five strains of *Sacch. cerevisiae*.

Other workers have elected to assess the ability of *Sacch. cerevisiae* to tolerate ethanol by determining the effect of the alcohol on the fermentative activity of cells. For example, Suto et al. (29) reported the ethanol tolerance of a *saké* strain of *Sacch. cerevisiae* as the ratio of the Q_{CO_2} values in the presence and absence of 15% ethanol. The method adopted by Nojiro and Ouchi (30) differed from that of Suto et al. (29) only in that the concentration of ethanol was increased to 18%. They found that the tolerances of strains they examined fell in the range 20-30%, and they were unable to find, somewhat surprisingly, differences in the tolerance of *saké* and distillery yeasts, as compared with brewer's and baker's yeasts.

Until the recent upsurge of interest in the subject consequent upon developments in high-gravity brewing of beer and the manufacture by fermentation of industrial ethanol, research on the physiological basis of ethanol tolerance in *Sacch. cerevisiae* proceeded in a decidedly desultory manner. Much of the early interest was sustained by a series of publications from W. D. Gray working in the University of Southern Illinois at Carbondale. He found that ethanol tolerance is not confined to any one genus or species of yeast (31) and that induced tolerance of glucose in *Sacch. cerevisiae*, brought about by sequential transfer into media containing higher concentrations of the sugar, was accompanied by a decrease in ethanol tolerance (32). Examination of a range of yeast species subsequently led Gray to report (33) that those which tolerate high concentrations of ethanol store less lipid and carbohydrate than less tolerant strains.

Troyer (34,35) later confirmed many of Gray's results, and also described more fully the increased sensitivity of *Sacch. cerevisiae* to
ethanol as the growth temperature is raised. The vitamin pantothenat
has been reported to confer additional ethanol tolerance on *Sacch.*
cerevisiae (36), although this effect may be related to the influenc€
of the vitamin on lipid synthesis (see section on "Role of Plasma-
Membrane Lipids in Ethanol Tolerance in *Saccharomyces Cerevisiae*".)

     The long-term aim in studies on ethanol tolerance in yeast is
to discover the molecular basis of the property. In view of the
denaturing effect of ethanol or proteins (26), one possible explanation
of tolerance is that it is manifested by those strains that have
proteins with an intrinsic ability to resist the denaturing effects
of ethanol. Data are not available to support or refute this hypothesis. However, if this were the basis of ethanol tolerance in
Sacch. cerevisiae it would resemble the basis of thermophily in
micro-organisms (37), and support the contention (38) that yeast
ethanol tolerance is under complex genetic control, and the failure
to select for ethanol tolerance during subculture of strains into
media containing increased concentrations of ethanol (27).

     A necessary prerequisite, however, to research on the molecula‡
basis of ethanol tolerance in *Sacch. cerevisiae* is the description o‡
the kinetics of ethanol formation by tolerant strains of this yeast,
and in particular to know of the maximum concentration of ethanol
that are realized both inside and outside the cell, and the manner
in which ethanol passes from the inside to the outside of the cell.
These considerations are dealt with in section 3, "Kinetics of
Ethanol Production by *Saccharomyces cerevisiae*", while the section o‡
"Role of Plasma-Membrane Lipids in Ethanol Tolerance in *Saccharomyce‡*
cerevisiae" is devoted to certain aspects of the molecular basis of
ethanol tolerance in a strain of *Sacch. cerevisiae*.

KINETICS OF ETHANOL PRODUCTION BY *SACCHAROMYCES CEREVISIAE*

     Considering the economic and scientific importance of the alco‑
holic fermentation of sugar-containing media by *Sacch. cerevisiae,*
it is decidedly puzzling to see how slowly information has accumulated concerning the physiological and kinetic basis of the fermentation. Probably the earliest definitive study was that by Rubner
(39) in 1912. However, the phraseology of his written account was
such as to deter students of ethanol tolerance, and it had to await
Otto Rahn's exegetic study of Rubner's conclusions (40) before most
workers became aware of his principal findings. Prominent among
these was that there exists a linear relationship between the declin€
in fermentation rate of *Sacch. cerevisiae* and the concentration of
ethanol included in the solution up to about 12% ethanol, after the
low but finite fermentation rate. Despite the importance of Rahn's
study, it attracted few fellow travellers to a study of the yeast

ethanol fermentation. Indeed, it was not until the 1960s that further publications on the subject began to appear, and the first two of these (41,42) were not in exactly the most accessible journals. Steinkraus and his colleagues then began to publish on the subject, and to establish some interesting findings despite the fact that they used grape juice as a medium. In the first of their publications (43), they established that, in the stationary phase of growth, the following relationship existed: $dP / dT = B (P_m - P)$ where P is the product concentration, P_m a stoicheiometric constant, and B another constant. Of significance is that, in this equation, terms appear for neither cell number nor cell growth, showing that ethanol is produced by cells for a period that extends after the time of cessation of cell multiplication. A study of ethanol production by a respiratory-deficient strain of *Sacch. cerevisiae* in continuous culture, using a glucose–salts–yeast extract medium, came from Aiba and his colleagues (44). They derived the following relationships:

$$\mu = \mu_0 \, e^{-k_1 p} \qquad \text{and}$$

$$\gamma = \gamma_0 e^{-k_2 p}$$

where p is the ethanol concentration in the medium, μ and γ are respectively the specific rates of growth and of ethanol production, k_1 and k_2 are empirical constants, and the subscript 0 denotes the respective value at zero ethanol concentration. The inhibitory effects of ethanol on values for μ and γ were shown, by Lineweaver-Burk plots, to be non-competitive. The formulae, when extrapolated to conditions of no substrate limitation (in the chemostat growth rate was limited by the availability of glucose), were in good agreement with equations derived previously for batch fermentations, although values for the coefficients were different.

Survival of a brewing strain of *Sacch. cerevisiae* carring out rapid fermentations of a honey-containing medium was reported in another paper by Steinkraus and his colleagues (45). The fermentations were accelerated by pitching the medium with 7. 10^8 cells per ml medium. When incubated at 30°C, only 2.5 - 3.0 hours were required to obtain an ethanol concentration in the medium of 9.5% (w/v), although after three hours only 2.1% of the yeast cells were viable. When the temperature was lowered to 15°C, six hours were required to obtain 9.5% ethanol, but the population remained more viable. Incremental addition of sugar to the medium, as opposed to including 25% sugar in the medium from the start of the fermentation, also permitted a greater retention of viability.

Until recently, researchers in this area shunned the problem of estimating the concentration of ethanol inside cells, information that is essential for a full physiological understanding of ethanol production and excretion by *Sacch. cerevisiae*. Returning to their rapid fermentations of honey-containing media, Nagodawithana and

TABLE III

LEAKAGE OF ETHANOL FROM *SACCHAROMYCES CEREVISIAE*
BY BUFFER WASHING

	Ethanol concentration (percent, w/v)	Release of intracellular ethanol (percent of total)
Culture filtrate	2.4	
First buffer washing	0.27	93.9
Second buffer washing	0.02	5.8
Third buffer washing	0.001	0.3
Fourth buffer washing	undetectable	0.0
Cell homogenate	undetectable	

Unpublished results of M.J. Beavan and A.H. Rose

The culture contained 1.6 mg dry wt ml^{-1}. The
population of cells used for buffer washing
contained 100 mg dry wt, and each buffer washing
was with 10 ml 67 mM KH_2PO_4.

Steinkraus (46) calculated that, with approximately 5.10^{10} ethanol
molecules inside each yeast cell, viability is retained and the
activity of ethanol dehydrogenase in cell extracts remains unaltered
However, higher intracellular ethanol concentrations, of the order
of $2. 10^{11}$ molecules per cell, were accompanied by loss of cell
viability and inhibition of ethanol dehydrogenase activity. These
workers determined concentrations of intracellular ethanol by removing cells from the fermentations, washing with buffer, followed by
sonication and ethanol estimations on the supernatant fluids.

Recently performed unpublished work by one of us (M.J.B.)
indicates that washing *Sacch. cerevisiae*, harvested by centrifugation from an anaerobically growing culture, causes rapid efflux of
ethanol (Table III).

Cells of *Sacch. cerevisiae* NCYC 431 were harvested from self-
induced anaerobic cultures, the culture filtrate containing 2.4%
(w/v) ethanol. The first washing of a 100 mg dry wt crop with 10
ml phosphate buffer leached out of the cell about 94% of the intracellular ethanol (Table III). The ease with which intracellular

ethanol is leached from cells by washing strongly suggests that
excretion in cultures is downhill, probably by diffusion, and that
estimation of intracellular ethanol must not include a buffer-washing
procedure. It should be emphasized that these data apply to late
exponential-phase cultures grown under conditions used in our laboratory. It remains to be seen whether they apply to cells from stationary-phase cultures.

     Further evidence for downhill exit of ethanol from *Sacch.*
cerevisiae came in a recent publication from Panchal and Stewart
(47). They studied production of ethanol by a strain of *Sacch.*
uvarum (soon to be recognized as synonymous with *Sacch. cerevisiae*;
D. Yarrow, personal communication) grown anaerobically in a partially
defined medium with sucrose as the carbon source, and supplemented
with the non-metabolizable polyol sorbitol. As the concentration of
sorbitol in the medium was raised, so the concentration of intracellular ethanol increased. Moreover, a decrease in cell viability
occurred when there were high concentrations of intracellular ethanol,
suggesting that intracellular accumulation of the alcohol might be
the cause of death of *Sacch. cerevisiae* in commercial fermentations.
The amount of glycerol produced increased with an increase in the
concentration of sorbitol in the medium, but glycerol diffused out
of the cells faster than ethanol.

     Once the experimental difficulties of determing the intra-
cellular concentration of ethanol have been appreciated, there
remains the need to express this as a meaningful value. Expressing
these values in molar terms may not have an explicit physiological
significance, since it assumes that all intracellular water is
freely available for solution of ethanol, an assumption which is
questionable. Such a means of expressing intracellular contents
of ethanol does, however, make possible an assessment of the relationship between intracellular and extracellular ethanol, and thereby begin to illuminate the manner in which ethanol leaves the yeast
cell.

     One of us (M.J.B.) devised a method for disrupting populations
of cells of *Sacch. cerevisiae* from a fermentation without subjecting
them to an osmotic stress. This involved slurrying the cells in
culture filtrate, and disrupting the slurry of cells in a Braun
homogenizor. Knowing the concentration of ethanol in the culture
filtrate and the packed volume of cells, and making the assumptions
that the volume of intercellular space in a packed cell volume is
26% of the total and that 1μg dry weight of cells is equivalent to
3 μl water in intact cells, it is possible to calculate the internal
molarity of ethanol. Data for *Sacch. cerevisiae* NCYC 431, a
moderately ethanol-tolerant strain (Table II), are presented in
Figure 2. In agreement with previously reported data, Figure 2
shows that production of extracellular ethanol runs closely parallel
with growth, and that ethanol continues to appear in the culture

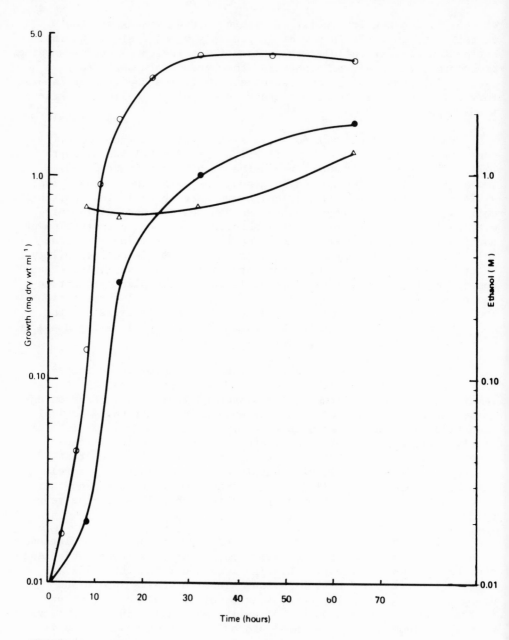

Figure 2. Time-course of growth (0) and accumulation of extracellular (●) and intracellular (Δ) ethanol by *Saccharomyces cerevisiae* NCYC 431. Intracellular ethanol concentrations were calculated by assuming that 1 μg dry weight yeast was equivalent to 3
μl water in live cells. Ethanol concentrations were determined by
gas-liquid chromatography.

filtrate after growth has largely ceased. Figure 2 also shows that
the concentration of intracellular ethanol rises only slightly during
the fermentation, being considerably greater than the extracellular
concentration early on in the fermentation but, from the onset of
the stationary phase of growth, attaining a value lower than that in
the culture filtrate.

The last of these results, implying that in the later stages
of the fermentation there is an active transport of ethanol from the
inside to the outside of the yeast cell, is, we believe, erroneous.
In arriving at values for the intracellular concentration of ethanol,
the assumption was made that 3 µl water are equivalent to each µg
of cell dry matter. Recently performed experiments in our laboratory
have indicated that this assumption is incorrect. Using radioactively labelled water and chloride, determinations have been made
of water freely available in the intercellular space and walls of
packed cells, and in the cytoplasm of cells. These determinations
have shown that a value of 3μ l mg dry wt^{-1} is too great, and that
the correct value declines considerably as the fermentation proceeds,
possibly due to accumulation of intracellular glycogen (48). While
we await further experimental data, these preliminary results would
indicate that the concentration of intracellular ethanol is extremely
high in the later stages of the fermentation, and that excretion is
probably always down a concentration gradient.

As data such as these become available on the relationship
between intracellular and extracellular concentrations of ethanol in
yeast fermentations, and on the manner in which ethanol leaves the
yeast cell, it will be possible to suggest experimental devices to
accelerate ethanol production by *Sacch. cerevisiae*. Such, we
believe, is the course that research on *Sacch. cerevisiae* should take
if this micro-organism is in the future to be the source of bulk
quantities of fuel and chemicals.

ROLE OF PLASMA-MEMBRANE LIPIDS IN ETHANOL TOLERANCE IN *SACCHAROMYCES
CEREVISIAE*

A study of the relationship between composition and function
in the plasma membrane of *Sacch. cerevisiae* has been in progress in
this laboratory for over a decade. Techniques have been devised for
bringing about specific enrichments of different lipids in the yeast
plasma membrane, and a study has been made of the effects which these
enrichments have on a variety of plasma-membrane properties (49).
The principal technique employed exploits the anaerobically induced
requirement in *Sacch. cerevisiae* for a sterol and an unsaturated
fatty acid (50,51). Since both requirements are fairly broad (52,
53), it has proved possible to grow a strain of *Sacch. cerevisiae*,
namely NCYC 366, anaerobically in appropriately supplemented media
such that the plasma membrane is enriched with the exogenously

supplied sterol to the extent of about 70% of the total sterol, and with residues of the exogenously supplied fatty acid to about 55% of the total residues in the membrane (54,55).

Recently, an examination was made of the effects of plasma-membrane lipid enrichments on the response of *Sacch. cerevisiae* to ethanol. The reasoning behind the approach made was that, since both plasma-membrane lipids and ethanol are, to different extents albeit, amphipathic molecules, it might be expected that there would be some interaction between membrane lipids and ethanol. Preliminary reports showed that loss of viability of populations of *Sacch. cerevisiae*, when suspended in phosphate buffer containing 1 M ethanol, was indeed influenced by the lipid composition of the plasma membranes. When membranes were enriched with linoleyl residues ($C_{18:2}$), the rate of drop in viability was always slower than for cells with membranes enriched in oleyl residues ($C_{18:1}$) (55). Moreover this protective effect of multiple unsaturated fatty-acyl residues was enhanced when the membranes contained a sterol with an unsaturated side chain (ergosterol, stigmasterol) rather than one with a fully saturated side chain (campesterol, cholesterol) (55).

The cells used in these experiments had been washed with buffer after harvesting, so that the bulk of the intracellular ethanol had been released. It is fair to assume, therefore, that the toxic effect of ethanol was a result of diffusion into cells of the comparatively high concentration (1M) in the suspending buffer. Biophysical studies have shown that, when ethanol enters a membrane, it causes a decrease in the fluidity in that membrane (56). Many membrane-bound proteins are thought to have precise requirements for membrane fluidity if they are to function optimally (57). The most plausible explanation for the protective effect of linoleyl residues, therefore, is that the decrease in fluidity caused by entry of ethanol into the yeast plasma membrane is more adequately compensated by the intrinsic fluidity caused by the presence of these double unsaturated residues than by oleyl residues. It has been shown, moreover, that, when plasma membranes of *Sacch. cerevisiae* are enriched with sterols with an unsaturated side chain, the membrane molecules assume a more compact structure than when enriched in sterols with saturated side chains (54). However, while these explanations appear plausible based on knowledge of membrane composition and behaviour, it is difficult to decide precisely which membrane proteins need to be fully active when *Sacch. cerevisiae* is suspended in non-nutrient buffer.

Further experiments in our laboratory (58) established that, when anaerobically growing cultures of *Sacch. cerevisiae* NCYC 366 were supplemented with 1.5 M ethanol, the increase in generation time of cells which this induced in cultures supplemented with ergosterol and linoleic acid (from 2.5 to 4.8 generations per hour) was smaller than with cultures supplemented with ergosterol and oleic acid (from 2.4 to 7.7 generations per hour).

TABLE IV

EFFECT OF ETHANOL ON RATES OF SOLUTE ACCUMULATION BY *SACCHAROMYCES CEREVISIAE* NCYC 366
WITH PLASMA MEMBRANES ENRICHED IN ERGOSTEROL AND EITHER OLEYL OR LINOLEYL RESIDUES

Fatty-acyl enrichment	Nature of solute	Concentration of solute (mM)	Rate of accumulation in absence of ethanol (nmol min^{-1} mg dry wt^{-1})	Rate of accumulation in presence of ethanol (nmol min^{-1} mg dry wt^{-1})	Percentage decrease in rate
Oleyl	Arginine	0.4	1.9	0.9	53
	Lysine	0.4	5.1	2.3	55
	Glucose	10.0	11.5	3.0	74
Linoleyl	Arginine	0.4	2.0	1.5	25
	Lysine	0.4	4.5	3.0	33
	Glucose	10.0	11.5	6.5	43

Ethanol (0.5 M) was incorporated in cell suspensions after 12 min incubation when measuring rates
of amino-acid uptake, and after 8 min when measuring rates of glucose uptake.

From Thomas and Rose (58).

TABLE V

ETHANOL CONTENTS OF *SACCHAROMYCES CEREVISIAE* NCYC 366 GROWN ANAEROB-
ICALLY IN THE PRESENCE OF ERGOSTEROL AND EITHER OLEIC OR LINOLEIC AC?

Method of extraction	Medium supplement	Ethanol content (M)
Braun disintegration	Oleic acid	0.64 ± 0.05
	Linoleic acid	0.35 ± 0.04
Perchloric acid	Oleic acid	0.66 ± 0.08
(23%, w/v)	Linoleic acid	0.39 ± 0.01
Perchloric acid	Oleic acid	0.65 ± 0.07
(0.33 N)	Linoleic acid	0.46 ± 0.07
Trichloroacetic acid	Oleic acid	0.61 ± 0.03
(6%, w/v)	Linoleic acid	0.46 ± 0.02

Molarity of ethanol in cells was calculated assuming
that 1 µg dry weight cells was equivalent to 3 µl water
in intact cells. From Thomas and Rose (58).

It is generally assumed that the rate of growth of batch cultures of micro-organisms is limited, to some extent at least, by the
rate of entry of solutes into cells. Experiments were therefore
carried out to establish the effect of fatty-acyl unsaturation in
plasma membranes of *Sacch. cerevisiae* NCYC 366 on rates of accumulation of a small range of nutrient solutes, in the presence and absence of ethanol (0.5M) (57). The results (Table IV) show that incor
porating ethanol into cell suspensions had, with three of the solutes
examined, a greater inhibitory effect when oleyl residues were enriched in plasma membranes than when the enrichment was with linolyel
residues. Incorporation of phosphate was not affected by the nature
of the fatty-acyl enrichment. It is presumed that one or more of the
proteins associated with mechanisms for uptake of each of these three
solutes has specific fluidity requirements, and that, in the presence
of ethanol, these are met to a greater extent in cells enriched with
linoleyl rather than with oleyl residues.

In view of the possible toxic effects of ethanol accumulated
intracellularly by *Sacch. cerevisiae*, it seemed possible that the
enhanced ability to survive when grown anaerobically in the presence
of linoleic acid, as compared with oleic acid (58), might be caused
partly at least, by an enhanced ability of ethanol to leak from cells
with plasma membranes enriched in linoleyl residues. An examination
was therefore made of ethanol contents of *Sacch. cerevisiae* NCYC 366,

grown anaerobically in media containing oleic or linoleic acid together with ergosterol, and harvested in the late exponential phase of growth (57). As shown in Table V, using any one of four methods for extracting ethanol from cells, ethanol contents were always slightly lower in cells enriched in linoleyl as compared with oleyl residues. It would seem a possibility, therefore, that enrichment with the doubly unsaturated fatty-acyl residues could be an important experimental goal in any study aimed at increasing excretion of ethanol from *Sacch. cerevisiae*.

ACKNOWLEDGEMENTS

We are grateful to Dr. G. G. Stewart for providing preprints of review articles on ethanol production by yeast.

REFERENCES

1. Koh, P.M. (1978) Chemical Engineer 85(5), 58.
2. Brachvogel, J.K. (1907). 'Industrial Alcohol'. 516pp. Crosby Lockwood & Son, New York.
3. Stone, J. (1974). 'Survey of Alcohol Fuel Technology'. An interim report to the Mitre Corporation of McLean, Virginia, U.S.A.
4. Bu'Lock, J.D. (1979). Symposium of the Society for General Microbiology 29, 309.
5. Ng, D.C.M., Kosaric, N., Russell, I. and Stewart, G.G. (1981). Advances in Applied Microbiology in press.
6. Jackman, E.A. (1976). Process Biochemistry 11(5), 19.
7. Rosen, K. (1978). Process Biochemistry 13(5), 25.
8. Harrison, J.S. and Graham, J.C.J. (1970). In 'The Yeasts', (A.H. Rose and J.S. Harrison, eds.), vol. 3, pg. 283.
9. Hofslund, E.F. (1979). In 'Kirk-Othmer Encyclopedia of Chemical Technology', vol. 7, pg. 849, John Wiley and Sons, New York.
10. Swings, J. and De Ley, J. (1977). Bacteriological Reviews 41, 1.
11. Kluyver, A.J. and Hoppenbrouwers, W.J. (1931). Archiv für Mikrobiologie 2, 245.
12. Rogers, P.L., Lee, K.J. and Tribe, D.E. (1979). Biotechnology Letters 1, 165.
13. Lee, K.J., Tribe, D.E. and Rogers, P.L. (1979). Biotechnology Letters, 1, 421.
14. Rogers, P.L., Lee, K.J. and Tribe, D.E. (1980). Biotechnology and Bioengineering in press.
15. Pasteur, L. (1879). 'Studies on Fermentation', translated by Frank Faulkner. 418 pp. MacMillan & Co., London.

16.   Sols, A., Gancedo, C. and Delafuente, G. (1971). In 'The
       Yeasts', (A.H. Rose and J.S. Harrison, eds.), vol. 2, pg. 271
       Academic Press, London.
17.   Atkinson, D.E. (1969). Current Topics in Cellular Regulation
       1, 29.
18.   Sols, A. and Marco, R. (1970). Current Topics in Cellular
       Regulation 2, 227.
19.   Rothstein, A., Jennings, D.H., Demis, C. and Bruce, H. (1959)
       Biochemical Journal 71, 99.
20.   Green, D.E., Murer, E., Hultin, H.O., Richardson, S.H., Salmon
       B., Brierley, G.P. and Baum, H. (1965). Archives of Bio-
       chemistry and Biophysics 122, 365.
21.   Mowbray, J. and Moses, V. (1976). European Journal of Bio-
       chemistry 66, 25.
22.   Gorringe, D.M. and Moses, V. (1980). International Journal
       of Biological Macromolecules 2, 161.
23.   Augustin, H.W., Kopperschlagen, G., Stefen, H. and Hoffman,
       E. (1965). Biochimica et Biophysica Acta 110, 437.
24.   Nogadawithana, T.W., Whitt, J.T. and Cutaia, A.J. (1977),
       Journal of the American Society of Brewing Chemists 35, 179.
25.   Navarro, J.M. (1980). Annals of Microbiology in press.
26.   Cohn, E.J., Gurd, F.R.N., Sungenor, D.M., Barnes, B.A., Brown,
       R.K., Derouaux, G., Gillespie, J.M., Kahnt, R.W., Lever, W.F.,
       Liu, C.H., Mittelman, D., Moutin, R.F., Schmid, K. and Uroma,
       E. (1950). Journal of the American Chemical Society 72, 465.
27.   Day, A., Anderson, E. and Martin, P.A. (1975). Proceedings
       of the European Brewery Convention, Nice, pg. 377. Elsevier.
28.   Inoue, T., Takaoka, Y. and Hata, S. (1962). Journal of
       Fermentation Technology, Osaka 40, 511.
29.   Suto, T., Furusaka, C. and Uemura, T. (1951). Journal of
       Fermentation Technology, Osaka 29, 10.
30.   Nojiro, K. and Ouchi, K. (1962). Journal of the Society of
       Brewing, Japan 27, 824.
31.   Gray, W.D. (1941). Journal of Bacteriology 42, 561.
32.   Gray, W.D. (1945). Journal of Bacteriology 49, 445.
33.   Gray, W.D. (1948). Journal of Bacteriology 55, 53.
34.   Troyer, J.R. (1953). Mycologia, 45, 20.
35.   Troyer, J.R. (1955). Ohio Journal of Science 55, 185.
36.   Fukai, S., Tani, Y. and Nishibe, T. (1955). Journal of
       Fermentation Technology, Osaka 33, 59.
37.   Ljungdahl, L.G. (1979). Advances in Microbial Physiology 19,
       149.
38.   Ismail, A.A. and Ali, M.M. (1971). Folia Microbiologica, Praha
       16, 350.
39.   Rubner, M. (1912). Archiv für Physiologie, Supplement, pp.
       1-392.
40.   Rahn, O. (1929). Journal of Bacteriology 18, 207.
41.   Frnz, B. (1961). Die Nahrung 5, 457.
42.   Aiyar, A.S. and Luedeking, R. (1963). Proceedings of the 57th

National Meeting of the American Institute of Chemical Engineers, September.

43. Holzberg, I., Finn, R.K. and Steinkraus, K.H. (1967). Biotechnology and Bioengineering 9, 413.
44. Aiba, S., Shoda, M. and Nagatani, M. (1968). Biotechnology and Bioengineering 10, 845.
45. Nagodawithana, T.W., Castellano, C. and Steinkraus, K.H. (1974). Applied Microbiology 28, 383.
46. Nagodawithana, T.W. and Steinkraus, K.H. (1976). Applied and Environmental Microbiology 31, 158.
47. Panchal, C.J. and Stewart, G.G. (1980) Journal of the Institute of Brewing 86, 207.
48. Chester, V.E. (1959). Nature, London 183, 902.
49. Rose, A.H. (1977). In "Alcohol, Industry and Research', (O. Forsander, K. Eriksson, E. Oura and P. Jounela-Eriksson, eds.), 179. State Alcohol Monopoly, Helsinki, Finland.
50. Andreasen, A.A. and Stier, T.J.B. (1953). Journal of Cellular and Comparative Physiology 41, 23.
51. Andreasen- A.A. and Stier, T.J.B. (1954). Journal of Cellular and Comparative Physiology 43, 271.
52. Light, R.J., Lennarz, W.J. and Bloch, K. (1962). Journal of Biological Chemistry 237, 1793.
53. Proudlock, J.W., Wheeldon, L.W., Jollow, D. and Linnane, A.W. (1968). Biochimica et Biophysica Acta 152, 434.
54. Hossack, J.A. and Rose, A.H. (1976). Journal of Bacteriology 127, 67.
55. Thomas, D.S., Hossack, J.A. and Rose, A.H. (1978). Archives of Microbiology 117, 239.
56. Ingram, L.O. (1976). Journal of Bacteriology 125, 670.
57. Haest, C.W.M., De Gier, J., Van Es, G.A., Verkleij, A.J. and Van Deenan, L.L.M. (1972). Biochimica et Biophysica Acta 288, 49.
58. Thomas, D.S. and Rose, A.H. (1979). Archives of Microbiology 122,49.

THE ROLE OF PROLINE IN OSMOREGULATION IN

SALMONELLA TYPHIMURIUM AND *ESCHERICHIA COLI*

László N. Csonka

Plant Growth Laboratory and Department of Agronomy and
Range Science, University of California at Davis
Davis, California 95616

INTRODUCTION

A variety of strategies have evolved for the regulation of the
internal osmotic strength of organisms, but the details of these
osmoregulatory mechanisms are poorly understood. In bacteria,
internal osmolarity is maintained mainly by the accumulation of
amino acids (3,10,16) and inorganic ions (4,9), such that it exceeds
the osmolarity of the growth medium. A discovery made a quarter of
a century ago by J. H. B. Christian suggested that proline has a
special role in osmoregulation: in media of inhibitory osmolarity
the growth and respiration rates of *Salmonella orianenburg* were
stimulated specifically by the addition of proline (5,6). Using
this observation as motivation, we have selected proline over-
producing mutants of *Salmonella typhimurium* and found that some, as
a result, have acquired an increased growth rate in media of inhibitory osmolarity (8; L. Csonka, manuscript in preparation). We
found that in these proline over-producing mutants, the intracellular
proline levels were regulated such that they increased with increasing osmotic stress. Here, we present experimental results which
suggest that in the over-producing mutants, and in wild type strain,
the proline permeases play an important role during osmotic stress
for the regulation of the intracellular proline levels.

RESULTS

As mentioned above, we have isolated mutants of *S. typhimurium*
which produce high levels of proline, and which, as a consequence
have acquired the phenotype of enhanced osmotolerance. In all these

533

mutants, we found that the intracellular proline levels were regulated such that they increased in response to osmotic stress. (L. Csonka, manuscript in preparation). Such regulation of proline levels occurred only in the over-producing mutants; in the wild type strain free proline was at undetectably low levels both in minimal medium and in media of inhibitory osmolarity. There are three possible mechanisms by which regulation of intracellular proline levels in the mutants might be accomplished: the synthesis of prolin might be stimulated as a consequence of osmotic stress, or the rate of synthesis might remain constant but the degradation of proline might be inhibited, or the ability of the cells to retain the amino acid might be increased.

In order to distinguish between these three alternatives, we have measured the proline levels (intracellular plus that excreted into the growth medium) produced by strain TL151 which carried the proline over-producing, osmotolerant mutation, *pro-74*, and a second mutation, *put A842::Tn5*, which blocked the degradation of proline. The results are presented in Table I.

TABLE I

The intracellular and extracellular proline levels in proline over-producing strain TL151 grown with various NaCl concentrations in the medium.

NaCl (M)	Free Proline Levels (nmoles/mg protein)		
	Intracellular	Extracellular	Total
0.0	174	624	798
0.2	381	588	969
0.4	673	208	881
0.6	874	227	1101
0.8	1265	294	1559

Strain TL151 (*putA⁻*, i.e. deficient in proline dehydrogenase) was grown for three doublings in medium 63 (7) with 20 mM glucose and the indicated concentration of NaCl. The cells were rapidly filtered and extracted as described (12). The proline content of the cell extracts was determined on an automatic amino acid analyzer the proline content of the growth medium was measured by the method of Bergman and Loxley (2).

As can be seen from the above results, the total amount of free proline (intracellular plus extracellular) produced by strain TL151 increased approximately two-fold as the NaCl concentration of the medium was increased from 0.0 M to 0.8 M. Since in this strain, the only known pathway of proline degradation is blocked, the increase in the amount of proline produced was due to a stimulation of the rate of biosynthesis. Furthermore, the concentration of proline found in the medium decreased with increasing osmotic stress, suggesting that the ability of cells to retain proline was enhanced in response to increasing osmotic stress.

This increased capacity to retain high intracellular proline levels could be brought about by two kinds of mechanisms: the leakage of proline through the membrane (by diffusion or carrier-mediated) might be diminished, or alternatively, a proline permease might be activated which would transport the proline leaked into the medium back into the cell. For reasons discussed below, we favor the second alternative.

Previously, two proline transport systems were shown to be functioning in *Salmonella typhimurium*. The major proline permease, the product of the *putP*+ gene is required for the uptake of proline when the organism utilizes that compound as the sole source of nitrogen or carbon (13). Mutants lacking this permease are resistant to the toxic proline analogue, L-azetidine-2-carboxylate (13). There is minor proline permease, encoded by the *proP*+ gene, which is activated in response to amino acid starvation (1).

We have discovered that there is a third proline permease which is active in media of elevated osmolarity. The presence of a functional proline permease can be established by two phenotypic characteristics: sensitivity of strains to proline analogues, or the minimum concentrations of proline required to sustain the growth of proline auxotrophic mutants. The phenotypes of strains carrying combinations of *putP*⁻ and *proP*⁻ mutations are summarized in Tables II and III.

TABLE II

The sensitivities of proline permease mutants to the proline analogues L-azetidine-2-carboxylate and 3,4-dehydro-D,L-proline.

Genotype	Minimal Medium		Minimal Medium + 0.15 M NaCl	
	Azt	DHP	Azt	DHP
putP+*proP*+	S	S	S	S
putP⁻*proP*+	R	S	S	S
putP+*proP*⁻	S	S	S	S
putP⁻*proP*⁻	R	R	S	S

Azt = 1 mM L-azetidine-2-carboxylate; DHP = 0.2 mM 3,4-dehydro-D,L-proline; S = sensitive to the anlogue; R = resistant to the analogue.

TABLE III

The proline requirements of proline auxotrophs
which have proline transport mutations.

Genotype	Minimal Medium		Minimal Medium + 0.15 M NaCl	
	0.1 mM	1 mM	0.1 mM	1 mM
proBA-47 putP⁺proP⁺	+	+	+	+
proBA-47 putP⁻proP⁺	+	+	+	+
proBA-47 putP⁺proP⁻	+	+	+	+
proBA-47 putP⁻proP⁻	−	+	+	+

+ denotes growth; - lack of growth.

        Thus, in minimal medium proline prototrophic putP⁻proP⁻ doubl
mutants are resistant to the proline analogues L-azetidine-2-carbo-
xylate (13) and 3,4-dehydro-D,L-proline. However, they are sensiti
to the analogues in the presence of an additional 0.15 M (or more)
NaCl. Similarly proline auxotrophic derivatives of putP⁻proP⁻
mutants, which in minimal medium cannot grow with 0.1 mM proline,
can grow in the presence of an additional 0.15 M NaCl. Similar results were observed when the osmolarity of the medium was increased
with 0.12 M K₂SO₄ or 0.26 M sucrose, indicating that the effect is a
general osmotic response rather than a specific effect elicited by
NaCl. The sensitivity to proline analogues of proline prototrophic
putP⁻proP⁻ mutants, and the ability of proline auxotrophic putP⁻
proP⁻ strains to grow with 0.1 mM proline in media of elevated
osmolarity suggest that there is a third proline permease which is
activated in response to osmotic stress.

        The sensitivity of putP⁻proP⁻ mutants to proline analogues in
media of elevated osmolarity was exploited to select mutants lacking the suggested third proline permease. Strain TL168, which
carried a deletion of the putP gene and a chromosomal rearrangement
(generated by the transposon Tn10) which inactivated the proP gene,
was used for the selection. Aliquots of cultures of strain TL168
containing ∿10⁸ cells were spread on minimal medium containing
0.3 M NaCl and 0.3 mM 3,4-dehydro-D,L-proline. Colonies resistant
to the analogue appeared at the approximate frequency of 1 per 10⁵
cells plated. In order to test whether the mutations damaged the
osmotically activated proline permease, a second mutation blocking
the proline biosynthetic pathway was introduced into fifty such
mutants. (This was done by transducing the mutants to tetracycline
resistance with a P22 lysate obtained from strain TT184 (pro-622::
Tn10).)   The tetracycline resistant transductants, which carried

the Tn*10* induced mutation blocking proline biosynthesis, were tested
for their ability to grow with 0.1 m*M* proline with 0.15 *M* NaCl. Of
the 50 tested, 43 were unable to do so; they needed 1 m*M* proline or
0.1 m*M* glycyl-proline for full growth, indicating that they were
probably deficient in the osmotically activated proline permease. We
are currently carrying out radioactive proline transport assays to
establish whether this is the case.

As we pointed out above, proline added to the culture medium
specifically stimulates the growth rate of enteric bacteria (5,6;
L. Csonka, manuscript in preparation). We tested which of the three
proline permeases are required for the stimulatory effect and we
obtained the results shown in Table IV.

TABLE IV

The stimulation of growth rate of proline transport
mutants by proline in the presence of 0.65 *M* NaCl.

Strain	Genotype	Growth rate with 0.65 *M* NaCl (generation/hour)	
		0.0 m*M* pro	0.5 m*M* pro
TL1	$putP^+proP^+proT^+$	0.21	0.38
TL135	$putP^-proP^+proT^+$	0.21	0.38
TL143	$putP^+proP^-proT^+$	0.21	0.32
TL145	$putP^-proP^-proT^+$	0.21	0.33
TL169	$putP^-proP^-proT^-$	0.23	0.24
TL170	$putP^-proP^-proT^-$	0.24	0.25

proT is the gene designation for the third, osmotically activated
proline permease.

Proline, at an external concentration of 0.5 m*M* caused approximately a two-fold stimulation of growth rate of the wild type
strain TL1 ($putP^+proP^+$) in the presence of 0.65 *M* NaCl. Equal
stimulation was observed in strain TL135 ($putP^-$), which lacked the
major proline permease, indicating that the major permease is not
required for the effect. The stimulatory effect is still evident,
although diminished in $proP^-$ strains. However, when in addition,
the third permease is inactivated (strains TL169 and TL170), proline is no longer stimulatory. Thus, the minor permease coded
by the $proP^+$ gene and the third osmotically activated proline permease seem to mediate the stimulatory effect of proline in media of
inhibitory osmolarity. (We have not yet constructed a single mutant
which is deficient only in the osmotically activated proline permease to determine the effect of the lesion in the absence of
$putP^-$ or $proP^-$ mutations.)

DISCUSSION

The observations of Christian (5,6) that proline added to culture media specifically stimulated the growth rate of *Salmonella orianenburg* in media of inhibitory osmolarity, and our findings (L. Csonka, 1980, manuscript in preparation) that mutations which result in proline over-production confer enhanced osmotolerance to *Salmonella typhimurium* suggest that, by some mechanism, high intracellular proline levels increase the ability of these organisms to tolerate osmotic stress. We found that *Salmonella typhimurium* has a proline transport system which is activated in response to osmotic stress (Tables II and III). In the wild type organism, a key component of the regulation of proline levels in response to osmotic stress may be the osmotically activated proline permease.

Why do high intracellular proline levels result in enhanced osmotolerance? One possible reason might be that proline acts as an osmotic balancer which maintains the osmolarity of the cytoplasm at a value equal to or greater than that of the exterior and thus acts to prevent osmotic dehydration. Measures (10) found that in a number of bacteria, including *Salmonella*, the concentration of proline (and glutamate) increases under osmotic stress. However, since these experiments were conducted using rich media which contained proline (and glutamate), it is possible that the increase in the intracellular levels of these compounds is due to increased uptake rather than increased *de novo* synthesis.

We found that in minimal medium (i.e. in the absence of exogenous proline) the proline content of the proline over-producing strain (TL151) was greater under osmotic stress than in its absence (Table I). Since, in the absence of osmotic stress 78% of the proline synthesized was found in the medium, and only 22% was intracellular, whereas in the presence of an additional 0.8 M NaCl, only 19% was in the medium and 81% in cells, we argued that osmotic stress enchanced the ability of cells to retain proline. It may be that the enhanced osmotolerant phenotype of proline over-producing strains is due to the fact that the over-production extends the range over which the cells can regulate their internal osmolarity, with the regulation being carried out by the proline permease(s).

There has been an alternate view proposed for the role of proline in osmoregulation by Schobert (14,15). According to her hypothesis, proline in addition to being an osmotic balancer, has special interactions with water and proteins which help maintain the stability and solubility of proteins in media of elevated osmolarity. This hypothesis has not been adequately tested, but should it be verified, it would be of importance because it would mean that in general, the selection of proline over-producing mutants of any organism might yield derivatives with increased osmotolerance.

SUMMARY

Previously we demonstrated that high intracellular proline levels conferred enhanced osmotolerance on *Salmonella typhimurium*. Stimulation of growth rate under conditions of osmotic inhibition could be brought about either by the addition of proline to the culture media or by mutations which result in proline over-production. Here, we report that there is a novel proline transport system in *S. typhimurium* which is activated in media of elevated osmolarity. This conclusion is based on the observation that *putP⁻ proP⁻* double mutants, which lack both of the known proline permeases are resistant in minimal medium to the toxic proline analogues 3,4-dehydro-D, L-proline and L-azetidine-2-carboxylate. However, they regain sensitivity to the analogues in media of elevated osmolarity. Selecting resistance to 3,4-dehydro-D, L-proline in media of elevated osmolarity, we obtained mutants of *putP⁻ proP⁻* strains which lack the osmotically activated proline permease. In these strains, exogenous proline could no longer alleviate osmotic inhibition.

ACKNOWLEDGEMENTS

I thank Raymond C. Valentine for stimulation and advice, and Sydney G. Kustu for helpful comments on the manuscript. This work was supported by the National Science Foundation under grant PFR 77-07301. Any opinions, findings, and conclusions or recommendations expressed in this publication are those of the author of the not necessarily reflect the view of the National Science Foundation.

REFERENCES

1. Anderson, R.R., R. Menzel, and J.M. Wood, 1980, Biochemistry and regulation of a second L-proline permease transport system L-proline permease transport system in *Salmonella typhimurium*. J. Bacteriol. $\underline{141}$, 1071-1076.

2. Bergman, I. and R. Loxley, 1970, New spectrophotometric method for the determination of proline in tissue hydrolysates. Anal. Chemistry $\underline{42}$, 702-706.

3. Brown, C.M. and S.O. Stanley, 1972, Environment-mediated changes in the cellular content of the 'pool' constituents and their associated changes in cell physiology. J. Appl. Biotechnol. $\underline{22}$, 363-389.

4. Christian, J.H.B. and J.A. Waltho, 1961, The sodium and potassium content of non-halophilic bacteria in relationship to salt tolerance. J. Gen. Microbiol. $\underline{25}$, 97-102.

5. Christian, J.H.B., 1955 The influence of nutrition on the water relations of *Salmonella orianenburg*. Aust. J. Biol. Sci. $\underline{8}$, 75-82.

6.   Christian, J.H.B., 1955b, The water relations of growth and
     respiration of *Salmonella orianenburg* at 30°. Aust. J. Biol.
     Sci. 8, 490–497.

7.   Cohen, G.N. and M.V. Rickenberg, 1956, Concentration specifiqu
     reversible des amino acides chez *E. coli*. Ann. Inst. Pasteur,
     Paris 91, 693–720.

8.   Csonka, L.N., 1979, The role of L-proline in response to
     osmotic stress in *Salmonella typhimurium*: selection of mutants
     with increased osmotolerance as strains which over-produce
     L-proline. In: Genetic Engineering of Osmoregulation. Ed.
     by D.W. Rains *et al.*, Plenum Press, New York, pp. 35–52.

9.   Epstein, W. and S.G. Schultz, 1965, Cation transport in
     Escherichia coli. V. Regulation of cation content. J. Gen.
     Physiol. 49, 221–234.

10. Measures, J.C., 1975, Role of amino acids in osmoregulation
     of non-halophilic bacteria. Nature 257, 398–400.

11. Menzel, R. and J. Roth, 1980, Identification and mapping of
     a second proline permease in *Salmonella typhimurium*. J.
     Bacteriol. 141, 1064–1070.

12. Pulman, D. and B. Johnson, 1978, Amino acid pools in members
     of the genus *Erwinia* grown in continuous culture. J. Gen.
     Microbiol. 108, 349–353.

13. Ratzkin, B., M. Grabnar, and J. Roth, 1978, Regulation of the
     major proline permease of *Salmonella typhimurium*. J. Bac-
     teriol, 133, 737–743.

14. Schobert, B., 1977, Is there an osmotic regulatory mechanism
     in algae and higher plants? J. Theor. Biol. 68, 17–26.

15. Schobert, B. and M. Tschesche, 1978, Unusual properties of
     proline and its interaction with proteins. Biochem. Biophys.
     Acta 541, 270–277.

16. Tempest, D.W., Meers, J.L., and Brown, C., 1970. Influence of
     environment on the content and composition of microbial free
     amino acid pools. J. Gen. Microbiol., 64:171–185.

DISCUSSION

TEMPEST: You did, of course, refer to the paper which we
published a number of years ago on bacterial amino-acid pools,
but in the Discussion section of that paper we also proposed
the mechanism whereby osmoregulation was effected. This, we
suggested, was essentially through the synthesis and intracellular accumulation of glutamic acid. With the Gram-negative
bacterial that we looked at we never found, as you did, an
accumulation of proline - only an accumulation of glutamate
and, as the counter-ion, potassium. The mechanism which we
proposed took into account a further observation that, when
organisms are suddently exposed to a high saline environment,
they excrete protons. Whether or not this is due to a sodium-
proton exchange I don't know. We only looked at the effect
of osmotic changes brought about by adding sodium chloride to
the medium. But there was an immediate acidification, which
means the intracellular hydrogen ion concentration decreased o

exposure of the cells to the saline environment. Now if one
looks at the enzyme glutamate dehydrogenase, one sees that its
activity is very pH dependent: it has almost no activity at
pH 6.8 and a maximum activity at pH 8.2. One can imagine that
if the internal hydrogen ion concentration is lowered (i.e.,
the internal pH is increased), this will promote glutamic acid
synthesis through an activation of glutamate dehydrogenase.
This will, in turn, channel the flow of carbon through to
2-oxoglutarate which, being a dicarboxylic acid, will be
accompanied by an accumulation of protons that will tend to
restore the internal H^+ concentration. This process will
continue, thereby progressively increasing the pool free
glutamate concentration, up to a point where osmotic balance
is re-established. Once this has happened the glutamate
dehydrogenase activity will be largely switched off. So we
suggest that it is by means of a homeostatic mechanisms for
regulating the internal H^+ concentration that osmoregulation
is effected through the synthesis and accumulation of glutamate. And potassium accumulates as the necessary counter ion.

Now if one looks at Gram-positive bacteria like *Bacillus
subtilis,* these already contain high concentrations of free
glutamate and potassium, even when growing in low-osmotic
environments. But when they are exposed to high saline environments they accumulate proline. However, the mechanism
surely is the same since proline is synthesized via glutamate.
Now the only thing that remains to be explained, as I see it,
is the reason why Gram-negative bacteria, like *Klebsiella
aerogenes,* cannot tolerate an environment containing more than
4% (w/v) sodium chloride. Here we suggested that this might
be because the intracellular concentrations of glutamate and
potassium are near to saturation. Of course, if the cells
could channel the excess glutamate through to proline they
should now be able to tolerate even higher concentrations of
sodium chloride.

CSONKA: Well, that is intriguing. One reason that our
mutants over-produce proline may be that they are trying to
make more glutamate, and we just gave them a channel into
which they can pour the glutamate. We deregulated proline
biosynthesis by some unknown mechanism, and the cells are
just pouring the glutamate into the proline drain. With regard
to the fact you mentioned about the role of glutamate dehydrogenase, we can actually test it. We have obtained, from
Sydney Kustu, mutants in which glutamate synthesis is blocked.
As you recall, there are two pathways of glutamate biosynthesis: one, involving GOGAT and the other involving GDH, both
of which convert αketoglutarate to glutamate by different
intermediates. So, one way to test your hypothesis is to take
away GDH, and if what you say is correct, the mutant should

not be able to over-produce glutamate, and it ought to be osmosensitive. The observation was that it could over-produce glutamate and was not osmosensitive. In fact, if you take away either GDH or GOGAT alone, the single mutants make just as much glutamate and are no more osmosensitive than the wild type. You have to take away both pathways to get a strain which cannot over-produce glutamate and which is not markedly osmosensitive. Annalisa Valentine in our lab also measured the potassium levels in these double mutants and found that they were not able to accumulate potassium in response to osmotic stress. So, it seems that the glutamate is there to balance the potassium that is accumulated as a result of osmotic stress.

TEMPEST: No, I would disagree with you here because this work to which I referred on amino acid pools was carried out at the same time that we were doing the GOGAT studies. So, quite naturally, we tested the pH activity profile of GOGAT and found it to be very similar to that of glutamate dehydrogenase

CSONKA: Oh, it is? I wasn't familiar with that. It needn't be glutamate dehydrogenase, but it may be either of the two enzymes.

TEMPEST: But you see it couldn't be, as John Measures suggested, that the potassium level is the activator of glutamic acid synthesis and accumulation since, with Gram-positive organisms, there is no increase in the cellular potassium content on exposing the cells to high saline environments.

Q.   Does glutamate accumulate in the culture medium?

A.   TEMPEST: I can only say that we did look at the extracellular fluids and these contained some glutamic acid – but not a large amount.

CSONKA; Sodium is not really sacred because we obtained similar results in the presence of potassium or sucrose. Granted there may be traces of sodium in the potassium buffer or in the water or in the glassware, but at least on a first approximation sodium is not essential to anything that we have seen.

TEMPEST: Well, yes; the acid test would be to stress cells with sucrose, and if one did not observe any acidification of the medium, then what I propose clearly must be wrong.

CSONKA: Well, what I can say to that is Wolfang Epstein has some data on potassium uptake and he finds, when he stresses the cells with sucrose, potassium levels go up just the same as if he stresses with sodium.

THE EFFECT OF *D*-GLUCOSE AND *D*-FRUCTOSE ON THE ACTIVITY OF β-GLUCOSI-

DASE IN *TRICHODERMA REESEI* C30 CELLULASE

Jonathan Woodward and Susan L. Arnold

Chemical Technology Division
Oak Ridge National Laboratory*
Oak Ridge, Tennessee   37830

One of the obstacles that needs to be overcome before the enzymatic hydrolysis of cellulose to glucose is realized commercially, β-glucosidase component of cellulase by glucose. As a result of this inhibition, cellobiose accumulates which, in turn, inhibits the other cellulase components and effects a drastic reduction in the rate of the enzymatic hydrolysis of cellulose. The effect of exogenously added *D*-glucose and *D*-fructose on the initial rates of cellobiose and ρ-nitrophenyl-β-*D*-glucoside (PNPG) hydrolysis, catalysed by the β-glucosidase component in *T. reesei* C30 cellulase, was determined. β-glucose inhibited the activity of this *D*-glucosidase competitively with K_i values of 0.5mM and 8.7mM when cellobiose or PNPG was used as the substrate respectively. The inhibition appeared to be pH dependent with maximum inhibition at pH 4.8. No inhibition was observed of this β-glucosidase, even at concentrations as high as 100mM which caused only 23% inhibition of enzyme activity. It is possible that a high rate of enzymatic cellulose hydrolysis could be maintained if glucose, as it is formed, is converted to fructose by a suitable preparation of glucose isomerase.

---

*Operated by Union Carbide Corporation under contract W-7405-eng-26 with the U.S. Department of Energy.

ETHANOL PRODUCTION IN FIXED-FILM BIOREACTORS EMPLOYING *ZYMOMONAS MOBILIS*

E.J. Arcuri, R.M. Worden, and S.E. Shumate II

Chemical Technology Division
Oak Ridge National Laboratory*
Oak Ridge, Tennessee 37830

Columnar reactors containing immobilized cells of *Zymomonas mobilis* were employed for the continuous production of ethanol from glucose. Two different immobilization strategies were employed in these investigations. In one case, cells were immobilized via flocculation, while in the other cells became entrapped in borosilicate glass fiber pads. The reactors were operated both in the fixed-bed and expanded-bed manner. Maximum ethanol productivities of 132.0 and 85.5 g of ethanol produced per ℓ of reactor volume·h were observed in the flocculant and fiber entrapped bioreactors, respectively. Data obtained from studies employing 5.0 and 10.0% (w/v) glucose concentrations will be presented, and problems encountered during the operation of the continuous, immobilized cell bioreactors will be discussed.

*Operated by Union Carbide Corporation under contract W-7405-eng-26 with the U.S. Department of Energy.

INDUCIBLE β-XYLOSIDE PERMEASE AS A CONSTITUENT OF THE XYLAN-DEGRADING ENZYME SYSTEM OF THE YEAST *CRYPTOCOCCUS ALBIDUS*

Z. Kratky and P. Biely

Institute of Chemistry
Slovak Academy of Sciences
Bratislava, Czechoslovakia

The yeast, *Crytococcus albidus,* depending on whether it is grown on xylan or glucose, differs remarkably in the ability to take up inducers of extracellular endo-1,4-β-xylanase synthesis. In washed, glucose-grown cells the initially low ability to take up xylobiose or methyl β-*D*-xylopyranoside, increases during incubation with these compounds after a lag-phase shorter than the induction time of the extracellular β-xylanase. Using of methyl β-*D*-[U-14C] xylopyranoside as a very slowly metabolizable inducer of xylobiose or methyl xyloside uptake is due to induction of an active transport system for methyl β-*D*-xyloside and β-1,4,-xylooligosaccharides. The system is called β-xyloside permease. The permease activity of induced cells decreases in the absence of β-xylanase inducers. The induction of permease as well as its inactivation (degradation) can be prevented with cycloheximide, thus both events appear to be dependent on *de novo* protein synthesis. In analogy with other active transport systems, β-xyloside permease function can be effectively blocked by inhibitors of energy metabolism in the cells.

The demonstrated example of induction of permease, for inducers and products of hydrolysis of an extracellular polysaccharide hydrolase, points to a new feature of induction of extracellular enzymes in eucaryotic microorganisms.

INDUCTION AND INDUCERS OF ENDO-1,4,-β-XYLANASE IN THE YEAST

CRYPTOCOCCUS ALBIDUS

P. Biely, Z. Kratky, M. Vrsanska, and D. Urmanicova

Institute of Chemistry
Slovak Academy of Sciences
Bratislava, Czechoslovakia

Extracellular endo-1,4-β-xylanase synthesis in the yeast
Cryptococcus albidus is largely inducible. During growth on wood
xylans the yeast produces the enzyme in amounts two orders of
magnitude greater than on other carbon sources, including xylose.
The enzyme can be induced in washed glucose-grown cells by xylan and
β-1,4-xylooligosaccharides. Among the oligosaccharides only xylobiose was not degraded extracellularly, therefore it appears to be
natural inducer of the enzyme. Xylobiose as a metabolisable inducer
is effective at low concentrations and constant availability to
cells. At high concentration of xylobiose the inductive effect is
less pronounced because of catabolic repression by degration products. Methyl β-*D*-xylopyranoside was found to serve as a non-
utilizable inducer of β-xylanase. The enzyme induced by the glycoside appears to be identical with that produced by the cells during
growth on xylan.

HORIZONTAL FIBER FERMENTER

Robert Clyde

Alfred University Research Foundation
Box 486
Alfred, New York 14802

It has been found that attaching yeast to a support results in
a reaction converting sugar to alcohol that is up to nine times that
when yeast is put in solution. Also investigators have found that
Zymomonas reacts two to three times faster than yeast. We have
found that *Z. mobilis* attaches quite readily to fibers. The advantage of flexible fibers is that biomass can be dislodged. Clogging is
the main problem with ceramic support columns. In vertical columns,
CO_2 generated at the bottom, travels all the way up the column,
dislodging bacteria, and biomass generated at the top of the column,
travels down, coating live cells. In a horizontal fermenter, CO_2
and biomass exit easier, and a way has been found to dislodge dead
cells, either with striker bars or ultrasonics. The striker bars
move back and forth and have internal heaters, so biomass is removed
from the, too, resulting in better heat transfer. The fibers can be
cotton, or, in the case where other bacteria convert cellulose to
sugar and sugar to alcohol in one step, a ceramic fiber is being
developed.

Figures are shown later. Chain 1 rotates the striker bars in
a clockwise rotation and chain 2 in a counter-clockwise, so the bars
interlock, giving the fibers several flexes and dislodging excess
biomass.

Another advantage of attaching organisms to a support is that
more alcohol tolerant ones can be attached at the end where alcohol
concentration is highest. The fermenter can be divided into compart-
ments by baffles, and different temperatures maintained in each
compartment to better promote the growth of that particular organism.
Solution can flow over the top of the baffle from one compartment
to the next. When attaching organisms, the solution could be kept
below the baffle and the striker bars provide gentle agitation.

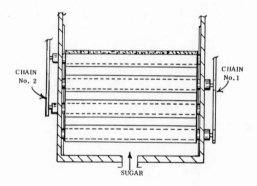

Figure 1.   Horizontal Fiber Fermenter – Top view.

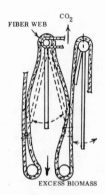

Figure 2.   Horizontal Fiber Fermenter – Side view.

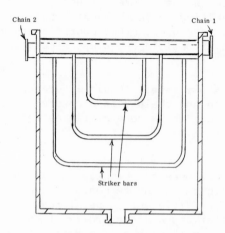

Figure 3.   Horizontal Fiber Fermenter – End view.

METHANOL AND CARBON MONOXIDE METABOLISM OF *BUTYRI-BACTERIUM METHYLO-TROPHICUM* THE MARBURG STRAIN

Lee H. Lynd and J.G. Zeikus

Department of Bacteriology
University of Wisconsin
Madison, Wisconsin 53706

Growth of *B. methylotrophicum* on methanol (100mM)/acetate (50mM) required CO_2 and exhibited: a chemical transformation stoichiometry of 10 methanol + $2CO_2 \rightarrow$ 3 butyrate: a cell yield of 7.8 g/mol methanol; and, a growth rate of 0.067 h^{-1}. Cultures adapted to grow on methanol with a CO atmosphere (100%) displayed: a 3-fold increase in growth yield; increased growth rate; no requirement for CO_2; and, production of acetate in lieu of butyrate. The maximum rate of CO oxidation displayed by cultures during mixotrophic growth on methanol/CO and 140 mmol/min/mg dry wt. *B. methlotrophicum* was adapted to grow in batch culture with a 100% CO atmosphere as the sole energy source. Fermentation parameters for growth on CO were: a chemical transformation stoichiometry of $4CO \rightarrow 2.2\ CO_2 + 0.6$ acetate; a growth yield of 2.9 g/mol CO; a final P.D.$_{666}$ of 0.8; and, a maximal CO-oxidation rate of 260 nmol/min/mg dry wt. *B-methylotrophicum* grew on a variety of substrates in the presence of one atmosphere CO. Under these conditions, >.9 atmospheres of CO were consumed during growth on H_2/CO_2 or methanol, while <0.4 and <0.2 atmospheres were consumed during growth $H_2/CO_2/CO$ increased greater than two-fold over that observed in the absence of CO. These data suggest that acetic acid or butyric acid production by *B. methylotrophicum* should be examined as a possible bioconversion technology for transformation of coal pyrolysis gas mixtures or simple one carbon compounds to larger molecular weight compounds.

REGULATION OF YEAST ALCOHOL DEHYDROGENASE ISOZYMES

Christopher Wills, Paul Kratofil, and Tracy Martin

University of California, San Diego
Department of Biology C-016
La Jolla, California 92093

The two major alcohol dehydrogenases of yeast are coded by separate nuclear genes, and show 95% amino acid homology. Nonetheless, the "constitutive" ADH, ADH-I, preferentially catalyzes the reaction acetaldehyde → ethanol, and the inducible ADH, ADH-II, preferentially catalyzes the reverse reaction. Linked and non-linked mutants rendering ADH-II constitutive have been isolated by Michael Ciriacy. An understanding of the regulation of these isozymes would greatly enhance our ability to control and understand the process of fermentation, and to isolate further regulatory mutants.

ADH-II is suppressed by high glucose on complete medium, by growth on glucose on minimal medium, or when the cells are converted to respiration-deficient (petite) mutants or grown under nitrogen. We have recently found that ADH-I is suppressed almost completely when the cells are grown on a non-fermentable substrate in medium buffered by phosphate to pH 8.

We have also observed that ADH-II shows a sharp derepression on minimal medium at a concentration of yeast extract (Difco) between 0.4 and 0.5%. After prolonged growth (4-5 days), ADH-I is repressed at this concentration, but at higher concentrations it is derepresed again. The derepression of ADH-II and repression of ADH-I is accompanied by a shift in the internal pH of the cell to 7 or below. A similar but less pronounced effect is seen with Bacto-peptone, also from Difco. Preliminary results suggest that a substance in the peptone or yeast extract is capable of derepressing ADH-II, and possibly repressing ADH-I, provided that the level of glucose in the medium is low. Cells grown only in the presence of yeast extract and peptone show only ADH-II.

UNI- AND DICARBON METABOLISM OF *METHANOSARCINA BARKERI* STRAIN MS IN DEFINED MEDIUM

J.A. Krzycki, J.H. Lobos, and J.G. Zeikus

Department of Bacteriology
University of Wisconsin
Madison, Wisconsin 53706

The contributions of C-2 and C-1 labelled acetate to CH_4 and CO_2 were examined in acetate adapted culture of *Methanosarcina barkeri* grown in mineral medium. The methyl group of acetate accounted for the majority of CH_4 produced; however, 15% of the C-2 of acetate was oxidized to $^{14}CO_2$. This oxidation correlated with the concurrent reduction of the carboxyl group. $^{14}CH_4$ was produced from ^{14}C-1 acetate in amounts slightly less than the values detected for ^{14}C-2 acetate conversion to CO_2. Acetate adapted cells were capable of simultaneous metabolism of both methanol and acetate during growth in a medium that contained 50 mM of each substrate. The rate of $^{14}CH_4$ generation from ^{14}C-2 acetate was logrithmic and faster than that observed during unitrophic growth on acetate. The rate of $^{14}CO_2$ production from ^{14}C-2 acetate was twice that of unitrophic cultures. After methanol depletion the rate of $^{14}CH_4$ production remained unchanged, while $^{14}CO_2$ production decreased two-fold. In mixotrophic growth studies with 120 mM methanol and 50 mM acetate the rate of $^{14}CH_2$ production from ^{14}C-2 acetate decreased several fold over that observed in unitrophic or in the equal (substrate) mixotrophic cultures. However, μ CH_4 decreased 2-fold which suggests that methanol toxcity was the cause of this effect. These results indicate: (1) a significant intramolecular redox process is possible during methanogenesis from acetate, the reducing equivalents generated from C_2 oxidation are utilized in part for C_1 reduction to CH_4; and, (2) energy metabolism from acetate by *M. barkeri* is not catabolite repressed by methanol, but the simultaneous catabolism of methanol and acetate depends on specific substrate concentrations and consumption rates.

We are currently attempting to isolate this substance from yeast extract. Preliminary fractionation of DE11 indicates that the

substance can be isolated, and that it forms a small part of the
highly heterogeneous collection of material in yeast extract. Further
results of this isolation will be reported on.

Supported by grants AMO3-76SF0034 from the Department of
Energy, NIAAA 1 RO1--AA94141 from NIH, PCM 7905 629 from NSF and
a grant from the University of California Appropriate Technology
Program.

ISOLATION OF ETHANOL-TOLERANT MUTANTS OF YEAST

BY CONTINUOUS SELECTION

S. W. Brown and S. G. Oliver

Biological Laboratory
University of Kent at Canterbury
Kent CT2 7NJ, U.K.

The ethanol tolerance of *Saccharomyces* species is an important constraint on the efficiency of the industrial production of ethanol by fermentation. The alcohol reduces the viability, growth rate and fermentation rate of the producing organism. The complexity of the effect make it difficult to isolate tolerant mutants by simple agar plate screening regimes. We have therefore turned to continuous selection in an attempt to isolate such mutants.

A haploid strain of *S. uvarum* was grown in continous culture under conditions in which its growth rate was limited by the ethanol concentration of the medium. This concentration was determined, via a feed-back control circuit, by the culture's fermentation rate. The CO_2 concentration in the effluent gases from the fermenter was continuously monitored using a flow-through infra-red analyser. The signal from this analyser was red to a potentiometric controller which caused ethanol to be pumped into the culture vessel if the CO_2 concentration exceeded a certain threshold value. The frequency of switching of the ethanol pump hence gave an indication of the adaptation of the culture to higher ethanol concentrations.

This system of continuous selection has led to the isolation of a range of mutants which remain viable in the presence of 12% w/v ethanol. The mutants selected were found to have higher fermentation rates than the wild-type strain and, moreover, their fermentation is more tolerant to the presence of ethanol.

INDUCTION AND REGULATION OF CELLULASE SYNTHESIS IN *TRICHODERMA* MUTANTS EA$_3$ 867 AND N$_2$-78

Y.S. Zhu, Y.Q. Wu, W. Chen, C. Tan, J.H. Gao, J.X. Fei, and C.N. Shih

Shanghai Institute of Plant Physiology
Academia Sinica, China

Two mutants, EA$_3$0367 and N$_2$-78 with high cellulase yields were obtained from wild strains of *Trichoderma pseudokoningii* Rifai, 1096 and MO$_3$, respectively by mutagenic treatments with linear accelerato ^{60}Co, U.V., NTG, DTS, etc. The mutants showed small colonies on agar plates with synthetic medium, and grew slowly, but on agar plates with peptone-yeast extract medium the small colonies became as large as wild strains. The cellulase activities on these mutants in koji extracts, shake flask culture filtrates, and enzyme preparations were distinctly higher than those of their parents. The mutan N$_2$-78 reached quite high activity level when cultured in shake flask on a simple medium containing milled straw, wheat bran, nutrient salts plus waste glucose molasses for 60 hours, and showed the highest cellulase saccharifying activities on CMC, filter paper and cotton, namely 255, 82 and 13.4 mg glucose/ml enzyme respectively, or 11, 4.3 and 6 times more than those of its parent MO$_3$.

The cellulase synthesis of EA$_3$-867 and N$_2$-78 was strongly induced by sophorose, isolated from pods of sophora japonica L., and inhibited by glucose, sugar phosphates, glycerol, organic acids, NAD, NADP and ATP. Therefore, cellulase synthesis of the mutants is regulated by the catabolite repression as well as the induction. The increase in cellulase production by both mutants results from the changes in the regulatory systems of cellulase synthesis, i.e., the mutants showed higher sensitivity to inducer and lower susceptibility to catabolite repression than those of their parents.

A cellulase preparation of *Trichoderma pseudokoningii* Rafai N -78 induced by sophorose was fractionated by DEAE-Sephadex A-50 and Sephadex G111 column chromatography, selective inactivation and polyacrylamide gel electrophoresis. The components C$_1$, C$_x$

and β-glucosidase were separated, and their molecular weights were estimated to be 67,000, 62,000 and 42,000 respectively. The homogeneity of C_1, which is glyco-protein complex and is rich in glycine, aspartic acid, threonine, serine, and glutamic acid, was verified by polyacrylamide gel electrophoresis, immuno-electrophoresis and ultracentrifugal analysis. The C_1 showed a strong synergistic action with C_x and β-glucosidase in the degradation of cotton, avicel and Walthes cellulose.

A poly(A)-RNA in N_2-78 mycelia induced by sophorose has been isolated by Oligo(dT)-cellulose affinity chromatography. Its content was distinctly higher than in the control. Moreover, a cell wall-bound ribosomes was observed in mycelia induced by sophorose with electron microscopy.

The cellulase of two mutants were utilized to isolate protoplasts from plant cells, to increase alcohol production, to make digestive medicines, to improve feed efficiencies in pig feeding, to partially replace alkaline treatment in textile production, and to improve quality in food industry.

REFERENCES

1. Cellulase Research Laboratory, Shanghai Institute of Plant Physiology, Academia Cinica and the Shanghai Distillery No. 2: Isolation of two mutant stains of *Trichoderma pseudokoningii* Rifai EA₃-867 and N_2-78 with high cellulase yields and comparison of their characteristics, Acta Microbiological Sinican 18(1): 270-338, 1978.

2. Zhu, Y.S., and C. Tan::Induction and regulation of cellulase formation in *Trichoderma* I. the Induction of Cellulase formation in *Trichoderma* EA₃-867 by sophorose. Acta Microbiologica Sinica 18(4) 320-331, 1978.

3. Zhu, Y.S. (Chu) and C. Tan: II. Induction of cellulase by sophorose in washed mycelia of *T. pseudokoningii* EA₃-867 and its catabolite repression. Acta phytophysiologia Sinica 4(1): 19-26, 1978.

4. Zhu, Y.S. (Chu) and C. Tan: III. The inductive formation of cellulase by glucose waste molasses and extracts of pods of *Sophora Japonica* L. Acta Phytophysiologia Sinica 4(11): 19-26, 1978.

5. Zhu, Y.S. (Chu): IV. Changes in regulatory mechanisms of cellulase synthesis of two mutants with high yields. Acta Phytophysiologia Sinica 4(2): 143-151, 1978.

6. Wu, Y.Q., Y.S. Zhu, W. Chen, J.H. Gao and J.X. Fei: V. The changes in nucleic acid metabolism of washed mycelia of *T. pseudokoningii* Rafai N_2-78 during inductive formation of cellulase. Acta Phytophysiologia Sinica. 5(4): 335-341.

7. Zhu, Y.S.,Y.Q. Wu, J.H. Gao and J.X. Fei: VI. Separation, purification and properties of cellulase components of *T. pseudokoningii* Rafai N_2-78 induced by sophorose, Acta Phytophysiologia Sinica 6(1): 1-9.

STUDIES ON THE PRODUCTION OF SCP AND 5'-MONONUCLEOTIDES
BY *CELLULOMONAS FLAVIGENA* AND *PSEUDOMONAS PUTIDA*
IN SUBMERGED CULTURE FROM PAPER PULP

Y.Q. Wu, C.A. Jing, J.X. Fei, D.L. Ma, and C.N. Shih

Shanghai Institute of Plant Physiology
Academia Sinica, China

A Strain of cellulose-decomposing bacterium 372-24D together with a saprophytic bacterium 372-24M were isolated from soil. On the basis of morphology, physiological properties and cellulolytic activity of these isolates, strain 372-24M was identified as *Cellulomonas flavigena* and strain 372-24M as *Pseudomonas putida*. They grew syntrophically in a liquid medium containing basal salts with paper pulp (73.3% cellulose) as sole carbon source. The cellulose was decomposed to the extent of 98% after 5-day culture. The cell protein yield was about 0.17 Kg per Kg of paper pulp used. The cell protein was rich in lysine, arginine, leucine and valine. After adjusting the pH of the culture broth to 10 and temperature to 60°C, one half of the cell RNAs could be degraded to mononucleotides by cell RNAase within 20 min. The products were isolated from the culture broth, purified and crystallized. They were identified at 5'-AMP, 5'-GMP, 5'-CMP and 5'-UMP. A complex process for the production of SCP and mononucleotides was developed.

REFERENCES

1. Cellulase Research Group Institute of Plant Physiology, Academia Sinica: Studies on the isolation and identification of a cellulose-decomposing bacterium with special reference to its association with a strain of Saprophytic bacterium. Acta Microbiologia Sinica. 18(2): 147-152, 1978.

2. Wu, Y.Q.,G.A. Jing, J.X. Fei and D.L. Ma: Studies on the production of single cell protein and 5'Mononucleotides by *Cellulomonas flavigena* and *Pseudomonas putida* in submerged culture from paper pulp. Acta Microbiologia Sinica 19(4): 400-407, 1979.

FERMENTATION SCIENCE: BASIC AND APPLIED RESEARCH NEEDS

ROUNDTABLE DISCUSSION

The purpose of this panel is to discuss some future research
needs and priorities in the area of fermentation science.

Participants:

Raymond C. Valentine, Chairman

Ralph S. Wolfe

David W. Tempest

Robert W. Detroy

Charles L. Cooney

Allen I. Laskin

Thressa C. Stadtman

Oskar R. Zaborsky

Each participant prepared these written comments which, along
with the discussion that follows, have been condensed to pub-
lishable form by Drs. Palmer Rogers and Robert Rabson.

Raymond C. Valentine, Chairperson
University of California at Davis

It is now clear that genetic engineering and recombinant DNA
technology will have major impacts on the area of fermentation
science. For example, genetic engineering is being used to construct
tailor-made organisms for synthesis of specific fuels and chemicals
from biomass. However, it should be emphasized that recombinant DNA
technology is simply a tool to solve problems and is not an end in
itself. It is also crucial to keep in mind that for solution of
real-world problems genetic engineering must be intimately linked
or integrated with other aspects of fermentation sciences.

Point 1: The Story of the Galapagos Tomato

Indeed, it may even be possible to form a marriage between
fermentation science and plant science, fields linked together
according to the following overall equation:

Genetic Engineering of Rate-Limiting Steps

$$\text{Solar Energy} \xrightarrow{\text{Green Plants}} \text{Biomass (Includes Food, etc.)} \xrightarrow{\text{Fermentation}} \text{Fuels, Chemicals}$$

While the right hand part of this equation has been emphasized at
this symposium, it is important to note that green plants which
function as "solar energy machines" contribute all of the fermentable
biomass.

To help make this point, I wanted to briefly tell the story
of the Galapagos tomato. Dr. Charles Rick, Department of Vegetable
Crops at the University of California, Davis has collected seeds of
tomatoes and related species from many areas of the world. He
suggested to Dr. Epstein's group also at Davis that the seeds he
collected from various plants in the Galapagos Islands might be
tolerant to salinity. Indeed, seed from a wild tomato collected
only three meters from high tide, produced plants that could survive
with their roots in full strength seawater, or flower and fruit when
subjected to 50% seawater. The fruit produced by this strain is
tiny, tough, and bitter, but fortunately the salt tolerance genes
of the Galapagos tomato could be successfully crossed to modern
varieties yielding hardy offspring.

559

Point 2: Osmotic Tolerant Fermentations

Buoyed by the success of the plant scientists in manipulating osmotic tolerance (Osm) genes we have set out to clone the Osm genes first in a simple bacterial system as a model for plants. Recent progress toward this goal will be discussed in this volume by László Csonka. Dr. Csonka has succeeded in constructing, using *in vivo* genetic engineering techniques, a conjugative plasmid conferring osmotic tolerance. The key point to mention here is that the osmotic tolerance plasmid works under fermentative conditions and thus might have applications for industrial fermentations. The Osm plasmid confers resistance to high sugar as well as high salt concentrations.

Point 3: Cloning Stress Tolerance Genes Deserves High Research Priority

The construction of an osmotic tolerance plasmid by Dr. Csonka opens the door to an important field of research deserving high priority--the manipulation and cloning of genes against environmental stresses including: osmotic tolerance (e.g., tolerance for high concentrations of sugars, starting materials, salinity, or end products); thermal tolerance; acid or alkali tolerance; ethanol tolerance and tolerance toward other toxic end products. Please refer to several papers in this volume dealing with these important topics.

Ralph Wolfe
University of Illinois

In the beginning there were methanogens; and they populated the earth; and they did so from the geothermal springs in Iceland, New Zealand and Yellowstone Park to the caecum, rumen and intestines of animals as well as in aquatic sediments. In fact, in any anaerobic habitat where vigorous biodegradation is going on methanogens will be found. In geothermal springs where hydrogen, carbon dioxide, and nitrogen are already in the volcanic gases, methanogens are not dependent on other microbes; elsewhere they live in communities and are dependent on a very complex biochemical microbial food chain. So these organisms, as we have seen today, are terminal organisms in the biodegrative food chain, the final products being methane, the most reduced carbon compound, and carbon dioxide, the most oxidized carbon compound.

Now I would like to propose for the future that we begin to mimic nature in the laboratory and that we start to construct microbial consortia. This will drive Dave Tempest up the wall because the one thing you don't want in a chemostat is wall growth composed of communities of organisms attached to each other. One of the best examples, as I have told some of you at this meeting, is the work of Lettinger in the Netherlands where he was challenged by the problem of treating wastes from a sugar beet factory. In this process the leaves are clipped off the sugar beet, and as the beet is then washed sugar leaches out. So there are thousands of liters of a very dilute solution of sugar coming out of the factory.

The normal way to treat such an effluent would be to aerobically trickle the effluent over the stones and oxidize the glucose away. Lettinger decided to try anaerobic treatment. After about 6 months in the laboratory he noticed that some of the fermentors developed small granular structures very much like kiefer grains. These small granules were like "integrated circuits" in that they contained all the organisms necessary for degrading glucose all the way to methane and carbon dioxide. He then scaled this process up to a pilot plant level and finally to a full scale treatment plant. Now all of the waste products from this sugar beet factory go through an anaerobic system where there's no energy input required. There is a gravity feed effluent from the factory that works its way up through the fluidized bed. The sugar is converted to methane which is collected and pumped back to the factory, providing 20% of the energy needs of the factory. Now I propose that somebody should start tearing those granules apart, studying what organisms are there and how to put them back together. Once simple experiments along this line are done, then we should be able to design specific catalysts for specific wastes. Sanitary engineers don't like this idea, but I think all we need is some imaginative people who are willing to invest the time with a little encouragement from the Department of Energy or National Science Foundation. Here we are trying to reverse past trends. For seventy-five years we've been tearing crude cultures apart to study pure cultures. Now its time to put them back together and study the microbial interaction in consortia at the chemical level. Now Ray mentioned a "marriage". I don't think there's any reason to go through a formal marriage with these organisms. All we're interested in is that they live together happily and carry out the degradation.

David Tempest
University of Amsterdam

Thank you, Ralph, for kindly providing me with an opportunity to point out that, following Lettinger's work, some people in my laboratory in Amsterdam set about developing a two-phase continuous flow culture system for the anaerobic digestion of carbohydrate wastes starting with these so-called "korreltjes" or integrated communities. This two-stage process now has found practical application in one of the sugar factories in the Netherlands where, so I am told, it is functioning very effectively.

But I do not wish to talk about this aspect of continuous fermentation, nor to dwell excessively on the obvious advantages of

continuous flow systems to large-scale processes. What I would
prefer to do is look critically at the motivations underlying devel-
ments in specific research areas and, in particular, that underlying
our current interest in possible new fermentation processes for fuel
and chemicals. For within this motivation, I suspect, resides at
least one consideration that is being overlooked and/or neglected.

Fundamental to what I wish to say is the realization that the
present-day "energy crisis" is not so much a consequence of some
overall shortage of fossil fuel, since many countries have huge
reserves of coal and shale oil; but of a lack of cheap crude oil.
And price is of the essence, since, at some level of cost, it would
become economic to liquify coal and/or recover the shale oil. Hence
it follows that, in devising alternative (biological) processes for
the generation of fuels and chemicals, these must be assessed not
only in terms of their technical feasibility, but also on the basis
of their economic viability. Alas, this latter aspect rarely seems
to have been expounded by those who would have us put our faith,
and money, into the development of ingenious novelties like the biophotolysis of water.

Bearing in mind the obvious economic strictures that must
circumscribe any new process for the production of fuel, and the
very large scale upon which such a process must operate to be useful
it is clear that a wide gulf currently exists between the theoretically possible and realistically practicable procedures for augment-
ing significantly our supplies of cheap fuel. But that should not
prevent us from recognizing the essential elements of the overall
problem, nor inhibit us from working on some specific components of
that problems.

In this latter connection I would like to draw your attention
yet again to the differences between batch culture and continuous
culture - not only at the operational level but, more importantly,
at the physiological level. Thus, it seems inescapable that future
ultra-large scale fermentation processes will need to operate in the
"continous-flow" mode. But it would be naive in the extreme to
assume that this could be effected by simply adding a medium pump
and overflow system to an existing batch system. The physiological
properties of organisms growing in chemostat environments necessaril
are very different from those growing in batch culture where there
is an excess of essential nutrient substances. These differences
must be understood and rationalized if they are to be exploited.
Not surprisingly, therefore, I would urge fermentation industries
and the relevant grant-giving bodies to invest far more extensively
in basic research into the behaviour of microorganisms in nutrient-
limited (chemostat) environments than has been the case hitherto.
We were asked to state our priorities; this is mine.

Robert Detroy
U.S. Department of Agriculture, Peoria

During this week, I have commented about aspects of generating
alternative chemicals and fuels from biomass; and I speak largely
from the point of view of our own laboratory. We are pretty much
involved in utilization of all types of biomass sources including
lignocellulosics, starch, hemicelluloses, etc. There are a few
things that I would like to mention.

The first one is really a plea for enhanced investigation into
intergrating the chemically and enzymatically treated cellulosics
and hemicellulosics, with a fermentation process whether it be with
yeast, *Zymononas*, or a thermophilic bacteria. As Dr. Zeikus
mentioned earlier, there are difficulties with some of the deleterious compounds that are generated from either forest or agricultural
residues that can really give some problems in terms of the types of
fermentation that are to be utilized. Thus, we have to investigate
in great detail the various liquid feedstocks that can be used either
for batch or for continuous fermentations.

A second item of importance is continued research on obtaining
high cellulase-producing, repression-resistant organisms whether with
conventional genetics, cell fusion or recombinant DNA technology.
As the Rutgers group and also Dr. Shoemaker have mentioned, they are
doing some very good work in terms of getting repression-resistant
organisms; and, of course, we will need these sorts of strains if
we are going to have a workable technique using an enzymatic process
for conversion. I also emphasize a plea for continued investigation
into the fundamental processes of lignin and cellulose solubilization and degradation. This is in view of application of these
processes to the generation of both feed and food stocks from cellulosic biomass. We, of course, need to know the precise enzymatic
role of fungi in lignin hydrolysis and also the possibility of
generating chemical intermediates from these recalcitrant polymers.

Other items for further investigation include, not only the
cloning of fermentative genes into prokaryotic and eukaryotic
organisms, but, more importantly, the ultimate expression and regulation of these genes in terms of end-product formation in the host
cells. A big part of this is going to be the construction of suitable new hybrid genes on plasmid vehicles employing the methods of
recombinant DNA technology. Enhanced support is needed for producing fermentation chemicals from thermophilic saccharifying organisms
which possess some unusually stable enzymes, i.e. the alcohol dehydrogenases and the cellulases. We need continued support in those
areas. Also, further investigation into the synthesis of chemicals
by other unique fermentation is another big item.

One of the things that the chemists frequently bring up is
that there are a lot of things that they feel we can make from
starch, cellulose and lignin. I think that we are going to have to
take a hard look at the types of chemical feedstocks that we might
be able to generate either through chemical processes or biological
processes which could serve not only as fuels but as alternative
chemical feedstocks in the chemical industry itself. Of course,
acrylic acid is one that we talked about along with butanol, fumaric
acid and glycerol as types of fermentation products that can act as
chemical feedstocks. Alcohol tolerance and osmoregulation which,
of course, has been touched on, is going to be very important.
Another plea would be for immobilized cell technology which I think
a lot of people feel could be competitive in the next two to three
years for conversion of carbohydrate feedstocks to alcohol. A
greater need is required for more research into either continuous
conversion or batch conversion by immobilized cells whether they be
Zymomonas or other microorganisms, i.e. stabilization of these cells
in the matrix whether it be fixed film or gel.

Charles Cooney
Massachusetts Institute of Technology

Looking at biotechnology from the engineering point of view,
one can ask a number of questions and try to pinpoint where the
future is going to be, what one should work on, what are the problems. There are a number of ways that you can look at it. You
can look at it from the point of view of the basic science, or as
an engineer and ask what are the engineering problems, what are the
bottlenecks? What costs money? What needs to be overcome? This
kind of approach can help define where the basic science effort
should be directed. We have had considerable discussion, and
rather exciting discussions on various aspects of bioprocesses for
fuels and chemicals production.

If you look at biological processes for fuels and chemicals
you will find that many of them fall into common categories. If
you look at the economics of these processes you find that there
are four major costs, one is raw material, another is capital investment, a third is energy and a fourth is labor and other minor
charges. Look at the raw material costs; typically, seventy percent
of the manufacturing costs is the cost of raw material. This gives
us a very important message; it says that if we are going to look
at bioprocesses it is imperative that we maximize the conversion
yield of raw material, whether it be lignocellulosic biomass, or
coal, or oil shale, or whatever, to the desired product. This
means that we need to understand the metabolic pathways; we need
to understand the regulation of these pathways, the microbial
physiology. For instance in work we are doing at MIT with *Clostridium thermosaccharolyticum*, we find that we can increase the yield

of ethanol from xylose from about one mole to about 1.6 or 1.7 moles of ethanol per mole of xylose. Is this good? What is the theoretical yield? How good can we get? Well, we know that the thermodynamic yield is about 1.9. But what is the mechanistic yield? We don't know! We don't know anything about the regulation of this pathway. This is true for many of the products that we might like to make; but we really don't understand how to get there and what the conversion yield might be. Therefore, the area of metabolic pathways and microbial physiology is wide open for some very interesting work, particularly in the anaerobic bacteria.

The next major cost item is capital investment. One of the reasons for developing alternative routes for fuel and chemical production is to make a profit, that is, to maximize the return on investment. One can ask how do you minimize the capital investment and minimize the profit margin and hence maximize the return on investment. This is done by maximizing productivity, e.g. kilograms of product per unit of reactor volume per time. There are some interesting approaches that one can take through biotechnology. First, to increase productivity it is necessary to maximize the specific activity of the cells, e.g. grams of product formed per gram of cell mass per hour. Genetic engineering is a very interesting and important tool to maximize the catalytic components within the cell and thereby maximize the specific activity. Once you have done that, you need to maximize the concentration of your catalyst, that is, maximize the cell concentration. A way of doing this is continuous culture. If you ask: how good can my continuous culture be? Well, to increase the productivity of a continuous culture, one must increase the cell density. If you then ask how high can I increase it, eventually you fill the fermentor with solid cells and there are about 250 grams of cells per liter. Now what you have is a packed bed of "immobilized" whole cells. Such a packed bed is a logical extension of continous culture with recycle. Therefore, one needs to integrate the use of genetic engineering with novel reactors to minimize the capital investment.

The next cost is energy. This typically represents 7 to 10 percent of total manufacturing costs and it is the goal here to reduce both the process and chemical energy of fermentations. There are a number of ways that one can minimize the energy import into biological processes. This can relate back to how the plant is grown. We are doing some work on the degradation of cellulosic corn wastes from corn mutants that are low in lignin; these appear to degrade faster and produce ethanol at a higher rate than using parental corn wastes. It follows that the use of genetic manipulation in the corn plant is beneficial to the biological process and results in lower pretreatment energy cost.

The last component is labor, which represents typically 4 to 5 percent of the cost. How do we minimize this cost? One approach

is the use of computer control and automation of steps in the fermentation process, which is likely to minimize a labor component in the
operation of a plant. And, of course, an additional method is to
minimize the labor component through the use of continuous culture.
Thus, an analysis of the basic economics of biological processes is
a very useful tool with which to pinpoint areas of research that will
be significant to the end goal.

Allen I. Laskin
Exxon Research and Engineering Company

You have heard talks touching on microbiology, microbial physiology, biochemistry, enzymology, molecular biology, biochemical
genetics, and bioengineering. All of these were in relation to
subjects that include starch and lignocellulose, xylan, hydrocarbon
oxidation, hydrocarbon biosynthesis, mesophilic organisms, thermophilic organisms, anaerobes, and aerobes. Some of the products that
we have heard talked about were methane, ethanol, butanol, acrylic
acid, and so on. Even so, we realize that we still have only been
hearing about parts of the whole problems; there are many other
technological hurdles. In the case of biomass conversion, for
example, there is the whole left side of the equation that Ray
Valentine presented (see above). All of the agricultural and agro-
nomic factors - as well as the methods of pretreatment of the lignocellulosics, of isolation and of separation of products, become
important elements in the overall process that have to be addressed.

What concerns me is my own preception of how we go about
selecting the specific research areas, specific topics and the
questions that we think should be answered. It seems to me that our
systems, and by that I mean the institutional systems and sometimes
the funding systems, encourage a great deal of fragmentation of our
efforts. People tend to look for specific little niches where they
can work, and also to respond to the pressures of developing data
very quickly so that they can have material for their next grant
application. What seems to be missing is the conviction that we
are really facing the critical questions. How can we determine what
the critical questions are? What we need, from my point of view,
is to look at the whole system. For example, in the case of biomass
there is the growing of the material, the collection, the product
mixes, the separations and so on, but in addition to that, what are
we going to do with the product once we have it ? Are there really
markets? Who is going to do the marketing? Many of us think that
we have a great idea and we are going to make a particular chemical
product from biomass, but how much time is spent trying to determine
whether this is a product that really is going to be useful and is
going to be marketable? Is it going to make, especially in this
country, a profit, so that someone will want to build the plant to
produce the product? Answers to these kinds of questions, arrived

at by looking at the whole picture, will help very much in determining what problems there are, specifically, that we need to work on.

In summary, I think that we need two kinds of information: one is the basic science, and the answers to the specific questions that my colleagues on the panel have been asking. But we also need basic information on the whole system that we are working with, in order to be sure that the problems we are picking are "correct", and that we can more confidently identify the specific components on which we want to work. This is the message I want to leave with you.

Thressa Stadtman
National Institutes of Health, Bethesda

I want to make a few remarks about the chemical transformations that take place in nature in the terminal portion of the carbon cycle and I will use methane generation as the example. Fermentations of a wide variety of compounds, such as heterocyclic compounds and all sorts of agricultural wastes produce acetate as a major endproduct. This simple substance that is very abundant in nature is a good substrate for several species of methane bacteria that you have been hearing about today. Some of these species convert acetic acid in very high yield to methane and carbon dioxide, the sole fermentation products. However, this, is a fermentation about which we don't know the intermediate(s), we know nothing about the catalysts, nobody has studied this reaction in any detail and therefore, we are in no position to intelligently exploit the process for large scale production of methane. Use of the more sophisticated techniques of immobilized enzymes for methane production from acetate is only a dream, at present. Ideally, solutions containing acetic acid obtained as by-products of fermentations of more complex substances could be passed over columns containing the enzymes required for production of methane. It is in this context that I would like to make a plea that some serious consideration be given to relatively long term investments for research in areas such as this.

A crash program is not what is needed. Instead one needs to assure people interested in working on a program of this type of some continuity of support for about five years as a minimum.

Another unkown area in the series of reactions comprising methanogeness is the overall conversion of carbon dioxide and molecular hydrogen to methane. In several of the reactions we know neither the intermediates nor the catalysts. Although we can carry out these reactions in fermentors using intact bacteria it's like a black box and if something goes wrong there is no way of knowing how to correct it. I like to work on the assumption that the more that is known about a process the better our position to rationally exploit it. And even if it never has any great economic impact in

solving our energy problems the worst effect funding of this resear
would have is to help rebuild some of our university microbiology
departments that have become solely department of virology and
eukaryotic genetics. These departments would certainly profit by
having some staff people doing this kind of research and reviving a
interest in fermentation biochemistry and physiology. I am illustr
ting my point merely with the methane fermentations, but, as you ha
heard today from Dr. Gottschalk, there are also numerous unknowns i
the clostridial fermentations that produce butanol and acetone. If
you wish to get the geneticists interested in isolation and charact
ization of catalysts and amplification of amounts of the desired
enzymes you must offer an incentive. We don't know anything about
the genetics of strictly anaerobic bacteria, how similar or how
different they are from other prokaryotes. And so, I would like to
emphasize that instead of using funds for some sort of rapid crash
program, many of these areas can really profit from more modest sum
spent over a longer period of time. This will most likely yield
badly needed basic information. One other point I should mention,
with which I have personal experience: some of the enzymes that are
involved in these methane-producing reactions are terribly oxygen
sensitive and there are numerous other proteins now known that are
destroyed by one whiff of oxygen. We can't really hope to exploit
such labile catalysts in an industrial system if we don't know the
chemistry of the oxygen inactivation reaction and have no way of
reversing it. Again, this is going to require a reasonable amount
of these oxygen-sensitive enzymes for a systematic study. Perhaps
if we learn how to handle just one of these O_2-sensitive proteins
it might help to understand many of the others. One can easily
think of alot of useful spin-off from a fundamental, careful study
of these anaerobic enzyme systems.

Oskar Zaborsky
National Science Foundation

I should like to raise some points of concern as well as to
give you some of my own views on biotechnology and fermentation. In
particular, I should like to bring to your attention and briefly
discuss four concerns. These are: (1) standardization, (2) education, (3) coordination and (4) "realism in research".

Standardization:

It is apparent to numerous individuals, including those in
research laboratories and some who are present at this conference,
that the nomenclature needs to be improved in several areas of biotechnology. Presently, researchers have considerable difficulty in
communicating in certain areas. Also, often subtleties of the
science and technology are not appreciated because of problems with
nomenclature. An obvious example of this problem is with the

nomenclature of cellulase enzymes. The terminology and literature
of cellulases is still confusing, and only experts who have devoted
years to this topic seem to be able to communicate with each other
(but at times with some difficulty). Likewise, on occasion, the
naming and reporting of microorganisms is a problem.

A second general problem exists with assays for insoluble
substrates. An example is cellulase enzymes in that numerous assays
exist but the results are difficult to compare easily. I might add
that reliable and simple assays are a universal need in understanding
and utilizing new advances in biotechnology. The problem exists not
only with cellulase enzymes and with cellulose as the substrate but
with every water-insoluble substrate, including hydrocarbons, lignin,
peat, and coal.

The third problem is the lack of substrate uniformity. Again,
I use cellulose as the example, but the same problem applies to
lignin, hemicellulose, peat or coal. A definite need exists for
standardized samples so that experiments from one investigator can
be routinely compared to those of another researcher. This problem
has been recognized and overcome in the petroleum industry and is
currently being addressed by the coal industry.

The fourth problem deals with insufficient data reporting. I
certainly don't advocate a prescribed way of reporting data, but,
there has to be more consistency in reporting data so that the degree
of information given in a paper is sufficient for one to understand
what other investigators have or have not done. Certainly, this is
not only a problem in biotechnology or fermentation but in other
areas as well. My plea is simply to recognize this as a problem.
Perhaps, then, we can do something about it. With regard to insufficient data reporting, our Europen colleagues seem to be ahead of
us in the U.S. in recognizing this as a problem.

Education:

We desperately need biotechnology training programs. All of
the biotechnologists I know, including myself, are basically self-
taught individuals. Everyone of us here who considers himself or
herself a biotechnologist has had to go through a training period
of many years, coming from such fields as chemical engineering, biochemistry, genetics, or, as in my case, chemistry. It is a long and
costly effort, and I strongly advocate appropriate programs in biotechnology for both advanced and vocational training.

Another element of education that I advocate is the establish-
ment of "biological resource facilities". I think that it is high
time to have several centers of specialized laboratory capabilities
available to academia and industry in such areas as tissue culture

cellulose hydrolysis, computerized identification of microbes, gene banks, and assay standardization procedures. Although biotechnolog is receiving wide attention at the moment, I believe that it is not advancing as fast as it could be because every investigator is doin his own thing (and at times doing it quite well), and because we don't seem to have good mechanisms for pulling the varied elements together in a coherent fashion--a point that Dr. Laskin has already mentioned. Other areas that might be appropriate for "biological resources facilities" are anaerobic fermentation, the isolation, characterization and stabilization of enzymes, biochemical reactor engineering, and renewable resources characterization. Of course, some organizations are presently fullfilling this role but not to any great extent (partly because of insufficient funds and the frag mentation of scientific endeavors).

With regard to educational program, I suggest additional sup-port for university-industry cooperative efforts. However, I urge that we not exclude the small business community from this effort. In fact, it is this community which has captured the early benefits from recombinant DNA research.

Coordination:

Coordination is like motherhood, and everyone is for it, including the other agencies represented at this meeting. However, we still need more coordination at the national level, and inter-national cooperation could also be improved. Although important steps have been taken to achieve more closely coordinated efforts i biotechnology, we need to do a better job in the future.

Realism in Research:

Now let me go to my final point--a topic that I describe as "realism in research". To illustrate what I mean by this phrase, let me select a few items that have been mentioned at this meeting.

Although one may use highly purified substrates for laborator research, considerable efforts should focus on substrates that exist in nature. In particular, lignocellulose as it exists in nature should be used instead of only purified or modified compo-nents. We don't find Avicel in nature, nor do we find an abundant supply of pure cellulose. Lignin is another substrate which has its own set of problems. In fact, we often seem to build a depen-dence, even an addiction, to certain kinds of substrates. With lignin, it is Kraft lignin--a material which does not exist in nature and whose large-scale supply is questionable. Other lignins e.g., autohydrolysis lignins, may be more appropriate to use as substrates. With regard to enzymes, let me simply point out a fact known to most of you; namely, that most enzymes in nature do not

exist in a soluble state. Thus, we ought to devote more attention
to these biocatalysts in a real-world setting, whether the enzymes
are imbedded in membranes or attached to various cellular bodies.
I also advocate that enzymic or microbial systems need to be examined
under non-ideal conditions which are more relevant to industrial
processing. More research should be conducted under chemostat environments. We should not fool ourselves by studying some of these
systems under conditions which are impossible to extrapolate to real-
world operating conditions. Certainly, I'm a defender of basic
research, and we need more support for the various disciplines.
However, in my opinion, the most critical deficiency of U.S. research is the lack of translating the vast amount of basic research
results generated each year into actual products or processes. In
spite of all the current rhetoric about the loss of productivity and
the demise of innovation in the U.S. during the last few years,
little or no financial or institutional support seems to exist for
this "intermediate" research.

Let me also make a few remarks about energy and material
balances in processes. To their credit, numerous speakers at this
conference gave an accounting of the energetics of the processes
which they discussed. Without information on the energy and material
balances of proposed processes, it is impossible to compare different
processes in a rational fashion. It is not enough to state that a
certain transformation takes place in nature, e.g., nitrogen fixation, and then to find out later that it takes an enormous amount
of biochemical energy to drive the reaction. In the case of
nitrogen fixation, the carbohydrate required for biological nitrogen
fixation of legumes is 10-17 kg of carbohydrate per kg of nitrogen
fixed. Of course, this is not to say that biological nitrogen
fixation is not important nor that it does not make a tremendous
contribution to the nitrogen balance of the world. In fact, biological nitrogen fixation accounts for close to 70% of all nitrogen
fixed on the planet. However, to neglect the fact that it takes
at least 25 molecules of ATP per N_2 fixed even under the most favorable conditions cannot be ignored when one is considering producing
ammonia fertilizer.

As I stated in the beginning of my presentation, my message
may be an oversimplification and harsh. I believe that facing the
real problems and needs in biotechnology and fermentation will result
in much better long-term support from both government and industry.

Summary of the Post-Roundtable Discussions

Following the round table discussion there was a period of
questioning and commenting from the floor. The discussion covered
a broad range of topics, some of which related to the round table,

others not. What follows is a summary of the key points that were
discussed at that time.

The question of standardization as raised by Dr. Zaborsky
received several comments. In an extended comment Dr. Mandels
offered the following:

"It is most desirable that cellulase assays should
be standarized and, in fact, Tarun Ghose (Indian
Institute of Technology, New Delhi), Bland Montenecourt
(Rutgers) and Douglas Eveleigh (Rutgers) are preparing
a document on Cellulase Assays for the Biotechnology
Commission, International Union of Pure and Applied
Chemistry. They have received input from most of the
active workers on cellulase and presently have a 93-
page draft which contains much useful information but
still does not fully answer the problems raised by
Dr. Zaborsky. I hope the final draft will come out
with some simple, clear-cut recommendations, but no one
should underestimate the difficulties of accomplishing
this. The basic problem is that cellulose is not one
substrate and cellulase in not one enzyme. Cellulose
particles are as variable as snowflakes, and everything
that happens to them, including enzyme action, changes
them and affects their susceptibility to enzyme action.
Cellulase is a mixture of enzymes that act synergistically, and sequentially, and are product inhibited. The
three organisms discussed here (*Clostridium*, *Trichoderma*
and *Sporotrichum*) attack cellulose by quite different
strategies utilizing different sets of enzymes; and
think of all the cellulolytic organisms that were not
discussed! Designing standardized assays for purified
cellulase components attacking model substrates is not
too difficult; and, in fact, there is little confusion
or controversy about the β-glucosidases because the
substrates are simple chemical compounds with the action
of the enzymes clearly understood. There are enormous
problems in designing simple assays for enzyme mixtures
acting on native cellulosics for use by biochemists
trying to understand synergism, microbiologists evaluat-
ing strains, chemical engineers optimizing fermentations,
and entrepreneurs trying to set up practical processes.
So perhaps it is too early to set these in concrete.
Bear with us."

Another issue concerning standardization suggested that someone
take the initiative to provide "real world" substrates such as a
standard sample of steam exploded wood for use by researchers.
Reference was made to the petroleum industry which has reference

samples of different types of crude oil of diverse origin.

One participant made the point about the dangers of overstan-
dardization of another kind. He used the example of the enormous
concentration of research on the bacterium *Escherichia coli* to the
detriment of work on a broader variety of microbial species. This
commenter praised the major accomplishments of genetic understanding
through the use of *E. coli* but suggested this standardization may
have been at the cost of limiting both the exploration of other
groups of organisms and possibly even some creativity.

This statement prompted a rejoinder from another participant
who indicated that *E. coli* research had indeed made a broad-based
contribution and could be used in the future to study the problems
relating to the theme of the symposium. This speaker went on to
give examples of topics where *E. coli* could be used experimentally
to provide important information.

The matter of integration of efforts among the various components of the system described by Dr. Valentine came in for discussion.
One participant suggested that the interactions during the symposium
itself reflected a situation in which the various interests are not
yet comfortable with one another. Another discussant pointed out
that the idea of these relationships and interactions was of relatively recent origin and that a primary meeting such as this could
not be expected to be thoroughly integrated. He went on to express
optimism that these ties would develop rapidly and strongly. Yet
another speaker pointed out that the levels of interaction must be
not only among workers in plant science responsible for biomass
production, microbiologists responsible for fermentations and the
engineers who do the processing, but also at the level of geneticists working closely with physiologists and biochemists to understand such questions of the genetics of alcohol tolerance.

The question was broached as to the roles of universities,
industry and government with respect to research and development
leading to the production of fuels and chemicals by fermentations.
Although the responses did not fully define these roles and relationships, a beginning was made.

Representatives from DOE and NSF attempted to portray the way
in which research funding is dependent on interactions with the
scientific community. In the case of research on fermentation, it
must be recognized that the current increasing interest by government and industry is a reaction to perceived opportunities for
replacement of anticipated shortages of petroleum. The very fact
that this symposium is being held attests to that interest. For
funding agencies and offices that depend upon unsolicited proposals,
it is then up to the research community to present good research

proposals and also make it known to the agencies what the critical research needs are. Without both of these inputs there is little a government agency can do in a field. Armed with both technical justification and proposal pressure it is possible for an agency staff to make the case for the importance of enhancing support within a particular area. Agencies will also cooperate with the scientific community in helping to define research needs ranging from the fundamental to the practical in various areas by the organization of workshops and other activities which result in critical assessments of specific areas. Clearly, if the relationship to a national problem is generally perceived there is added weight in making the case for incremental funding. The overall view is that dialogues between the funding agencies and the research community are critical elements for building the technical base for future technologies.

The relationships between government and industry and industry and universities was not discussed in any detail but it is recognized that these are of major importance for early and effective deployment of the coming generations of new biotechnologies.

LIST OF PARTICIPANTS

Akedo, Massey — Massachusetts Institute of Technology, Cambridge, MA 02139

Alexander, James K. — Hahnemann Medical College, Philadelphia, PA 19102

Anderson, Arthur W. — Barc, Inc. San Jose, CA 95112

Ankwanda, En'Sem — National University of Zaire, Zaire

Arcuri, Edward J. — Oak Ridge National Laboratory, Oak Ridge, TN 37830

Armentrout, Richard — University of Cincinnati College of Medicine, Cincinnati, OH 45267

Atkins, Marsha — Howard University, Washington, D.C. 20059

Bakshi, Kiran — Gulf Science and Technology Co, Pittsburgh, PA 15238

Bandurski, Robert S. — Michigan State University, East Lansing MI 48824

Bartsch, Robert G. — University of California, San Diego La Jolla, CA 92093

Battley, E.H. — State University of New York, Stony Brook, NY 11974

Bay, Agnes — Howard University, Washington, D.C. 20059

Bellamy, W. Dexter — Cornell University, Ithaca, NY 14853

Bennetta, William — Chemical Week, San Francisco, CA 94126

Benson, Spencer — Cancer Biology Program, Frederick, MD 21701

Bergstrom, Sheryl — California Institute of Technology, Pasadena, CA 91103

Botsford, James L. — New Mexico State University, Las Cruces, NM 88001

Bradley, Clifford — National Center for Appropriate Technology, Butte, MT 59701

Brock, Richard D. — C.S.I.R.O. Australia, Washington, D.C. 20036

Brown, Ross — University of Florida, Gainesville, FL 32611

Burr, Benjamin — Biology Department, Brookhaven National Laboratory, Upton, NY 11973

Burr, Frances A. — Biology Department, Brookhaven National Laboratory, Upton, NY 11973

Busche, Robert M.

E.I. DuPont de Nemours and Co., Inc., Wilmington, DE 19898

Cailleau, Max

Elf Bio Recherche, Paris, France

Carreira, Laura H.

University of Georgia, Athens, GA 30606

Clyde, Robert

Alfred University Research Foundation, Alfred, NY 14802

Cooney, Charles

Massachusetts Institute of Technology, Cambridge, MA 02139

Cranford, Bruce

U. S. Department of Energy, Washington, D.C. 20585

Csonka, Laszló

University of California, Davis, CA 9561(

Detroy, Robert

U. S. Department of Agriculture, Peoria, IL 61604

Easter, Susan

Texaco Inc., Beacon, NY 12508

Edwards, David L.

Scripps Clinic and Research Foundation, La Jolla, CA 92037

Ehrlich, Kenneth C.

Gulf South Research Institute, New Orlear LA 70186

Ellefson, William L.

University of Illinois, Urbana, IL 61801

Eriksson, Karl-Erik

Swedish Forest Products Research Laboratory, Stockholm, Sweden

Eveleigh, Douglas E.

Cook College Rutgers University, New Brunswick, NJ 08903

Faber, Marcel

HRI, Lawrenceville, NJ 08648

Falkehag, Ingemar

Renewing Systems, Mt. Pleasant, SC 29464

Fennell, Pamela

Howard University, Washington, D.C. 20059

Ferchak, John

University of Pennsylvania, School of Med., Philadelphia, PA 19104

Finnerty, W.R.

University of Georgia, Athens, GA 30602

Fraenkel, Dan

Harvard Medical School, Boston, MA 02115

Francis, A.J.

Dept. of Energy and Environment, Brookhaven National Lab, Upton, NY 11973

Frederick, Lafayette

Howard University, Washington, D.C. 20059

Freer, Shelby N.

USDA, Northern Regional Research Center, Peoria, IL 61604

French, Dexter

Iowa State University, Ames, IA 50010

Gaskins, Joseph E.

Atlanta University, Atlanta, GA 30314

Ghosh, Arati

Rutgers Medical School, Piscataway, NJ 08854

Glover, George

Monsanto Co., St. Louis, MO 63166

Goldberg, Robert

Dept. of Energy/Environment, Brookhaven National Lab, Upton, NY 11973

Gottschalk, Gerhard

University of Gottingen, Gottingen, West Germany

Gottschalk, Milton

Rohm and Haas, Bristol, PA 19007

Graves, Craig

Howard University, Washington, D.C. 20059

Greer, Helen

Harvard University, Cambridge, MA 02138

Gum, E.K., Jr.

General Foods Corp., White Plains, NY 107

Hadley, Raymond H.

Cornell University, Ithaca, NY 14853

Hamill, Thomas	Power Authority State-NY, New York, NY 10019
Hansford, Geoffrey	Lehigh University, Bethelehem, PA 18015
Hayward, Albert G.	Atlanta University, Atlanta, GA 30314
Heyrman, Roger	Power Authority State-NY, New York, NY 10019
Hill, Ray A.	Community College of Baltimore, Baltimore, MD 21215
Hind, Geoffrey	Brookhaven National Laboratory, Upton, NY 11973
Hira, Ayub U.	Mueller Associates, Baltimore MD 21227
Hollaender, Alexander	Associated Universities, Inc., Washington, D.C. 20036
Jackson, David A.	Genex Corporation, Rockville, MO 20852
Jackson, Lynda	Howard University, Washington, D.C. 20059
Jones, Johnnye Mae	Hampton Institute, Hampton, VA 23668
Johnston, Robert F.	Johnston Associates, Inc., Princeton, NJ 08540
Kablaoui, M.S.	Texaco Inc., Beacon, N.Y. 12508
Kirk, T. Kent	U.S. Department of Agriculture, Madison, WI 53705
Kohlhaw, Gunter	Purdue University, West Lafayette, IN 47907
Krampitz, Lester	Queens College, Flushing, NY 11365
Kratky, Zdenek	McGill University, Montreal, Canada
Krulwich, Terry Ann	Mount Sinai School of Medicine, New York, NY 10029
Krzycki, Joseph	University of Wisconsin-Mison, WI 53706
Kushner, Leslie	Case Western Reserve Univ., Cleveland, OH 44106
Ladisch, Michael R.	Purdue University, West Lafayette, IN 47906
Larson, Eric H.	Allied Chemical, Solvay, NY 13209
Laskin, Allen	Exxon Res. and Eng. Co., Linden, NJ 07036
Leadbetter, Edward R.	The University of Connecticut, Storrs, CT 06268
Ledbetter, Myron C.	Biology Dept., Brookhaven Natl. Lab., Upton, NY 11973
Lin, Edmund C.C.	Harvard Medical School, Boston, MA 02115
Ljungdahl, Lars G.	University of Georgia, Athens, GA 30602
Lynd, Lee	University of Wisconsin-Madison, Madison, WI 53706
Maas, G.E.	Texaco, Inc., Beacon, NY 12508
Mah, Robert A.	University of California, Los Angeles, CA 90024
Maisch, Weldon F.	Archer Daniels Midland Co., Decatur, IL 62526
Mandels, Mary	U.S. Army Natick Laboratory, Natick, MA 01760

Mason, Barbara   Cal-OSHA, Berkeley, CA 94709
Mayfield, John   Atlanta University, Atlanta, GA 30314
McDonald, C.C.   EI DuPont De Nemours and Co., Wilmington,
                                   DE 19898
Meeusen, Ronald   Rohm and Haas Company, Spring House, PA
                                   19477
Melles, Sahle   Howard University, Mt. Rainier, MD 20822
Mitchell, Robert   University of Pennsylvania, Philadelphia,
                                   PA 19104
Montenecourt, Bland   Cook College, Rutgers University, New
                                   Brunswick, NJ 08903
Moura, Isabel   (Univ. Lisbon-Portugal), Athens, GA 30602
Moura, José J.G.   (Univ. Lisbon-Portugal), Athens, GA 30602
Mulloney, Joseph A.   Mueller Associates, Baltimore, MD 21227
Murrell, W.G.   C.S.I.R.O., North Ryde, New South Wales,
                                   Australia
Napier, R.A.   Celanese Chem. Co., Corpus Christie, TX
                                   78408
Nasim, Anwar   Ntl. Res. Council-Canada, Ontario, Canad
Notani, Nihal   Brookhaven National Laboratory, Upton,
                                   NY 11973
Oliveira, Olga   Brookhaven National Laboratory, Upton,
                                   NY 11973
Oliver, Stephen G.   University of Kent at Canterbury, Kent,
                                   England
Olson, John M.   Biology Dept., Brookhaven Natl. Lab.,
                                   Upton, NY 11973
Peck, Harry   University of Georgia, Athens, GA 30601
Person, Stanley   Penn State University, University Park,
                                   PA 16802
Pfeiffer, Richard   LSL Biolafitte, Princeton, NJ 08540
Phillips, Janice   Lehigh University, Bethlehem, PA 18015
Pramer, David   The State University of New Jersey,
                                   Piscataway, NJ 08854
Pringle, Leon   Hampton Institute, Hampton, VA 23668
Pulkrabek, Peter   Enzo Biochem, New York, NY 10010
Rabson, Robert   U.S. Department of Energy, Washington,
                                   D.C. 20545
Reddy, C.A.   Michigan State University, East Lansing,
                                   MI 48823
Reilly, Peter J.   Iowa State University, Ames, IA 50011
Ridley, Esther   Morgan State University, Baltimore, MD
                                   21239
Rogers, Palmer   U.S. Department of Energy, Washington,
                                   D.C. 20545
Romanoff, Elijah R.   National Science Foundation, Washington,
                                   D.C. 20550
Rose, Anthony H.   University of Bath, Bath, England
Ross, Michael J.   Genentech Inc., S. San Francisco, CA
                                   94080

Rubanoff, Beverly	Texaco Research Center, Beacon, NY 12508
Sall, Theodore	Ramapo College, Woodcliff Lake, NJ 07675
San Pietro, Anthony	Indiana University, Bloomington, IN 47405
Scott, Kevin	Howard University, Washington, D.C. 20059
Setlow, Richard B.	Brookhaven National Laboratory, Upton NY 11973
Shanmugam, K.T.	University of Florida, Gainesville, FL 32611
Shapiro, James A.	University of Chicago, Chicago, IL 60637
Shih, Jason C.H.	North Carolina State University, Raleigh, NC 27650
Shoemaker, Sharon P.	Cetus Corporation, Berkeley, CA 94710
Siegelman, H.W.	Brookhaven National Laboratory, Upton, NY 11973
Silver, Richard	Gulf Science and Technology Company, Pitsburgh, PA 15230
Simon, Martha N.	Biology Dept., Brookhaven National Laboratory, Upton, NY 11973
Smith, R.E.	University of Guelph, Ontario, Canada
Snipes, Wallace	Penn State University, University Park, PA 16802
Stadtman, T.C.	NIH, Bethesda, MD 20205
Stafford, Darrel W.	Univ. of North Carolina-Chapel Hill, Chapel Hill, NC 27514
Sternberg, David	Genex Laboratories, Rockville, MD 20852
Stevenson, Enola	Atlanta University, Atlanta, GA 30314
Stokes, Barry	California Inst. of Technology, Pasadena, CA 91109
Tait, Robert C.	University of California-Davis, Davis, CA 95616
Tempest, David W.	University of Amsterdam, Amsterdam, The Netherlands
Thomas, Charles A., Jr.	Scripps Clinic and Research Foundation, La Jolla, CA 92037
Tornabene, Thomas	Solar Energy Research Institute, Golden, CO 80401
Tsuchiya, H.M.	Univ. of Minnesota, Minneapolis, MN 55455
Tusé, Daniel	SRI International, Menlo Park, CA 94025
Uzodinma, John E.	Jackson State University, Jackson, MS 39217
Valent, Barbara S.	Cornell University, Ithaca, NY 14853
Valentine, Raymond	University of California, Davis, CA 95616
Walker, Alice	Howard University, Washington, D.C. 20059
Wan, Nick	Texaco Inc., Beacon, NY 12508
Watkins, S.H.	Crown Zellerbach Pioneering Research, Washington, D.C.
Weiner, Henry	Purdue University, West Lafayette, IN 47907

Williams, Norma   Howard University, Washington, D.C.
                                       20059
Wills, Christopher   University of California-San Diego,
                                       La Jolla, CA 92093
Wolfe, Ralph   University of Illinois, Urbana, IL 61801
Wolford, Lionel T.   Columbian Chemicals Company, Swartz,
                                       LA 71281
Wood, Willis   Michigan State University, East Lansing,
                                       MI 48824
Woodward, Jonathan   Oak Ridge National Laboratory, Oak Ridge,
                                       TN 37830
Zaborsky, Oskar R.   National Science Foundation, Washington,
                                       DC 20550
Zeikus, J.G.   University of Wisconsin, Madison, WI 5370
Zhu, Yu Sheng   University of Maryland, Baltimore, MD 212
Zimmer, Steve   F. Eberstadt and Co., New York, NY 10006
Zinder, Stephen H.   Cornell University, Ithaca, NY 14853
Zuber, Hans   Institut für Molekularbiologie/Biophysik
                                       Zurich, Switzerland

INDEX